DIFFERENTIAL DIAGNOSIS IN CYTOPATHOLOGY

The cytologic method of pathology is now one of the most widely used diagnostic modalities worldwide. This new and practical text in cytopathology is an organ-based guide for professionals in which malignant and benign tumors are the predominant focus, but the full spectrum of infectious and inflammatory disorders will also be presented in detail, and in both adult and pediatric populations. Coverage is not limited to findings from only the light microscope but also includes many examples of other genetic, molecular, and immunologic diagnostic modalities, giving pathologists diagnostic and clinical criteria needed when formulating a diagnosis and differential diagnosis. This book is illustrated with more than 2,000 full-color photomicrographs and accompanied by a CD-ROM of all images in a downloadable format. *Differential Diagnosis in Cytopathology* proves to be the most comprehensive text in a market in which no other has focused exclusively on essential diagnostic criteria.

Dr. Paolo Gattuso is Professor and Director of Anatomic Pathology at Rush Medical College in Chicago, Illinois.

Dr. Vijaya B. Reddy is Professor and Associate Chair of the Department of Pathology at Rush Medical College in Chicago, Illinois.

Dr. Shahla Masood is Professor and Chair of the Department of Pathology and Laboratory Medicine at the University of Florida College of Medicine in Jacksonville, Florida.

To my wife Nancy and my children Vincent and Francesca
Paolo Gattuso

To my husband Jagan Mohan for his unfailing love and support
Vijaya B. Reddy

To my family Drs. Ahmad, Ali, and Sina Kasraeian
Shahla Masood

DIFFERENTIAL DIAGNOSIS IN CYTOPATHOLOGY

Edited by

Paolo Gattuso
Rush Medical College

Vijaya B. Reddy
Rush Medical College

Shahla Masood
University of Florida College of Medicine

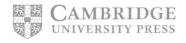

CAMBRIDGE
UNIVERSITY PRESS

CAMBRIDGE UNIVERSITY PRESS
Cambridge, New York, Melbourne, Madrid, Cape Town, Singapore, São Paulo, Delhi

Cambridge University Press
32 Avenue of the Americas, New York, NY 10013-2473, USA

www.cambridge.org
Information on this title: www.cambridge.org/9780521873383

First published 2010

Printed in China

A catalog record for this publication is available from the British Library.

Library of Congress Cataloging in Publication Data

Differential diagnosis in cytopathology / edited by Paolo Gattuso, Vijaya B.
Reddy, Shahla Masood.
   p. ; cm.
  Includes bibliographical references and index.
  ISBN 978-0-521-87338-3
  1. Cytodiagnosis. 2. Diagnosis, Differential. I. Gattuso, Paolo. II. Reddy, Vijaya B. III. Masood, Shahla.
IV. Title.
  [DNLM: 1. Cytodiagnosis – methods. 2. Biopsy, Fine-Needle – methods. 3. Diagnosis, Differential.
QY 95 D538 2009]

RB43.D54 2009
616.07′582–dc22   2008044142

ISBN 978-0-521-87338-3 hardback

Contents

List of Contributors

Syed Z. Ali, M.D.
Associate Professor of Pathology and Radiology
Associate Director of Cytopatholgy
The Johns Hopkins Hospital
Baltimore, Maryland

Rose Anton, M.D.
Assistant Professor of Pathology
Weill Medical Center of Cornell University
New York, New York
Pathologist
The Methodist Hospital
Houston, Texas

Güliz A. Barkan, M.D.
Assistant Professor of Pathology
Loyola University School of Medicine
Maywood, Illinois

Joan F. Cangiarella, M.D.
Associate Professor of Pathology
Director of Cytopathology, Vice Chair
New York University School of Medicine
New York, New York

Odile David, M.D.
Assistant Professor of Pathology
Director of Cytopathology
University of Illinois College of Medicine
Chicago, Illinois

Rosa M. Dávila, M.D.
Staff Pathologist
Missouri Baptist Medical Center
St. Louis, Missouri

Antonino Di Certo, M.D.
Director of General Surgery
Oppido Mamertina
Reggio Calabria, Italy

Tarik M. Elsheikh, M.D.
Director of Pathology, PA Labs
Ball Memorial Hospital
Muncie, Indiana

Kristin Galan, M.D.
Surgical Pathology Fellow
Rush University Medical Center
Chicago, Illinois

Paolo Gattuso, M.D.
Professor of Pathology
Director of Anatomic Pathology
Rush Medical College
Chicago, Illinois

Shriram Jakate, M.D.
Professor of Pathology
Director of Laboratory
Rush Medical College
Chicago, Illinois

Umesh Kapur, M.D.
Assistant Professor of Pathology
Loyola University School of Medicine
Maywood, Illinois

Lester J. Layfield, M.D.
Professor of Pathology
Director of Anatomic Laboratory
Huntsman Cancer Hospital
Salt Lake City, Utah

Pascale Levine, M.D.
Assistant Professor of Pathology
New York University School of Medicine
New York, New York

Shahla Masood, M.D.
Professor of Pathology and Chair of Pathology
University of Florida College of Medicine
Jacksonville, Florida

Claire W. Michael, M.D.
Professor of Pathology
Director of Cytopathology Laboratory
University of Michigan Health System
Ann Arbor, Michigan

Anil V. Parwani, M.D., Ph.D.
Division Director, Pathology Informatics
Staff Pathologist, Shadyside Hospital
UPMC Shadyside Hospital
Pittsburgh, Pennsylvania

Telma C. Pereira, M.D.
Assistant Professor of Pathology
Drexel University College of Medicine
Pathologist
Allegheny General Hospital
Pittsburgh, Pennsylvania

Marilin Rosa, M.D.
Assistant Professor of Pathology
University of Florida College of Medicine
Jacksonville, Florida

Reda S. Saad, M.D.
Associate Professor of Pathology
Drexel University College of Medicine
Pathologist
Allegheny General Hospital
Pittsburgh, Pennsylvania

Jan F. Silverman, M.D.
Chairman and Director of Anatomic Pathology Laboratory
Professor of Pathology
Drexel University College of Medicine
Pittsburgh, Pennsylvania

Aylin Simsir, M.D.
Associate Professor of Pathology
New York University School of Medicine
New York, New York

Luan D. Truong, M.D.
Professor of Pathology and Laboratory Medicine
Weill Medical College of Cornell University
New York, New York
Adjunct Professor of Pathology and Medicine
Baylor College of Medicine
Houston, Texas
Chief of Nephropathology
The Methodist Hospital
Houston, Texas

Eva M. Wojcik, M.D.
Professor and Chair of Pathology
Loyola University School of Medicine
Maywood, Illinois

Lourdes R. Ylagan, M.D.
Assistant Professor of Pathology and Immunology
Washington University School of Medicine
St. Louis, Missouri

Mohammad M. Yousef, M.D.
Cytopathology Fellow
The University of Michigan
Ann Arbor, Michigan

Jing Zhai, M.D., Ph.D.
Staff Pathologist
Department of Pathology
Cedars-Sinai Medical Center
Los Angeles, California

Preface

Advances in science and technology in recent years have revolutionized our approach to the diagnosis and management of various disease entities. Similarly there has been significant change in the fundamental concept of delivery of health care. Emphases are now directed to find the most efficient ways to deliver personalized medicine and to improve the quality of patient care. Integrated care has resulted in better treatment planning and improved patient satisfaction, and minimally invasive diagnostic and therapeutic models have replaced excisional biopsies and open surgical procedures.

Pathologists have played a central role in the realization of delivery of personalized patient care. Their efforts in the development, validation, and implementation of various technologies have been central in providing appropriate diagnostic, prognostic, and predictive information. The discipline of cytopathology has also played a critical role in responding to the changing trends in health care. Aside from learning more about morphologic features and diagnostic pitfalls, cytopathologists have been actively engaged in using advanced technologies on cytologic preparations in an effort to maximize the efficiency of the practice of cytopathology. Currently cytologic preparations are routinely used in ancillary studies in order to offer the most accurate information about the nature and biology of a disease process.

Practice of cytopathology is exciting and challenging. A good cytopathologist must be a good surgical pathologist. In many ways, cytopathology practice is similar to looking through the keyhole and being able to see the entire room. It takes imagination, knowledge, and courage to do so. We believe that *Differential Diagnosis in Cytopathology* will offer the knowledge and the vision necessary for the practice of cytopathology.

Differential Diagnosis in Cytopathology is designed to offer a systematic, concise, and organized approach to addressing differential diagnosis in cytopathology and the application of possible ancillary studies to help reach the correct diagnosis. *Differential Diagnosis in Cytopathology* is unique because of the remarkably simple language used and the quality of the images.

Each chapter has a uniform format. Every entity discussed features several sections: clinical findings, cytologic features, special stains, immunohistochemistry, modern techniques for diagnosis, differential diagnosis, and take home messages, or "pearls."

The book is designed to fulfill the needs of pathology residents, cytopathology Fellows, cytotechnologists, and the academic/pathology community in cytologic diagnosis of the female genital tract, exfoliative pulmonary cytology, body cavity fluids (peritoneal, pleural) CSF and intra-ocular cytology, gastrointestinal tract, urine cytology, cytopathology of the breast, fine needle aspiration of tumors of unknown origin, soft tissue and bone, thyroid gland, kidney and adrenal gland, head and neck, salivary glands, liver, pancreas, prostate, lymph nodes, gonads and cytopathology of the central nervous system.

This multiauthored publication is representative of the fine work of many key opinion leaders in the discipline of cytopathology who have spent a great deal of time in the preparation of their chapters. We greatly appreciate their contributions and their sincere effort in this process.

Paolo Gattuso, MD
Vijaya B. Reddy, MD
Shahla Masood, MD

Acknowledgments

The editors gratefully acknowledge Mrs. Mira Davis, who spent innumerable hours typing and organizing the manuscript. She was instrumental in communicating with all the contributors and ensuring the timeliness of the project. Our thanks to Mr. Allan Ross, Executive Editor at Cambridge University Press, and Ms. Shelby Peak, Production Controller at Cambridge University Press, for their assistance in the production of this book.

1

Pap Smear

Lourdes R. Ylagan

Chlamydia trachomatis
Neisseria gonorrhea
Syphilis
Pubic louse or "crab"
Contaminants in Pap smear
Alternaria alternata
Asterosclereids
Plant matter
Trichomes
Carpet beetle part
Pollen

INTRODUCTION

Although this chapter on Pap smears will closely follow the recommendations set forth by the current Bethesda System, it is not by any means a replacement of the standard text on Pap smear cytology. It, however, should be a good resource for the experienced cytomorphologist for possibilities of various differential diagnoses, which may present in Pap smears

Any interpretation of cytologic material, including Pap smears starts with the procurement, processing, and presentation of the criteria for an adequate sample. The minimum cellularity of squamous cells on conventional Pap smears is anywhere between 8,000 and 12,000 cells and between 5,000 and 20,000 cells in liquid-based media (Bethesda 2001). The presence of at least ten well-preserved endocervical or squamous metaplastic cells, which implies adequate sampling of the transformation zone, is also important. This criteria is only negated if the woman has had a known history of a hysterectomy. Having satisfied all criteria for an adequate sample, the 2001 Bethesda System suggests a uniformity in laboratory reporting of Pap smears by adhering to a proscribed and standardized method of reporting, which includes: (i) the type of specimen obtained; (ii) a statement on the specimen adequacy and any reason for an unsatisfactory specimen; (iii) the general category of lesions; and (iv) interpretations of results. The reader is referred to the current publication of Bethesda 2001 for a more complete listing of the classification system

REACTIVE CHANGES

Clinical Features
▓ Common cytologic pattern, which can be due to repair, atrophy, prolapsed uterus, radiation changes, and infectious processes
▓ Could be due to numerous infectious process such as trichomonas, bacterial vaginosis, Chlamydia, gonorrhea, HPV, candida, and herpes
▓ Commonly clinically treated and Pap smear repeated after treatment
▓ Most cases are symptomatic and is a presenting concern to the patient

Cytologic Features
▓ A prominent or subtle neutrophilic exudate
▓ Maybe associated with common infectious processes: candida, trichomonas, Gardnerella vaginosis, etc.
▓ Cells are commonly found in cohesive sheets and tile-like or honeycomb configuration
▓ Nuclei are enlarged (1 to 1.5× the size of an intermediate cell nucleus), can be binucleated, nuclear outlines are round, smooth and uniform, vesicular, and hypochromatic to mildly hyperchromatic
▓ Multiple or single nucleoli in most of the cells in the sheets

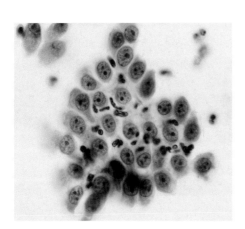

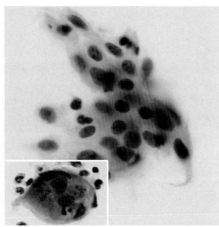

1-1A. Reactive changes *(opposite, left)*. With neutrophils (Papanicolaou stain)

1-1B. Reactive changes due to atrophy *(opposite, right)*. (Papanicolaou stain)

1-1C. Reactive changes due to Radiation *(below, top)*. (Papanicolaou stain)

1-1D. Reactive changes due to IUD *(below, middle)*. (Insets are reactive endometrial cells) (Papanicolaou stain)

■ Cytoplasm could be polychromatic, vacuolated with a small perinuclear halo

1-1E. Tubal metaplasia *(below, bottom)*. (Papanicolaou stain)

Special Stains and Immunohistochemistry
■ The cytologic features of most infectious agents are well-defined and usually do not need special stains in a Papanicolaou-stained slide

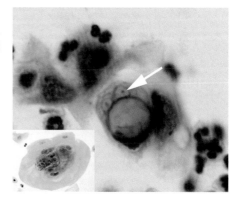

Modern Techniques for Diagnosis
■ PCR testing for both chlamydia and gonorrhea

Differential Diagnosis
■ Typical repair associated with atrophy with and without inflammation
  ➤ Age >50 years, anovulatory syndromes or history of bilateral oophorectomy for treatment of breast cancers
  ➤ Presence of squamous metaplastic cells or parabasal cells are more common
  ➤ Presence of naked nuclei secondary to autolysis called "blue blobs"
  ➤ Presence of granular or degenerated background
  ➤ ± Parakeratotic cells and histiocytes
  ➤ Lack of maturing squamous epithelium

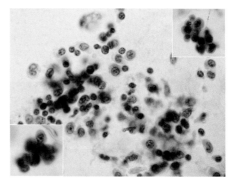

■ Reactive cellular changes associated with radiation
  ➤ History of cervical or endometrial malignancy, status post-radiation
  ➤ Markedly enlarged cells with preserved nuclear to cytoplasmic ratio
  ➤ Presence of bizarre cell shapes with multinucleation and polychromasia
  ➤ Presence of cytoplasmic and nuclear vacuolization (arrow)
■ Reactive cellular changes associated with IUD
  ➤ History of IUD placement or recent removal
  ➤ Presence of endometrial cells
  ➤ Presence of small vacuolated cells or histiocytes
  ➤ Presence of nuclear degeneration and prominent nucleoli

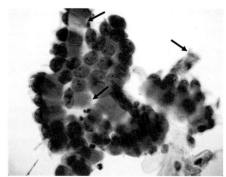

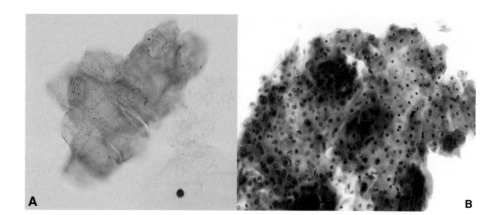

1-1F. Hyperkeratosis and Parakeratosis. (A) and (B) (Papanicolaou stain)

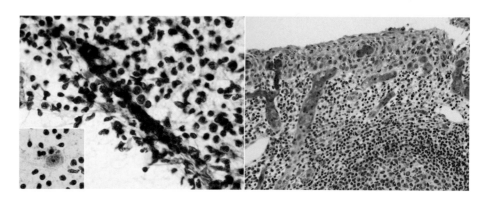

1-1G. Lymphocytic cervicitis. (Papanicolaou stain)

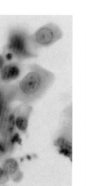

1-1H. Endocervical cell atypia. (Papanicolaou stain)

■ Other nonneoplastic or metaplastic changes that could be seen in association with these reactive changes
➤ Tubal metaplasia
Very common in reactive endocervices and is composed of endocervical cells with well-defined terminal bars and ciliated borders (arrows)
➤ Hyperkeratoses and parakeratoses
Commonly associated with prolapse, but could also harbor a squamous intraepithelial lesion (SIL)
➤ Lymphocytic cervicitis
Commonly associated with Chlamydia trachomatis *infection than any other venereal infection*
➤ Reactive endocervical cells
Commonly have sheets of endocervical cells with multiple nucleoli or prominent chromocenters

PEARLS

★ The search for an infectious agent and an adequate correlation with clinical history is imperative in the diagnosis

LOW-GRADE SQUAMOUS INTRAEPITHELIAL LESIONS (LGSIL)

Clinical Features
■ Could be found as a raised warty or flat lesion in the vulva, vagina, or cervix that is acetowhite by acetic acid application upon colposcopy
■ Includes histologic diagnoses of mild dysplasia (CIN 1) or koilocytic changes

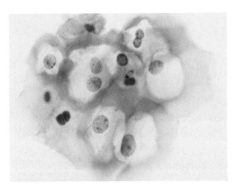

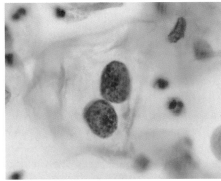

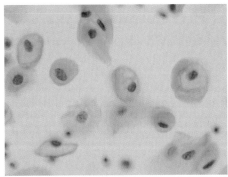

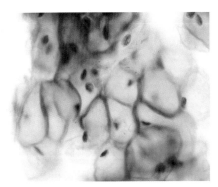

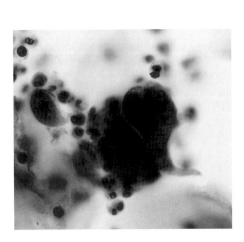

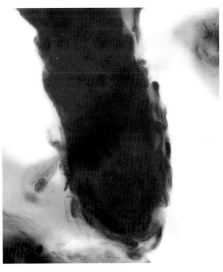

1-2A. Koilocytes (LGSIL) *(top, left).*

1-2B. Low-grade squamous intraepithelial lesion *(top, right).* (Papanicolaou stain)

1-2C. Navicular cells of pregnancy *(middle).* (Papanicolaou stain)

1-2D. Trophoblasts and Arias-Stella change of pregnancy *(bottom, left).* (Papanicolaou stain)

1-2E. Atypical parakeratosis *(bottom, right).* (Papanicolaou stain)

Cytologic Features

■ Singly dispersed or groups of cells with abundant cytoplasm and a dense perinuclear clearing or halo around a nucleus

■ Others may not have a distinct halo around the nucleus, but still have abundant cytoplasm

■ Nucleus is at least 2 to 3× the size of an intermediate cell nucleus, can be binucleated, with some variation in size from cell to cell

■ Nucleus is hyperchromatic with irregularly granular chromatin and can have irregular nuclear contours

■ Usually have no conspicuous nucleoli

Special Stains and Immunohistochemistry

■ Not necessary if the cytologic features are observed as above

Modern Techniques for Diagnosis
- Noncontributory

Differential Diagnosis
- Glycogenated or navicular cells of pregnancy
  - Lacks nuclear enlargement and hyperchromasia
  - Presence of small nuclei the same size as an intermediate cell nucleus
  - A perinuclear halo without perinuclear cytoplasmic condensation around the nuclei
- Atypical squamous cells of undetermined significance (ASCUS)
  - Presence of nuclear enlargement up to 3× the size of an intermediate cell nucleus with some degree of hyperchromasia
  - Lacks the irregular granular chromatin and nuclear contour irregularity of a LGSIL lesion

PEARLS

★ Despite the morphologic changes described above, these lesions can harbor both low-and high-grade human papilloma viral types

ARIAS-STELLA CHANGE OF PREGNANCY

Clinical Features
- A history or pregnancy is present. Very early postpartum changes can also present with Arias-Stella changes in the epithelial and stromal cells that can be interpreted as atypical glandular cells, NOS

Cytologic Features
- Marked cellular enlargement, marked nuclear atypia including nuclear enlargement, pleomorphic nuclei, and prominent nucleoli. The nuclear to cytoplasmic ratio is unchanged

Special Stains and Immunohistochemistry
- CD10 may be helpful in the differentiation between Arias-Stella cell of trophoblastic origin versus a clear cell carcinoma, which was found to be negative in one study
- Cyclin E expression, on the other hand, has been seen mostly in clear cell adenocarcinoma of mullerian origin and would be negative in clear cell tumors of renal primary. A combination of these markers would be useful

Modern Techniques for Diagnosis
- Noncontributory

Differential Diagnosis
- A clear cell adenocarcinoma of mullerian origin may be cytologically difficult to differentiate and may present in young women, therefore, a tissue biopsy and serum B-HCG levels would be necessary to exclude one from the other
- Radiation effect – a history of radiation or pregnancy are the main differentiating factors

⋆ A history of recent pregnancy is of paramount importance
⋆ May be the first presenting finding in a young woman with a tubal or extrauterine pregnancy, such that a serologic B-HCG level may be necessary
⋆ May also be the presenting finding in women with molar pregnancies

ATYPICAL SQUAMOUS CELLS

Clinical Features
▦ Patients may not have a distinct or specific clinical symptom
▦ May represent the first indication of a smoldering squamous intraepithelial lesion

Cytologic Features
▦ "ASC refers to cytologic changes suggestive of SIL, which are qualitatively and quantitatively insufficient for a definitive interpretation of an SIL lesion" (Bethesda 2001)
▦ This is not a distinct diagnostic entity, but a "waste-basket" category reserved for those cases for which a definitive diagnosis of SIL could not be reached. An ASCUS rate of 5.2% (mean) and 4.5% (median) was seen in 768 participating cytology laboratories across the United States in 1996. This entity includes both ASCUS and ASC-H for cases in which atypical squamous metaplastic cells have features that fall short of a high grade squamous intraepithelial lesion (HGSIL)

Special Stains and Immunohistochemistry
▦ In-situ hybridization techniques for the detection of episomic and integrated HPV DNA. A positive test indicates the presence of one or more high risk HPV types: 16, 18, 31, 33, 35, 39, 45, 51, 52, 56, 58, and 68
▦ ProExC® by Tripath imaging is a new antibody, which stains cells undergoing aberrant S-phase induction as would be seen in highly and inappropriately proliferative

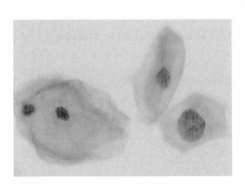
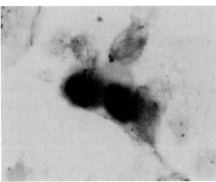
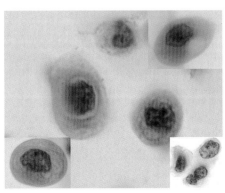
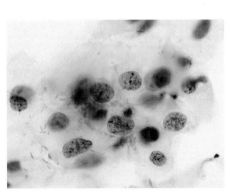

1-3A. *(top, left).* Atypical squamous cells of undetermined significance (ASCUS) (Papanicolaou stain)

1-3B. *(top, right).* In situ hybridization technique for detecting high-risk HPV infection (Papanicolaou stain)

1-3C. *(bottom, left).* Atypical squamous cells – cannot exclude HGSIL (ASC-H) with ProExC® (Papanicolaou stain)

1-3D. *(bottom, right).* LGSIL without koilocytosis (Papanicolaou stain)

squamous epithelium. This could potentially differentiate HGSIL from ASC-H lesions, which are similar in size to squamous metaplastic cells

Modern Techniques for Diagnosis
▧ Digene hybrid capture method for the detection of high-risk HPV viral types 16, 18, 31, 33, 35, 39, 45, 51, 52, 56, 58, and 68. A positive test indicates the presence of one or more high-risk HPV types. This does not test for the presence of low-risk HPV DNA. This test is based in Salt Lake City, Utah, to which all specimens are sent for testing

Differential Diagnosis
▧ LGSIL without koilocytosis
➤ Squamous cells considered ASCUS lack the hyperchromasia and irregular granularity of chromatin present in most LGSIL lesions. However, when in doubt, some type of HPV DNA testing is now mandatory

PEARLS
★ NOT a specific diagnostic entity and should only be reserved for those cases for which a diagnosis of SIL cannot be made morphologically

HIGH-GRADE SQUAMOUS INTRAEPITHELIAL LESIONS (HGSIL)

Clinical Features
▧ May present as raised or flat excoriated lesions with punctuate hypervascularity and mosaicism on colposcopy in the vulva, vagina, or cervix
▧ Includes histologic diagnoses of moderate (CIN 2) or severe dysplasia (CIN 3) lesions

Cytologic Features
▧ Singly dispersed, sheets, linearly arranged and syncytial aggregates of cells with high nuclear to cytoplasmic ratios
▧ Cells are considerably smaller in size and can be 1 to 1.5× the size of an intermediate cell nucleus
▧ Cytoplasm can vary from delicate, to polychromatic and metaplastic, to densely keratinized
▧ Hyperchromatic nuclei with irregular granular chromatin and prominent nuclear convolutions
▧ Inconspicuous nucleoli

Special Stains and Immunohistochemistry
▧ Noncontributory

Modern Techniques for Diagnosis
▧ Biomarkers of proliferation and cell cycle dysregulation such as p16INK4, cyclin E, and Ki-67 have been used in histologic specimens to gauge the thickness of dysplastic epithelium, but these antibodies have not found its usefulness in Pap smear cytologic screening

Differential Diagnosis
▧ Endometrial cells
➤ Cells are usually found in clusters or as in a ball, typically called "exodus" cells and may be seen during the first fourteen days of menstrual cycle

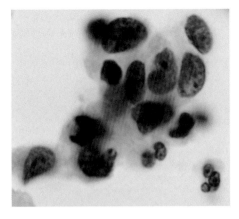

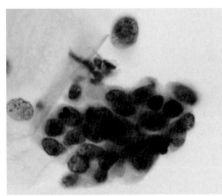

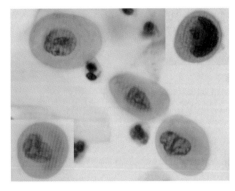

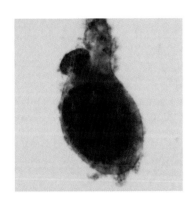

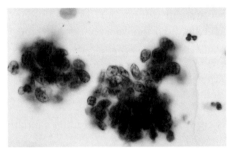

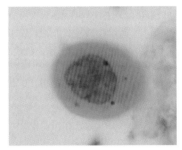

1-4A. High-grade squamous intraepithelial lesion (HGSIL) *(top, left).* (Papanicolaou stain)

1-4B. HGSIL with lacy cytoplasm *(top, right).* (Papanicolaou stain)

1-4C. HGSIL with metaplastic-appearing cytoplasm *(middle, left).* (Papanicolaou stain)

1-4D. HGSIL with densely keratinized cytoplasm *(middle, right).* (Papanicolaou stain)

1-4E. Benign endometrial cells *(bottom, left).* (Papanicolaou stain)

1-4F. ASC-H *(bottom, right).* (Papanicolaou stain)

➤ Cytoplasm is usually lacy and lacks the metaplastic or orangeophilic and keratinized cytoplasm of HGSIL
▪ ASC-H
➤ Typically, the cells in ASC-H are few and far between and may not have all of the features of a HGSIL lesion

PEARLS

★ HGSIL maybe associated with an endocervical adenocarcinoma in situ

HIGH-GRADE SQUAMOUS INTRAEPITHELIAL LESIONS INVOLVING ENDOCERVICAL GLANDS

Clinical Features
▪ Usually does not have a clinically visible lesion, but is generally associated with a HGSIL lesion with punctuate hypervascularity and mosaicism on colposcopy in the cervix

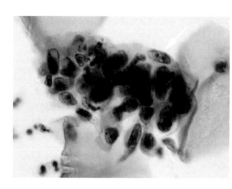

1-5. HGSIL involving endocervical glands. (Papanicolaou stain)

Cytologic Features
■ Cellular features similar to that seen in HGSIL lesions, but typically have a flattening of the nuclei at the edge of the cluster (arrow)
■ Columnar cells at the edge of the clusters may mimic an adenocarcinoma in situ of the endocervix

Special Stains and Immunohistochemistry
■ Not necessary if the cytologic features are observed as above

Modern Techniques for Diagnosis
■ Noncontributory

Differential Diagnosis
■ Adenocarcinoma in situ of the endocervix
➤ Presence of abundant feathery borders in the hyperchomatic crowded groups of an AIS lesion

PEARLS

✶ Although not a commonly diagnosed entity in cytology, it can be seen in liquid-based cytologic preparations

KERATINIZING SQUAMOUS CELL CARCINOMA

Clinical Features
■ Clinical history of SIL lesions without follow-up biopsy or patient lost to follow-up, patients with clinical history of HIV or patients who did not have a regular Pap smear screening test
■ Clinically presents with irregular bleeding
■ May present as large fungating lesions of the vulva, vagina, or cervix

Cytologic Features
■ Singly dispersed orangeophilic cells in varying sizes and shapes including caudate and spindled cells colloquially called "tadpole cells"
■ Nuclei can be variable in size, but generally dense and hyperchomatic or pyknotic with densely packed chromatin
■ Inconspicuous nucleoli
■ Can be seen with a background tumor diathesis and marked acute inflammation

Special Stains and Immunocytochemistry
■ Noncontributory in cytology

Modern Techniques for Diagnosis
■ Noncontributory

1-6. Keratinizing squamous cell carcinoma. (Papanicolaou stain)

Differential Diagnosis
■ Keratinizing squamous cell carcinoma from other sites such as skin, but the cytologic features are the same

PEARLS

✶ The morphologic feature commonly used to identify these lesions is the presence of keratin "pearls" or more commonly "tadpole cells" in cytology
✶ Tumor diathesis

NONKERATINIZING SQUAMOUS CELL CARCINOMA

Clinical Features
- Clinical history of SIL lesions without follow-up biopsy or patient lost to follow-up, patients with clinical history of HIV or patients who did not have a regular Pap smear screening test
- Clinically presents with irregular bleeding
- Can have large fungating lesions of the vulva, vagina, or cervix

Cytologic Features
- Mostly, cells are arranged in synctitia or cellular aggregates
- Nuclei shows hyperchomatic granular chromatin, with prominent nucleoli (red arrows)
- Commonly associated with cells typical of HGSIL lesions
- Tumor diathesis commonly present

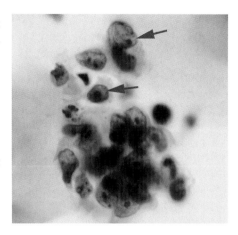

1-7. Nonkeratinizing squamous cell carcinoma. (Papanicolaou stain)

Special Stains and Immunocytochemistry
- Not contributory if the cytologic features are observed as above

Modern Techniques for Diagnosis
- Noncontributory

Differential Diagnosis
- Endocervical adenocarcinoma in situ
  - ➤ Typically would not have tumor diathesis
  - ➤ Typically would not have prominent nucleoli
  - ➤ Typically have elongated columnar nuclei with finely granular chromatin
- HGSIL involving endocervical glands
  - ➤ Typically would not have tumor diathesis, but would be otherwise very difficult to differentiate from nonkeratinizing SCCa (a comment section with this differential would be appropriate)

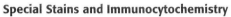

PEARLS

✷ Is the invasive counterpart of a HGSIL lesion typically identified in cytology by the presence of prominent nucleoli

PAPILLARY SQUAMOTRANSITIONAL CELL OR PAPILLARY SQUAMOUS CELL CARCINOMA OF THE CERVIX

Clinical Features
- Clinically have fungating or warty mass in the cervix, which on histology may have both an exophytic and endophytic pattern

Cytologic Features
- Three-dimensional, arborizing, papillary clusters with well-defined fibrovascular cores surrounded by basal and parabasal type cells, which may be aligned horizontally
- These tumors can present with a spectrum of cytologic features from those that are predominantly transitional or urothelial, like those seen in the bladder,

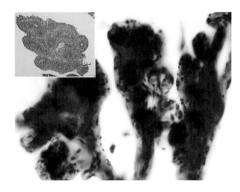

1-8. Papillary squamotransitional cell carcinoma of the cervix. (Papanicolaou stain)

to a mixture of squamous and transitional to predominantly squamous in appearance
▨ Nuclear features of HGSIL are typical in these papillary clusters with a high nuclear to cytoplasmic ratio and nuclear contour irregularities
▨ Mitotic figures are common
▨ Absence of tumor diathesis and koilocytosis and a lack of maturation or keratinization of these basal or parabasal type squamous cells

Special Stains and Immunocytochemistry
▨ Immunohistochemical stains for uroplakin III, p63, and p16 show some of the tumors to be immunoreactive
▨ Whether the tumor is mostly transitional or predominantly squamous, they are typically positive for both CK7 and CK20

Modern Techniques for Diagnosis
▨ Noncontributory

Differential Diagnosis
▨ Metastatic urothelial cell carcinoma of the urinary bladder
➤ Typically would have tumor diathesis

PEARLS

★ These tumors are typically aggressive regardless of the type of cellular differentiation found in the tumor
★ Some have been found to be HPV 16 positive
★ This diagnosis cannot be made on cytology alone
★ The cytologic features would be indistinguishable from a nonkeratinizing squamous cell carcinoma by Pap smear cytology alone

ADENOCARCINOMA IN SITU OF ENDOCERVIX

Clinical Features
▨ May not present with any specific symptoms

Cytologic Features
▨ Endocervical cells arranged in picket fence arrangement or in a pseudostratified manner with nuclear crowding and feathering
▨ Cytoplasm is lacy and foamy with ill-defined borders
▨ Nuclei are hyperchromatic, elongated, oblong in shape and show fine granular pattern
▨ Inconspicuous nucleoli

Special Stains and Immunocytochemistry
▨ p16 can be used for detection of endocervical adenocarcinoma and its precursor lesions on histologic preparations, but has not found its usefulness in cytologic preparations

Modern Techniques for Diagnosis
▨ May need to do either a hybrid capture method for HPV typing or in situ hybridization for HPV if there is a question of atypical glandular cells and a definitive diagnosis is necessary, as in the case of current pregnancy. Although there is no

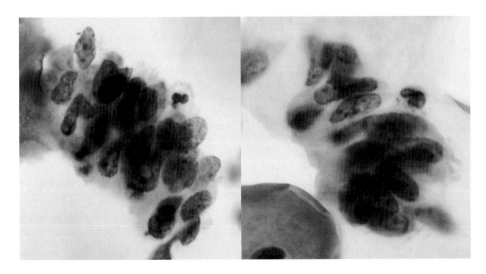

1-9. Adenocarcinoma in situ. (feathering artifact) (Papanicolaou stain)

current recommendation for the performance of HPV testing in presumed AIS lesions of the endocervix, 42% of cases with atypical glandular cells harbor high risk HPV types

Differential Diagnosis
- Tubal metaplasia
  - ➤ Typically have cells with ciliated borders
  - ➤ Usually seen as sheets in well-organized honeycomb pattern without nuclear overlapping
- High grade squamous intraepithelial lesion involving endocervical glands
  - ➤ Typically have a flattening of the cells at the edge of the cluster

PEARLS

✶ Is a diagnostic entity in Pap smear cytology, which prototypically has a distinct cytologic feature of a "feathering" pattern
✶ Picket fence arrangement may also be seen in benign endocervical epithelium
✶ HPV 18 is the most common high risk HPV type seen in cases of adenocarcinoma in situ

ENDOCERVICAL ADENOCARCINOMA

Clinical Features
- Patients may present with profuse clear vaginal discharge

Cytologic Features
- Singly dispersed flat sheets or clusters of cells, which still maintain some degree of polarity
- Polychromatic dense but not keratinized cytoplasm
- Nuclei are 2 to 3 × the size of an intermediate cell nucleus, with irregular chromatin or chromocenters
- Typically have large prominent cherry red nucleoli (red arrows)
- Tumor diathesis may be present

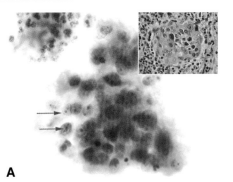

A

1-10A. Endocervical adenocarcinoma, and histologic section. (inset) (Papanicolaou stain and H and E)

Special Stains and Immunocytochemistry
- Noncontributory

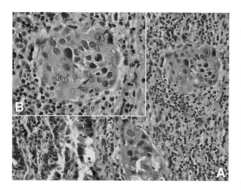

1-10B. Endocervical adeno-carcinoma histologic section.
(A) low power of invasive adenocarcinoma, (B) High power of invasive area with prominent nucleoli (red arrows) (H & E histologic section)

Modern Techniques for Diagnosis
▮ P16INK antibody, in combination with other markers, may be used to distinguish between a cervical adenocarcinoma (diffuse positivity) and an endometrioid-type endometrial adenocarcinoma (negative or focally positive)

Differential Diagnosis
▮ Endometrial adenocarcinoma or other metastatic carcinoma
➤ If metastatic, typically no tumor diathesis

PEARLS

★ It can be related to prenatal Diethylstilbestrol (DES) exposure in utero

ENDOMETRIAL CELLS

Clinical Features
▮ May be found in the first fourteen days of the menstrual cycle in premenopausal women and is considered a benign finding
▮ If the woman is >40 years of age, in addition, a comment that a significant lesion maybe present in the endometrium
▮ The Pap smear is generally not a sensitive test for screening lesions of the endometrium

Cytologic Features
▮ May be seen as a ball of cells consisting of a central core of endometrial stromal cells surrounded by a single layer of cuboidal or columnar endometrial epithelium. This structure is called "exodus" in cytology
▮ May be seen as singly dispersed and small clusters of cells in three-dimensional aggregates with round to oval nuclei, and fine granular chromatin with or without nucleoli
▮ Cytoplasm can be vacuolated, lacy, or nonexistent and nonkeratinized
▮ Nuclei are small and about the same size as an intermediate cell nucleus

Special Stains and Immunocytochemistry
▮ Not necessary if the cytologic features are observed as above

Modern Techniques for Diagnosis
▮ Noncontributory

Differential Diagnosis
▮ Well-differentiated endometrial adenocarcinoma
➤ Usually occurs in postmenopausal women or in patients with unopposed estrogen therapy
▮ High-grade squamous intraepithelial lesion
➤ Would typically have associated cells with dense cytoplasm in varying degrees of keratinization

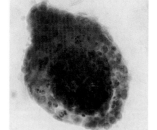

1-11. "Exodus". (Papanicolaou stain)

PEARLS

★ When singly dispersed, can mimic a HGSIL lesion

ENDOMETRIAL ADENOCARCINOMA

Clinical Features
▮ Typical presentation is postmenopausal bleeding

Cytologic Features

▪ Singly dispersed, clusters or large three-dimensional aggregates of small to large cells with lacy to vacuolated cytoplasm, some with intraepithelial neutrophils

▪ Nuclei may vary in size from small to large angulated and convoluted, with irregularly granular chromatin, some with parachromatin clearing

▪ Presence of nucleoli is ±, but usually large and prominent if present in high grade FIGO grade III/III tumors

▪ Depending on type of endometrial adenocarcinoma, other cytologic findings such as psammoma bodies may be present

▪ Finely granular or watery background and tumor diathesis

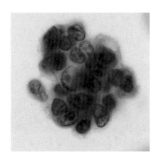

1-12A. Endometrial adenocarcinoma, low grade. (Papanicolaou stain)

Special Stains and Immunocytochemistry

▪ Noncontributory

Modern Techniques for Diagnosis

▪ Noncontributory

Differential Diagnosis

▪ Endometrioid or papillary serous adenocarcinoma of either cervical or ovarian origin
➤ The primary origin of the lesion may not be evident on the basis of the cytologic diagnosis

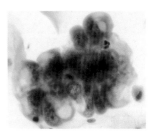

1-12B. Endometrial adenocarcinoma, high grade. (Papanicolaou stain)

PEARLS

✦ Is NOT a diagnosis that can be definitively made in cytology alone. Radiographic features and a tissue biopsy are generally necessary to avoid an unnecessary hysterectomy

EXTRAUTERINE MALIGNANCIES

PAPILLARY SEROUS ADENOCARCINOMA FROM EITHER OVARY, FALLOPIAN TUBE, AND ENDOMETRIUM

Clinical Features

▪ Patients may not present with any specific symptomatology

▪ Others may present to the clinician with abdominal bloating and ascites

Cytologic Features

▪ As would be seen in peritoneal washings of patients with papillary serous adenocarcinomas of the ovary, large papillary groupings with or without a distinct fibrovascular core

▪ Malignant-appearing cells with vacuolated cytoplasm, surrounding psammoma bodies can be seen

▪ Nuclei can be round, irregular, or angulated and indented or pushed to one side of the cytoplasm

▪ Presence of nucleoli can be ±

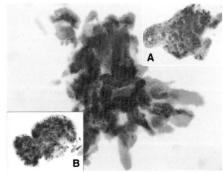

Special Stains and Immunocytochemistry

▪ Immunohistochemical stains for Wilms' Tumor 1 (WT-1) has been found to be expressed in primary ovarian papillary serous adenocarcinomas and may help differentiate from a primary endometrioid tumor

Modern Techniques for Diagnosis

▪ Noncontributory

1-13A. Papillary serous adenocarcinoma with areas of clear cell differentiation. (Papanicolaou stain)

Differential Diagnosis

■ Primary papillary serous carcinomas of ovarian, endometrial, fallopian vs. cervical origin would have similar cytologic features. However, the background is clean in metastatic tumors

PEARLS

☆ The presence of psammoma bodies in cytology does not necessarily mean a malignant neoplasm, but should prompt for the search of one

SMALL CELL, UNDIFFERENTIATED OR "OAT CELL" CARCINOMA

Clinical Features

■ May present as a primary tumor of the cervix with bulky, polypoid mass and is highly aggressive

■ In spite of its morphologic similarity to its lung counterpart is not a metastasis from lung

Cytologic Features

■ The smear shows bare-naked nuclei, with prominent nuclear molding, and fine granular chromatin without nucleoli

■ A nuclear streaming artifact maybe seen as is commonly found in the lung

Special Stains and Immunocytochemistry

■ Neuroendocrine markers such as chromogranin and synaptophysin maybe necessary to confirm the diagnosis and exclude a high-grade squamous intraepithelial lesion. CD56 (neural adhesion molecule) has been shown to be more sensitive (88%, $n = 25$), than synaptophysin (64%) or chromogranin (14%) in a recent study.

■ C-kit expression has been seen in some cases (43%, $n = 21$) of small cell carcinomas of the cervix

■ Typically associated with HPV 18

Modern Techniques for Diagnosis

■ Noncontributory, as both HGSIL lesions and small cell carcinomas could be positive for high-risk HPV types especially HPV 18 in small cell carcinoma. Proliferative markers such as Ki-67 and P16INK are of no prognostic or diagnostic value

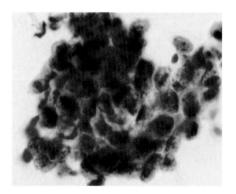

1-13B. Small cell, undifferentiated, or "oat cell" carcinoma.
(Papanicolaou stain)

Differential Diagnosis

■ HGSIL
    ➤ Typically would have cells with dense cytoplasm with varying degrees of keratinization
■ Squamous cell carcinoma with small cells
    ➤ This is a much older terminology and is not a commonly used diagnosis in surgical biopsies without supporting immunohistochemistry to rule out a neuroendocrine malignancy. Most cases of *squamous cell carcinoma with small cells* that are nonneuroendocrine tumors are now put in the category of nonkeratinizing squamous cell carcinomas

PEARLS

☆ A high-grade neoplasm, whose prognosis is comparatively worse than a non-keratinizing squamous cell carcinoma, typically presents in younger women and is commonly associated with HPV 18

MALIGNANT MIXED MÜLLERIAN TUMORS

Clinical Features
▧ Is a rare malignant neoplasm of the uterine corpus which presents with a large bulging mass of the uterus which may protrude through the cervical os
▧ Mostly seen in postmenopausal woman presenting with uterine bleeding
▧ Typically highly aggressive with frequent recurrences and metastasis within five years of diagnosis

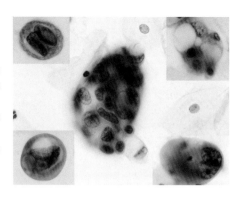

1-13C. Malignant mixed müllerian tumor (MMMT). (Papanicolaou stain)

Cytologic Features
▧ By definition, the histologic finding consists of a malignant stromal and epithelial component. The epithelial component is typically endometroid, but could have a mixture of papillary serous or squamous component. The stromal component may be homologous and consists of malignant smooth muscle and fibroblast or heterologous and may be chondrosarcoma, osteosarcoma, or rhabdomyosarcoma. The cytologic changes found would then be any of the above elements, but would typically have a malignant sarcomatous component and a malignant epithelial component in varying amounts

Special Stains and Immunocytochemistry
▧ Not necessary if the cytologic features are observed as above
▧ A definitive diagnosis is based on histologic architecture rather than cytologic features

Modern Techniques for Diagnosis
▧ Noncontributory

Differential Diagnosis
▧ High-grade sarcoma
  ➤ Would typically not have a malignant epithelial component
▧ High-grade endometrial adenocarcinoma
  ➤ Would typically not have a malignant stromal component

PEARLS

✶ An uncommon neoplasm arising from the uterus and even more uncommon from the cervix

MALIGNANT MIXED EPITHELIAL TUMORS, ADENOSQUAMOUS CARCINOMAS

Clinical Features
▧ Patients may present with both endometrial and cervical lesions or one of the other. Sometimes this tumor is lumped under the Endometrial adenocarcinomas with squamous differentiation, but a true mixed tumor or collision tumor has been seen

Cytologic Features
▧ True mixed epithelial carcinomas will have an equal distribution of both the squamous cell carcinoma which maybe well differentiated or keratinizing to

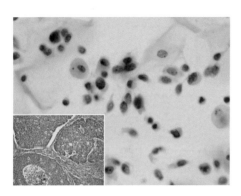

1-13D. Adenosquamous carcinoma. (Papanicolaou stain)

poorly differentiated or non-keratinizing as well as cells with true glandular differentiation
- Because of its uncommon nature, a cervical and endometrial biopsy maybe necessary to make the diagnosis

Special Stains and Immunocytochemistry
- A CK 5/6 and 34BE12 may be useful for documentation of the squamous component of the neoplasm

Modern Techniques for Diagnosis
- Non-contributory

Differential Diagnosis
- Endometrial adenocarcinoma with squamous differentiation
- Collision tumor of both endometrial adenocarcinoma and a cervical squamous cell carcinoma
  ➤ Both of these neoplasms could not be distinguished on a Pap smear cytologic diagnosis alone. Typically, a hysterectomy is done to document this type of lesion

PEARLS

⭑ True collision tumors and endometrial adenocarcinomas with squamous differentiation are very rare tumors and difficult to definitively diagnose on a Pap smear alone

HIGH-GRADE SARCOMAS

Clinical Features
- Patients present with bulky endometrial or myometrial masses, sometimes with diffuse enlargement of the uterus. These are usually picked up on computed tomography (CT) or ultrasound (US). In children, a protruding mass in the vaginal vault may be an indication of a sarcoma botryoides

Cytologic Features
- A difficult diagnosis to pick up in a Pap smear
- Singly dispersed or cohesive groups of large, pleomorphic, and bizarre cells with abundant polychromatic cytoplasm, variable-sized nuclei, some with marked nuclear convolutions, irregularly granular chromatin, and multiple nucleoli or chromocenters

Special Stains and Immunocytochemistry
- Not necessary if the cytologic features are observed as above

Modern Techniques for Diagnosis
- Noncontributory

Differential Diagnosis
- Stromal component of a malignant mixed müllerian tumor (MMMT)
  ➤ Typically would have both a malignant epithelial and stromal component

PEARLS

⭑ A positive Pap smear cytology of a pure uterine sarcoma is very rare. Even when abnormal cells are found, it may be difficult to give a definitive diagnosis of uterine sarcoma based solely upon its cytomorphologic characteristic on Pap smears

MALIGNANT LYMPHOMA

Clinical Features
▪ May present in a Pap smear of a patient with a history of leukemia/lymphoma. May also be a presenting finding of a Burkitt's lymphoma or a diffuse large cell lymphoma

Cytologic Features
▪ A monomorphic population of either small, intermediate sized, or large lymphocytes without appreciable tingible body macrophages

Special Stains and Immunocytochemistry
▪ Leukocyte common antigen (LCA), CD20, CD19, Kappa, and Lambda
▪ Although a Kappa and Lambda immunostain may not predict monoclonality in a cytologic specimen, a tissue core biopsy with immunohistochemistry and flow cytometry should be done to confirm the cytologic impression

Modern Techniques for Diagnosis
▪ Flow cytometric studies
▪ Molecular studies, PCR

Differential Diagnosis
▪ Lymphocytic cervicitis
  ➤ Lymphocytes may show variability in size and shape with tingible body macrophages in the smears

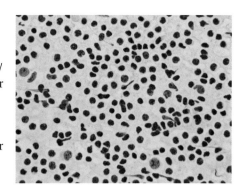

1-13E. Lymphoma. (Papanicolaou stain)

PEARLS

★ Ancillary testing such as flow cytometry and immunohistochemistry is the key to the diagnosis of a primary lymphoma or involvement by lymphoma of the cervix

METASTASES BY DIRECT EXTENTION AND DISTANT SPREAD

BREAST ADENOCARCINOMA

Clinical Features
▪ Clinical history of breast carcinoma is usually present
▪ There is usually no presenting illness, and malignant cells are usually found incidentally in a routine Pap smear

Cytologic Features
▪ Singly dispersed small cells with vacuolated cytoplasm pushing the nucleus to the side, angulating it, with inspissated material in the vacuoles, called "signet-ring" cells (red arrow)
▪ Nuclei are about the same size as a neutrophil, have fine to granular chromatin and inconspicuous nucleoli

Special Stains and Immunocytochemistry
▪ Gross cystic disease fluid protein-15 or mammaglobin could be used to confirm the cytologic impression

Modern Techniques for Diagnosis
▪ Noncontributory

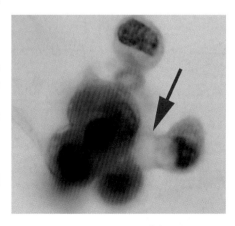

1-14A. Metastatic breast adenocarcinoma. (Papanicolaou stain)

Differential Diagnosis
■ HGSIL
➤ Typically, the cytoplasm would have some degree of keratinization or orangeophilia
■ Endometrial adenocarcinoma
➤ Typically, difficult to distinguish from a metastatic breast carcinoma without other ancillary immunohistochemical techniques
■ Metastatic gastric carcinoma
➤ Typically difficult to distinguish from metastatic breast carcinoma
➤ Needs immunohistochemistry for confirmation

PEARLS

☆ A metastatic lobular breast carcinoma verses metastatic gastric carcinoma to the cervix can be difficult to distinguish and may need immunohistochemistry for identification of the primary tumor

PAGET'S DISEASE OF THE VULVA

Clinical Features
■ Presents either as an erythematous or raised eczematous lesion of the vulva
■ Clinical history of adenocarcinoma of müllerian origin is the most common association, but adenocarcinoma may be found in association with a primary Bartholin's gland or adnexal adenocarcinoma of skin origin
■ The lesion is not an HPV-mediated disease

Cytologic Features
■ Singly dispersed and poorly cohesive groups of large nonkeratinized cells with vacuolated cytoplasm with inspissated material (arrows), finely granular chromatin and small nucleoli. Paget cells can be found in a cell-in-cell arrangement. There can be an associated HGSIL

Special Stains and Immunohistochemistry
■ Immunohistochemical stains show that the Paget cells are strongly immunoreactive for low-molecular-weight cytokeratins, CEA and EMA shows CK7 (B) and CK20 (C) staining

Modern Techniques for Diagnosis
■ Noncontributory

Differential Diagnosis
■ Adenocarcinoma of rectal primary
■ Urothelial or transitional cell carcinoma of the bladder

PEARLS

☆ Most cases are originally diagnosed as HGSIL or AGUS on Pap smears
☆ Biopsy is the mainstay of diagnosis

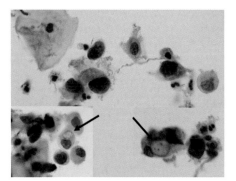

1-14B. Paget's disease of the vulva. (Papanicolaou stain)

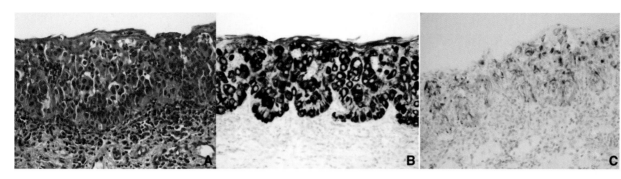

1-14C. Paget's disease of the vulva. (A) Hematoxylin and eosin stain, (B) CK7 and C. CK20. (Papanicolaou stain)

GASTRIC ADENOCARCINOMA

Clinical Features
- Clinical history of gastric carcinoma is usually present

Cytologic Features
- Singly dispersed small cells with vacuolated cytoplasm pushing the nucleus to the side, angulating it, with inspissated material in the vacuoles, called "signet-ring" cells
- Nuclei are about the same size as a neutrophil, have fine to granular chromatin and inconspicuous nucleoli

Special Stains and Immunocytochemistry
- Immunohistochemical stains for CDX2, MUC1, CK20, ERP, and Hep Par-1 has been used to differentiate a metastatic gastric from breast signet ring adenocarcinomas with a sensitivity of staining for CDX2 (90%), CK20 (60%), and Hep Par-1 (50%) for gastric primaries and MUC1 (100%) and ERP (80%) in breast primaries
- GCDFP-15 or mammaglobin may also be useful in the differentiation between primary gastric versus breast primary

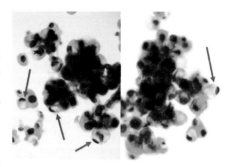

1-14D. Gastric carcinoma. Signet ring cells (arrows) (Papanicolaou stain)

Modern Techniques for Diagnosis
- Noncontributory

Differential Diagnosis
- Metastatic breast adenocarcinoma
  - ➤ Needs immunohistochemistry for confirmation of primary neoplasm

PEARLS

★ Cervical cytology is an uncommon yet probable site for the initial presentation of patients with gastric carcinomas

COLON ADENOCARCINOMA

Clinical Features
- Clinical history of rectal or colonic adenocarcinoma with direct extension to the vagina
- May also present concurrent with a history of radiation in the pelvis for treatment of stage III or IV colon adenocarcinoma

Cytologic Features
- Palisading aggregates of cells with elongated nuclei with irregularly granular chromatin without nucleoli are observed usually in a background of dirty necrosis and marked acute inflammation. These aggregates could be interpreted as "feathering."

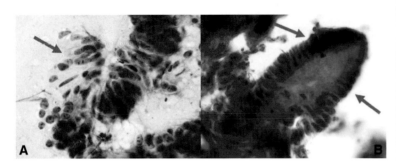
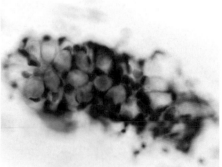

1-14E. Colonic carcinoma with *(top, left)*. (A) and without (B) "feathering" (Papanicolaou stain)

1-14F. Rectovaginal fistula *(top, right)* With benign colonic glands. (Papanicolaou stain)

But a substantial number of groupings would also have palisaded nuclei with a nice clean border around them

Special Stains and Immunocytochemistry
■ Immunohistochemical stains for CEA (monoclonal) and CK20 may be necessary to confirm the cytologic impression

Modern Techniques for Diagnosis
■ Noncontributory

Differential Diagnosis
■ Endocervical adenocarcinoma in situ or invasive endocervical adenocarcinoma
  ➤ Typically have no tumor diathesis if the lesion is primary to the endocervix
■ Rectovaginal fistula or colonic neovagina
  ➤ Tumor diathesis is not present, and benign glandular colonic epithelium is present instead

PEARLS

★ A complete clinical history of colonic adenocarcinoma is imperative for the diagnosis

UROTHELIAL CELL CARCINOMA

Clinical Features
■ Clinical history of bladder cancer with subsequent radiation therapy for stage III or IV cancers

Cytologic Features
■ Singly dispersed and clusters of cells with uniformly round to oval nuclei, fine granular chromatin without nucleoli in a background of tumor diathesis

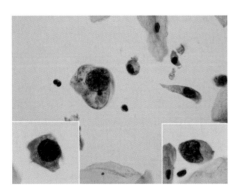

Special Stains and Immunocytochemistry
■ Uroplakins and CK20 is typically positive in metastatic transitional cell carcinomas of the urinary bladder

Modern Techniques for Diagnosis
■ Noncontributory

Differential Diagnosis
■ Papillary transitional cell carcinoma of the cervix
  ➤ Typically would be CK7 positive and CK20 negative
■ Endocervical adenocarcinoma in situ with associated HGSIL
  ➤ Typically would not have tumor diathesis

1-14G. Urothelial cell carcinoma. (Papanicolaou stain)

✴ A complete clinical history of urothelial carcinoma is imperative for the diagnosis

MALIGNANT MELANOMA

Clinical Features
▨ May present as a primary cervical tumor or metastasis from other sites

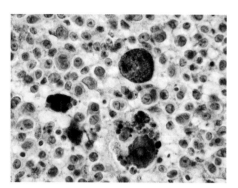

Cytologic Features
▨ Singly dispersed plasmacytoid cells in varying sizes with amphophilic to metachromatic cytoplasm with enlarged, at times binucleated nuclei, frequently with centrally placed nucleoli
▨ The cells may have deep pigmentation or not

Special Stains and Immunocytochemistry
▨ Melan A and HMB-45 are the most commonly used immunostains to confirm the cytologic impression

1-14H. Malignant melanoma.
(Papanicolaou stain)

Modern Techniques for Diagnosis
▨ Noncontributory

Differential Diagnosis
▮ Invasive endocervical adenocarcinoma
➤ Typically are nonpigmented, but would need to use immunohistochemistry to rule out a melanoma if the patient has a history of melanoma

✴ The cells of malignant melanoma may be epithelioid or spindled and may be pigmented or not. Immunohistochemical stains should help in the definitive diagnosis

MICROORGANISMS IN PAP SMEAR

CANDIDA

Clinical Features
▨ Patients typically present with itchy, inflamed skin and mucous membranes often with a thick white cottage cheese-like discharge. Predisposing factors include HIV infection, diabetes, chemotherapy suppression, and broad-spectrum antibiotics

Cytological Features
▨ This shows the yeast and pseudohyphae forms of the fungi

Special Stains and Immunohistochemistry
▨ The Papanicolaou stain is an adequate stain for the identification of fungi in Pap smears and can be seen in both conventional and liquid based media

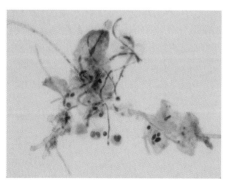

Modern Techniques for Diagnosis
▨ Noncontributory

1-15A. Candida. (Papanicolaou stain)

Differential Diagnosis

■ *Candida (Torulopsis) glabrata* – Morphologically consists only of the yeast form. Although not commonly seen in Pap smears, speciation to support its presence may represent a more diffuse or disseminated infection involving the cervix in this otherwise opportunistic infection

■ *Geotrichum candidum* – Morphologically consists only of the hyphae form. This organism is not commonly seen in Pap smears unless as part of a generalized infection, and perhaps if were not for its morphologic similarity to *Candida albicans* would not be mentioned in association with Pap smears, in general

PEARLS

★ Although fungi are fairly common occurrence in Pap smear cytology, both *Candida glabrata* and *Geotrichum candidum* may also herald a disseminated infection

HERPES

Clinical Features

■ Anogenital painful ulcers, which starts out as blisters, which take several weeks to heal are common presenting symptoms. Reinfection and reactivation of either HSV-1 and HSV-2 may be less painful due to antibody production from latent infections. Pap smear diagnosis during pregnancy is important to prevent direct vertical passage to the neonate that can present with a potentially fatal infection

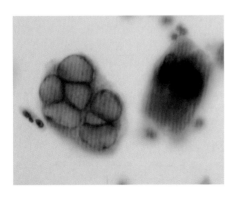

1-15B. Herpes. (Papanicolaou stain)

Cytologic Features

■ Shows an enlarged multinucleated cell with prominent nuclear molding with chromatin condensation and margination in the nuclear rim producing glassy nuclei

Special Stains and Immunohistochemistry

■ HSV-1 and HSV-2 immunocytochemical stains can be used in equivocal cases where the classical cytopathic effect seen in Papanicolaou stain may not be easily identified

Modern Techniques for Diagnosis

■ Noncontributory

Differential Diagnosis

■ Multinucleated endocervical cells. However, they lack the intranuclear inclusions

PEARLS

★ Diagnosis in Pap smear cytology especially in pregnancy is important so that an elective cesarean section can be explored as an option to the mother

CYTOMEGALOVIRUS

Clinical Features

■ Are usually seen in association with immune deficiencies as in HIV infection, chemoradiation, and in patients on steroidal therapy. It is rarely seen in Pap smears and is more commonly seen in urine specimens or endothelial or stromal cells in tissues.

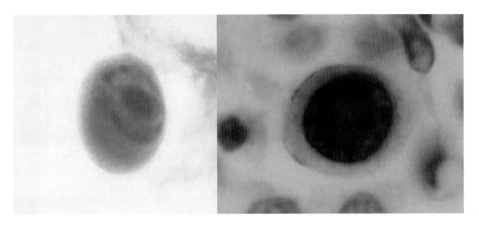

1-15C. CMV. (A) Papanicolaou and (B) IP stain

However, infection in the endocervical glandular and squamous epithelium of the cervix has been reported. Coinfection with HPV is not common

Cytologic Features
▥ This shows the prototypically enlarged cell with an enlarged nuclei and centrally placed prominent nucleoli with an "owl's-eye" or "bulls-eye" cytomorphology

Special Stains and Immunohistochemistry
▥ Immunohistochemical stains for CMV may be used in equivocal cases

Modern Techniques for Diagnosis
▥ Noncontributory

Differential Diagnosis
▥ Differentiation from HSV can be difficult

PEARLS

★ May present as a Pap smear finding even in immunocompetent and asymptomatic hosts. And because of its potential significance in women of childbearing age, identification of this viral cytopathic effect is crucial

TRICHOMONADS

Clinical Features
▥ Typically causes a frothy greenish discharge with putrid odor. Itching, painful urination and abdominal pain are common presenting symptoms. When symptomatic, the vagina and cervix have punctate small hemorrhages, which grossly looks like a strawberry, hence is clinically dubbed the "strawberry cervix". Many can be asymptomatic

Cytologic Features
▥ These organisms are typically found either singly dispersed or in aggregates, as in this case, in the cytoplasm of one of the squamous epithelial cells. They are typically "pear shaped" and have eosinophilic granules in their cytoplasm. An axostyle where the flagellae is attached is typically seen (arrows)

Special Stains and Immunohistochemistry
▥ A wet prep mount at the clinic is enough to document the presence of this fast-moving flagellate organism. The organisms can also be seen using the

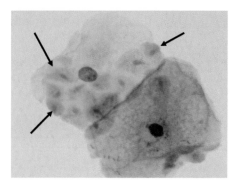

1-15D. Trichomonads. (Papanicolaou stain)

Papanicolaou-stained slide prepared from either conventional or liquid-based media. Typically, an associated marked acute inflammation is seen that a thorough search for the organism is warranted if there is exuberant marked acute inflammation consisting mainly of neutrophils on a Pap smear. At times, "cannon-ball" or "golf-ball" cells are seen in association with this organism

Modern Techniques for Diagnosis
■ Noncontributory

Differential Diagnosis
■ Amoebiasis
  ➤ Amoebiasis maybe seen in Pap smears in women with concurrent diarrhea at the time of the Pap smear. These organisms are about the same size as trichomonads, parabasal cell nuclei, or neutrophils. They do not have a visible axostyle, but the organelles in amoebas may be mistaken for the granules in trichomonas

PEARLS

★ This infection, including amebiasis is very easily treatable with metronidazole, that its identification in Pap smear is imperative

LEPTOTHRIX

Clinical Features
■ Does not have a clinical presenting symptom by itself, but is commonly associated with trichomonads. The presence of Leptothrix in a Pap smear heralds the presence of trichomonads (75–80%), but the reverse is not true. Trichomonads can be seen without Leptothrix

Cytologic Features
■ These are long, filamentous bacteria that are about half the diameter of candida, but with clear segmentations. They can be seen in association with bacterial vaginosis and trichomoniasis

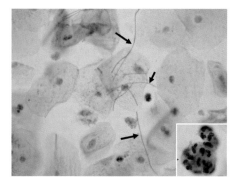

1-15E. Leptothrix. (arrows) are commonly associated with trichomonads and "golf-ball" cells (Papanicolaou stain) (inset)

Special Stains and Immunohistochemistry
■ Noncontributory

Modern Techniques for Diagnosis
■ Noncontributory

Differential Diagnosis
■ May be confused with certain forms of Dorderlein's bacillus

PEARLS

★ Presence of this long, filamentous bacterium should prompt a search for trichomonads, which are treatable symptomatic infections

GARDNERELLA VAGINALIS

Clinical Features
▨ Commonly seen in sexually active women of childbearing age and presents with a frothy vaginal discharge with "fishy" odor. There is usually no associated acute inflammation unless also associated with other infections such as trichomonads, candida, or HPV

Cytologic Features
▨ A prototypical "clue-cell" is seen whereby coccoid to somewhat short bacilloid organisms are found completely covering the squamous epithelium. This is due to the shift in the vaginal flora from mildly acidic where the normal vaginal bacterial flora is predominantly composed of the lactobacilli to basic where a plethora of coccoid microorganisms exponentially grow

Special Stains and Immunohistochemistry
▨ Noncontributory

Modern Techniques for Diagnosis
▨ Noncontributory

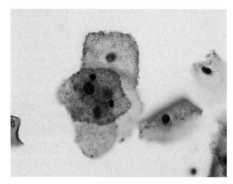

1-15F. Gardnerella vaginalis. (clue cells) (Papanicolaou stain)

Differential Diagnosis
▨ Microorganisms that have been described to comprise this spectrum include: Peptostreptococcus, *Mycoplasma hominus*, Mobilincus, and *Ureaplasma urealyticum*

PEARLS

☆ Can be related to frequent douching and subsequent gradual loss of hydrogen-peroxide producing lactobacilli as a natural vaginal flora

ACTINOMYCES

Clinical Features
▨ Usually associated with women on IUD or other foreign body such as tampons. Usually does not cause any clinical symptoms and may be present without any acute inflammation

Cytologic Features
▨ The organisms form a fuzz-ball that is very dense in the center and thinned out in the periphery whereby one can see the filamentous bacteria. The filaments formed by this bacterium are thinner than either candida or Leptothrix. It is the same organism found in the crevices of tonsils which has been dubbed "sulfur granules" because they are somewhat whitish yellow in color

Special Stains and Immunohistochemistry
▨ Noncontributory

Modern Techniques for Diagnosis
▨ Noncontributory

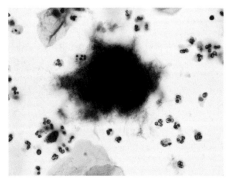

1-15G. Actinomyces. (Papanicolaou stain)

Differential Diagnosis

■ A number of organisms, including candida, nocardia, dermatophytes, bacterial aggregates, and foreign substances such as sulfa drug crystals may resemble actinomyces

PEARLS

☆ Actinomyces is usually a normal commensal organism in tonsils

☆ In IUD users, it can cause serious infection of the pelvis, ovary and uterus, such that routine identification of the organism is still important in Pap smears

☆ Removal of the intrauterine device and treatment with trimethoprim and sulfamethoxazole (Bactrim®) effectively gets rid of the infection

SCHISTOSOMA HAEMATOBIUM

Clinical Features

■ Schistosome eggs and miracidia are usually found in urine in patients living in areas where the organism is indigenous such as Egypt or Madagascar and can present with visible lesions in the cervix characterized by erosion and induration. A vaginal or cervical biopsy and Pap smear can also show the eggs of the Schistosomes. Presumably the adult organisms have found its way from the bladder to the vagina and cervix and lay their eggs in these soft tissues. Can be the most common cause of squamous cell carcinoma of the bladder in some people of those parts of the world

Cytologic Features

■ The eggs of *Schistosoma haematobium* measure somewhere between 120 and 180 μm by 40–70 μm. It is enough to be seen at a low 100× light microscopic magnification. The eggs have a terminal spine as opposed to *Schistosoma mansoni* where the spine is found laterally. The miracidia is the hatched form of the organism and is diffusely ciliated

Special Stains and Immunohistochemistry

■ Noncontributory

Modern Techniques for Diagnosis

■ Noncontributory

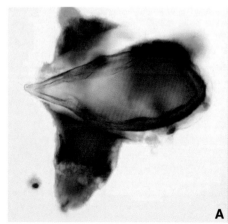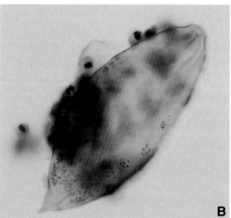

1-15H. Schistosoma haematobium egg. (A and B and miracidium (A)) (Papanicolaou stain)

Differential Diagnosis
- Other schistosomes: *S. mansoni, S. japonicum and S. haematobium*

★ Must be kept in mind in Pap smears of new immigrants coming from those parts of the world where the organism is indigenous

NEISSERIA GONORRHEA

Clinical Features
- Venereal infection
- Abundant, purulent vaginal exudate
- Urethra and perivaginal glands commonly infected

Cytologic Features
- Bean-shaped gram-negative diplococci
- The microorganisms often are seen on the surface of squamous cells
- Better seen on air-dried areas of the smears (edges of the glass slide)
- Large numbers of microorganisms can be appreciated within swollen polymorpho-nuclear leucocytes

Special Stains and Immunohistochemistry
- Gram-negative diplococci

Differential Diagnosis
- Other cocci microorganisms
- Chlamydial microorganisms
- Phagocytosed debris

Modern Techniques for Diagnosis
- A PCR test for chlamydia and gonorrhea using a cervical swab or urine sample is available using Roche Diagnostics' AMPLICOR® PCR platform.
- Becton Dickenson's ProbeTec CT by Gen-probe®
- Hybrid capture 2 CT/NG by Digene®

★ Along with *Chlamydia trachomatis*, is the most common and easily treatable cause of infertility in women, that a clinical suspicion and immediate testing based on clinical suspicion at the doctor's office should be done

★ *Chlamydia trachomatis* and *Neisseria gonorrhea* are two infectious agents that do not have a clear cytopathic effect and for which the Pap smear is NOT the diagnostic modality of choice

CHLAMYDIA TRACHOMATIS

Clinical Features
- *Chlamydia trachomatis* is the most common cause of pelvic inflammatory disease (PID) in young women of child-bearing age. The organism has been considered a bacterium with both DNA and RNA but considered to have similar properties to a viral pathogen as it does not have the ability to produce its own source of ATP

and therefore, an obligate intracellular organism. It is difficult to identify morphologically on Pap smears as it does not induce any typical cytopathic change in the cells. However, it induces a lymphocytic or chronic inflammatory change within the cervix causing a "follicular cervicitis" consisting of well-formed germinal centers with plasma cells and lymphocytes. Because of this difficulty in Pap smear diagnosis, other diagnostic strategy is used, such as antigen detection, immunoflourescence and polymerase chain reaction such as: (1) Amplicor Chlamydia trachomatis/Neisseria gonnorhea by Roche Diagnostics®, (2) BD ProbeTec CT by Gen-probe®, and (3) hybrid capture 2 CT/NG by Digene® are all appropriate tests used reaching 80–95% detection rates

Cytologic Features
▪ Prototypical cytologic features seen on Pap smears, therefore, include a plasmacytoid to lymphocytic infiltrate with capillary networks

Special Stains and Immunohistochemisty
▪ Noncontributory

Modern Techniques for Diagnosis
▪ A PCR test for chlamydia and gonorrhea using a cervical swab or urine sample is available using Roche Diagnostics' AMPLICOR® PCR platform
▪ Becton Dickenson's ProbeTec CT by Gen-probe®
▪ Hybrid capture 2 CT/NG by Digene®

Differential Diagnosis
▪ Noncontributory

PEARLS

★ Along with *Neisseria gonorrhea*, is the most common and easily treatable cause of infertility in women, that a clinical suspicion and immediate testing based on clinical suspicion at the doctor's office should be done

SYPHILIS

Clinical Features
▪ This disease is generally accepted as a generalized infection, which is usually divided into stages for which inclusion in a Pap smear chapter is done mainly for completeness and perhaps only detected, if at all, clinically during its primary phase. Venereal syphilis may present in the mucus membranes of the vagina, vulva, and intertriginous areas as a painless ulcer or chancre with a smooth base and a rolled, raised firm edge. Clinical suspicion at this point may warrant a scrape test of the ulcer base and visualization under dark-field microscopy to show the spirochetes of Treponema pallidum (the organism causing syphilis). Unless suspected at the outset of the infection, may be difficult to diagnose clinically during its secondary and tertiary stages, as this disease typically mimics most other diseases by its clinical symptomatology

Cytologic Features
▪ Unless suspected, and a scrape test is not done, may be missed entirely at the time of initial clinical presentation. There are no prototypical cytopathic changes other than visualization of the organism by dark-field microscopy

Special Stains and Immunohistochemistry
▨ Special silver stains may be helpful

Modern Techniques for Diagnosis
▨ Noncontributory

Differential Diagnosis
■ Other spirochetal organisms: *Borrelia burgdorferi* (Lyme disease), *B. recurrentis* (relapsing fever)

★ A clinical diagnosis done best at the bedside

PUBIC LOUSE OR "CRAB"

Clinical Features
▨ Lice are arthropod vectors, which are typically seen in association with hairy parts of the body such as hair, beard, and of course, the pubis. Pubic lice sometimes are seen in Pap smears of women in endemic areas and characteristically present themselves with a pruritic bite wound in the skin

Cytologic Features
▨ Nits can be seen attached to the hair shaft, but more commonly, the arthropod itself. Pubic lice can be seen with the naked eye as 1–2 mm long. The arthropod itself has three pairs of legs with a claw on each end

Special Stains and Immunohistochemistry
▨ Noncontributory

Modern Techniques for Diagnosis
▨ Noncontributory

Differential Diagnosis
■ Other arthropods such as:
➤ *Pediculosis humanus* (body louse)
➤ *Ctenocephalides* spp. (dog or cat flea)
➤ *Tunga penetrans* (jigger flea)
➤ *Triatoma* spp. (reduviid or kissing bug)
➤ *Cimex* spp. (bed bug)

★ Pubic louse can be passed on through sexual transmission from person-to-person, but can also be passed on from bedding and towels from an infected individual
★ An over-the-counter medication used to treat head louse can be used to treat the infection
★ Anyone in contact with the person and all family members should also be informed so they can be treated and the linens and towels discarded or washed

CONTAMINANTS IN PAP SMEAR

ALTERNARIA ALTERNATA

Clinical Features
■ Typically considered a nonpathogenic fungal contaminant in a Pap smear, but has been described as a once emerging pathogen in the immunocompromised host causing infections of the bone, nasal sinuses, ear, eye, skin, and soft tissues

Cytologic Features
■ Alternaria is an uncommon Pap smear contaminant, here shown to have hyphal budding. It is commonly referred to as a "snow-shoe" or "club-shaped" fungus. It forms dark, erect, septate conidiophores, either simple or branched, bearing large, catenulate (in chains), muriform brown conidia

Special Stains and Immunohistochemistry
■ Masson–Fontana stain can be used to demonstrate the melanin-like brown pigment in the fungal cell wall, but is generally unnecessary

Modern Techniques for Diagnosis
■ Noncontributory

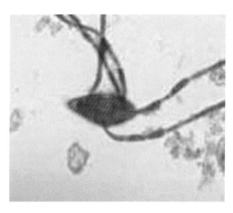

1-16A. Alternaria alternata.
(Papanicolaou stain)

Differential Diagnosis
■ Other Phaeohyphomycoses with similar cytomorphology such as
  ➤ Curvularia species
  ➤ Bipolaris species
  ➤ Exserohilum species
■ Dactylaria species

PEARLS

★ Very uncommonly identified, so take a photomicrograph

ASTEROSCLEREIDS

Clinical Features
■ Asterosclereids are uncommon contaminant found in Pap smears that are derived from higher plant parts such as flowers and seeds. Growing plants absorb water containing silica. Silification of plant cell walls and intercellular spaces happen from condensation of water in these spaces. Water lilies, which belong to the genus Nymphaeaceae, in particular, are endogenous to ponds. Laticiferous cells are found in the peduncle of the flower and are commonly associated with the vascular bundles. At one point, they are thought to function as a supporting structure, but more recently, sclereids are thought to act as condensers of water vapor

Cytologic Features
■ The classic cytologic features are demonstrated in Figure 1-16B.
■ This asterosclereid structure found in a Pap smear of a nineteen-year-old woman: Papanicolaou stain (left) and in polarized light (right), attests to the silification of this plant cell structure, which seems to have "holes" (arrows) in its center structure, which speaks to its function as a possible water condenser

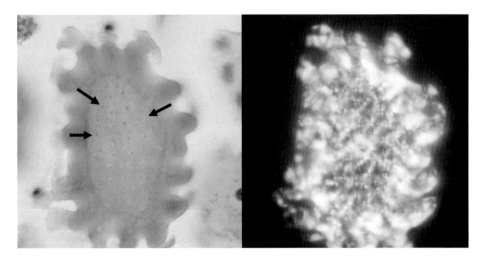

1-16B. Asterosclereids. (Pap stained and polarized) (Papanicolaou stain)

Special Stains and Immunohistochemistry
- Noncontributory

Modern Techniques for Diagnosis
- Noncontributory

Differential Diagnosis
- Parasitic infectious agents
- Foreign bodies

★ Again, very uncommonly identified, so take a photomicrograph

PLANT MATTER

Clinical Features
- Noncontributory

Cytologic Features
- Several acellular fluid filled sacs with poorly defined cell walls were seen in this Pap smear

Special Stains and Immunohistochemistry
- Noncontributory

Modern Techniques for Diagnosis
- Noncontributory

Differential Diagnosis
- Other plant cellular parts such as sclereids, plant fibers, plant epidermis, etc.
  ➤ Plant cellular parts usually does not have a distinguishable nuclei as they are usually structural or protective layers of plant parts the same way superficial squamous cells lose their nuclei in human skin

1-16C. Vegetable matter.
(Papanicolaou stain)

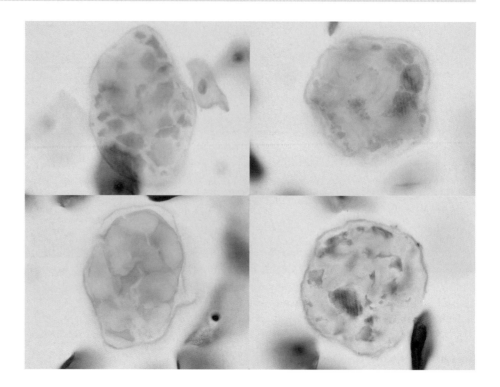

★ These come in unusual and interesting shapes and sizes in cytology

TRICHOMES

Clinical Features
■ Trichomes are higher plant particles which are also unusual Pap smear contaminant

Cytologic Features
■ Trichomes can come in many shapes, but this one has eight separate tentacles

Special Stains and Immunohistochemistry
■ Noncontributory

Modern Techniques for Diagnosis
■ Noncontributory

Differential Diagnosis
■ Mites and other species of ticks. See list of arthropods on XVI. K. under pubic louse – these organisms, however, have a central body core, which is not present in Trichomes

1-16D. Trichomes. (Papanicolaou stain)

★ Can be alarming when you first see it as they can look like arthropods, but should not have a complex bodily structure

CARPET BEETLE PART

Clinical Features
▨ Noncontributory

Cytologic Features
▨ Typically are elongated structures with regularly repeating spines and a spearhead tip

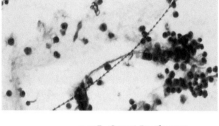

1-16E. Carpet Beetle part.
(Papanicolaou stain)

Special Stains and Immunohistochemistry
▨ Noncontributory

Modern Techniques for Diagnosis
▨ Noncontributory

Differential Diagnosis
■ Nothing else looks like that

PEARLS
★ More commonly seen in the days when Pap smears where taken using cotton-tipped swabs and wooden spatulas

POLLEN

Clinical Features
▨ Noncontributory

Cytologic Features
▨ Can be found in different sizes and forms from oval to round shapes

Special Stains and Immunohistochemistry
▨ Noncontributory

Modern Techniques for Diagnosis
▨ Noncontributory

Differential Diagnosis
■ Parasite eggs of *Enterobius vermicularis* have the same smooth shape and can be mistaken for pollen. However, parasite eggs measure approximately 50 × 130 microns and a typical intermediate cell nuclei approximately 6–7 microns in diameter. Pollens, depending on type, are the same size as or slightly bigger than intermediate cell nuclei

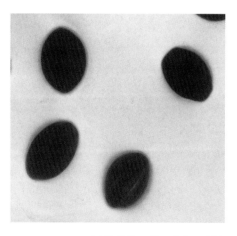

PEARLS
★ The best way to differentiate parasite eggs from pollen is to make a size comparison with an inflammatory cell such as a lymphocyte and neutrophil or with an intermediate cell nucleus

1-16F. Pollen. (Papanicolaou stain)

REFERENCES

REACTIVE CHANGES

Chien CR, Ting LL, Hsieh CY, Lai MS. Post-radiation Pap smear for Chinese patients with cervical cancer: a ten-year follow-up. *Eur J Gynaecol Oncol.* 2005;26(6):619–22.

Demay, R. The Pap smear. *The Art and Science of Cytopathology, Exfoliative Pathology.* ASCP Press, Copyright 1996, pp. 61–205.

Halford JA. Cytological features of chronic follicular cervicitis in liquid-based specimens: a potential diagnostic pitfall. *Cytopathology.* 2002; 13(6):364–70.

Halse TA, Musser KA, Limberger RJ. A multiplexed real-time PCR assay for rapid detection of *Chlamydia trachomatis* and identification of serovar L-2, the major cause of *Lymphogranuloma venereum* in New York. *Mol Cell Probes.* 2006; 20(5):290–7.

Kiviat NB, Paavonen JA, Wolner-Hanssen P, Critchlow CW, Stamm WE, Douglas J, Eschenbach DA, Corey LA, Holmes KK. Histopathology of endocervical infection caused by *Chlamydia trachomatis*, herpes simplex virus, *Trichomonas vaginalis*, and *Neisseria gonorrhoeae*. *Hum Pathol.* 1990; 21(8):831–7.

Malik SN, Wolkinson EJ, Drew PA, Hardt NS. Benign cellular changes in Pap smears. Causes and significance. *Acta Cytol.* 2001; 45(1):5–8.

Williamson BA, DeFrias D, Gunn R, Tarjan G, Nayar R. Significance of extensive hyperkeratosis on cervical/vaginal smears. *Acta Cytol.* 2003; 47(5):749–52.

LOW-GRADE SQUAMOUS INTRAEPITHELIAL LESIONS

Demay, R.. The Pap smear. *The Art and Science of Cytopathology, Exfoliative Pathology.* ASCP Press, 1996, pp. 61–205 (Chapter 6).

Solomon D, Nayar R. *The Bethesda System for reporting Cervical Cytology.* 2nd ed., 2004, pp. 91–98.

ARIAS-STELLA CHANGE OF PREGNANCY

Chhieng DC, Elgert P, Cangiarella JF, Cohen JM. Significance of AGUS Pap smears in pregnant and postpartum women. *Acta Cytol.* 2001; 45(3):294–9.

Kabayashi TK, Okamoto H. Cytopathology of pregnancy-induced cell patterns in cervicovaginal smears [review]. *Am J Clin Pathol.* 2000; 114 Suppl:S6–20.

Michael CW, Esfahani FM. Pregnancy-related changes: a retrospective review of 278 cervical smears. *Diagn Cytopathol.* 1997; 17(2):99–107.

Ordi J, Romagosa C, Tavassoli FA, Nogales F, Palacin A, Condom E, Torne A, Cardesa A. CD10 expression in epithelial tissues and tumors of the gynecologic tract: a useful marker in the diagnosis of mesonephric, trophoblastic, and clear cell tumors. *Am J Surg Pathol.* 2003; 27(2):178–86.

Session DR, Lee GS, Choi J, Wolgemuth DJ. Expression of cyclin E in gynecologic malignancies. *Gynecol Oncol.* 1999; 72(1):32–7.

ATYPICAL SQUAMOUS CELLS

Clavel C, Masure M, Levert M, Putaud I, Mangeonjean C, Lorenzato M, Nazeyrollas P, Gabriel R, Quereux C, Birembaut P. Human papillomavirus detection by the hybrid capture II assay: a reliable test to select women with normal cervical smears at risk for developing cervical lesions. *Diagn Mol Pathol.* 2000; 9(3):145–50.

Demay, R.The Pap smear. *The Art and Science of Cytopathology, Exfoliative Pathology.* ASCP Press, 1996, pp. 61–205 (chap 6).

Solomon D, Nayar R. *The Bethesda System for reporting Reporting Cervical Cytology*, 2nd ed., 2004, pp. 91–98.

HIGH-GRADE SQUAMOUS INTRAEPITHELIAL LESIONS

Demay, R. The Pap smear. *The Art and Science of Cytopathology, Exfoliative Pathology.* ASCP Press, 1996, pp. 61–205 (Chapter 6).

Keating JT, Cviko A, Reithdorf S, Rietdorf L, Quade BJ, Sun D, Duensing S, Sheets EE, Munger K, Crum CP. Ki-67, cyclin E, and p16INK4 are complimentary surrogate biomarkers for human papilloma virus-related cervical neoplasia. *Am J Surg Pathol.* 2001; 25(7):884–91.

Keating JT, Ince T, Crum CP. Surrogate biomarkers of HPV infection in cervical neoplasia screening and diagnosis [review]. *Adv Anat Pathol.* 2001; 8(2):83–92.

Solomon D, Nayar R. *The Bethesda System for Reporting Cervical Cytology.* 2nd ed., 2004, pp. 91–98.

HIGH-GRADE SQUAMOUS INTRAEPITHELIAL LESIONS INVOLVING ENDOCERVICAL GLANDS

Selvaggi SM. Cytologic features of high grade squamous intraepithelial lesions involving endocervical glands on thin-layer cytology. *Acta Cytol.* 2005; 49(6):689–90.

KERATINIZING SQUAMOUS CELL CARCINOMA

Demay, R. The Pap smear. *The Art and Science of Cytopathology, Exfoliative Pathology.* ASCP press, Copyright 1996, pp. 61–205 (Chapter 6).

Solomon D, Nayar R. *The Bethesda System for Reporting Cervical Cytology.* 2nd ed., 2004, pp. 91–98.

NONKERATINIZING SQUAMOUS CELL CARCINOMA

Demay, R. The Pap smear. *The Art and Science of Cytopathology, Exfoliative Pathology.* ASCP Press, 1996, pp. 61–205 (Chapter 6).

Selvaggi SM. Cytologic features of high grade squamous intraepithelial lesions involving endocervical glands on thin-layer cytology. *Acta Cytol.* 2005; 49(6):689–90.

Solomon D, Nayar R. *The Bethesda System for Reporting Cervical Cytology.* 2nd ed., 2004, pp. 117–8.

PAPILLARY SQUAMOTRANSITIONAL CELL OR PAPILLARY SQUAMOUS CELL CARCINOMA OF THE CERVIX

Al-Nafussi AI, Al-Yusif R. Papillary squamotransitional cell carcinoma of the uterine cervix: an advanced stage disease despite superficial location: report of two cases and review of the literature [review]. *Eur J Gynaecol Oncol.* 1998; 19(5):455–7.

Drew PA, Hong B, Massol NA, Ripley DL. Characterization of papillary squamotransitional cell carcinoma of the cervix. *J Low Genit Tract Dis.* 2005; 9(3):149–53.

Ng WK. Thin-layer (liquid-based) cytologic findings of papillary squamotransitional cell carcinoma of the cervix. Review of cases over a 4-year period with emphasis on potential diagnostic pitfalls [review]. *Acta Cytol.* 2003; 47(2):141–8.

Robinson CE, Sarode VR, Albores-Saavedra J. Mixed papillary transitional cell carcinoma and adenocarcinoma of the uterine cervix: a clinicopathologic study of three cases. *Int J Gynecol Pathol.* 2003; 22(3):220–5.

Vesoulis Z, Erhardt CA. Cytologic diagnosis of vaginal papillary squamotransitional cell carcinoma. A case report. *Acta Cytol.* 2001; 45(3):465–9.

ADENOCARCINOMA IN SITU OF ENDOCERVIX

Barreth D, Faught W, Schepansky A, Johnson G. The relationship between atypical glandular cells of undetermined significance on Pap smear and a clinically significant histologic diagnosis. *J Obstet Gynaecol Can.* 2004; 26(10):867–70.

Negri G, Egarter-Vigl E, Kasal A, Romano F, Haitel A, Mian C. p16INK4a is a useful marker for the diagnosis of adenocarcinoma of the cervix uteri and its precursors: an immunohistochemical study with immunocytochemical correlations. *Am J Surg Pathol.* 2003; 27(2):187–93.

Roberts JM, Thurloe JK, Biro C, Hyne SG, Williams KE, Bowditch RC. Follow-up of cytologic predictions of endocervical glandular abnormalities: histologic outcomes in 123 cases. *J Low Genit Tract Dis.* 2005; 9(2):71–7.

Saqi A, Gupta PK, Erroll M, Babiac A, Blackmun D, Mansukhani M, Vasquez M. High-risk human papillomavirus DNA testing: a marker for atypical glandular cells. *Diagn Cytopathol.* 2006; 34(3):235–9.

ENDOCERVICAL ADENOCARCINOMA

Negri G, Egarter-Vigl E, Kasal A, Romano F, Haitel A, Mian C. p16INK4a is a useful marker for the diagnosis of adenocarcinoma of the cervix uteri and its precursors: an immunohistochemical study with immunocytochemical correlations. *Am J Surg Pathol.* 2003; 27(2):187–93.

O'Neill CJ, McCluggage WG. p16 expression in the female genital tract and its value in diagnosis. *Adv Anat Pathol.* 2006; 13(1):8–15.

Vang R, Vihn TN, Burks RT, Barner R, Kurman RJ, Ronnett BM. Pseudoinfiltrative tubal metaplasia of the endocervix: a potential form of in utero diethylstilbestrol exposure-related adenosis simulating minimal deviation adenocarcinoma. *Int J Gynecol Pathol.* 2005; 24(4):391–8.

ENDOMETRIAL CELLS

Browne TJ, Genest DR, Cibas ES. The clinical significance of benign-appearing endometrial cells on a Papanicolaou test in women 40 years or older. *Am J Clin Pathol.* 2005; 124(6):834–7.

Simsir A, Carter W, Elgert P, Cangiarella J. Reporting endometrial cells in women 40 years and older: assessing the clinical usefulness of Bethesda 2001. *Am J Clin Pathol.* 2005; 123(4):571–5.

Thrall MJ, Kjeldahl KS, Savik K, Gulbahce HE, Pambuccian SE. Significance of benign endometrial cells in papanicolaou tests from women aged > or = 40 years. *Cancer.* 2005: 25; 105(4):207–16.

ENDOMETRIAL ADENOCARCINOMA

Haidopoulos DA, Stefanidis K, Rodolakis A, Pilalis A, Symiakaki I, Diakomanolis E. Histologic implications of Pap smears classified as atypical glandular cells. *J Reprod Med.* 2005; 50(7): 539–42.

Saad RS, Takei H, Liu YL, Silverman JE, Lipscomb JT, Ruiz B. Clinical significance of a cytologic diagnosis of atypical glandular cells, favor endometrial origin, in Pap smears. *Acta Cytol.* 2006; 50(1):48–54.

Scheiden R, Wagener C, Knolle U, Dippel W, Capesius C. Atypical glandular cells in conventional cervical smears: incidence and follow-up. *BMC Cancer.* 2004; 4:37.

Selvaggi SM. Background features of endometrial carcinoma on ThinPrep cytology. *Diagn Cytopathol.* 2005; 33(3):162–5.

Simsir A, Hwang S, Cangiarella J, Elgert P, Levine P, Sheffield MV, Roberson J, Talley L, Chhieng DC. Glandular cell atypia on Papanicolaou smears: interobserver variability in the diagnosis and prediction of cell of origin. *Cancer.* 2003: 25; 99(6):323–30.

EXTRAUTERINE MALIGNANCIES: PAPILLARY SEROUS ADENOCARCINOMA FROM EITHER OVARY, FALLOPIAN TUBE, AND ENDOMETRIUM

Park JY, Kim HS, Hong SR, Chun YK. Cytologic findings of cervicovaginal smears in women with uterine papillary serous carcinoma. *J Korean Med Sci.* 2005; 20(1):93–7.

Hwang H, Quenneville L, Yaziji H, Gown AM. Wilms tumor gene product: sensitive and contextually specific marker of serous carcinomas of ovarian surface epithelial origin. *Appl Immunohistochem Mol Morphol.* 2004; 12(2):122–6.

Egan JA, Ionescu MC, Eapen E, Jones JG, Marshall DS. Differential expression of WT1 and p53 in serous and endometrioid carcinomas of the endometrium. *Int J Gynecol Pathol.* 2004; 23(2):119–22.

Al Hussaini M, Stockman A, Foster H, McCluggage WG. WT-1 assists in distinguishing ovarian from uterine serous carcinoma and in distinguishing between serous and endometrioid ovarian carcinoma. *Histopathology.* 2004; 44(2):109–15.

EXTRAUTERINE MALIGNANCIES: SMALL CELL, UNDIFFERENTIATED OR "OAT CELL" CARCINOMA

Albores-Saavedra J, Latif S, Carrick KS, Alvarado-Cabrero I, Fowler MR. CD56 reactivity in small cell carcinoma of the uterine cervix. *Int J Gynecol Pathol.* 2005; 24(2):113–7.

Ciesla MC, Guidos BJ, Selvaggi SM. Cytomorphology of small-cell (neuroendocrine) carcinoma on ThinPrep cytology as compared to conventional smears. *Diagn Cytopathol.* 2001; 24(1):46–52.

Horn LC, Hentschel B, Bilek K, Richtr CE, Einenkel J, Leo C. Mixed small cell carcinomas of the uterine cervix: prognostic impact of focal neuroendocrine differentiation but not of Ki-67 labeling index. *Ann Diagn Pathol.* 2006; 10(3):140–3.

Ohwada M, Wada T, Saga Y, Tsunoda S, Jobo T, Kuramoto H, Konno R, Suzuki M. C-kit overexpression in neuroendocrine small cell carcinoma of the uterine cervix. *Eur J Gynaecol Oncol.* 2006; 27(1):53–5.

Stoler MH, Mills SE, Gersell DJ, Walker AN. Small-cell neuroendocrine carcinoma of the cervix. A human papillomavirus type 18-associated cancer. *Am J Surg Pathol.* 1991; 15(1): 28–32.

Zhou C, Hayes MM, Clement PB, Thomson TA. Small cell carcinoma of the uterine cervix: cytologic findings in 13 cases. *Cancer.* 1998 25; 84(5):281–8.

MALIGNANT MIXED MULLERIAN TUMORS

Casey MB, Caudill JL, Salomao DR. Cervicovaginal (Papanicolaou) smear findings in patients with malignant mixed Mullerian tumors. *Diagn Cytopathol.* 2003; 28(5):245–9.

Clement PB, Zubovits JT, Young RH, Scully RE. Malignant mullerian mixed tumors of the uterine cervix: a report of nine cases of a neoplasm with morphology often different from its counterpart in the corpus [review]. *Int J Gynecol Pathol.* 1998; 17(3):211–22.

Sharma NK, Sorosky JI, Bender D, Fletcher MS, Sood AK. Malignant mixed mullerian tumor (MMMT) of the cervix [review]. *Gynecol Oncol.* 2005; 97(2):442–5.

MALIGNANT MIXED EPITHELIAL TUMORS, ADENOSQUAMOUS CARCINOMAS

Serrano MF, El-Mofty SK, Gnepp DR, Lewis JS Jr. Utility of high molecular weight cytokeratins, but not p63, in the differential diagnosis of neuroendocrine and basaloid carcinomas of the head and neck. *Hum pathol.* 2008 Apr; 39(4):591–8.

Stefansson IM, Salvesen HB, Akslen LA. Loss of p63 and cytokeratin 5/6 expression is associated with more aggressive tumors in endometrial carcinoma patients. *Int J Cancer.* 2006 mar 1; 118(5):1227–33.

HIGH-GRADE SARCOMAS

Nickie-Psikuta M, Gawrychowski K. Different types and different prognosis-study of 310 uterine sarcomas. *Eur J Gynaecol Oncol.* 1993; 14 Suppl:105–13.

Wang X, Khoo US, Xue WC, Cheung AN. Cervical and peritoneal fluid cytology of uterine sarcomas. *Acta Cytol.* 2002; 46(3):465–9.

Wang X, Khoo US, Xue WC, Cheung AN. Cervical and peritoneal fluid cytology of uterine sarcomas. *Acta Cytol.* 2002; 46(3):465–9.

MALIGNANT LYMPHOMA

Chan JK, Loizzi V, Magistris A, Hunter MI, Rutgers J, DiSaia PJ, Berman ML. Clinicopathologic features of six cases of primary cervical lymphoma. *Am J Obstet Gynecol.* 2005; 193(3 pt. 1): 866–72.

Dursun P, Gultekin M, Bozdag G, Usubutum A, Uner A, Celik NY, Yuce K, Ayhan A. Primary cervical lymphoma: report of two cases and review of the literature. *Gynecol Oncol.* 2005; 98(3):484–9.

METASTASES BY DIRECT EXTENTION AND DISTANT SPREAD: BREAST ADENOCARCINOMA

Bhargava R, Beriwal S, Dabbs DJ. Mammaglobin vs GCDFP-15: an immunohistologic validation survey for sensitivity and specificity. *Am J Clin Pathol.* 2007; 127(1):1–11.

Flynn M, Singh N, Howitt R. An unusual case of concurrent metastatic breast carcinoma and endometrial adenocarcinoma detected on a routine cervical smear. *Cytopathology.* 2005; 16(3):157–8.

Green KM, Turyan HV, Jones JB, Hoda RS. Metastatic lobular carcinoma in a ThinPrep Pap test: cytomorphology and Differential Diagnosis. *Diagn Cytopathol.* 2005; 33(1):58–9.

Haji BE, Kapila K, Francis IM, Temmim L, Ahmed MS. Cytomorphological features of metastatic mammary lobular carcinoma in cervicovaginal smears: report of a case and review of literature [review]. *Cytopathology.* 2005; 16(1):42–8.

Watson MA, Dintzis S, Darrow CM, Voss LE, DiPersio J, Jensen R, Fleming TP. Mammaglobin expression in primary, metastatic, and occult breast cancer. *Cancer Res.* 1999; 59(13):3028–31.

PAGET'S DISEASE OF THE VULVA

Boardman CH, Webb MJ, Cheville JC, Lerner SE, Zincke H. Transitional cell carcinoma of the bladder mimicking recurrent paget's disease of the vulva: report of two cases, with one occurring in a myocutaneous flap. *Gynecol Oncol.* 2001; 82(1):200–4.

Costello TJ, Wang HH, Schnitt SJ, Ritter R, Antonioli DA. Paget's disease with extensive involvement of the female genital tract initially detected by cervical cytosmear. *Arch Pathol Lab Med.* 1988; 112(9):941–4.

Gu M, Ghafani S, Lin F. Pap smears of patients with extramammary Paget's disease of the vulva. *Diagn Cytopathol.* 2005; 32(6):353–7.

Guarner J, Cohen C. Vulvar Paget's disease. Cytologic and immunohistologic diagnosis of a case. *Acta Cytol.* 1988; 32(5):727–30.

Orlandi A, Piccione E, Francesconi A, Spagnoli LG. Simultaneous vulvar intraepithelial neoplasia and Paget's disease: report of two cases. *Int J Gynecol Cancer.* 2001; 11(3):224–8.

GASTRIC ADENOCARCINOMA

Bhargava R, Beriwal S, Dabbs DJ. Mammaglobin vs GCDFP-15: An immunohistologic validation survey for sensitivity and specificity. *Am J Clin Pathol.* 2007; 127(1):1–11.

Chu PG, Weiss LM. Immunohistochemical characterization of signet-ring cell carcinomas of the stomach, breast, and colon. *Am J Clin Pathol.* 2004; 121(6):884–92.

Fan Z, van de Rijn M, Montgomery K, Rouse RV. Heppar 1 antibody stain for the Differential Diagnosis of hepatocellular carcinoma: 676 tumors tested using tissue microarrays and conventional tissue sections. *Mod Pathol.* 2003; 16(2):137–44.

McGill F, Adachi A, Karimi N, Wadler S, Kim ES, Greston WM, Kleiner GJ. Abnormal cervical cytology leading to the diagnosis of gastric cancer [review]. *Gynecol Oncol.* 1990; 36(1): 101–5.

Okadome M, Saito T, Tsukamoto N, Nishi K, Nishiyama N, Nagata E. Endometrial scraping cytology in women with extragenital malignancies. *Acta Cytol.* 2006; 50(2):158–63.

Selvaggi LE, Di VAgno G, Loverro G, Masotina A, Cramarossa D, Napoli A, Resta L. Abnormal cervical PAP smear leading to the diagnosis of gastrointestinal cancer without cervico-vaginal metastases. *Eur J Gynaecol Oncol.* 1993; 14(5):398–401.

Watson MA, Dintzis S, Darrow CM, Voss LE, DiPersio J, Jensen R, Fleming TP. Mammaglobin expression in primary, metastatic, and occult breast cancer. *Cancer Res.* 1999; 59(13):3028–31.

COLON ADENOCARCINOMA

Childs AJ, Burke JJ 2nd, Perry MY, Check WE, Gallup DG. Recurrent colorectal carcinoma detected by routine cervicovaginal papanicolaou smear testing. *J Low Genit Tract Dis.* 2005; 9(4):236–8.

Sozen I, Small L, Kowalski M, Mayo SW, Hurwitz CA. Adenocarcinoma of the cervix metastatic from a colon primary and diagnosed from a routine pap smear in a 17-year-old woman: a case report. *J Reprod Med.* 2005; 50(10):793–5.

UROTHELIAL CELL CARCINOMA

Epstein NA. The cytologic appearance of metastatic transitional cell carcinoma. *Acta Cytol.* 1977; 21(6):723–5.

Johnson TL, Kini SR. Cytologic features of metastatic transitional cell carcinoma. *Diagn Cytopathol.* 1993; 9(3):270–8.

MALIGNANT MELANOMA

Deshpande AH, Munshi MM. Primary malignant melanoma of the uterine cervix: report of a case diagnosed by cervical scrape cytology and review of the literature. *Diagn Cytopathol.* 2001; 25(2):108–11.

Gupta S, Sodhani P, Jain S. Primary malignant melanoma of uterine cervix: a rare entity diagnosed on fine needle aspiration cytology – report of a case. *Cytopathology.* 2003; 14(3):153–6.

Schlosshauer PW, Heller DS, Koulos JP. Malignant melanoma of the uterine cervix diagnosed on a cervical cytologic smear. *Acta Cytol.* 1998; 42(4):1043–5.

Takehara M, Ito E, Saito T, Nishioka Y, Kudo R. Primary malignant melanoma of the uterine cervix: a case report. *J Obstet Gynaecol Res.* 1999; 25(2):129–32.

MICROORGANISMS IN PAP SMEAR: CANDIDA

Marks MI, Langston C, Eickhoff TC. Torulopsis glabrata–an opportunistic pathogen in man. *N Engl J Med.* 1970; 19;283(21):1131–5.

Sheehy TW, Honeycutt BK, Spencer JT. Geotrichum septicemia. *JAMA.* 1976; 8;235(10):1035–7.

Takei H, Ruiz B, Hics J. Cervicovaginal flora. Comparison of conventional pap smears and a liquid-based thin-layer preparation. *Am J Clin Pathol.* 2006; 125(6):855–9.

HERPES

Brown EL, Morrow R, Krantz Em, Arvin Am, Prober CG, Yasukawa LL, Corey L, Wald A. Maternal herpes simplex virus antibody avidity and risk of neonatal herpes. *Am J Obstet Gynecol.* 2006; 195(1):115–20.

Mark KE, Kim HN, Wald A, Gardella C, Reed SD. Targeted prenatal herpes simplex virus testing: can we identify women at risk of transmission to the neonate? *Am J Obstet Gynecol.* 2006; 194(2):408–14.

Sacks SL, Griffiths PD, Corey L, Cohen C, Cunningham A, Dusheiko gm, Self S, Spruance LR, Wald A, Whitley RJ. HSV-2 transmission [review]. *Antiviral Res.* 2004; 63 Suppl 1:S27–35.

Wald A.Genital HSV-1 infections. *Sex Transm Infect.* 2006; 82(3):189–90.

CYTOMEGALOVIRUS

Daxnerova Z, BErkova Z, Kaufman RH, Adam E. Detection of human cytomegalovirus DNA in 986 women studied for human papillomavirus-associated cervical neoplasia. *J Low Genit Tract Dis.* 2003; 7(3):187–93.

Huang JC, Naylor B. Cytomegalovirus infection of the cervix detected by cytology and histology: a report of five cases. *Cytopathology*. 1993; 4(4):237–41.

Hunt JL, Baloch Z, Judkins A, LiVolsi VA, Montone KT, Gupta PK. Unique cytomegalovirus intra-cytoplasmic inclusions in ectocervical cells on a cervical/endocervical smear. *Diagn Cytopathol*. 1998; 18(2):110–12.

Sekhorn HS, Press RD, Schmidt WA, Hawley M, Rader A. Identification of cytomegalovirus in a liquid-based gynecologic sample using morphology, immunohistochemistry, and DNA real-time PCR detection. *Diagn Cytopathol*. 2004; 30(6):411–17.

TRICHOMONADS

Audisio T, Pigini T, de Riutort SV, Schindler L, Ozan, Tocalli C, Bertolotto P. Validity of the papanicolaou smear in the diagnosis of Candida spp., *Trichomonas vaginalis*, and bacterial vaginosis. *J Low Genit Tract Dis*. 2001; 5(4):223–225.

Gupta RK, Naran S, Lallu S, Fauck R. Diagnosis of Entamoeba histolytica in a routine cervical smear. *Diagn Cytopathol*. 2003; 29(1):13.

Samuelson, J. Why metronidazole is active against both bacteria and parasites. *Antimicrobial Agents Chemother*., 1999; 43(7):1533–41.

Takei H, Ruiz B, Hicks J. Cervicovaginal flora. Comparison of conventional pap smears and a liquid-based thin-layer preparation. *Am J Clin Pathol*. 2006; 125(6):855–9.

Wolner- hanssen P, Krieger JN, Stevens CE, Kiviat NB, Koutsky L, Critchlow C, DeROuen T, Hillier S, Holmes KK. Clinical manifestations of vaginal trichomoniasis. *JAMA*. 1989; 261(4):571–6.

LEPTOTHRIX

Bibbo M, Harris MJ. *Acta Cytol*. 1972; 16(1):2–4.

GARDNERELLA VAGINALIS

Audisio T, Pigii T, de Riutort SV, Schindler L, Ozan M, Tocalli C, Bertolotto P. Validity of the papanicolaou smear in the diagnosis of Candida spp., *Trichomonas vaginalis*, and bacterial vaginosis. *J Low Genit Tract Dis*. 2001; 5(4):223–225.

Georgijevic AV, Sisovic JR, Djukic SV, Bujko MJ. Colposcopic and cytologic findings among women with abnormal vaginal flora. *J Low Genit Tract Dis*. 2002; 6(3):155–161.

Ness RB, Hillier SL, Richter HE, Soper DE, Stamm C, McGregor J, Bass DC, Sweet RL, Rice P. Douching in relation to bacterial vaginosis, lactobacilli, and facultative bacteria in the vagina. *Obstet Gynecol*. 2002; 100(4):765

Tolosa JE, Chaithongwongwatthana S, Daly S, Maw WW, Gaitan H, Lumbiganon P, Festin M, Chipato T, Sauvarin J, Goldenberg RL, Andrews WW, Whitney CG. The International Infections in Pregnancy (IIP) study: variations in the prevalence of bacterial vaginosis and distribution of morphotypes in vaginal smears among pregnant women. *Am J Obstet Gynecol*. 2006; 195(5):1198–204.

ACTINOMYCES

Bonacho I, Pita S, Gomez-Besteiro MI. The importance of the removal of the intrauterine device in genital colonization by actinomyces. *Gynecol Obstet Invest*. 2001; 52(2):119–23.

DeMay R. The Pap test. *American Society of Clinical Pathology*, 1st ed., 2005. p 102.

SCHISTOSOMA HAEMATOBIUM

Leutscher P, Raharisolo C, Pecarrere JL, Ravaoalimalala VE, serieye J, Rasendramino B, Vennervald B, Feldmeier H, Esterre P. Schistosoma haematobium induced lesions in the female genital tract in a village in Madagascar. *Acta Trop*. 1997; 66(1): 27–33.

Winn W, Allen S, Janda W, Koneman E, Procop G, Schreckenberger P, Woods G. *Koneman's Color Atlas and Textbook of Diagnostic Microbiology*. 6th ed. Lippincott Williams and Wilkins, pp. 1254, 1275–1276.

NEISSERIA GONORRHEA

Ghanem KG, Koumans EH, Johnson RE, Sawyer MK, Papp JR, Unger ER, Black CM, Markowitz LE. Effect of specimen order on Chlamydia trachomatis and Neisseria gonorrhoeae test performance and adequacy of Papanicolaou smear. *J Pediatr Adolesc Gynecol*. 2006; 19(1):23–30.

Heller CJ. Neisseria gonorrhoeae in Papanicolaou smears. *Acta Cytol*. 1974; 18(4):338–40.

CHLAMYDIA TRACHOMATIS

Winn W, Allen S, Janda W, Koneman E, Procop G, Schreckenberger P, Woods G. *Koneman's Color Atlas and Textbook of Diagnostic Microbiology*, 6th ed. Lippincott Williams and Wilkins, pp. 1128–1129.

SYPHILIS

Winn W, Allen S, Janda W, Koneman E, Procop G, Schreckenberger P, Woods G. *Koneman's Color Atlas and Textbook of Diagnostic Microbiology*. 6th ed. Lippincott Williams and Wilkins, pp. 1254, 1275–1276.

PUBIC LOUSE OR "CRAB"

Winn W, Allen S, Janda W, Koneman E, Procop G, Schreckenberger P, Woods G. *Koneman's Color Atlas and Textbook of Diagnostic Microbiology*, 6th ed. Lippincott Williams and Wilkins, pp. 1434–1435 and color plates A-3.

CONTAMINANTS IN PAP SMEAR: ALTERNARIA ALTERNATA

Ersahim C, Yong S, Wojcik EM. Alternaria spp. in the Pap test of a 25 year-old woman. *Diagn Cytopathol.* 2006; 34(5):349–50.

ASTEROSCLEREIDS

Angeles G, Owens SA, Ewers FW. Fluorescence shell: a novel view of sclereid morphology with the confocal laser scanning microscope. *Microsc Res Tech.* 2004; 1; 63(5):282–8.

Bozarth SR. Diagnostic Opal Phytoliths from pods of selected varieties of common beans (Phaseolus vulgaris). *American Antiquity.* 1990; 55(1): 98–104.

DeMay RM. *Practical Principles of Cytopathology.* ASCP Press. American Society of Clinical Pathology, p. 378.

Schneider EL. The floral anatomy of Victoria Schomb (Nymphaeaceae). *Botanical J Linnean Soc.*1976; 72: 115–148.

Schell WA, Pasarell L, Salkin IF, McGinnis MR. Bipolaris, Exophilia, Scedosporium, Sporothrix, and other dematiaceous fungi. *Manual of Clinical Microbiology.* 6th ed., Washington, DC: American Society of Microbiology. 1995, pp. 825–846.

Kwon-Chung KJ, Bennett JE. Phaeohyphomycosis. *Medical Mycology.* Williams and Wilkins; 1992, pp. 620–694.

PLANT MATTER

DeMay RM. *Practical Principles of Cytopathology.* ASCP Press, American Society of Clinical Pathology, p. 378.

TRICHOMES

DeMay RM. *Practical Principles of Cytopathology.* ASCP Press. American Society of Clinical Pathology. p. 378.

Winn W, Allen S, Janda W, Koneman E, Procop G, Schreckenberger P, Woods G. *Koneman's Color Atlas and Textbook of Diagnostic Microbiology*. 6th ed. Lippincott Williams and Wilkins, pp. 1434–1435 and color plates A-3.

CARPET BEETLE PART

Bechtold E, Staunton CE, Katz SS. Carpet beetle larval parts in cervical cytology specimens. *Acta Cytol.* 1985; 29(3):345–52.

DeMay RM. *Practical Principles of Cytopathology.* ASCP Press. American Society of Clinical Pathology, p. 378.

POLLEN

DeMay RM. *Practical Principles of Cytopathology.* ASCP Press. American Society of Clinical Pathology. p. 378.

Winn W, Allen S, Janda W, Koneman E, Procop G, Schreckenberger P, Woods G. *Koneman's Color Atlas and Textbook of Diagnostic Microbiology*, 6th ed. Lippincott Williams and Wilkins, pp. 1254, 1275–1276.

2

Exfoliative Pulmonary Cytology

Claire W. Michael

Chemotherapy
Radiation therapy
Malignant neoplasms
  Squamous cell carcinoma/epidermoid carcinoma (SQCC)
  Invasive bronchogenic adenocarcinoma (ADC)
  Bronchioalveolar carcinoma (BAC)
  Neuroendocrine tumors
  Anaplastic large cell carcinoma
  Hematopoietic malignancies (HPM)
Miscellaneous rare tumors
  Amyloidosis
Salivary gland analog tumors

METHODS OF EXFOLIATIVE RESPIRATORY CYTOLOGY

Sputum
- Consists mostly of mucus admixed with cellular and noncellular elements
- Candida, actinomyces, and other oral and pharyngeal contaminants as squamous (sq) epithelium are commonly present
- Can be easily obtained from patients with spontaneous production such as chronic smokers
- Can be induced by allowing the patient to breath a nebulized hypertonic saline solution for thirty minutes
- Best in diagnosing centrally located tumors
- Three consecutive sputum samples to diagnose carcinoma and five consecutive samples to exclude it
- Using five samples, the detection rate of disease is 90–95%
- Sensitivity is highest for detecting squamous cell carcinoma (SQCC), and reliability for typing of tumor is highest for small cell carcinoma
- Postbronchoscopy sputum has the highest diagnostic rate of all respiratory sampling techniques and is equally sensitive for central and peripheral lesions
- Adequate sample should contain numerous alveolar macrophages and adequate number of cells. Squamous cells should not be the predominant finding
- While not cost-effective as a screening method for SQCC, it remains an effective method for early detection of carcinoma/occult carcinoma in high-risk populations such as that of heavy smokers and in those with occupational risk

BRONCHOSCOPIC SPECIMENS (BRUSH, WASH, AND LAVAGE)

- Indicated for
  - Abnormal sputum cytology
  - Patients presenting with cough, hemoptysis, localized wheezes, bronchial obstruction, and a chest x-ray suspicious for tumor
  - Central lesions on chest x-ray and three consecutive negative sputum samples
  - Peripheral lesions
  - Evidence of severe diffuse lung disease
  - Inoperable or high-risk patients who need pathologic confirmation prior to initiating treatment
- Bronchial brushings (BBr) and washings (BW)
  - Sample mucosal and submucosal lesions that can be directly visualized by the bronchoscope
  - Allow mapping of sites involved with tumor

░ Brushings retrieve fragments of well-preserved tissue for diagnosis
  ➤ Alone has a diagnostic sensitivity of 70% and up to 90% when combined with other bronchoscopic samples
░ Washing may allow typing of some tumors that could not be accurately typed by brushing
░ Recent data suggest that BBr rather than brushing in conjunction with biopsy is more cost-effective, particularly when a lesion is well visualized
░ Bronchial alveolar lavage (BAL) is obtained by physically placing the bronchoscope in a segmental bronchus and injecting 2–100 mL of warm saline. The fluid is then aspirated and the process repeated four to five times
  ➤ Samples the epithelial lining cells of the distal airway spaces, inflammatory cells, histiocytes, and any foreign material or microorganisms residing within the alveolar spaces. Normal airway flora that have been pushed down by the endoscope may also be sampled
  ➤ Useful in the workup of opportunistic infections, interstitial lung disease, lung transplant patients, and peripheral lung masses
  ➤ Has a 68% sensitivity for detecting cancer and specificity of 80%

PULMONARY NATIVE CELLS: FROM NORMAL TO REACTIVE

SQUAMOUS (SQ) CELLS

░ Most commonly arise from the mouth and seen in sputum specimens
░ Numerous Sq cells in sputum imply saliva contamination rather than adequate deep cough sputum. They may also be seen in bronchoscopic specimens as an oral contaminant

Clinical Features
░ Atypia resulting in false positive diagnoses may be seen in Sq cells of oral origin due to buccal irritation, pemphigus disease, leukoplakia, and other mucosal injury
░ Atypia may also be seen in Sq metaplasia associated with a wide spectrum of conditions, such as chronic smoking, chronic bronchitis, bronchiectasis, lining of an abscess wall, center of pulmonary infarct, tracheostomy site, background of viral pneumonia, pulmonary fibrosis, or response to radiation and chemotherapy

Cytologic Features
░ Majority of Sq cells of oral origin are superficial keratinized cells similar to those seen in cervical smears. Occasionally these cells exhibit slight atypia
░ Immature metaplasia resembles that of cervix. The cells present as sheets of polygonal cells, sometimes with angulated borders. They are uniform in size and shape and exhibit regular nuclei with evenly distributed chromatin and normal nuclear to cytoplasmic (N/C) ratio
░ The cytoplasm is basophilic in immature forms and eosinophilic in the more mature cells
░ The atypia may appear in sheets or single cells and present as variation in size and shape and slight increase in N/C ratio. Depending on the cause of metaplasia, the cell may contain a vesicular nucleus with prominent nucleolus or a dark nucleus resembling SQCC

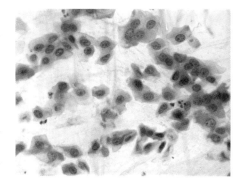

2-1. Squamous metaplasia. Squamous metaplasia in a bronchial washing from a patient with organizing pneumonia. The cells are polygonal in shape and contain vesicular nuclei with a small nucleoli. (Papanicolaou stain)

Special Stains and Immunohistochemistry
░ Noncontributory

Modern Techniques for Diagnosis
░ Noncontributory

Differential Diagnosis

■ Leukoplakia
  ➤ Anucleated Sq cells with intense orangeophilia
■ Pemphigus
  ➤ Highly abnormal cells with dense cytoplasm, enlarged nuclei with prominent nucleoli, evenly distributed chromatin, and thick but regular nuclear membrane
■ Tracheostomy
  ➤ Nuclear fragmentation, karyorrhexis, and karyolysis
■ Contaminant vegetable matter
  ➤ Regular spatial arrangement
  Quadrangular shape
  Thick cell walls
■ Pseudo-orangeophilia
  ➤ Occurs in the context of coagulative necrosis and may affect both benign and malignant cells
  ➤ Cells exposed to radiation or chemotherapy may acquire dense orange cytoplasm and nuclear atypia
  ➤ Glandular epithelium may appear as orangeophilic spindled cells
■ Well-differentiated/keratinizing SQCC
  ➤ Single cells with dense eosinophilic refractile (Papanicolaou stain) or bright robin blue cytoplasm (modified Giemsa stain), dark pyknotic nucleus, and a perinuclear halo
  ➤ Cells variable in shape and attain bizarre shapes
  ➤ Background of keratin, necrosis, and tumor diathesis
  ➤ Monolayer or two-dimensional sheets of malignant cells may be present particularly in brushings

PEARLS

✶ Atypical Sq cells present in small numbers
✶ Evidence of reactive changes in the background
✶ Necrotic background that lacks keratin suggests pseudoorangeophilia

TRACHEOBRONCHIAL LINING CELLS

■ Bronchial cells are pseudostratified ciliated columnar cells interspersed with goblet cells
  ➤ Line the tracheobronchial tree
  ➤ Bronchial cells are characterized by their columnar shape, a terminal bar at the luminal border to which cilia are attached. The cells are basally attached to a basement membrane. The nuclei are usually basal but can vary in location particularly in women where the nucleus migrate north during the cycle. The nucleoli are small
  ➤ Ciliated cells can shed as single cells or clusters
  ➤ They are the most common cells in BBr and BW
  ➤ As bronchial cells become irritated or undergo reactive changes, they will exhibit more prominent nucleoli, may become multinucleated, may undergo hyperplasia in the reserve cells (creola bodies), or lose their cilia (ciliocytophthoria)
■ Goblet cells are interspersed among the bronchial cells in the ratio of 1:5 or 1:6 along the bronchial tree. They are less frequent in the trachea and occur at the ratio of 1:10. Their number may increase as a reactive response to irritation in settings such as chronic smoking, asthma, bronchitis etc.
  ➤ Goblet cells have basally located nuclei similar to those of the bronchial cells. Their cytoplasm is distended with mucin that may compress the nuclei

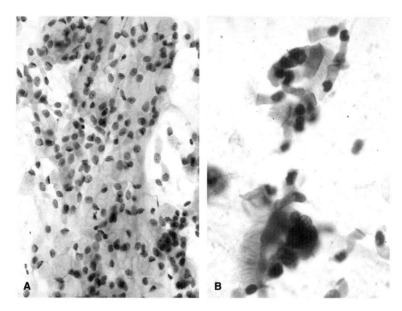

2-2A. Bronchial epithelium. Bronchial brush showing tall, columnar ciliated cells with basally located nuclei in a loosely cohesive sheet interspersed with goblet cells with signet ring appearance and intracytoplasmic pink mucin. (Papanicolaou stain)

2-2B. Bronchial epithelium. Reactive bronchial cells may become multinucleated and hypertrophied as shown on the lower portion of the image. (Papanicolaou stain)

▓ Basal cells, also known as reserve cells, are small round cells usually seen beneath the ciliated cells as small clusters with nuclei similar to those of bronchial cells

REACTIVE AND REPARATIVE BRONCHIAL CELL CHANGES

Clinical Features
▓ Insult to the bronchial mucosa such as bronchiectasis, pneumonial, toxic fumes, or radiation and chemotherapy may induce changes that vary in severity from simple reactive changes to repair with or without atypia
▓ Chronic irritation such as smoking and chronic bronchitis

Cytologic Features
▓ With reactive changes, the bronchial cells get shorter and become rectangular (boxcars). The nuclei become larger causing a slightly higher N/C ratio. The chromatin is clumpier and the nucleoli are more prominent. Slight nuclear membrane irregularity can be detected
➢ Multinucleated bronchial cells retain their basal nuclei and terminal bar with cilia
  • The number of nuclei can vary from two to numerous. Their presence could be nonspecific although they increase in number as part of the reactive change or in response to the presence of malignancy
➢ Ciliocytophthoria rarely occurs as a result of injury or viral infection
  • The bronchial cell sheds its ciliary tuft
➢ Reparative changes are similar to those seen in other areas of the body and are characterized by:
  • Monolayer sheets of evenly spread cells
  • Uniformly enlarged nuclei and prominent nucleoli/macronucleoli
  • Normal N/C ratio
  • Vesicular marginated chromatin
  • Dense cytoplasm and well-defined cell borders
  • Overall monotonous appearance
➢ Atypical repair may be present in cases with severe injury and can be difficult to distinguish from carcinoma

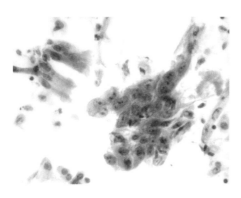

2-3. Bronchial epithelium undergoing repair. A monolayer sheet of reactive bronchial cells with markedly enlarged cells, vesicular enlarged nuclei and prominent nucleoli when compared to those on the left corner. Notice the even distribution of cells and the well defined cell borders. (Papanicolaou stain)

- The cells lose their uniform monotonous appearance and become somewhat overlapping and pleomorphic with coarser and less vesicular chromatin

Special Stains and Immunohistochemistry
- ▓ Noncontributory

Differential Diagnosis
- ▓ Adenocarcinoma (ADC)
  - ➤ Sheets of pleomorphic cell population
  - ➤ Large cells with variable amount of delicately vacuolated cytoplasm
  - ➤ Enlarged nuclei with high N/C ratio
  - ➤ Rosettes and acinar structures suggest gland formation
- ▓ Nonkeratinizing SQCC
  - ➤ Cells with dense cytoplasm and obvious pleomorphism
  - ➤ Lack of monotony separates it from typical repair

Special Stains and Immunohistochemistry
- ▓ Noncontributory

Modern Techniques
- ▓ Noncontributory

PEARLS

- ⋆ Features supportive of benign changes
  - Cohesive sheets
  - Presence of cilia at the periphery of cell sheets
  - Variable degrees of atypia within the same sheet with transition to normal (particularly helpful in atypical repair)
  - Lack/very few mitotic forms or apoptotic figures
  - Smooth nuclear membranes
  - History or cytologic findings of a coexisting reactive process
- ⋆ Features supportive of malignancy
  - High number of mitotic figures
  - Necrosis
  - Discohesion
  - Cellular crowding and irregular distribution

GOBLET CELL HYPERPLASIA

Clinical Features
- ▓ Chronic irritation such as smoking

Cytologic Features
- ▓ Monolayer sheets and small aggregates with no cellular overlap
- ▓ Bland nuclei with small nucleoli that resemble those of bronchial cells
- ▓ Nuclei may be indented by mucin resulting in a signet ring appearance

Special stains and immunohistochemistry
- ▓ Noncontributory

Modern techniques
- Noncontributory

Differential diagnosis
- Signet ring cell carcinoma
  - Sheets with disorderly arrangement and overlapping of cells
  - Clusters with depth of focus
  - Relatively larger nuclei with prominent nucleoli
  - Nuclear membrane irregularity (irregular indentation by mucin)

PEARLS

★ The presence of ciliated cells admixed with and bordering the signet ring cells is a clue to their bronchial origin

RESERVE CELL HYPERPLASIA

Clinical Picture
- Chronic irritation

Cytologic features
- Most commonly seen in brushes of ulcerated mucosa or from aggressive brushing
- Rarely seen in sputum and may be degenerated
- Small groups of dark cohesive small cells with uniform nuclei and high N/C ratio
- Frequently in partial continuity of ciliated cells
- Nucleoli may be prominent in cases with severe irritation

Special Stains and Immunohistochemistry
- Ki-67 may help separating reserve cell hyperplasia (low Ki-67 mean) from small cell carcinoma (high Ki-67 mean)
- p63 may have a role in separating reserve cells (consistently positive) from small cell carcinoma

Modern Techniques for Diagnosis
- Noncontributory

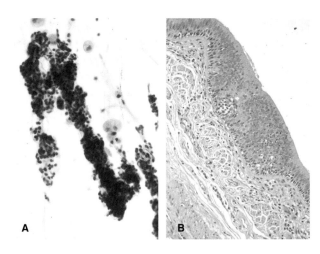

2-4A. Reserve (basal) cell hyperplasia. Bronchial wash with clusters of tightly cohesive small blue cells with high N/C ratio mimicking small cell carcinoma. Notice the lack of discohesion or single atypical cells. (Papanicolaou stain)

2-4B. Reserve (basal) cell hyperplasia. Bronchial biopsy showing areas of hyperplasia. (H&E stain)

Differential Diagnosis

■ Small cell carcinoma
➤ Dimorphic pattern of small tightly cohesive sheets in a background of numerous single cells, doublets, and triplets
➤ Extensive molding
➤ Apoptotic bodies or frank necrosis
➤ Increase mitotic figures
➤ Chromatin smearing on conventional smears

PEARLS

☆ Features suggestive of reserve cells:
• Few tightly cohesive clusters
• No single cells
• Small dark cells (nucleus similar in size to bronchial cells)
• Adjacent ciliated cells
• Lack of mitosis or necrosis

BRONCHIAL CELL HYPERPLASIA (CREOLA BODIES)

Clinical Features
■ Originally described in asthmatic patients and coined the term "Creola bodies" in honor of the first patient in whose sputum contained numerous such clusters
■ Attributed to excessive shedding of detached hyperplastic clusters
■ Can be also seen in a variety of pulmonary conditions such as viral pneumonia, chronic bronchitis, etc.

Cytologic Features
■ Since ciliated cells cannot divide, the underlying immature cell undergo hyperplasia in response to irritation
■ Form papillary-like growth devoid of vascular cores
■ Exfoliate in abundance in sputum and other bronchoscopic samples
■ Immature cells form the center of cluster surrounded by ciliated bronchial cells

Special Stains and Immunohistochemistry
■ Noncontributory

Modern Techniques for Diagnosis
■ Noncontributory

2-5A. Creola body *(left)*. Creola body appearing as a tight cellular cluster bordered by and in partial continuity with ciliated bronchial cells. Within the cluster, interspersed goblet cells can also be identified. (Papanicolaou stain)

2-5B. Creola body *(right)*. Creola body that is more difficult to identify due to the high cellularity. In focal areas, the terminal bars and cilia can be identified. Notice the absence of single atypical cells in the background. (Papanicolaou stain)

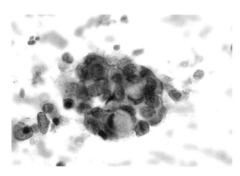
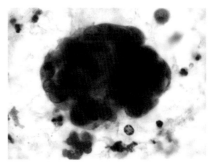

Differential Diagnosis

■ Adenocarcinoma
  ➤ Both clusters and single abnormal cells
  ➤ Discohesion
  ➤ Macronucleoli
  ➤ Coarse chromatin, irregular nuclear membranes, and high N/C ratio

PEARLS

★ Features supportive of a benign process:
  • Cilia at the circumference or in partial continuum with the cellular spheres
  • Cellular palisading at the periphery of clusters
  • Detection of goblet cells within the cluster
  • A monomorphic population of very compact cellular groups with extensive molding and absence of atypical single cells
  • Cells exhibit normal N/C ratio, with no macronucleoli or mitotic figures

ALVEOLAR LINING CELLS

PNEUMOCYTE TYPE I

▨ Flat small cells with long cell processes
▨ Normally line over 90% of the alveolar wall
▨ Does not proliferate or show reactive changes
▨ Not recognized in bronchial lavage

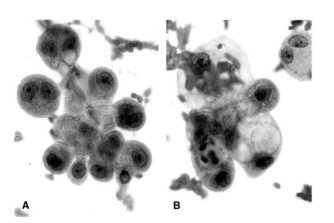

A   B

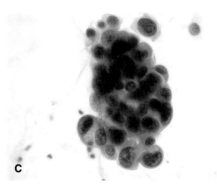
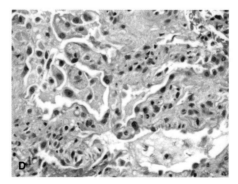

C   D

2-6A. Pneumocyte type II hyperplasia *(top, left)*. Pneumocyte type II hyperplasia presenting as clusters of atypical cells with enlarged slightly hyperchromatic nuclei and prominent nucleoli. Notice the protruding cells with hobnail appearance at the periphery of the clusters. The cluster on the right contains huge intracytoplasmic vacuoles distending the cell and distorting its morphology. (Papanicolaou stain)

2-6B. Pneumocyte type II hyperplasia *(top, right)*. Pneumocyte type II hyperplasia from a patient with ARDS presenting with more pronounced atypia. A scalloping border can still be detected along with intercellular windows. No single abnormal cells in the background, which also exhibited features of repair and other reactive changes. (Papanicolaou stain)

2-6C. Pneumocyte type II hyperplasia *(bottom, left)*. Histologic section of lung with diffuse alveolar damage showing pneumocyte type II hyperplasia lining the alveolar septa and protruding into the alveolar spaces. (H&E stain)

2-6D. Pneumocyte type II hyperplasia *(bottom, right)*. Histologic section of lung with diffuse alveolar damage showing pneumocyte type II hyperplasia lining the alveolar septa and protruding into the alveolar spaces. (H&E stain)

PNEUMOCYTE TYPE II

- Normally occur interspersed between the pneumocyte type I cells
- Rounded cells with central nuclei
- Also known as granular cells due to the presence of cytoplasmic granules
- Secretes surfactant
- Ultrastructurally surfactant granules appear as laminated bodies
- When exfoliated singly, they are indistinguishable from macrophages

PNEUMOCYTE TYPE II HYPERPLASIA

Clinical Features
- Proliferate as a regenerative response following pulmonary injury
- Mostly encountered in organizing pneumonia, pulmonary fibrosis, infarct/ embolism
- Develops three to seven days following injury and persists throughout the organizing phase
- Can be highly proliferative during the organizing phase of diffuse alveolar damage (DAD)/Adult respiratory disease
- Viral infection
- Thermal injury
- Radiological presentation
  - ➤ Most commonly as a diffuse or reticular consolidation
  - ➤ Rarely as a localized lesion, for example, localized organizing pneumonia

Cytologic features
- Atypical pneumocytes exfoliate as single cells or as clusters
- Sparse atypical cells are the most common presentation
- Numerous clusters can occur and may be difficult to separate from ADC
- Background of coexisting conditions such as therapy-related changes, infectious agents, repair, neutrophils, and hemosiderin-laden macrophages particularly in patients with DAD
- Enlarged cells easily seen at low magnification
- Clusters with scalloped edges reflecting the hobnail appearance in histology
- Variable amount of cyanophilic cytoplasm that may be granular or vacuolated
- Vacuoles range from fine to large and distended, distorting the cell shape
- Slit spaces or windows are frequently seen between cells
- N/C ratio is relatively high and can be variable between individual cells and clusters
  - Single or multiple nuclei, some attaining angulated or lobulated shapes
  - Round or oval macronucleoli
  - Variable chromatin from uniform to clumped

Special stains and Immunohistochemistry
- Noncontributory

Modern techniques
- Noncontributory

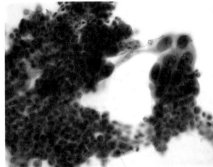

2-7. Atypical repair in a BAL from a patient with ARDS.
Notice how the highly atypical cells blend with cells showing more typical reparative features. (Papanicolaou stain)

Differential Diagnosis
- Adenocarcinoma
  - ➤ Small and large papillary-like groups with depth of focus admixed with large sheets and many single cells

> Smooth (common) cell borders
> Evidence of discohesion
> Variable-sized cytoplasmic vacuoles that are rarely prominent or distended
> Monomorphous population of atypical cells
> High N/C ratio
> Nuclear atypia with irregular membranes and hyperchromasia

PEARLS

✸ Features supporting hyperplasia
- Except for DAD, the atypical clusters are usually few
- With DAD, the atypical features may exhibit a wide spectrum within the same cluster. The same sheet may show features of repair transitioning into sever atypia
- Scalloped borders and intercellular windows
- Prominent distending cytoplasmic vacuoles
- Multinucleation more common in hyperplasia than adenocarcinoma

✸ Diagnosis of carcinoma should be considered very cautiously in a patient who is presenting with acute distress or is febrile
- Majority are benign on follow-up

CELLS WITHIN ALVEOLAR SPACES

PULMONARY (ALVEOLAR) MACROPHAGES

▣ Two-thirds are derived from bone marrow and one-third from tissue histiocytes at the alveolar wall

▣ Clean alveolar spaces from foreign material that was not cleared by the ciliated cells

▣ Variably sized histiocytes with eccentric reniform nuclei

▣ Specialized histiocytes may harbor different types of particles

▣ Their presence is important to determine that a sputum sample is produced by a deep cough rather than just a spit (saliva)

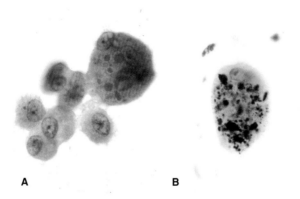

2-8A. Pulmonary macrophages
Dust cells appearing as small-sized histiocytes with a sprinkle of dust within their cytoplasm. Also noted is a larger hemosiderin laden macrophage with globular cytoplasmic golden brown pigment. (Papanicolaou stain)

2-8B. Pulmonary macrophages
Macrophage with irregularly shaped black anthracotic pigment. (Papanicolaou stain)

A   B

HEMOSIDERIN-LADEN MACROPHAGES

▣ Alveolar macrophages that contain hemosiderin pigment
> Hemosiderin appears as irregular refractile globular particles that vary in size
> Stains greenish brown with modified Giemsa stain and golden brown with Papanicolaou

■ Commonly seen in patients with congestive heart failure (heart failure cells)
■ Conditions causing hemorrhage, for example, vasculitis, Goodpasture's syndrome, DAD, trauma, and idiopathic pulmonary hemosiderosis

Special Stain – Immunohistochemistry
■ Iron stain could be applied to identify and count the macrophages
■ Mainly used to separate idiopathic pulmonary hemosiderosis from infectious pathology

CARBON-LADEN HISTIOCYTES (DUST CELLS)

■ Common in all types of pulmonary specimens
■ Key for sputum specimen adequacy
■ Number increased in smokers and those exposed to highly polluted air (miners)
■ Carbon appears as small globular nonrefractile pigment with little variation in size
■ Stains black to dark brown with both Papanicolaou and modified Giemsa stains

VACUOLATED HISTIOCYTES

■ Cytoplasmic vacuoles from engulfed mucin (muciphages)
  ➤ Positive with mucin stains such as Periodic acid-Schiff (PAS) or mucicarmine
■ Cytoplasmic vacuoles from engulfed lipid (lipophages), for example, aspiration pneumonia
  ➤ Details to follow
■ Amiodarone treatment
  ➤ Cytoplasm is distended by numerous fine clear vacuoles
  ➤ Details to follow

MULTINUCLEATED GIANT CELLS

■ Nonspecific histiocytes commonly seen in smokers
■ Nuclei per cell range from two to fifty and are scattered within the cytoplasm
■ Nuclei have normal chromatin and inconspicuous nuclei
■ Their presence may indicate certain pathology

Differential Diagnosis
■ Multinucleated bronchial cells
  ➤ Basal nuclei
  ➤ Terminal bar and cilia
  ➤ Response to irritation or injury
■ Megakaryocytes
  ➤ Normally reside in the capillary bed
  ➤ Even number of dark nuclei with connecting DNA strand
■ Giant cell reaction
  ➤ Reaction to a host of foreign material such as keratin, mucin, amyloid, corpora amylacea, ferruginous bodies, aspirated food, etc.
  ➤ May be numerous and obscure the presence of the eliciting substance
  ➤ Component of a granulomatous reactions, for example, sarcoidosis, Wegener's granulomatosis, fungal infection, or mycobacterium
  ➤ Phagocytosis may be prominent in conditions such as foreign body reaction
■ Viral Infection
  ➤ Infected cells exhibit characteristic inclusions

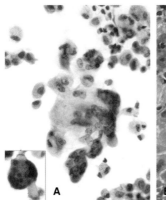 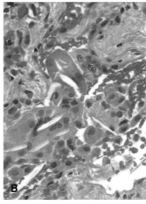

2-9A. Foreign body histiocytes. BAL from a patient with pulmonary infiltrate showing multi-nucleated histiocytes with polarized reniform nuclei consistent with foreign body giant cells. Insert showing a giant cell engulfing a non-asbestos ferruginous body. (Papanicolaou stain)

2-9B. Foreign body histiocytes. Correlating lung biopsy showing histiocytic reaction to nonpolarizable foreign body amid mild interstitial fibrosis. (H&E stain)

➤ Giant cell interstitial pneumonia
▢ Malignant neoplasms with giant cell component
  ➤ Pleomorphic ADC and giant cell carcinoma
  ➤ Rare metastatic tumors such as choriocarcinoma, sarcoma, and seminoma with a granulomatous component

PEARLS

✴ When to look for an etiology?
- Numerous giant cells
- Exhibit elongated reniform nuclei (epithelioid)
- Occur in aggregates
- Hyperchromatic nuclei
- Nuclei are polar, in a horse-shoe or a ring arrangement
- Refractile or asteroid bodies within the cytoplasm

INFLAMMATORY CELLS

▢ Can be seen in various bronchoscopic preparations
▢ Pathologically significant when increased particularly in BAL

ACUTE INFLAMMATION/NEUTROPHILS

▢ Can be significantly increased in bacterial pneumonia, acute bronchitis, and pulmonary abscess
▢ Sputum with significant increase in acute inflammation can be considered adequate even in the absence of dust cells, provided that it is not contaminated by saliva
▢ Can be increased in other conditions such as:
  ➤ Cigarette smoking
  ➤ Viral pneumonia
  ➤ Idiopathic pulmonary fibrosis
  ➤ Myeloid leukemia
  ➤ Autoimmune disease such as rheumatoid arthritis
▢ Could be a component of a background necrosis associated with malignancy

LYMPHOCYTES

- May normally be present in small numbers as small mature lymphocytes
- May be increased in a variety of inflammatory conditions such as
  - Chronic lymphocytic bronchitis (bronchial brushes). Morphologically, this is similar to follicular cervicitis consisting of a polymorphous population of mature and immature lymphocytes admixed with tingible body macrophages
  - Amiodarone lung
  - Hypersensitivity pneumonitis
  - Idiopathic pulmonary fibrosis
  - Sarcoidosis
  - Sjögren syndrome
  - Tuberculosis
- May indicate lymphoma/leukemia
  - Mucosal/bronchial associated lymphoma (bronchial brush and wash)
  - Other lymphomas (all bronchoscopic samples depending on the extent of the lymphoma and its relation to the bronchial walls)

EOSINOPHILS

- Increased in patients with asthma
  - Associated with Cruschmann's spirals and creola bodies
- Increased with parasitic or fungal infections
- May be significantly increased in eosinophilic pneumonia

MISCELLANEOUS FINDINGS

CRUSCHMANN'S SPIRALS

Clinical Features
- Increased mucus production such as chronic smoking
- Bronchial obstruction such as asthma and chronic bronchitis
- Represent inspissated mucous casts arising from deep bronchioles
- Can be seen in other parts of the body in conditions associated with inspissated mucin

Cytologic Features
- Central dark core surrounded by a filamentous structure in a corkscrew like manner
- Associated with numerous eosinophils in asthmatic patients

Special Stains and Immunohistochemistry
- Noncontributory

Modern Techniques for Diagnosis
- Noncontributory

Differential Diagnosis
- None

PEARLS

★ Their presence may argue for reactive changes in cases with florid bronchial or pneumocyte hyperplasia

CHARCOT–LEYDEN CRYSTALS

Clinical Picture
▥ Conditions associated with eosinophilia such as asthma, allergic bronchopulmonary aspergillosis, etc.

Cytologic Features
▥ Orangeophilic structures with bipyramidal, needle-like or rhomboid appearance
▥ Indicate increased breakdown of eosinophils in vivo (usually increased in older specimens than freshly prepared ones)
▥ Formed by condensation of eosinophilic granules

Special Stains and Immunohistochemistry
▥ Noncontributory

Modern Techniques for Diagnosis
▥ Noncontributory

Differential Diagnosis
▥ Foreign body debris

PEARLS

★ In some cases, particularly older specimens, these crystals may be the only clue for the once present eosinophils

CORPORA AMYLACEA

Clinical Features
▥ Usually an incidental finding with no clinical significance
▥ More frequent in older patients
▥ May be seen in patients with congestive heart failure, pulmonary infarction, or chronic bronchitis

2-10. Curschmann's spiral. Cruschmann's spiral with a dark core surrounded by a filamentous structure in a corkscrew-like manner. (Papanicolaou stain)

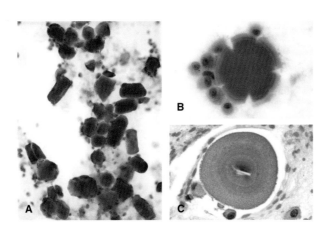

2-11A. Corpora amylacea. BAL presenting as numerous rounded hyaline material. (Papanicolaou stain)

2-11B. Corpora amylacea. Single corpora showing classic cracking artifact and annular rings. Notice the surrounding macrophages. (Papanicolaou stain)

2-11C. Corpora amylacea. Corpora in a cell block nicely showing the concentric rings, radiating arrays, and a central slightly calcified nidus. (H&E stain)

Cytologic Features

- Round to oval glycoprotein bodies with well-defined smooth borders
- Stain densely amphophilic with Papanicolaou stain
- Concentric laminations but not calcified
- Radiating array arising from a central nidus
- Calcification of central nidus occasionally
- May be phagocytosed by giant cells
- Frequently cracks during preparation

Special Stains and Immunohistochemistry

- Positive for PAS stain
- Weekly positive with Congo red stain
- Positive particles with Berlin Blue
- Positive for epithelial membrane antigen and PE-10, suggesting that it is composed of surfactant apoprotein

Modern Techniques for Diagnosis

- Noncontributory

Differential Diagnosis

- Alveolar proteinosis
- Amyloid
- Psammoma bodies

PEARLS

★ Lamination, regular shapes, and frequent cracking are the best clues

PSAMMOMA BODIES AND CALCOSPHERITES

Clinical Features

- Psammoma bodies
  - ➤ Are usually associated with bronchoalveolar carcinoma (BAC)
  - ➤ Could also be associated with other types of papillary ADC
- Calcospherites
  - ➤ Less likely to be associated with malignancy
  - ➤ Seen in chronic pulmonary disease such as tuberculosis and pulmonary microlithiasis

Cytologic Features

- Both are concentrically laminated and calcified bodies
- Psammoma bodies are surrounded by cells while calcospherites are naked

Special Stains and Immunohistochemistry

- Not contributory

Modern Techniques for Diagnosis

- Not contributory

Differential Diagnosis

- Corpora amylacea
  - ➤ Weakly birefringence

> ➤ PAS positive
> ➤ Central nidus with radiating array
> ➤ Calcification if present, is only central

PEARLS

⭐ Calcification is the characteristic feature

PULMONARY ALVEOLAR MICROLITHIASIS

Clinical Features

▪ Extremely rare condition characterized by intraalveolar calcium deposits

▪ Affects all ages although peaks in the second decade

▪ May be inherited by an autosomal recessive gene

▪ Symptoms are absent in about 50% of patients and are at discrepancy with radiological findings usually performed for workup of different reasons

▪ Symptoms may include dyspnea, cough, chest pain, and asthma in order of frequency

▪ Radiological findings are considered diagnostic

> ➤ Involves the lower lobes, middle, then upper lobes progressively
> ➤ Chest X-ray reveals a "sand storm" pattern as a result of the numerous calcium deposits. Advanced stages produce a "white lung" picture with disappearance of the boundaries between the heart and lungs. At the periphery the lungs are separated by a thin black line representing subpleural air cysts
> ➤ CAT scan shows preserved interlobar septa and lobules
> ➤ Sintiscan with ^{99}Tc reveals a diffuse increase uptake

Cytologic Features

▪ Numerous microliths can be seen in sputum (spontaneous or induced), bronchial washes, and in BAL

▪ Microliths are round to oval, irregularly concentric, and laminated. They consist of calcium salts

Special Stains and Immunohistochemistry

▪ Not contributory

Modern Techniques of Diagnosis

▪ Diagnostic radiological pattern

▪ Electron microscopy of microlith fragments reveal spectra for calcium and phosphorous with 2:1 ratio peak intensities consistent with Ca_2PO_3

Differential Diagnosis

▪ Other causes of calcospherites (see above)

PEARLS

⭐ Rare disease and should only be considered in the presence of
  • Numerous microliths
  • Appropriate radiological findings

FERRUGINOUS BODIES

Clinical Features
- Generic term for any type of mineral fibers that has been inhaled and sheathed with golden brown iron complex
- While asbestos is the most common mineral fiber, other particles such as fiberglass, carbon fibers, silicates, metal oxides, and other minerals could cause ferruginous bodies
- Asbestos bodies are the hallmark of asbestos exposure
- Even a rare fiber suggests that a higher load is present in the patient's lung

Cytologic Features
- Asbestos bodies are characterized by the presence of clear colorless central fiber of uniform thickness surrounded by a sheathe of golden brown beaded protein complex and bulbous tips
- Other ferruginous bodies may resemble asbestos bodies but the core is usually not uniform and may be black or yellow in color
- Frequently phagocytosed by macrophages

Special Stains and Immunohistochemistry
- Iron stain identifies the coating protein sheath

Modern Techniques for Diagnosis
- Tissue analysis for mineral composition could assist in identifying asbestos bodies

Differential Diagnosis
- Nonasbestos ferruginous bodies
  - Silicates form more irregular bodies with distinctive yellow core. Other forms may be broader and less regular than asbestos bodies
  - Carbon fibers have distinctive black cores and range from very thin to broad and platlike forms
  - Metal oxides have uniform diameter and segmented coating similar to asbestos. However they have dark brown to black cores

PEARLS

★ Clear and uniform central core is characteristic of asbestos

2-12A. Ferruginous bodies.
Asbestos body with its distinct clear colorless central fiber of uniform thickness surrounded by a sheathe of golden brown beaded protein complex and bulbous tips. (Papanicolaou stain)

2-12B. Ferruginous bodies.
Nonasbestos ferruginous body showing many features similar to the one on the left, however notice the lack of the clear uniform central fiber. (Papanicolaou stain)

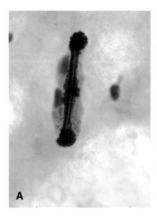
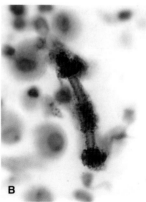

ELASTIN FIBERS

Clinical Features
- Tissue destruction, for example, infarct, bronchiectasis, abscess
- May be the result of aggressive brushing

Cytologic Features
- Elongated fibers, usually curved and frayed
- Pick up the stain poorly
- Somewhat refractile

Special Stains and Immunohistochemistry
- Noncontributory

Modern Techniques for Diagnosis
- Noncontributory

Differential Diagnosis
- Long fungal hyphae, for example, aspergillus
- Filamentous food particles
- Cotton fibers

PEARLS

★ Elastin fibers lack septations or cell walls

PULMONARY-RELATED DISEASES

PULMONARY ALVEOLAR PROTEINOSIS

Clinical Features
- Unusual diffuse autoimmune lung disease characterized by accumulation of abnormal phospholipoproteinacous material within the alveolar spaces
- Can occur as a primary disease or secondary to a variety of conditions such as infection, malignancy and exposure to dust such as cotton, linen, silica, etc.
- Granulocyte-macrophage colony-stimulating factor (GM-CSF) deficiency may have a role
- Patients present with the following symptoms in order of frequency: progressive dyspnea, dry cough, and low-grade fever

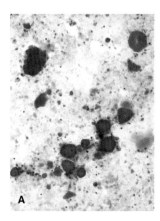 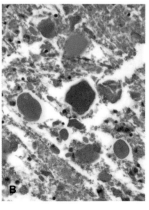

2-13A. Alveolar proteinosis. BAL presenting as variably shaped amorphous material and slightly granular background. (Papanicolaou stain)

2-13B. Alveolar proteinosis. Cell block showing similar amorphous irregularly shaped material in a thick granular background. (H&E stain)

▪ Extensive bilateral consolidation on chest X-ray that is usually disproportionate to the patient's mild symptoms. The consolidation may be patchy and perihilar in up to 50%, giving a "bat's wing pattern." Other patterns reflecting consolidation of air space include poorly defined acinar nodules and ground glass opacification. CAT scan demonstrates thickened interlobular septa in addition to the consolidation producing the so called "crazy paving" pattern

▪ These patients are considered at a higher risk of developing pulmonary infections

▪ Treated by repeat total lung lavage

Cytologic Features

▪ Grossly opaque fluid retrieved by BAL that is milky white to gray

▪ Thick amorphous slightly irregular extracellular material (lipoproteinaceous) that is basophilic by modified Giemsa stain and cyanophilic or amphophilic by Papanicolaou stain. This material exhibits a granular quality in cell blocks and histologic sections and in some instances may mimic *Pneumocystis carinii*

▪ Histiocytes are reduced in number and highly vacuolated

Special Stains and Immunohistochemistry

▪ Extracellular material positive for PAS stain and resists digestion

▪ Strongly positive to Oil Red O stain

▪ Negative for mucicarmine Alcian blue, and congo red

▪ Negative for GMS stain

Modern Technique for Diagnosis

▪ Increased circulating autoantibodies against GM-CSF

▪ Ultrastructural analysis demonstrates concentric laminated annular structures (lamellar bodies)

Differential Diagnosis

▪ Amyloid
  ➤ Congo red positive with apple-green birefringence
▪ Mucin
  ➤ Positive for mucicarmine and PAS
▪ Corpora amylacea
  ➤ Strongly positive to PAS and weakly positive to congo red
  ➤ Concentric rings
  ➤ Central nidus with radiating array
  ➤ Frequently cracks during preparation
  ➤ Frequently surrounded or ingested by multinucleated histiocytes

PEARLS

★ Corpora amylacea may not show clear concentric rings and at times could be difficult to separate from proteinosis
  • Clinical and radiological presentation is different

SARCOIDOSIS

Clinical Features

▪ Multiorgan disease of unknown etiology

▪ Frequently affects lung but also affects other organs such as lymph nodes, spleen, liver, skin, eye, and so forth

▪ Diagnosis confirmed by the histologic finding of noncaseating granulomas

▪ Acute sarcoidosis presents with abrupt onset of pulmonary symptoms associated with fever, fatigue, and weight loss

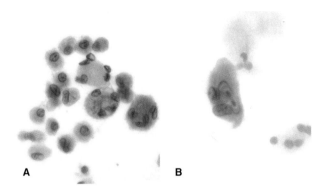

2-14A. Epithelioid histiocytes
BAL from a patient with sarcoidosis. The number of multinucleated histiocytes with peripheral reniform nuclei is high. (Papanicolaou stain)

2-14B. Epithelioid histiocytes
Multinucleated histiocyte with an asteroid body may be identified on rare cases. (Papanicolaou stain)

▨ Chronic sarcoidosis has more insidious onset of chronic respiratory disease and few constitutional symptoms

▨ Radiological findings include bilateral hilar and mediastinal lymphadenopathy as well as nodular or reticulonodular pulmonary interstitial infiltrate. On high-resolution CT, the nodules are bilateral and symmetrical with a characteristic perilymphatic distribution. They are most numerous along the pulmonary bronchi and vessels

Cytologic Features

▨ While the findings in BAL and sputum are not diagnostic, they are useful in establishing the diagnosis and ruling out infection and neoplasia

▨ Characteristically, the BAL exhibits a clean background with numerous lymphocytes and scattered multinucleated histiocytes and epithelioid histiocytes

▨ The histiocytic nuclei demonstrate reactive features such as nuclear enlargement, open chromatin and one to two nucleoli

▨ The lymphocytes usually constitute about 50% of the inflammatory component and are predominantly T lymphocytes with a CD4/CD8 ratio of 4 or more

▨ Neutrophils tend to be few in number

Modern Techniques for Diagnosis

▨ Flow cytometry for BAL fluid establishing CD4/CD8 ratio

Differential Diagnosis

▨ Infections such as tuberculosis
  ➤ Lymphocytic count is about 15% with a CD4/CD8 ratio about 2
  ➤ Acid fast bacilli detected in about 40% of active cases with Ziel–Neelson
  ➤ Positive cultures for *Mycobacterium tuberculosis*
▨ Rheumatoid granulomas
  ➤ Lung nodules are rare and usually in severe cases
  ➤ Frequently associated with pleuritis and effusion
  ➤ Epithelioid histiocytes are few and appear as elongated fibroblast-like cells with elongated nuclei that have one end more tapered than the other hence coined "carrot-like" shape
  ➤ Histiocytes may stain orangeophilic and contain dark nuclei due to degenerative changes and should not be mistaken for SQCC
  ➤ Necrotic debris in the background

PEARLS

★ Do not confuse degenerative and reactive atypia with carcinoma

PULMONARY INFARCT/EMBOLISM

Clinical Features
▪ Recent history of pulmonary infarction or embolism
▪ Rarely, an infarct is not clinically recognized, yet the exfoliated cells are seen in bronchoscopic samples during the patient work up for other reasons

Cytologic Features
▪ Rare diagnostic problem in exfoliative cytology and mainly encountered when an aspirate is performed for a mass in a clinically unrecognized infarct
▪ The atypical cells represent reactive pneumocyte II hyperplasia (at the periphery of the regenerating infarct) and squamous metaplasia (occurring at the center of the infarct)
▪ Reactive bronchial and pneumocyte II cells form clusters with enlarged and atypical nuclei. The chromatin may be irregularly clear and nucleoli may be prominent. This picture can be confused with ADC
▪ Sq metaplastic cells will appear as single cells or sheets of atypical orangeophilic cells with enlarged, hyperchromatic nuclei. This picture can be confused with SQCC
▪ Fresh blood, inflammation, and numerous hemosiderin-laden macrophages would be seen in the early phase. These findings disappear as the organization of the infarct proceeds

Special Stains and Immunohistochemistry
▪ Noncontributory

Modern Techniques for Diagnosis
▪ Once an infarct is suggested, modern radiological techniques could establish the diagnosis

Differential Diagnosis
▪ Squamous cell carcinoma
  ➤ The abnormal cells are more frequent
  ➤ Cells are better preserved with less smudging of nuclei
  ➤ Necrotic rather than a hemorrhagic background
▪ Adenocarcinoma
  ➤ Clusters have more depth of focus
  ➤ No cilia or features suggestive of pneumocyte hyperplasia
  ➤ High cellularity

PEARLS

★ The atypical cells are usually few in number, in a background of reactive changes
★ The same cluster may exhibit a spectrum of changes ranging from normal to reactive to atypical
★ The atypia is worse at second and third weeks and improves with time

LUNG TRANSPLANT PATIENTS

Clinical features
▪ Posttransplant patients undergoing routine surveillance
▪ Posttransplant patients with pulmonary symptoms and are worked up to rule out rejection or infection

Cytologic Features

▢ BAL is the procedure of choice to rule out infection

▢ Cytologic findings do not accurately predict rejection when compared with correlating biopsies

▢ BAL usually contains numerous histiocytes and has a clean background

▢ Increase neutrophils are seen in the first three months posttransplant. Beyond that period it may indicate infection such as bacterial pneumonia

▢ Increased lymphocytes are seen in long-term patients

▢ Lymphocytosis with decreased CD4/CD8 ratio may indicate rejection or viral pneumonia

▢ Mixed inflammatory infiltrate can be seen in chronic rejection

▢ Cytologic findings consistent with reactive changes such as pneumocyte hyperplasia are occasionally seen

Special Stains and Immunohistochemistry

▢ Noncontributory

Modern Techniques for Diagnosis

▢ Measuring T lymphocyte lectin-dependent cell-mediated cytotoxicity (LDCMC), natural killer cytotoxicity (NKC) and cytokine levels in BAL may have a role in predicting rejection

▢ Rejection associated with increase of LDCMC and NKC

▢ Infection associated with significant increase of NKC

Differential Diagnosis

▪ Other causes for lymphocytosis such as viral infection

▪ Pneumocyte hyperplasia versus carcinoma

PEARLS

★ Don't confuse reactive pneumocytic hyperplasia with a neoplastic process

ASPIRATION PNEUMONIA

Clinical Features

▢ Aspiration of exogenous lipid such as mineral oils

▢ Children with history of infections, asthmatic bronchitis, laryngomalacia, or gastroesophageal reflux

▢ History of neurological impairment or lipid storage disease, for example, Niemann-Pick

▢ Radiologically it presents as pulmonary infiltrate with features similar to infection or malignancy

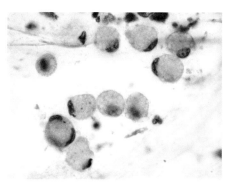

2-15. Aspiration pneumonia. BAL from a patient with aspiration pneumonia (lipoid) showing histiocytes with numerous variable-sized vacuoles and frequently eccentric reniform or crescent-shaped nuclei. (Papanicolaou stain)

Cytologic Features

▢ Presence of vacuolated histiocytes with fluffy variably sized vacuoles

➤ Score Oil Red O to predict aspiration

• Count 100 macrophages and score the intensity of stain per cell from 0 to 4+

• Aspirators tend to have a score from 100 to 300

• Not specific to aspiration pneumonia and similar score could be encountered in other conditions in adults

• May have a more significant role in neonates

Special Stains and Immunohistochemistry
- Vacuoles positive for Oil Red O smears (to be performed on air-dried smears)

Modern Techniques
- Noncontributory

Differential Diagnosis
- See vacuolated histiocytes

PEARLS

✶ Watch out on oil Red O, do not confuse positive lipid droplets with hemosiderin pigment
- Lipid appears as larger and more globular droplets

RESPIRATORY INFECTIONS

Clinical Picture
- Patients are usually in distress with shortness of breath, cough, and fever
- X-ray usually reveals a localized coin-shaped one or more nodules except for lobar pneumonia where it could show complete white out of a lobe
- Some infections are more prevalent in specific circumstances
  - ➤ Candidiasis more prevalent in acute leukemia and rare in acquired immunodeficiency syndrome (AIDS)
  - ➤ *Pneumocystis carinii* and cytomegalovirus (CMV) more prevalent in AIDS and rare in leukemic patients
  - ➤ Fungal infections can frequently be traced to an exposure or residence in a particular geographic location

Cytologic Features
- BAL has the highest sensitivity in the detection of infectious agents
- While some organisms can be identified morphologically, most infections require cultures or molecular methods to identify or subspeciate the organism
- Cytologic features vary depending on the causative agent and will be discussed separately below

BACTERIAL PNEUMONIA

- Most pulmonary samples will contain numerous neutrophils and cell debris in the background. Bacterial colonies may be detected. Immunocompromised patients may present with few neutrophils
- Cytology is of limited value in the diagnosis of bacterial pneumonia with the exception of *Legionella* and *Mycobacterium* due to the frequent presence of commensal organisms usually present in the upper airways. Patients with endotracheal tubes also have colonization by multiple organism
  - ➤ Cultures are also of limited value

ACTINOMYCES AND CANDIDA

- Can be normally seen in exfoliative cytology specimens since they normally inhabit the tonsils. Frequently they are pushed down by the bronchoscope and retrieved back with the samples

▓ Their presence can be significantly reduced if the first BAL aliquot is separately processed

MYCOBACTERIAL INFECTION

Clinical Features
▓ *M. tuberculosis* and *M. avium* intracellulare constitute most of the infections. AIDS patients may harbor both types of organisms

Cytologic Features
▓ Bronchoscopic cytology has a minor role in the diagnosis of mycobacterial infection
▓ Smears from non-AIDS patients contain lymphocytes (about 15–30%) and few neutrophils (about 4%), scattered multinucleated histiocytes, and a necrotic background. AIDS patients usually present with sparse inflammatory component and the smears contain mostly foamy histiocytes
▓ Intracellular acid fast bacilli will appear as negative spaces within the histiocytic cytoplasm on air-dried smears "negative image." In addition, during smearing some of the histiocytes break causing these bacilli to spread in the background

Special Stains and Immunohistochemistry
▓ *M. tuberculosis* is acid fast and will stain positive with Ziel–Neelson method
▓ Atypical mycobacteria is weakly acid fast and will stain positive with Fite stain

Modern Techniques for Diagnosis
▓ Fluorescence staining of smears are now widely used
▓ CD4:CD8 ratio of 2
▓ Enzyme-linked immunospot (ELISPOT) assay to detect IFN-γ secreting lymphocytes in BAL fluid

Differential Diagnosis
■ Nocardia
  ➤ Usually acquired by inhalation of soil saprophytes
  ➤ Morphologically similar to actinomyces
  ➤ Delicately branched gram-positive filaments
  ➤ Weakly acid fast and stains with Fite stain
  ➤ In contrast to *Mycobacterium*, it is an extracellular organism
■ *Legionella*
  ➤ Nonspore forming, narrow, gram-negative rods that may form filaments
  ➤ Stain positive with Dieterle or Warthin-Starry silver impregnation procedure
  ➤ Can be weakly acid fast and stain with Fite stain
■ Cultures from BAL or detection by immunofluroscence are diagnostic
  ➤ Smears exhibit marked neutophilia and significant necrotic debris
■ Sarcoidosis
  ➤ More lymphocytosis and neutrophilia
  ➤ CD4:CD8 ratio of 4
  ➤ No organisms detected

PEARLS

★ Clinical and microbiology correlation

FUNGAL INFECTIONS

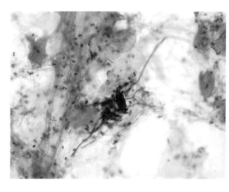 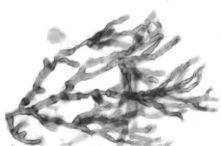

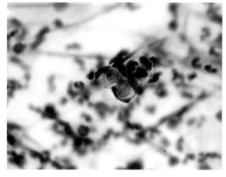

2-16. Alternaria *(left)*. Alternaria in a bronchial wash appearing as a fusiform structure with horizontal line and natural brown pigmentation. (Papanicolaou stain)

2-17. Aspergillus *(right)*. Aspergillus in a BAL of a patient with a cavitary lesion appearing as thin, septated, and uniform hyphae branching at 45°. (Papanicolaou stain)

2-18. Blastomyces *(opposite)*. Blastomyces presenting in BAL as single broad-based budding cells in a suppurative background. (Papanicolaou stain)

2-19A. Cryptococcus *(left)*. Cryptococcus presenting in BAL as narrow-based single-budding cells surrounded by a hallo in a necrotic background. (Papanicolaou stain)

2-19B. Cryptococcus *(middle)*. Cryptococcus demonstrating positive staining of the thick capsule. (Mucicarmine stain)

2-19C. Cryptococcus *(right)*. Cryptococcus demonstrating positive staining of the thick capsule. (PAS stain with digestion)

Clinical Features

▣ Most commonly encountered in immunocompromised patients although some may present in otherwise healthy patients who experienced massive inhalation of the organisms

▣ While Aspergillus species are ubiquitous and found world wide, certain fungal infections are prevalent in particular geographic locations

➤ Coccidioidomycosis, also known as San Joaquin valley fever, grows optimally in the hot, dry climates (desert) and is endemic in southwestern United States, northern and central Mexico, and in regions in central and south America

➤ Blastomyces dermatitidis also known as North American Blastomycosis or Gilchrist's disease occurs in the Mississippi and Ohio River Valleys, around the Great Lakes and in the southeast USA

➤ *H. capsulatum* is a natural inhabitant in the soil and endemic in south-central United States, particularly in the Mississippi and Ohio valleys

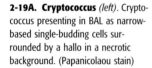

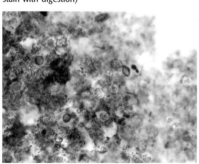 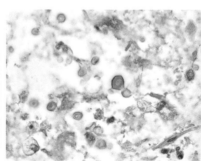 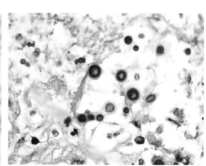

> Paracoccidioidomycosis is endemic in tropical and subtropical regions of Latin America

Cytologic Features

▓ Most of them can be morphologically detected on routine stains and consequently confirmed by silver stains

▓ Morphological features of fungi are not characteristic enough for cytological typing and speciation should be done by cultures. This is particularly true in *Pseudoallescheria boydii* and *Fusarium* that could look identical morphologically to Aspergillus

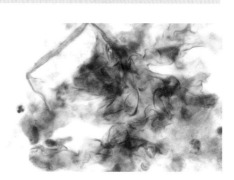

2-20. Zygomycetes. Zygomycetes in a BAL of patient with history of diabetes mellitus appearing as broad hyphae that are folded and branching at 90°. The hyphae walls are thin and the center is relatively clear. Septae are infrequent and not easily identified. (Papanicolaou stain)

▓ Morphologic characteristic

> Alternaria – extracellular
  • A stain contaminant appears as large fusiform structure with horizontal lines. It has natural brown pigmentation

> *Candida albicans* – extracellular
  • Small 4 μm tear drop budding yeast and pseudohyphae
  • Stains eosinophilic with routine Papanicolaou stain

> Aspergillus species – extracellular
  • 3–6 μm hyphae with uniform thickness and septae at regular intervals
  • Dichotomous branching, that is, width of the branch is the same as that of the original hyphae. Branching occurs at 45°
  • Hyphal size may appear larger with treatment
  • Fruiting heads and conidia are seldom encountered in bronchoscopic samples and indicate in vivo exposure of the mycetoma to air e.g. erosion of a bronchial wall
  • May be associated with calcium oxalate crystals (needle like and birefringent), especially *A. niger*
  • Easily detected by Papanicolaou as well as modified Giemsa stain and toluidine-based stains
  • Could induce a necrotizing granulomatous reaction
  • Definitive diagnosis is based on culture and immunohistochemistry

> Blastomycosis
  • Oval yeast-like cells measuring 8–15 μm in diameter
  • Single broad-based budding
  • Have a thick refractile wall
    • Stains positive with GMS and PAS
    • Negative with Fontana-Masson stain
  • Usually induce a suppurative granulomatous reaction
  • Stains eosinophilic or basophilic on Papanicolaou stain
  • Appear as basophilic spheres on air-dried, modified Giemsa stain–stained smears without any internal detail
  • Definitive diagnosis is based on cultures and immunohistochemistry/direct immunofluroscence
  • Serologic testing is not reliable

> Cryptococcus species
  • 4–6 μm in diameter with single, narrow-based budding
  • Eosinophilic on Papanicolaou stain and may be refractile
  • Positive to Fontana-Masson stain
  • Mucinous capsule appears as a halo. This capsule thickness could reach five times that of the fungal cells
  • Positive for mucicarmine, DPAS and Alcian blue
  • Capsule-deficient cryptococcus may be seen in immunocompetent patients
  • Mucin stains are negative
  • Fontana-Masson positive
  • Culture or immunohistochemistry may be needed for definitive diagnosis

➤ *H. capsulatum* – intracellular
  - Is not usually detected by bronchoscopic specimens except in patients exposed to massive inhalation where the fungal cells are packed within the intra-alveolar histiocytes and hence detected by BAL
    - 2–4 μm in diameter, spherical to oval, single-budding cells
  - Often seen as clusters within histiocytes
➤ Coccidioides immitis
  - Mature spheres measuring 30–100 μm in diameter and can measure up to 200 μm and contain numerous endospores. Spheres may rupture releasing the endospores
  - Refractile cell wall measuring 1–2 μm in thickness that stains only with GMS
➤ Endospores measure 2–5 μm in diameter each
  - Positive with PAS
  - Negative with GMS
  - Immature spheres lack endospores
  - Induces acute suppurative and/or necrotizing granulomatous reaction and may be associated with eosinophilic radiating Splendore-Hoeppli material
  - Definitive diagnosis requires culture, serology, or immunofluorescence
➤ Paracoccidioides brasiliensis
  - Spherical yeast cells that vary markedly in size between 5 and 30 μm, with multiple budding
  - Thick, refractile double-contoured cell wall
  - Negative for mucin stains
➤ Zygomycetes (Mucorales)
  - Broad-based hyphae, 5–25 μm in diameter
  - Hyphae have thin walls and frequently appear twisted or folded, with clear centers
  - Irregular branching pattern at 90° angle
  - Septation is absent or inconspicuous
  - Morphology cannot distinguish the different types of zygomycetes

Special Stains and Immunohistochemistry
▪ Please refer to specific types

Modern Techniques for Diagnosis
▪ Panfungal polymerase chain reaction assay has reportedly been promising in detecting aspergillus DNA
▪ Definitive diagnosis in most types is established with culture and/or immuno-histochemistry

Differential Diagnosis
▪ Elastin fibers may simulate fungal hyphae but they lack internal structure or branching
▪ Talc powder may mimic spores and could be GMS positive; however, it lacks the internal structure or the empty center seen with spores

PEARLS

★ Because of the uncertainty in typing fungal forms by morphology alone it is recommended that they are reported as ''fungal forms morphologically consistent with ...''
★ The background particularly in cases with *Aspergillus mycetoma* may contain highly atypical sq metaplasia

PNEUMOCYSTIS JIROVECI (PJ, FORMERLY PNEUMOCYSTIS CARINII)

Clinical Features
▥ Most common infection in immunocompromised patients
▥ Clinical picture of pneumonia

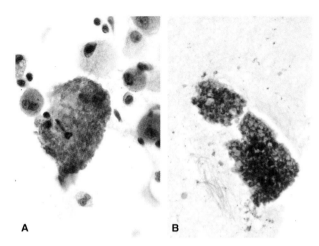

A   B

2-21A. Pneumocystis jiroveci (Carinii). BAL showing foamy eosinophilic cast containing the unstained small cysts of the organism. (Papanicolaou stain)

2-21B. Pneumocystis jiroveci (Carinii). Cell block section stained with GMS outlining the cyst walls appearing as cup-shaped and crescent-shaped structures

Cytologic Features
▥ Eosinophilic exudates produced by the organism are detected as foamy casts on smears
▥ The foamy appearance is a result of the presence of small cysts about the size of a RBC that are not staining with Papanicolaou stain
▥ Modified Giemsa stain detects the internal trophozoites as small dark blue dotlike structures
▥ GMS stains the cyst walls that appear as circular, cup-shaped and crescent shaped structures. Central dense dots are also seen sometimes and they represent collapsed cyst wall and not trophozoites

Special Stains and Immunohistochemistry
▥ Organism best seen by routine stains and reflex staining with silver stains is not cost-effective
▥ Immunostains with monoclonal antibodies produce variable results

Modern Techniques for Diagnosis
▥ PCR performed on BAL was reported to have 100% specificity and negative predictive value

Differential Diagnosis
▥ Clustered nonpigmented RBC could mimic the foamy cast but will stain negative with silver stain
▥ Mucin

PEARLS

★ Smears from treated patients may have fewer number of cysts, and the casts may appear rather granular than foamy

VIRAL INFECTIONS

Clinical Features
■ Symptomatic patients manifest clinically significant symptoms
■ Occasionally Virus cytopathic effect may be detected on smears from asymptomatic patients

Cytologic Features
■ Some of the viral infections can be identified by the cytopathic effect and characteristic inclusions in the infected cells
■ CMV is the most commonly detected virus in cytology
■ CMV is frequently identified in immunocompromised patients. In AIDS patients the infected cells could be numerous while in the non-AIDS patients may have more severe associated reactive changes with rare infected cells demanding meticulous screening
■ Special features:
➤ CMV – cytoplasmic inclusions appearing as small granules
• Intranuclear inclusions appearing as a refractile eosinophilic material surrounded by a halo "owl's eye"
• Infected cells may be multinucleated
➤ Herpes simplex/varicella-zoster-intranuclear inclusions, appearing as a homogeneous ground-glass material
• May have multinucleation
➤ Measles – causes giant cell pneumonia
• Large multinucleated cells with intracytoplasmic and intranuclear large eosinophilic inclusions
➤ Adenovirus – two types of intranuclear inclusions
• Basophilic intranuclear inclusion that occupies the entire nucleus and causes a smudgy appearance
• Ground glass inclusions similar to herpes virus
➤ Respiratory syncytial virus – giant cell pneumonia
• Large multinucleated cells
• Cytoplasmic inclusions are difficult to detect microscopically

Special Stains and Immunohistochemistry
■ Specific antiviral antibodies for immunostains are available

2-22A. Viral infections. A multinucleated cell with enlarged, molded ground-glass nuclei due to intranuclear herpes simplex virus inclusion. (Papanicolaou stain)

2-22B. Viral infections. Enlarged binucleated cell with "owl eye" appearance due to intranuclear somewhat eosinophilic cytomegalovirus inclusions surrounded by a halo. (Papanicolaou stain)

2-22C. Viral infections. Slightly enlarged cell with smudgy chromatin and high N/C ratio due to intranuclear adenovirus inclusion. (Papanicolaou stain)

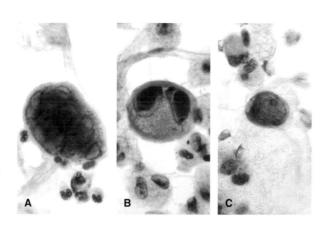

Modern Techniques for Diagnosis
- In situ hybridization and PCR

★ Viral infection may be superimposed on other infections
★ Some virus infections cause severe necrotizing pneumonia and require screening for those cells within the necrotic debris

THERAPY-RELATED CHANGES

AMIODARONE LUNG

Clinical Features
- History of treatment with amiodarone for ventricular or supraventricular arrhythmia
- Symptoms of toxicity are nonspecific and may include dyspnea, cough, fatigue, and muscle weakness
- Moderate amount of sputum may be expectorated
- Diffuse bilateral pulmonary infiltrate is usually seen radiologically involving more than one lobe with alveolar and/or interstitial pattern

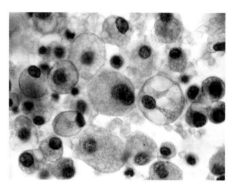

2-23. Amiodarone therapy changes. BAL form patient with history of amiodarone therapy showing numerous highly vacuolated histiocytes. The vacuoles are clear and distended with well-defined borders. (Papanicolaou stain)

Cytologic Features
- BAL with numerous highly vacuolated histiocytes
- Vacuoles are clear and distended with defined borders
- Osmiophilic membrane-bound inclusions containing laminated whorls are usually demonstrated in many types of cells including bronchial cells, histiocytes, and pneumocytes. These inclusions are consistent with phospholipidosis
- These findings are not diagnostic of toxicity and are only indicative of the treatment
- Biopsy-proven interstitial fibrosis and inflammation are essential to establish the diagnosis of toxicity

Special Stains and Immunohistochemistry
- Noncontributory

Modern Techniques for diagnosis
- Noncontributory

Differential Diagnosis
- Lipoid/aspiration pneumonia
  - ➤ Vacuoles with less-defined borders
  - ➤ Positive for Oil Red O stain

★ Verify history of treatment

2-24. Degenerated bronchial epithelium *(left)*. Degenerated bronchial epithelium with pseudo-orangeophilia mimicking squamous cells. They still retain their columnar shape although the cilia are difficult to identify. (Papanicolaou stain)

2-25. Chemotherapy changes *(right)*. Cellular enlargement and cytoplasmic eosinophilia mimicking squamous cell carcinoma. Notice the syncytial appearance and degenerated nuclear chromatin in many nuclei. (Papanicolaou stain)

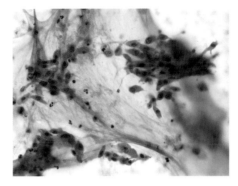
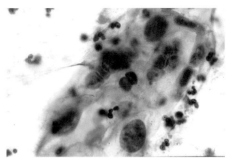

CHEMOTHERAPY

Clinical Features
- Undergoing treatment for malignancy
- Changes appear within few weeks of initiating therapy
- Subsides within a month after its cessation

Cytologic Features
- Changes are seen within single cells and cellular groups
- Markedly enlarged cells (cytomegaly)
- Proportionately enlarged nuclei resulting in a relatively normal N/C ratio
- Irregular nuclear membranes and chromatin distribution
- Usually few heterogeneous atypical cells (unless superimposed by other pathology)
- The atypical cells scattered among normal cells within the same aggregate
- Cells may have cilia or terminal bars
- Rectangular configuration
- Dense vacuolated cytoplasm (vacuoles may be large)
- Cytoplasmic eosinophilia
- Smudged chromatin with poor nuclear detail

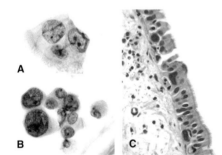

2-26A. Busulfan therapy. Bronchial brush showing cytomegalic cells with markedly enlarged nuclei and occasional prominent nucleoli. The chromatin is either washed out or smudged. Notice the rectangular configuration of cells in the top left image "box cars." (Papanicolaou stain)

2-26B. Busulfan therapy. Correlating bronchial biopsy. (H&E stain)

2-26C. Busulfan therapy. Bronchial epithelium undergoing repair. A monolayer sheet of reactive bronchial cells with markedly enlarged cells, vesicular enlarged nuclei and prominent nucleoli when compared to those on the left corner. Notice the even distribution of cells and the well defined cell borders. (Papanicolaou stain)

RADIATION THERAPY

Clinical Features
- Patients undergoing treatment for malignancy
- Acute therapy changes develop within six months from initiating the treatment
- Chronic therapy changes may persist for years probably due to induced changes in the DNA

Cytologic Features
Acute Changes
- Cytomegaly with preserved N/C ratio
- Fragile cytoplasm that streams and blends with the background appearing as ill-defined borders
- Prominent cytoplasmic vacuoles

▧ Neutrophils ingestion
▧ Syncytium of cells with blurred cell borders
▧ Enlarged nuclei with irregular wrinkled membranes and chromatin condensation
▧ Multinucleation common

Chronic Changes
▧ Similar to chemotherapy changes

Special Stains and Immunohistochemistry
▧ Noncontributory

Modern Techniques for Diagnosis
▧ Noncontributory

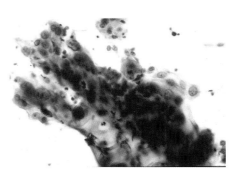

2-27. Radiation therapy change in a BW. Syncytium of atypical cells with washed out nuclei and chromatin smudging. Notice the large vacuoles and neutrophils ingestion. (Papanicolaou stain)

Differential Diagnosis
▧ ADC or SQCC
  ➤ Numerous atypical cells
  ➤ Homogeneous population of atypical cells
  ➤ Mitotic figures
  ➤ Coarse chromatin and good nuclear detail
  ➤ High N/C ratio

PEARLS

★ If atypia is too good to be true, it may not be true carcinoma

MALIGNANT NEOPLASMS

The exfoliative cytologic features of pulmonary neoplasms are quite similar to those seen on fine needle aspiration. Therefore only information relevant to sputum and bronchoscopic sampling is discussed in this chapter. For more detailed description, please refer to Chapter 14.

Clinical features
▧ The radiological findings and clinical features are usually helpful in predicting the type of pulmonary carcinoma, namely small cell carcinoma (SCLC) versus nonsmall cell carcinoma (NSCLC), for example, a centrally located mass with extensive lymphadenopathy is most probably a SCLC, while a peripherally located nodule is more consistent with NSCLC
▧ Guidelines for diagnosis of lung carcinoma recommend obtaining the diagnosis by the easiest and least invasive method as dictated by the patient's presentation. Sputum sampling is considered the quickest and least invasive sample followed by bronchoscopic samples including BBr, BW, and BAL
▧ Sputum sampling has a relatively high detection rate of cancer with a pooled specificity of 0.99, and a pooled sensitivity of 0.66 with higher sensitivity for central lesions than peripheral ones (0.71 vs. 0.49). Typing accuracy for SCLC vs. NSCLC is 97.7%. In one study, accurate typing for epidermoid carcinoma and SCLC was 92.1% versus only 55.3% for undifferentiated carcinoma
▧ Pooled diagnostic sensitivity for bronchial brushing is 0.59, for bronchial wash is 0.48 and BAL is 0.43, while that of bronchial biopsy is 0.74. The combined sensitivity of all three methods is 0.88

▧ The pooled sensitivity for a peripheral mass less than 2 cm is 0.33 versus 0.62 for those above 2 cm in size

▧ A variety of tumors were reportedly detected in sputum including mesothelioma. These tumors either invaded the bronchial mucosa and therefore shed their cells in sputum or were amenable to bronchoscopic sampling or had a lepidic growth pattern

▧ Tumors with lymphangitic spread could present with highly cellular sputum comprised of tightly cohesive cellular balls regardless of the tumor type

SQUAMOUS CELL CARCINOMA/EPIDERMOID CARCINOMA (SQCC)

Clinical features

▧ High association with smoking and high-risk occupations

▧ Most commonly a central mass that invades the bronchial wall and lends itself to sputum and bronchoscopic sampling

▧ The only pulmonary neoplasm with an in situ or preinvasive component that can be cytologically detected

▧ Occult cases with negative radiological findings have been reportedly detected by sputum and further localized by bronchoscopic sampling

Cytologic Features

▧ Sputum tends to represent the more differentiated keratinizing SQCC, while bronchoscopic samples tend to select less differentiated or nonkeratinizing carcinoma

▧ SQCC detected in sputum may represent pulmonary or head and neck origin, for example, larynx. Laryngeal carcinoma tends to be very well differentiated

➤ Keratinizing SQCC presents as numerous abnormal sq cells in small clusters or singly scattered. The cells contain abnormal dark nuclei and dense orangeophilic cytoplasm. The single cells have variety of shapes such as spindles, round, oval, trapezoids, and so forth. Sq pearls may be detected with similar abnormal cellular features

2-28. Squamous cell carcinoma in sputum *(top, left)*. Squamous cell carcinoma in sputum. Variably sized and shaped squamous cells with hyperchromatic nuclei, atypical keratinization (dense orangeophilia), and background of necrosis. Notice how the cells are hanging around the mucus strands. (Papanicolaou stain)

2-29A. Poorly differentiated non-keratinizing squamous cell carcinoma *(top, right)*. Poorly differentiated non-keratinizing squamous cell carcinoma presenting as a geographic sheet of malignant cells with enlarged nuclei, low N/C ratio, clumpy chromatin and macronucleoli. Notice the well-defined cell borders in many of the cells in contrast to the syncytial appearance of adenocarcinoma. (Papanicolaou stain)

2-29B. Nonkeratinizing squamous cell carcinoma in sputum *(bottom, left)*. Nonkeratinizing squamous cell carcinoma in sputum. The cells are very poorly differentiated (third type cells) with very dense cyanophilic cytoplasm and hyperchromatic irregular nuclei. Notice the wrapping of cells around each other in an attempt to form pearls. (Papanicolaou stain)

2-30. Atypical squamous cell *(bottom, right)*. Atypical squamous cell in a background of severe inflammation from a patient with tracheostomy. (Papanicolaou stain)

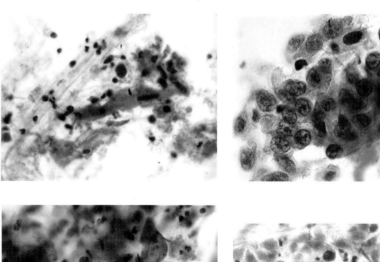

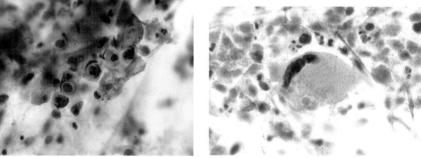

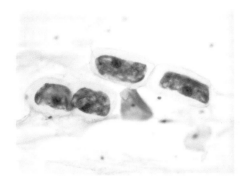 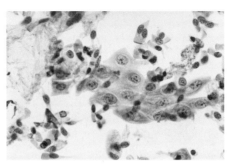

2-31. Plant cells *(left)*. Plant cells in sputum mimicking squamous cells. Notice the thick cell wall. (Papanicolaou stain)

2-32. Typical repair from a bronchial wash of a patient with ARDS *(right)*. Typical repair from a bronchial wash of a patient with ARDS. The reparative cells are presenting in a monolayer sheet of monotonous cells that are evenly distributed within the sheet. The cells are moderately enlarged with vesicular large nuclei with prominent nucleoli and normal N/C ratio. The cell borders are well defined and there is slight cellular streaming in one direction. (Papanicolaou stain)

➤ Nonkeratinizing SQCC exfoliate as basophilic cells with refractile dense cytoplasm. Larger cohesive groups may be seen particularly in bronchial brushes and washes. It may be difficult to differentiate from ADC due to lack of differentiation. The following are features helpful in recognizing sq differentiation and evidence of aborted keratinization

- Dense refractile cytoplasm with well-defined cell borders
- Because keratinization starts at the periphery of the cell and proceeds inwards, the premembranous area appears denser, while the perinuclear area appears more lacy and textured. The two areas are separated by a refractile ring representing the area where keratinization was aborted giving the microscopic appearance of endoectoplasmic demarcation. When the cell is displayed laterally this refractile line appears as a long corkscrew filament across the cytoplasm otherwise known as "Herxheimer's spirals"
- Few cells forming small clusters with a whorled appearance represent primitive attempt to form sq pearls

Special Stains and Immunohistochemistry

▦ Sq cells are strongly reactive to pancytokeratin, low- and high-molecular keratin stains including cytokeratin 5/6. High percentage is positive to p63

▦ SQCC of lung is characteristically negative for WT-1 and the majority are negative for TTF-1

Modern Techniques for Diagnosis

▦ Electron microscopy demonstrates intercellular desmosomal junctions

▦ Image analysis suggests that nuclear quantitative features could help in separating invasive from noninvasive cells

▦ Detection of alterations of the p16 gene using multiplex PCR and loss of heterozygosity in invasive and preinvasive lesions exfoliated in sputum specimens

▦ Detection of microsatellite instability

Differential Diagnosis

▦ Atypical sq cells in the background of viral infections, granulomatous disease particularly aspergillus infection, necrotizing pneumonia, pulmonary infarction, or secondary to an infiltrating malignancy

▦ Posttracheostomy sq atypia

➤ Few cells with evidence of degenerative atypia

▦ Plant matter, for example, contaminating food particles from mouth

➤ Well-defined and rigid cell outlines

➤ Cell walls (not present in human cells)

▦ Radiation and chemotherapy changes causes cytoplasmic eosinophilia and nuclear atypia

➤ Few cells with smudged nuclei and no chromatin detail

➤ Multinucleation and occasional syncytium formation

➤ Cytoplasmic large vacuoles and neutrophils ingestion

➤ Cytoplasmic fragility and breakdown in some cells

- Pseudokeratosis induced by coagulative necrosis
- Dysplastic sq cells
    - Mild dysplasia presents as few small clusters of mildly atypical sq cells with mild degree of pleomorphism. The nuclei are slightly enlarged, with relatively fine chromatin and smooth nuclear borders
    - Severe dysplasia presents as higher number of abnormal cells both as small clusters and single cells, with more obvious pleomorphism, high N/C ratio, coarse nuclear chromatin, and irregular nuclear membrane
- Typical and atypical repair could be confused with nonkeratinizing carcinoma
    - Both present as two-dimensional sheets
    - Both exhibit well-defined cell borders
- Repair presents with highly monotonous cells arranged in monolayer sheets with well-defined cell borders (like a pizza divided but not separated)
    - Nuclear chromatin is vesicular and marginated imparting a well-defined nuclear border
    - No cellular overlap
    - Prominent nucleoli
    - In atypical repair there may be nuclear overlap or more prominent nuclear atypia. However, these atypical areas frequently blend with areas of typical repair within the same sheet. Also other evidence of reactive changes and sheets of typical repair could be detected in the background

PEARLS

⋆ Well-differentiated sq carcinoma may present with subtle cytologic atypia particularly those of head and neck origin
⋆ Be very cautious in making a diagnosis of carcinoma in the absence of single abnormal cells

INVASIVE BRONCHOGENIC ADENOCARCINOMA (ADC)

Clinical Features
- Associated with smoking history, however, less strongly than small and SQCC
- Rate is increasing lately particularly among women
- Majority are peripheral lesions
- Radiologically it may present as a solitary nodule, multiple nodules or pulmonary infiltrate

Cytologic Features
- Better detected by bronchoscopic sampling than sputum. Cells appear larger in BAL than in sputum due to absence of degenerative changes
- In BAL, ADC is mainly confused with large cell undifferentiated carcinoma but not with small cell carcinoma
- Exfoliates as single cells, small clusters, papillary groups, or trabeculae depending on the degree of differentiation
- May present as syncytial aggregates or sheets particularly in BBr
- The nuclei are enlarged with irregular but relatively vesicular chromatin and irregular nuclear membranes
- Nucleoli are prominent (more prominent than those seen in PD SQCC)
- The cytoplasm can be vacuolated or nonvacuolated; however, it generally is more transparent than that of SQCC and the cytoplasmic borders are not well defined
- Vacuoles when present tend to be fine

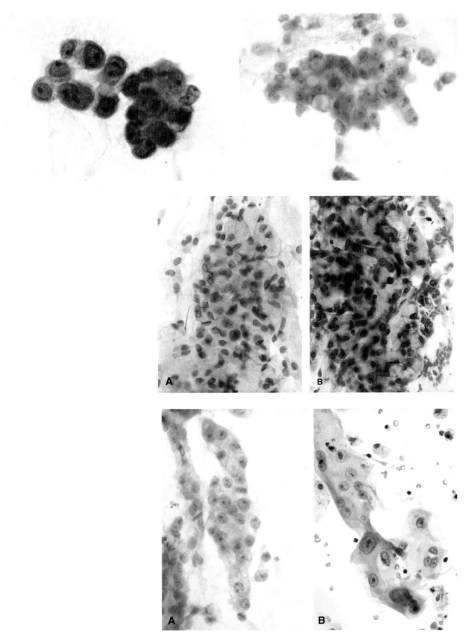

2-33A. Well-differentiated adenocarcinoma *(top, left)*. Well-differentiated adenocarcinoma in a bronchial wash presenting as a tight cluster with depth of focus as well as loose cells attempting to form acini. The cells are enlarged with high N/C ratio and macronucleoli. While the chromatin is relatively vesicular, coarseness and irregular distribution can still be detected. (Papanicolaou stain)

2-33B. Moderately differentiated adenocarcinoma *(top, right)*. Moderately differentiated adenocarcinoma presenting as a syncytial sheet of highly atypical cells. The cell borders are indistinct and the cells are irregularly distributed within the sheet. The nuclei are relatively vesicular, but the irregular distribution of chromatin can be detected. (Papanicolaou stain)

2-34A. Signet ring cells carcinoma versus goblet cells *(middle, left)*. Bronchial brush from a chronic smoker showing a sheet with numerous evenly arranged signet ring cells with small eccentric crescent or round nuclei consistent with goblet cell. Notice the admixed bronchial cells. (Papanicolaou stain)

2-34B. Signet ring cells carcinoma versus goblet cells *(middle, right)*. Bronchial brush from a woman with a lung mass showing signet ring cells that are haphazardly arranged and contain hyperchromatic relatively enlarged nuclei when compared with goblet cells. (Papanicolaou stain)

2-35A. Repair like architecture *(bottom, left)*. Poorly differentiated adenocarcinoma in a repair-like sheet. While the nuclei appear vesicular the chromatin is slightly clumpy, the nuclei are not very monotonous and the cells are not as evenly distributed as in typical repair. (Papanicolaou stain)

2-35B. Repair like architecture *(bottom, right)*. Syncytial sheet of most likely squamous metaplastic cells in a repair-like configuration from a BAL of a patient with ARDS. Notice the degenerative changes in some of the nuclei. (Papanicolaou stain)

▨ The N/C ratio can be variable but tends to be high
▨ The nuclei tend to be polarized or basal in location within the cytoplasm
▨ Attempt to form glands in the form of small acinar structures is a clue

Special Stains and Immunohistochemistry
▨ In many cases intracytoplasmic mucin can be detected by mucicarmine or PAS with digestion
▨ Frequently positive to epithelial stains such as CEA, MOC31, B72.3 and so forth
▨ Up to 80% are positive to TTF-1
▨ Other antibodies such as ER/PR, mammoglobin, cytokeratin 7 and 20, PSA and so forth are helpful in establishing metastatic versus primary ADC and in many cases the primary origin

Modern Techniques for Diagnosis
▨ Electron microscopy could detect mucin droplets in poorly differentiated cases

Differential Diagnosis

■ ADC exfoliated as tight clusters

➤ Bronchial cell hyperplasia/creola bodies are characterized by relatively monomorphic compact cellular groups with normal N/C ratio, extensive molding, cellular palisading at the periphery, the presence of cilia at the border or in partial continuum with the cellular group, and goblet cells dispersed among the cells forming the periphery. There are no mitotic figures or discohesion

➤ Pneumocyte type II hyperplasia is characterized by the presence of tightly cohesive groups with scalloped borders, intercellular windows and prominent vacuoles that may distort the cells. The cells may be heterogeneous with uneven chromatin and prominent nucleoli (unusual atypia for ADC), and the N/C ratio remains relatively low. Few single cells with similar morphology may be seen in the background

➤ Chemotherapy and radiation therapy may cause exfoliation of few clusters and single cells with variable degree of atypia. Generally the nuclei are smudged with little chromatin detail. Cells with similar atypia and definite cilia could establish the benign origin of cells

➤ BAC will be discussed below

➤ Metastatic adenocarcinoma may exfoliate as tight clusters particularly in those with lymphangitic spread. ADC with large vacuoles are more likely to be of metastatic than primary origin. History is very important in these cases and immunostaining could assist in the differential

■ ADC exfoliating as two-dimensional or monolayer sheets

➤ Reactive bronchial cells seen on-face will show variable degrees of atypia within the same sheet with transition to normal forms. The finding of similar atypical cells with definite cilia establishes the reactive nature. The nuclear membranes are smooth and there are no or very rare mitotic figures. Examination of the background reveals evidence of a reactive process such as infection

➤ Repair presents as truly monolayer sheets. The cells are evenly distributed with well-defined cells borders. The nuclei are enlarged (up to six times that of normal) with very pale and marginated chromatin and prominent nucleoli. Streaming of cells in one direction is sometimes seen. Atypical repair can be more difficult to establish as a benign process due to the more pronounced cellular atypia, overlapping of cells, and coarser chromatin. However, at low magnification, the overall appearance of the cohesive sheet is still that of repair. Frequently these atypical reparative cells blend with areas exhibiting typical repair. The finding of a reactive background such as creola bodies and pneumocyte hyperplasia can be a helpful clue to their benign nature. Inflammatory background by itself is not enough since it can also be present with carcinoma

➤ Large cell neuroendocrine carcinoma (LCNE) can frequently be difficult to distinguish from adenocarcinoma. The presence of feather-like clusters with cells surrounding fine capillaries and small oval acinar structures with palisading nuclei are helpful features suggesting LCNE. Once suspected immunostains confirming neuroendocrine origin will establish the diagnosis

➤ Poorly differentiated SQCC presents as geographic sheets of highly atypical cells with hyperchromatic nuclei and prominent nucleoli. Generally the nuclei tend to be less vesicular and the nucleoli are less prominent than those of ADC. The cytoplasm is dense (although degenerative vacuoles may be seen) with well-defined cell border rather than the syncytial appearance of ADC sheets. The borders of the cellular groups are made of cytoplasm in SQCC while in the majority of ADC the basally located nuclei form the border of the group

➤ Granular cell tumor may rarely arise in the trachea and if it invades the mucosa could be detected by sputum or tracheal brushing or washing. The cells are arranged in monolayer sheets with little overlap. They have abundant and characteristically granular cytoplasm that may be fragile and breaks during processing releasing the granules in the background and leaving behind bare slightly oval nuclei. Intact cells have low N/C ratio, abundant cytoplasm and eccentric uniform round to oval nuclei. S-100 stain would establish the diagnosis

★ Be cautious in diagnosing ADC in patients presenting with acute distress or in the presence of few atypical cells unless the diagnostic features are indisputable
★ The presence of large vacuoles distorting the cells is usually seen in benign lesions and occasionally in metastatic ADC
★ Contaminants such as Protoctista or food particles may resemble ADC

BRONCHOALVEOLAR CARCINOMA (BAC)

Clinical Features
■ Defined by the latest WHO classification as a tumor that is comprised entirely of a lepidic pattern of growth without any evidence of interstitial or stromal invasion
■ The five-year survival is 100%
■ Approximately 50% of patients are asymptomatic at the time of diagnosis
■ Patients with extensive disease may complain of cough, sputum production, chest pain, fever, and hemoptysis
■ Radiological presentation is variable. Peripheral nodule is detected in 40% of patients. Remaining patients present with multicentric nodules or extensive airway disease involving an entire lobe and a clinical impression of unresolving pneumonia. This is a reflection of the characteristic lepidic growth along the alveolar walls
■ Bronchorrhea or abundant sputum is evidence of abundant mucin production a symptom unique to mucin producing BAC

Cytologic Features
■ Most of the features described in the literature are not based on the current WHO classification and included cases with pleural invasion or pleural effusion and in some cases metastasis

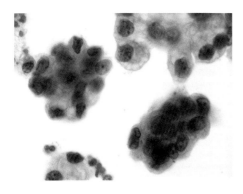
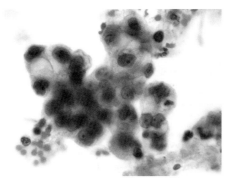
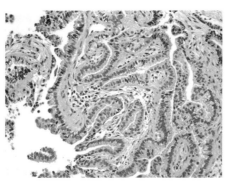

2-36A. Bronchoalveolar carcinoma nonmucinous type *(left).* Bronchoalveolar carcinoma nonmucinous type presenting as 3-D clusters with depth of focus, cellular overlap, and crowding. The nuclei are enlarged with slight hyperchromasia and chromatin clumping. Nuclear membrane irregularity and nuclear grooves can be detected. The cytoplasm is finely vacuolated with only rare large vacuoles distorting the cells. The cluster outline is scalloped and hob nailing can be present but less pronounced than that of pneumocyte hyperplasia. (Papanicolaou stain)

2-36B. Bronchoalveolar carcinoma with subtle nuclear atypia *(right).* Notice the 3-D configuration, nuclear membrane irregularity and loose cohesion. (Papanicolaou stain)

2-36C. Bronchoalveolar carcinoma *(opposite).* Histologic section of bronchoalveolar carcinoma showing the growth of malignant cells along the alveolar septa and the papillary enfolding within the alveolar spaces. (H&E stain)

■ Based on a recent study as well as the author's experience the following features are more consistent with a bronchoalveolar growth pattern rather than a true BAC

■ Because of its growth pattern as papillary enfoldings, these clusters are easily exfoliated and detected in sputum and other bronchoscopic samples

> Contrary to the flat sheets frequently seen on FNA, numerous tight clusters are the characteristic in sputum and bronchoscopic samples. The diagnostic yield is highest in sputum followed by BAL

- Papillary clusters are three times more common in BAC pattern than invasive ADC
- Small uniform cells with striking uniformity
- Cytoplasm may be pink and abundant with fine vacuoles (Mucinous type) or scant to moderate basophilic (Clara cell type)
- Nuclei are slightly enlarged and oval with finely granular chromatin
- Optically clear nuclei could be seen
- Prominent nucleoli are detected in up to 10%
- Psammoma bodies may be detected although not common
- Single abnormal cells are few

Special Stains and Immunohistochemistry

■ Noncontributory

Modern Techniques for Diagnosis

■ Noncontributory

Differential Diagnosis

■ Invasive adenocarcinoma

> Less papillary groups and more evidence of discohesion such as loose clusters and single cells

> More pronounced cellular pleomorphism with prominent nuclei, coarse chromatin and irregular nuclear membranes

■ Pneumocyte type II hyperplasia

> May be impossible to separate from BAC particularly in the acute phase of lung injury where the atypia may approach that of radiation therapy changes. The atypia usually subsides in repeated BAL within six weeks while that of BAC will persist

> Intercellular windows and prominent distorting vacuoles

> Hob-nailing nuclei

> Evidence of reactive changes such as repair may be noted in the background

PEARLS

★ Do not make the diagnosis on few clusters even if the atypia is severe

NEUROENDOCRINE TUMORS

■ These are classified by the latest WHO classification as

1. Typical carcinoid
2. Atypical carcinoid
3. Large cell neuroendocrine carcinoma (LCNE)
4. Small cell carcinoma (SCC)

■ The most commonly detected neuroendocrine tumor by exfoliative cytology is SCC that grows as a central mass and invades the bronchial mucosa

■ Carcinoids grow as endobronchial tumors; however, they can only be sampled if the overlaying mucosa is ulcerated

■ LCNE are rarely detected in exfoliative cytology

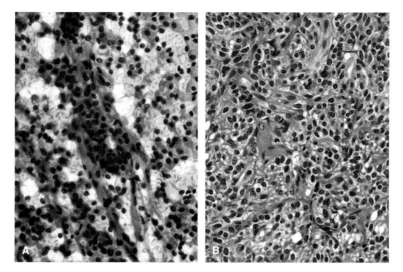

2-37A. Typical carcinoid *(left)*. Highly cellular bronchial brush containing numerous small plasmacytoid cells with moderate amount of cyanophilic cytoplasm. The nuclei have a salt-and-pepper appearance and small nucleoi. Notice the prominent capillaries intermingled with the cells. No mitotic or apoptotic figures noted. (Papanicolaou stain)

2-37B. Typical carcinoid *(right).*) Tissue resection of the carcinoid showing organoid architecture surrounded by capillaries. (H&E stain)

▨ Except for LCNE, they are capable of producing a broad spectrum of hormones including serotonin and peptide hormones, and most of them produce paraneoplastic syndromes

▨ All exhibit neuroendocrine features by light microscopy, electron microscopy (dense core granules), and immunohistochemistry

TYPICAL AND ATYPICAL CARCINOID

Clinical Features
▨ 1–2% of lung tumors
▨ Not associated with smoking
▨ Mean age of diagnosis, fifty-five years
▨ Most common lung tumor in childhood
▨ 60–80% central and 20–40% peripheral

Cytologic Features
▨ Typical carcinoid
  ➤ Highly cellular smears
  ➤ Monotonous population of round to fusiform cells
  ➤ Cohesive clusters, loosely cohesive sheets, and single cells
  ➤ Acinar structures, papillae, cords of cells and interconnecting trabeculae (less commonly seen in exfoliative cytology)
  ➤ Prominent capillary structures
  ➤ Plasmacytoid cells with eccentrically located nuclei
  ➤ Nuclei are slightly enlarge with finely granular (salt and pepper) chromatin
  ➤ Moderate amount of cytoplasm and low N/C ratio
  ➤ No chromatin smearing
  ➤ Mitotic figures are extremely rare in cytology
▨ Atypical carcinoid
  ➤ Features are similar to typical carcinoid
  ➤ Slight to moderate nuclear pleomorphism
  ➤ More prominent nucleoli
  ➤ Occasional mitotic and or apoptotic figures
▨ Spindle cell carcinoid
  ➤ Less likely detected in bronchial samples since it is more commonly peripheral
  ➤ Can be typical or atypical

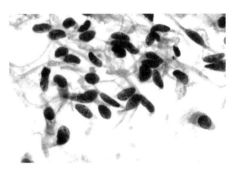

2-38. Typical carcinoid, spindle cell variant. Numerous spindled cells with basal oval nuclei and wispy cytoplasm admixed with bronchial ciliated cells. The nuclei have salt and pepper chromatin and are approximately 1.5 × that of the adjacent bronchial nuclei. (Papanicolaou stain)

➢ Monotonous population of long fusiform cells forming arches and coma shapes
➢ Occurs singly or in small aggregates
➢ Nuclei are oval to elongated, measuring from 10 to 20 μm on their long axis and from 5 to 10 μm on their short axis
➢ Finely granular chromatin
➢ Small nuclear indentations
➢ Single small inconspicuous nucleoli
➢ Lack of nuclear molding or chromatin smearing
➢ Prominent capillaries

Special Stains and Immunohistochemistry
■ Reactive to neuroendocrine markers including chromogranin, Synaptophysin, NSE and CD56
■ Demonstration of argyrophilic granules by Grimelius stain

Modern Techniques
■ Electron microscopy could reveal neuroendocrine granules

Differential Diagnosis
■ Bronchial epithelium
  ➢ Oval bland nuclei very close in size to that of carcinoid
  ➢ Identify terminal bars and cilia
■ Other neuroendocrine lesions
  ➢ Separation based on degree of pleomorphism, mitotic activity, and extent of necrosis
■ Lymphoma
  ➢ Exclusively a single cell population with few aggregates
  ➢ Thin rim of basophilic cytoplasm
  ➢ Lymphoglandular bodies particularly on modified Giemsa stain
  ➢ Cell size and nuclear features vary depending on type of lymphoma
  ➢ Nuclear membrane irregularity with grooves or protrusions
■ Metastatic small cell neoplasms, for example, breast or prostate carcinoma
  ➢ Clinical history is invaluable
  ➢ Appropriate immunostains PSA, ER and PR etc.
  ➢ Positive mucin stains (more than focal stain is not characteristic of carcinoid)
■ Spindle cell neoplasms versus spindle cell carcinoid
  ➢ Nuclear pleomorphism may not be prominent
  ➢ Immunostains
  ➢ Clinical history

PEARLS

☆ Lymph node status is not helpful since 5–15% of typical carcinoid and 40–50% of atypical carcinoid present with local lymph node metastasis
☆ Rarely carcinoid may present as a mucin producing neoplasm
  • Salt-and-pepper nuclei
  • Organoid and trabecular growth around prominent vessels

LARGE CELL NEUROENDOCRINE CARCINOMA

Clinical Picture
■ High-grade carcinoma
■ Strong association with smoking

■ Mean age is sixty-four years
■ No ectopic hormonal production

Cytologic Features

■ Large polygonal to oval cells; three times that of a resting lymphocyte
■ Some evidence of discohesion
  ➤ Variable size and shape and may present as
    • Large vesicular nucleus and prominent nucleoli mimicking ADC
    • Stippled nucleus and occasional nucleoli mimicking SCC
■ Obvious mitotic figures
■ Obvious necrosis
■ Nuclear molding variable
■ Delicate capillaries surrounded by palisading cells with a feather-like pattern

Special Stains and Immunohistochemistry

■ Positive staining with neuroendocrine markers
■ Dense core granules by electron microscopy

Differential Diagnosis

■ Adenocarcinoma
  ➤ Coarser chromatin
  ➤ Feather-like aggregates should raise the possibility of LCNE and should not be confused with papillae
  ➤ Papillary ADC tend to have several feathery groups and tight clusters while LCNE exhibit rare feathery aggregates and no tight clusters
■ Small cell carcinoma
  ➤ Dimorphic population of monomorphic small cells, not larger than three times that of resting lymphocytes
  ➤ Aggregates admixed with discohesive cells
  ➤ Extensive cell molding within the aggregates
  ➤ Doublets and short cords in the background
  ➤ More pronounced chromatin smearing

PEARLS

★ When cytologic features are intermediate between ADC and SCC think of LCNE

SMALL CELL CARCINOMA (SCC)

Clinical Features

■ High-grade neoplasm
■ Strong association with smoking
■ Mean age sixty years
■ Arises from the major bronchi and spread fast to mediastinal lymph nodes
■ Ectopic hormone production

Cytologic Features

■ Small cells, three times that of a resting lymphocyte
■ Scant or no cytoplasm
■ Hyperchromatic nuclei with irregular nuclear membranes and no nucleoli
■ The cells in sputum are somewhat degenerated and characteristically hang along the mucus strands and appear as short cords of extensively molded cells
■ The cells in BBr and BW are well preserved, appear larger, and present as a dimorphic population of cellular groups and a background of discohesive cells, doublets, and triplets

2-39A. Small cell carcinoma in sputum. Groups of tightly cohesive small rounded to ovoid cells with prominent molding in a background of short cords of molded cells (doublets and triplets). The cells have no apparent cytoplasm, the nuclei are hyperchromatic with no evident nucleoli. (Papanicolaou stain)

2-39B. Small cell carcinoma in sputum. Short cords of tightly molded small cells with finely speckled chromatin hanging along the mucin strands. (Papanicolaou stain)

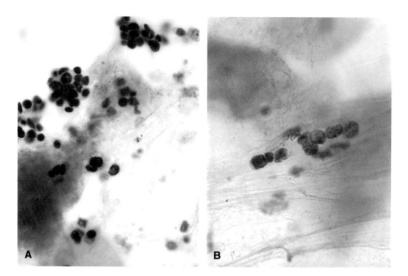

- Extensive molding
- Chromatin smearing as a result of manual crushing artifact
- Pleomorphic, hyperchromatic, stippled nuclei with no nucleoli
- Obvious mitotic activity
- Necrotic background

Special Stains and Immunohistochemistry
- All neuroendocrine tumors react to neuroendocrine markers with variable degrees: chromogranin, Synaptophysin, NSE, and CD56. Carcinoids tend to react with more frequency than LCNE and SCC reflecting the better differentiation of the former
- SCC is reactive to TTF-1 in 60% of cases

Modern Techniques for Diagnosis
- Electron microscopy illustrates dense core granules

Differential Diagnosis
- Very poorly differentiated carcinoma
  - ➤ No reaction to neuroendocrine markers
- Lymphoma or reactive lymphocytosis
  - ➤ Extensive discohesion in SCC may render it difficult to separate from lymphocytic lesions
  - ➤ No reaction to pancytokeratin or neuroendocrine markers
  - ➤ Positive reaction to lymphocytic markers
- Basal cell hyperplasia
  - ➤ Small tight cohesive clusters of dark cells
  - ➤ Sometimes in partial continuity with bronchial epithelium
  - ➤ No single cells in the background

PEARLS

★ Well-preserved and fixed SCC cells may appear larger in size, may have a thin rim of basophilic cytoplasm or an occasional inconspicuous nucleolus

ANAPLASTIC LARGE CELL CARCINOMA (ALCC)

Clinical Features
- Comprises 10–20% of all lung carcinomas
- Aggressive carcinoma with strong association with smoking

- Mean age around sixty years
- Represents a very poorly differentiated carcinoma by light microscopy
- Most manifest evidence of differentiation by electron microscopy, indicating that it represents a poorly differentiated state rather than a specific entity

Cytologic Features
- Large undifferentiated cells with high degree of discohesion
- Predominantly single pleomorphic cells with eccentric nuclei
- Cellular groups appear as syncytial groups
- Neutrophils ingestion can be prominent
- Moderate eosinophilic or basophilic cytoplasm
- Large and highly atypical nuclei with macronucleoli
- Chromatin vary from coarse to finely granular
- Tumor diathesis
- Giant cells may be seen and if they exceed 25% it is termed giant cell carcinoma

Special Stains and Immunohistochemistry
- Over 50% coexpress both cytokeratin, EMA, and vimentin
- Over 50% express the pulmonary ADC phenotype of positive CK7 and TTF-1 and negative CK5
- May variably react to a variety of differentiation antibodies such as CEA, B72.3, and NSE

Modern Techniques for Diagnosis
- Electron microscopy may illustrate evidence of differentiation

Differential Diagnosis
- Poorly differentiated adenocarcinoma
  - ➤ Cellular and nuclear areas significantly larger in adenocarcinoma
  - ➤ Nucleolar area is larger in ALCC
  - ➤ ADC cells are larger and rounder
  - ➤ ALCC are more ellipsoid and convoluted
- Atypical repair
  - ➤ Monolayer sheets with well-defined cell borders despite the occasional overlap
  - ➤ Occasional cells may be atypical but the overall appearance is well organized and indicative of repair
  - ➤ Vesicular chromatin
  - ➤ No discohesion
- Metastatic tumors presenting as single large cells, for example, melanoma, germ cell tumor, large cell lymphoma, or even sarcoma
  - ➤ Use immunostains whenever possible especially when a history of a previous tumor is available

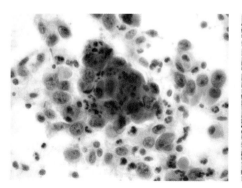
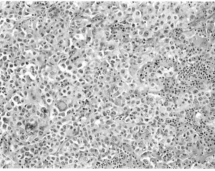

2-40A. Large cell anaplastic carcinoma *(left)*. Large cell anaplastic carcinoma in bronchial wash presenting as a loosely cohesive aggregate and many discohesive cells. The cells are highly pleomorphic with enlarged nucleo, high N/C ratio, and macronucleoli. Notice the numerous ingested intracytoplasmic neutrophils. (Papanicolaou stain)

2-40B. Large cell anaplastic carcinoma *(right)*. Large cell anaplastic carcinoma, histologic section showing a sheet of anaplastic cells with high degree of pleomorphism, multinucleated cells, and lack of differentiation. (H&E stain)

2-41A. Primary lung melanoma *(left)*. Primary lung melanoma in a bronchial wash presenting as small discohesive groups of high atypical large cells with eccentric nuclei and prominent nucleoli. (Papanicolaou stain)

2-41B. Primary lung melanoma *(right)*. Cell block section showing positive reaction to HMB-45, confirming the melanoma diagnosis. (HMB-45 stain)

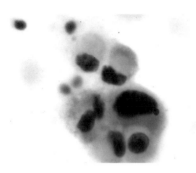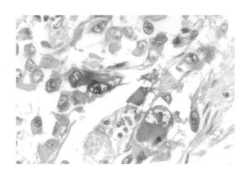

HEMATOPOIETIC MALIGNANCIES (HPM)

Clinical Features
▥ Primary pulmonary hematopoietic tumors are less common than metastatic ones

Cytologic Features
▥ Hodgkin and non-Hodgkin lymphoma including bronchial associated lymphoma, multiple myeloma, and others have been reported on BBr and BW
▥ Cytologic features depend on the type of HPM
　➤ Lymphoma
　　• Cellular lymphocytic monotonous infiltrate of cells
　　• Relatively rounded cells with scant basophilic cytoplasm
　　• Some types may exhibit nuclear grooves or prominent nucleoli
　　• Relatively vesicular chromatin
　　• Lymphoglandular bodies
　➤ Multiple myeloma (MM)
　　• Discohesive population of single cells
　　• Eccentric nuclei with cartwheel chromatin pattern
　　• Single, double, or multinucleated cells
　　• Perinuclear huff

Special Stains and Immunohistochemistry
▥ Variable depending on lymphoma type

Modern Techniques for Diagnosis
▥ Immunophenotyping by flow cytometry
▥ Identification of molecular alterations related to the specific type of lymphoma can be done using BAL specimens

2-42. Mucosal associated lymphoma in a bronchial wash *(left)*. Presenting as numerous atypical small lymphocytes, some have cleaved nucleoli. The lymphocytes are intimately associated with the reactive bronchial cell. (Papanicolaou stain)

2-43. Large cell lymphoma *(right)*. Large cell lymphoma in a bronchial wash presenting as monotonous population of large atypical cells with scant cytoplasm and highly convoluted nuclei. (Papanicolaou stain)

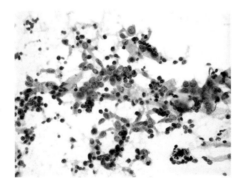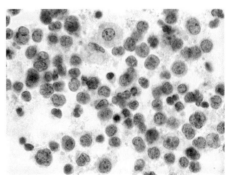

Differential Diagnosis
- Reactive lymphocytosis
  - ➤ Polymorphous population of lymphocytes
  - ➤ Cellularity is relatively lower
  - ➤ Tingible body macrophages
- Small cell carcinoma
  - ➤ Coarser chromatin
  - ➤ More ovoid cells and no visible cytoplasm
  - ➤ No nucleoli
- Non-small cell carcinoma (NSCC)
  - ➤ Large cell lymphoma and MM may be mistaken for NSCC
  - ➤ Few gland-like groups may be seen in MM

PEARLS

★ Some types of lymphoma such as bronchial associated or follicular may have few tinglible body macrophages

MISCELLANEOUS RARE TUMORS

AMYLOIDOSIS

Clinical Features
- Could be part of systemic amyloidosis or a component of lymphoma or carcinoid
- Primary amyloidosis tends to arise in the tracheobronchial tree
- Rarely detected in bronchoscopic samples and is most likely to be picked by bronchial brushing or washing

Cytologic Features
- Flocculent material or irregularly shaped fragments with scalloped and pointed borders
- Stain eosinophilic to cyanophilic with Papanicolaou stain
- May be accompanied by giant cell reaction

Special stains and Immunohistochemistry
- Positive to congo red stain with apple green birefringence
- Weekly reactive to PAS

Modern Techniques for Diagnosis
- Electron microscopy demonstrates a crossed β-pleated sheets that can be seen by x-ray diffraction

Differential Diagnosis
- Alveolar proteinosis
- Corpora amylacea
- Mucin
  - ➤ Film of watery and stringy material
- Chondroid material
  - ➤ Filamentous dense texture
  - ➤ Scattered lacunae
- Basement membrane material, for example, adenoid cystic carcinoma
  - ➤ Rigid cylindrical structures surrounded by small blue cells
  - ➤ Smooth borders
  - ➤ May show branching

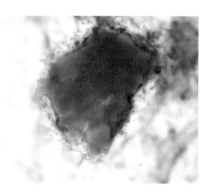

2-44. Amyloid. Amyloid in bronchial washing from a patient with previous diagnosis of systemic amyloidosis. The smear contains numerous irregular or rounded fragments of amorphous thick eosinophilic and occasionally cyanophilic material. (Papanicolaou stain)

⋆ Can be easily overlooked unless included in the differential

SALIVARY GLAND ANALOG TUMORS

Clinical Features
▪ Rarely occur in the lung
▪ Arises in the tracheobronchial tree
▪ Most common ones are adenoid cystic tumor and mucoepidermoid carcinoma

Cytologic Features
▪ Features are similar to those seen in FNA
▪ Cylindrical extracellular matrix is a characteristic feature for adenoid cystic tumor
▪ Mucoepidermoid presentation will vary depending on the grade

Special Stains
▪ The hyaline material is positive to PAS but negative to mucicarmine and congo red
▪ Positive mucin stain in well-differentiated mucoepidermoid carcinoma

Modern Techniques for Diagnosis
▪ Noncontributory

Differential Diagnosis
▪ Bronchogenic adenocarcinoma
▪ Squamous cell carcinoma

⋆ Extracellular matrix

REFERENCES

METHODS OF EXFOLIATIVE RESPIRATORY CYTOLOGY
Agusti C, Xaubet A, Monton C, Sole M, Soler N, Carrion M, Rodriguez-Roisin R. Induced sputum in the diagnosis of peripheral lung cancer not possible endoscopically. *Respir Med* 2001;95(10):822–828.

Bechtel JJ, Kelley WR, Petty TL, Patz DS, Saccomanno G. Outcome of 51 patients with roentgeno-graphically occult lung cancer detected by sputum cytologic testing: a community hospital program. *Arch Intern Med* 1994;154(9):975–980.

Erozan YS, Frost JK. Cytopathologic diagnosis of lung cancer. *Sem Oncol* 1974; 1(3):191–198.

Koss LG, Melamed MR, Goodner JT. Pulmonary cytology: a brief survey of diagnostic results from July 1st, 1952 until December 31st, 1960. *Acta Cytol* 1964; Mar-Apr; 8:104–113.

Matsuda M, Horai T, Doi O, Kodama K, Tateishi R. Diagnosis of squamous cell carcinoma of the lung by sputum cytology: with special reference to correlation of diagnostic accuracy with size and proximal extent of resected tumor. *Diagn Cytopathol* 1990;6(4):248–251.

Risse EK, van Hof MA, Laurini RN, Vooijs PG. Sputum cytology by the Saccomanno method in diagnosing lung malignancy. *Diagn Cytopathol* 1985;1(4):286–290.

BRONCHOSCOPIC SPECIMENS (BRUSH, WASH, AND LAVAGE)
Bibbo M, Fennessy JJ, Lu CT, Straus FH, Variakoji SD, Wied GL. Bronchial brushing technique for the cytologic diagnosis of peripheral lung lesions: a review of 693 cases. *Acta Cytol* 1973;17(3):245–251.

Daniele RP, Elias JA, Epstein PE, Rossman MD. Bronchoalveolar lavage: role in the pathogenesis, diagnosis, and management of interstitial lung disease. *Ann Intern Med* 1985; 102(1):93–108.

De Gracia J, Bravo C, Miravitlles M, Tallada N, Orriols R, Bellmunt J, Vendrell M, Morell F. Diagnostic value of bronchoalveolar lavage in peripheral lung cancer. *Am Rev Respir Dis* 1993;147(3):649–652.

DeFine LA, Saleba KP, Gibson BB, Wesseler TA, Baughman R. Cytologic evaluation of bronchoalveolar lavage specimens in immunosuppressed patients with suspected opportunistic infections. *Act Cytol* 1987;31(3):235–242.

Garg S, Handa U, Mohan H, Janmeja AK. Comparative analysis of various cytohistological techniques in diagnosis of lung diseases. *Diagn Cytopathol* 2007:35(1):26–31.

Jewell J. Diagnostic value and cost effectiveness of bronchial brushings in the diagnosis of bronchial malignancies. *Cytopathology* 2005;16(1):52–53.

Johnston WW, Bossen EH: Ten years of respiratory cytopathology at Duke University Medical Center: II. The Cytopathologic diagnosis of lung cancer during the years 1970–1974, with a comparison between cytopathology and histopathology in the typing of lung cancer. *Acta Cytol* 1981b;25(5):499–505.

Linder J, Radio SJ, Robbins RA, Ghapouri M, Rennard SI. Bronchoalveolar lavage in the cytologic diagnosis of carcinoma of the lung. *Acta Cytol* 1987;31(6):796–801.

Peikert T, Rana S, Edell ES. Safety, diagnostic yield, and therapeutic implications of flexible bronchoscopy in patients with febrile neutropenia and pulmonary infiltrates. *Mayo Clin Proc* 2005;80(11):1414–1420.

Stanley MW, Henry-Stanley MJ, Iber C. *Bronchoalveolar lavage: cytology and clinical applications.* New York: Igaku-Shoin, 1991, pp. 50–57.

Solomon DA, Solliday NH, Gracey DR. Cytology in fiberoptic bronchoscopy: comparison of bronchial brushing, washing, and post-bronchoscopy sputum. *Chest* 1974;65(6):616–619.

PULMONARY NATIVE CELLS: FROM NORMAL TO REACTIVE

Berman JJ, Murray RJ, Lopez-Plaza IM. Widespread post-tracheostomy atypia simulating squamous cell carcinoma: A case report. *Acta Cytol* 1991;35(6):713–716.

Cahan WG, Melamed MR, Frazell EL. Tracheobronchial cytology after laryngectomy for carcinoma. *Surg Gynecol Obstet* 1966;123(1):15–21.

Nunez V, Melamed M, Cahan W. Tracheo-bronchial cytology after laryngectomy for carcinoma of larynx II. *Acta Cytol* 1966;10(1):38–48.

Nasiell M. Metaplastic and atypical metaplasia in the bronchial epithelium: a histopathologic and cytopathologic study. *Acta Cytol* 1966;10(6):421–427.

TRACHEOBRONCHIAL LINING CELLS

Nasiell M. The general appearance of the bronchial epithelium in bronchial carcinoma: a histopathological study with some cytological viewpoints. *Acta Cytol* 1963;Mar-Apr 7:97–106.

Saito Y, Imai T., Sato M, Ota S, Kanma K, Takahashi S, Usuda K, Sagawa M. Cytologic study of tissue repair in human bronchial epithelium. *Acta Cytol* 1988;32(5):622–628.

GOBLET CELL HYPERPLASIA

Laucirica R, Ostrowski ML. Cytology of nonneoplastic occupational and environmental diseases of the lung and pleura. *Arch Pathol Lab Med.* 2007 Nov;131(11):1700–1708.

RESERVE CELL HYPERPLASIA

Grefte MMJ, Salet-Van de Pol MRJ, Gemmink JH, Bulten J, Hanselaar AG, de Wilde PC. Quantitation of Ki-67 expression in the differential diagnosis of reserve cell hyperplasia vs. small cell lung carcinoma. *Acta Cytol* 2004;48(5):608–612.

Sheikh HA, Fuhrer K, Cieply K, Yousem S. p63 expression in assessment of bronchioalveolar proliferations of the lung. *Modern Pathology* 2004;17(9):1134–1140.

BRONCHIAL CELL HYPERPLASIA (CREOLA BODIES)

Johnston W. Cytologic diagnosis of lung cancer: Principles and problems. *Pathol Res Pract* 1986;181(1):1–36.

Naylor B, Railey C. A pitfall in the cytodiagnosis of sputum of asthmatics. *J Clin Pathol* 1964; Jan;17:84–89.

Naylor B. The shedding of the mucosa of the bronchial tree in asthma. *Thorax* 1962;Mar;17:69–72.

ALVEOLAR LINING CELLS

Bedrossian CWM, Delly LV. Cytopathology of non-neoplastic pulmonary disease. *Laboratory Medicine* 1983;14:86–95.

Crapanzano JP, Zakowski MF. Diagnostic dilemmas in pulmonary cytology. *Cancer (Cancer Cytopathol)* 2001;93(6):364–375.

Grotte D, Stanley MW. Swanson PE, Henry-Stanley M, Davies S. Reactive type II pneumocytes in bronchoalveolar lavages fluid from adult distress syndrome can be mistaken for cells of adenocarcinoma. *Diagn Cytopathol* 1990;6(5):317–322.

Johnston WW. Type II pneumocytes in cytologic specimens: a diagnostic dilemma. *Am J Clin Pathol* 1992;97(5):608–609.

Naryshkin S, Young NA. Respiratory cytology: a review of non-neoplastic mimics of malignancy. *Diagn Cytopathol* 1993;9(1):89–97.

Stanley MW, Henry-Stanley M, Gajl-Peczalska KJ, Bitterman PB. Hyperplasia of type II pneumocytes in acute lung injury: cytologic findings of sequential bronchoalveolar lavage. *Am J Clin Pathol* 1992;97(5):669–677.

Thivolet-Béjui F. Cytological pitfalls in bronchopulmonary tumors. *Diag Cytopathol* 1997; 17(6):412–416.

Yazdy AM, Tomashefski JF, Yagan R, Kleinerman J. Regional alveolar damage (RAD): A localized counterpart to diffuse alveolar damage. *Am J Clin Pathol* 1989;92(1):10–15.

Zaman SS, Van Hoeven KH, Slott S, Gupta PK. Distinction between bronchioloalveolar carcinoma and hyperplastic pulmonary proliferations: a cytologic and morphometric analysis. *Diagn Cytopathol* 1997;16(5):396–401.

CELLS WITHIN ALVEOLAR SPACES

Chalon J, Tang CK, Gorstein F, Turndorf H, Katz JS, Klein GS, Patel C. Diagnostic and prognostic significance of tracheobronchial epithelial multinucleation. *Acta Cytol* 1978;22(5):316–320.

Copeland AR, O'Tool K, Chadburn A, Greenbaum E. Megakaryocytes in bronchial brush cytology. A case report. *Acta Cytol* 1993;37(3):400–442.

Costabel U, Matthys H, Guzman J, Freudenberg N. Multinucleated cells in bronchoalveolar lavage. *Acta Cytol* 1985;29(2):189–190.

Hector MF. Sputum cytology in two cases of Wegener's granulomatosis. *J Clin Pathol* 1976; 29(3):259–263.

Kim CC, Saleba K, Baughman RP, et al. Iron staining on bronchoalveolar lavage smears for detecting occult pulmonary hemorrhage: is it reliable? *Acta Cytol* 1989;33(5):716.

Michael CW, Flint A. The cytologic features of Wagener's granulomatosis. *Am J Clin Pathol* 1998;110(1):10–15.

Nasiell M, Roger V, Nasiell K, Enstad I, Vogel B, Bisther A. Cytologic findings indicating pulmonary tuberculosis: the diagnostic significance of epithelioid cells and Langerhans giant cells found in sputum or bronchial secretions. *Acta Cytol* 1972;16(2): 146–151.

Tabatowski K, Roggli VL, Fulkerson WJ, Langley RL, Benning T, Johnston WW. Giant cell interstitial pneumonia in a hard-metal worker: cytologic-histologic and analytical electron microscopic investigation. *Acta Cytol* 1988;32(2):240–246.

Valincenti FJ, Mcmaster KRm, Daniell C. Sputum cytology of giant cell interstitial pneumonia. *Act Cytol* 1979;23:217–221.

INFLAMMATORY CELLS

Michael CW, Richardson PH, Boudreaux CW. Pulmonary lymphoma of the mucosa-associated lymphoid tissue type: report of a case with cytological, histological, immunophenotypical correlation, and review of the literature. *Ann Diagn Pathol* 2005;9(3):148–152.

Tassoni EM. Pools of lymphocyte: significance in pulmonary secretions. *Acta Cytol* 1963;May-June;7:168–173.

MISCELLANEOUS FINDINGS

Bornstein J, Stinson-Carter T, Kaufman RH. Cruschmann's spiral in an endocervical brushing. *Acta Cytol* 1987;31(4):530–532.

Frost JK, Gupta PK, Erozan YS, Carter D, Hollander DH, Levin ML, Ball, WC Jr. Pulmonary cytologic alterations in toxic environmental inhalation. *Human Pathol* 1973;4(4):521–536.

Novak PM, Kumar NB, Naylor B. Cruschmann's spirals in cervicovaginal smears: prevalence, morphology, significance and origin. *Acta Cytol* 1984;28(1):5–8.

Walker KR, Fullmer CD. Progress on study of respiratory spirals. *Acta Cytol* 1970;14(7):396–398.

CHARCOT-LEYDEN CRYSTALS

Chen KT. Cytology of allergic bronchopulmonary aspergillosis. *Diagn Cytopathol* 1993;9(1):82–85.

Sakula A. Charcot-Leyden crystals and Cruschmann's spirals in asthmatic sputum. *Thorax* 1986;41(7):503–507.

CORPORA AMYLACEA

Michael CW, Naylor B. Amyloid in cytologic specimens: differential diagnosis and diagnostic pitfalls. *Acta Cytol* 1999;43(5):746–755.

Yamanouchi H, Yoshinouchi T, Watanabe R, Fujita J, Takahara J, Ohtsuki Y. Immunohistochemical study of a patient with diffuse pulmonary corpora amylacea detected by open lung biopsy. Case Reports. *Intern Med* 1999;38(11):900–903.

Schmitz B, Pfitzer P. Acellular bodies in sputum. *Acta Cytol* 1985;28(2):118–125.

PSAMMOMA BODIES AND CALCOSPHERITES

DeMay RM. Exfoliative respiratory cytology. In: RM DeMay, ed. *The Art and Science of Cytopathology, Exfoliative Cytology.* First edition. Chicago, ASCP, 1996, pp. 218.

Unterman DH, Reingold IM. The occurrence of psammoma bodies in papillary adenocarcinoma of the lung. *AJC P.*1972; 57(3):297–302.

PULMONARY ALVEOLAR MICROLITHIASIS

Mariotta S, Ricci A, Papale M, De Clementi F, Sposato B, Guidi L, Mannino F. Pulmonary alveolar microlithiasis: report on 576 cases published in the literature. *Sarcoidosis Vasc Diffuse Lung Dis* 2004;21(3):173–181.

FERRUGINOUS BODIES

Greenberg SD. Cytopathology of asbestos-associated pulmonary disease. *Diagn Cytopathol* 1985;1(3):177–182.

Roggli VL, Coin PG, MacIntyre NR, Bell DV. Asbestos content of bronchoalveolar lavage fluid: a comparison of light and scanning electron microscopic analysis. *Acta Cytol* 1994;38(4):502–510.

Roggli VL. Asbestos bodies and nonasbestos ferruginous bodies. In: Roggli VL, Greenberg SD, Pratt PC, ed. *Pathology of asbestos-associated diseases.* Boston, MA, Little, Brown and Company, 1992, pp. 39–75.

Roggli VL, Piantadosi CA, Bell DY. Asbestos bodies in bronchoalveolar lavage fluid: a study of 20 asbestos-exposed individuals and comparison to patients with other chronic interstitial lung disease. *Acta Cytol* 1986;30(5):470–476.

Vathesatogkit P, Harkin TJ, Addrizzo-Harris DJ, Bodkin M, Crane M, Rom WN. Clinical correlation of asbestos bodies in BAL fluid. *Chest* 2004;126(3):966–971.

ELASTIN FIBERS

DeMay RM. Exfoliative respiratory cytology. In: RM DeMay, ed. *The art and ccience of cytopathology, exfoliative cytology.* First edition. Chicago, ASCP, 1996, pp. 218.

Shales DM, Lederman M, Chemielewski R, Tweardy D, Wolinsky E. Elastin fibers in the sputum of patients with necrotizing pneumonia. *Chest* 1983;83(6):885–889.

PULMONARY-RELATED DISEASES

Bonfield TL, John N, Malur A, Barna BP, Culver DA, Kavuru MS, Thomassen MJ. Elevated monocyte chemotactic proteins 1, 2, and 3 in pulmonary alveolar proteinosis are associated with chemokine receptor suppression. *Clin Immunol* 2005;114(1):79–85.

Burkhalter A, Silverman JF, Hopkins MBIII, Geisinger KR. Bronchoalveolar lavage cytology in pulmonary alveolar proteinosis. *Am J Clin Pathol* 1996;106(4):504–510.

Crocker HL, Pfitzner J, Doyle IR, Hague WM, Smith BJ, Ruffin RE. Pulmonary alveolar proteinosis: two contrasting cases. *Eur J* 2000;15(2):426–429.

Mermolia M, Rott T, Debeljak A. Cytology of bronchoalveolar lavage in some rare pulmonary disorders: pulmonary alveolar proteinosis and amiodarone toxicity. *Cytopathology* 1994;5(1):9–16.

Michael CW, Naylor B. Amyloid in cytologic specimens: differential diagnosis and diagnostic pitfalls. *Acta cytol* 1999;43(5):746–755.

Shah PL, Hansell D, Lawson PR, Reid KBM, Morgan C. Pulmonary alveolar proteinosis: clinical aspects and current concepts on pathogenesis. *Thorax* 2000;55(1):67–77.

Sosolik SC, Gammon RR, Julius CJ, Ayers LW. Pulmonary alveolar proteinosis: a report of two cases with diagnostic features in bronchoalveolar lavage specimens. *Acta Cytol* 1998;42(2):377–383.

SARCOIDOSIS

Check IJ, Gowitt GT, Staton GJ. Bronchoalveolar lavage cell differential in the diagnosis of sarcoid interstitial lung disease. Likelihood ratios based on computerized database. *Am J Clin Pathol* 1985;84(6):744–747.

DeMay RM. Exfoliative respiratory cytology. In: RM DeMay, ed. *The art and science of cytopathology, exfoliative cytology.* First edition. Chicago, ASCP, 1996, pp. 223.

Greco S, Marruchella A, Massari M, Saltini C. Predictive value of BAL cellular analysis in differentiating pulmonary tuberculosis and sarcoidosis. *Eur Respir J* 2005;26(2):360–361.

Grenier P, Valeyre D, Cluzel P, Brauner MW, Lenoir S, Chastang C. Chronic diffuse interstitial lung disease: diagnostic value of chest radiography and high-resolution CT. *Radiology* 1991;179(1):123–132.

Müller NL, Kullnig P, Miller RR. The CT findings of pulmonary sarcoidosis: analysis of 25 patients. *AJR Am J Roentgenol* 1989;152(6):1179–1182.

Welker L, Jorres RA, Costabel U, Magnussen H. Predictive value of BAL cell differentials in the diagnosis of interstitial lung disease. *Eur Respir J* 2004;24(6):1000–1006.

Zaman SS, Elashami A, Gupta PK. Bronchoalveolar lavage cytology in pulmonary sarcoidosis. *Acta Cytol* 1995;39(6):1117–1123.

PULMONARY INFARCT/EMBOLISM

Scoggins WG, Smith RH, Frable WJ, O'Donohue WJ. False positive cytological diagnosis of lung carcinoma in patients with pulmonary infarcts. *Ann Thorac Surg* 1977;24(5):474–480.

LUNG TRANSPLANT PATIENTS

Ohori NP. Epithelial cell atypia in bronchoalveolar lavage specimens from lung transplant recipients. *Am J Clin Pathol* 1999;112(2):204–210.

Selvaggi SM. Bronchoalveolar lavage in lung transplant patients. *Acta Cytol* 1992;36(5):674–679.

Shennib HL, Serrick AG, Giaid A. Altered nonspecific lymphocyte cytotoxicity in bronchoalveolar lavage of lung transplant recipients: can it be used in monitoring rejection or infection? *Transplantation* 1996;62:1262–1267.

Snell GI, Levvy BJ, Zheng L, Baily M, Orsida B, Lucas L, Whitford HM, Kotsimbos TC, Williams, TJ. Evermolius alters the bronchoalveolar lavage and endobronchial biopsy immunologic profile post-human lung transplant. *Am J of Transplant* 2005;5(6):1446–1451.

Toroke AH, Bewig B, Haverich A. Bronchoalveolar lavage in lung transplantation: state of the art. *Clin Transplant* 1999;13(2):131–157.

Ward C, Snell GI, Zheng L, Orsida B, Whitford H, Williams TJ, Walters EH. Endobronchial biopsy and bronchoalveolar lavage in stable lung transplant recipients and chronic rejection. *Am J Respir Crit Care Med* 1998;158(1):84–91.

ASPIRATION PNEUMONIA

Collins KA, Geisinger LR, Wagner PH, Blackburn KS, Washburn LK. The cytologic evaluation of lipid-laden alveolar macrophages as an indicator of aspiration pneumonia in young children. *Arch Pathol Lab Med* 1995;119(3):229–231.

Colombo JL, Hallberg TK. Pulmonary aspiration and lipid-laden macrophages: in search of gold (standards). *Pediatr Pulmonol* 1999;28(2):79–82.

Corwin RW, Irwin RS. The lipid-laden alveolar macrophages as a marker of aspiration in parenchymal lung disease. *Am Rev Respir Dis* 1985;132(3):576–81.

Cullen MR, Balmes JR, Robins JM, Smith GJ. Lipoid pneumonia caused by oil mist exposure from a steel rolling tandem mill. *Am J Ind Med* 1981;2(1):51–58.

Knauer-Fisher S, Ratjen F. Lipid-laden macrophages in bronchoalveolar lavage fluid as a marker for pulmonary aspiration. *Pediatr Pulmonol* 1999;27(6):419–422.

Nicholson AG, Wells AU, Hooper J, Hansell DM, Kelleher A, Morgan C. Successful treatment of endogenous lipoid pneumonia due to Niemann-Pick type B disease with whole-lung lavage. *Am J Respir Crit Care Med* 2002;165(1):128–131.

MYCOBACTERIAL INFECTION

Bentz JS, Carroll K, Ward JH, Elstad M, Marshall CJ. Acid-fast-positive legionella pneumophila: a possible pitfall in the cytologic diagnosis of mycobacterial infection in pulmonary specimens. *Diagn Cytopathol* 2000;22(1):45–48.

Greco S, Marruchella A, Massari M, Saltini C. Predictive value of BAL cellular analysis in differentiating pulmonary tuberculosis and sarcoidosis. *Eur Respir J* 2005;26(2):360–361.

Jafari C, Ernst M, Kalsdorf JM Jr, Greinert U, Diel R, Kristen D, Marienfeld K, Lalvani A, Lange C. Rapid diagnosis of smear-negative tuberculosis by bronchoalveolar lavage enzyme linked immunospot. *Am J Respir Crit Care Med* 2006;174(9):1048–1054.

Maygarden SJ, Flanders EL. Mycobacteria can be seen as ''negative images'' in cytology smears from patients with acquired immunodeficiency syndrome. *Mod Pathol* 1989;2(3):239–243.

Nasiell M, Roger V, Nasiell K. Cytologic findings indicating pulmonary tuberculosis. *Acta Cytol* 1972;16(2):146–151.

Tani EM, Schmitt FCL, Oliveria ML, Gobetti SM, Decarlis RM. Pulmonary cytology in tuberculosis. *Acta Cytol* 1987;31(4):460–463.

FUNGAL INFECTIONS

Al-Abbadi MA, Russo K, Wilkinson EJ. Pulmonary mucormycosis diagnosed by bronchoalveolar lavage: a case report and review of the literature. *Pediatr Pulmonol* 1997;23(3):222–225.

DiTomasso JP, Ampel NM, Sobonya RE, Bloom JW. Bronchoscopic diagnosis of pulmonary coccidioidomycosis. Comparison of cytology, culture, and transbronchial biopsy. *Diagn Microbiol Infect Dis* 1994;18(2):83–87.

Fischler DF, Hall GS, Gordon S, Stoler MN, Nunez C. Aspergillus in cytology specimens: a review of 45 specimens from 36 patients. *Diagn Cytopathol* 1997;16(1):26–30.

Kapur U, Yong SL, Wojcik EM. Blastomyces associated with granulomatous inflammation in a bronchial lavage. *Diagn Cytopathol* 2005;33(6):399–400.

Lemos LB, Baliga M, Taylor BD, Cason ZJ, Lucia HL. Bronchoalveolar lavage for diagnosis of fungal disease. Five years' experience in a southern United States rural area with many blastomycosis cases. *Acta Cytol* 1995;39(6):1101–1111.

Maesaki S, Kohno S, Mashimoto H, Araki J, Asai S, Hara K. Detection of Cryptococcus neoformans in bronchial lavage cytology: report of four cases. *Intern Med* 1995;34(1):54–57.

Oren I, Goldstein N. Invasive pulmonary aspergillosis. *Curr Opin Pulm Med* 2002,8(3):195–200.

Seyfarth HJ, Nenoff P, Winkler J, Krahl R, Haustein UF, Schauer J. Aspergillus detection in bronchoscopically acquired material. Significance and interpretation. *Mycoses* 2001;44(9–10):356–360.

Travis WD, Colby TV, Koss MN, Rosado-de-Christenson ML, Müller NL, King Jr TE. Lung infections. In: King DW, ed. *Non-Neoplastic Disorders of the Lower Respiratory Tract*. First edition. Washington, DC, American Registry of pathology and the Armed Forces Institute of Pathology: 2002; pp. 539–728.

Williamson JD, Silverman JF, Mallak CT, Christie JD. Atypical cytomorphologic appearance of Cryptococcus neoformans: a report of five cases. *Acta Cytol* 1996;40(2):363–370.

PNEUMOCYSTIS JIROVECI (PJ, FORMERLY PNEUMOCYSTIS CARINII)

Leibovitz E, Pollack H, Moore T, Papillas J, Gallo L, Krasinski K, Borkowsky W. Comparison of PCR and standard cytological staining for detection of Pneumocystis carinii from respiratory specimens from patients with or at high risk for infection by human immunodeficiency virus. *J Clin Microbiol* 1995;33(11):3004–3007.

Nassar A, Zapata M, Little JV, Siddiqui MT. Utility of reflex Gomori methenamine silver staining for Pneumocystis jirovecii on bronchoalveolar lavage cytologic specimens: a review. *Diagn Cytopathol* 2006;34(11):719–723.

Pinlaor S, Mootsikapun P, Pinlaor P, Phunmanee A, Pipitgool V, Sithithaworn P, Chumpia W, Sithithaworn J. PCR diagnosis of Pneumocystis carinii on sputum and bronchoalveolar lavage samples in immunocompromised patients. *Parasitol Res* 2004;94(3):213–218.

Wiwanitkit V. Study of the cost-effectiveness of three staining methods for identification of Pneumocystis carinii in bronchoalveolar lavage fluid. *Trop Doc* 2005;35(1):23–25.

Wazir JF, Macrorie SG, Coleman DV. Evaluation of the sensitivity, specificity, and predictive value of monoclonal antibody 3F6 for the detection of Pneumocystis carinii pneumonia in bronchoalveolar lavage specimens and included sputum. *Cytopathology* 1994;5(2):82–89.

VIRAL INFECTIONS

Bayon MN, Drut R. Cytologic diagnosis of adenovirus bronchopneumonia. *Acta Cytol* 1991;35(2):181–182.

Crosby JH, Pantazis CG, Stigall B. In situ DNA hybridization for confirmation of herpes simplex virus in bronchoalveolar lavage smears. *Acta Cytol* 1991;35(2)248–250.

Fajac A, Stephan F, Ibrahim A, Gautier E, Bernaudin JF, Pico JL. Value of cytomegalovirus detection by PCR in bronchoalveolar lavage routinely performed in asymptomatic bone marrow recipients. *Bone Marrow Transplant* 1997;20(7):581–585.

Harboldt SL, Dugan JM, Tronic BS. Cytologic diagnosis of measles pneumonia in a bronchoalveolar lavage specimen. A case report. *Acta Cytol* 1994;38(3):403–406.

Iwa N, Sasaki CT, Yutani C, Wakasa K. Detection of cytomegalovirus DNA in pulmonary specimens: Confirmation by in situ hybridization in two cases. *Diagn Cytopathol* 1992;8(4):357–360.

Macasact F, Holley KE, Smith TF, Key TF. Cytomegalovirus inclusion body in bronchial brushing material. *Acta Cytol* 1977;21(2):181–182.

Naib ZM, Stewart JA, Dowdle WR, Casey HL, Marine WM, Nahmias AJ. Cytological features of viral respiratory tract infections. *Acta Cytol* 1968;12(2):162–170.

Travis WD, Colby TV, Koss MN, Rosado-de-Christenson ML, Müller NL, King Jr TE. Lung infections. In: King DW, ed. *Non-neoplastic disorders of the lower respiratory tract*. First edition.

Washington, DC, American Registry of pathology and the Armed Forces Institute of Pathology: 2002; pp. 539–728.

THERAPY-RELATED CHANGES

Akoun GM, Gauthier-Rahman S, Milleron BJ, Perrot JY. Amiodarone-induced hypersensitivity pneumonitis. Evidence of an immunological cell-mediated mechanism. *Chest* 1984;85(1):133–135.

Coudert B, Bailly F, Lombard JN, Andre F, Camus P. Amiodarone pneumonitis. Bronchoalveolar lavage findings in 15 patients and review of the literature. *Chest* 1992;102(4):1005–1012.

Fraire AE, Guntupalli KK, Greenberg SD, Cartwright J Jr, Chasen MH. Amiodarone pulmonary toxicity: a multidisciplinary review of current status. *South Med J* 1993;86(1):67–77.

CHEMOTHERAPY

Bedrossian CWM. Iatrogenic and toxic injury. In: Dail DH, Hammar SP, eds. *Pulmonary pathology*. New York, NY: Springer-VerlagNY Inc., 1988, pp. 511–534.

Koss LG, Melamed MR, Mayer K. The effect of busulfan on human epithelia. *Am J Clin Pathol* 1965;44(4);385–397.

Luna MA, Bedrossian CWM, Lichtiger B, Salem PA. Interstitial pneumonitis associated with bleomycin therapy. *Am J Clin Pathol* 1972;58(5):501–510.

MALIGNANT NEOPLASMS

Gupta RK. Value of sputum cytology in the diagnosis and typing of bronchogenic carcinomas, excluding adenocarcinomas. *Acta Cytol* 1982;26(5):645–648.

Liang XM. Accuracy of cytologic diagnosis and cytotyping of sputum in primary lung cancer: analysis of 161 cases. *J Surg Oncol* 1989;40(2):107–111.

Nakajima M, Manabe T, Yagi S. Appearance of mesothelioma cells in sputum: a case report. *Acta Cytol* 1992;36(5):731–736.

Rivera MP, Detterbeck F, Mehta AC. Diagnosis of lung cancer: the guidelines. *Chest* 2003;123(1 Suppl):129S–136S.

Schreiber G, McCrory DC. Performance characteristics of different modalities for diagnosis of suspected lung cancer: Summary of published evidence. *Chest* 2003;123(1 Suppl):115S–128S.

Shanies HM, Mehta DC, Robert TL. Diagnosis of lymphangitic carcinoma to lung by sputum cytology: case report. *Angiology* 1995;46(11):1035–1038.

SQUAMOUS CELL CARCINOMA/EPIDERMOID CARCINOMA (SQCC)

Auerbach O, Stout AP, Hammond EC, Garfinkell L. Changes in bronchial epithelium in relation to cigarette smoking and in relation to lung cancer. *New J Med* 1961;265:253–267.

Bechtel JJ, Kelley WR, Petty TL, Patz DS, Saccomanno G. Outcome of 51 patients with roentgenographically occult lung cancer detected by sputum cytologic testing: a community hospital program. *Arch Intern Med* 1994;154(9):975–980.

Chen JT, Chen YC, Wang YC, Tseng RC, Chen CY, Wang YC. Alterations of the p16^{INKA4A} gene in resected nonsmall cell lung tumors and exfoliated cells within sputum. *Int J Cancer* 2002;98(5):724–731.

Erozan YS, Pressman NJ, Donovan PA, Gupta PK, Frost JK. A comparative cytopathologic study of noninvasive and invasive squamous cell carcinoma of the lung. *Anal Quant Cytol* 1979;1(1):50–56.

Frost JK. The Cell in Health and Disease. An Evaluation of Cellular Morphologic Expression of Biologic Behavior. In: G.I. Wied, ed. *Monographs in Clinical Cytology*, Second Edition. Basel, S Krager, 1986, pp. 165–186.

Frost JK, Gupta PK, Erozan YS, Carter D, Hollander DH, Levin ML, Ball Jr WC. Pulmonary cytologic alterations in toxic environmental inhalation. *Hum Pathol* 1973; 4(4):521–536.

Matsuda M, Nagumo S, Horai T, Yoshino K. Cytologic diagnosis of laryngeal and hypopharyngeal squamous cell carcinoma in sputum. *Acta Cytol* 1988;32(5):655–657.

Miozzo M, Sozzi G, Musso K, Pilotti S, Incarbone M, Pastorino U, Pierotti MA. Microsatellite alterations in bronchial and sputum specimens of lung cancer patients. *Cancer Res* 1996:56(10);2285–2288.

Ritter JH, Wick MR, Reyes A, Coffin CM, Dehner LP. False-positive interpretations of carcinoma in exfoliative respiratory cytology. Report of two cases and a review of underlying disorders. *Am J Clin Pathol* 1995;104(2):133–140.

Saccomanno G. Carcinoma in situ of the lung: its development, detection, and treatment. *Sem Resp Med* 1982;4:156–160.

Tao LC, Chamberlain DW, Delarue NC, Pearson FG, Donat EE. Cytologic diagnosis of radiographically occult squamous cell carcinoma of the lung. *Cancer* 1982;50(8):1580–1586.

INVASIVE BRONCHOGENIC ADC

Fedullo AJ, Ettensohn DB. Bronchoalveolar lavage in lymphangitic spread of adenocarcinoma to the lung. *Chest* 1985;87(1):129–131.

Hirokawa M, Shimizu M, Kanahara T, Manabe T. Plant cells mimicking adenocarcinoma in sputum. *Acta Cytol* 1998;42(5):1306–1307.

Kaminsky DA, Leiman G. False-positive sputum cytology in a case of pulmonary infarction. *Respir Care* 2004;49(2): 186–188.

Linder J, Radio SJ, Robbins RA, Ghafouri M, Rennard SI. Bronchoalveolar lavage in the cytologic diagnosis of carcinoma of lung. *Acta Cytol* 1987;31(6):796–801.

Martinez-Giron R, Ribas-Barcelo A. Pitfall in sputum cytology: Protoctista resembling adenocarcinoma cells. *Diagn Cytopathol* 2007;35(1):32–33.

Mermolja M, Rott T. Cytology of endobronchial granular cell tumor. *Diagn Cytopathol* 1991; 7(5):524–526.

Naryshkin S, Young NA. Respiratory cytology: a review of non-neoplastic mimics of malignancy. *Diagn Cytopathol* 1993;9(1):89–97.

Radio SJ, Rennard SI, Kessinger A, Vaughan WP, Linder J. Breast carcinoma in bronchoalveolar lavage. A cytologic and immunohistochemical study. *Arch Pathol Lab Med* 1989;113(4):333–336.

Smith JH, Frable WJ. Adenocarcinoma of the lung: cytologic correlation with histologic types. *Acta Cytol* 1974;18(4):316–320.

Thivolet-Bejui F. Cytological pitfalls in bronchopulmonary tumors. *Diagn Cytopathol* 1997; 17(6):412–416.

BRONCHOALVEOLAR CARCINOMA

Beasley MB, Brambilla E, Travis WD. The 2004 World Health Organization Classification of lung tumors. *Semin Roentgenol* 2005;40(2):90–97.

Casey K, Winterbauer RH. Persistent pulmonary infiltrate and bronchorrhea in a young woman. *Chest* 1997;111(5):1442–1445.

Ohori NP, Santa Maria EL. Cytopathologic diagnosis of bronchioalveolar carcinoma: does it correlate with the 1999 World Health Organization definition? *Am J Clin Pathol* 2004; 122(1):14–16.

Gupta RK. Value of sputum cytology in the differential diagnosis of alveolar cell carcinoma from bronchogenic adenocarcinoma. *Acta Cytol* 1981;25(3):255–258.

Lozowski W, Hajdu SI. Cytology and immunocytochemistry of bronchioloalveolar carcinoma. *Acta Cytol* 1987;31(6):717–725.

Roger V, Nasiell M, Linden M, Enstad I. Cytologic differential diagnosis of bronchiolo-alveolar carcinoma and bronchogenic adenocarcinoma. *Acta Cytol* 1976;20(4):303–307.

Sestini P, Rottoli L, Gotti G, Miracco C, Luzi P. Bronchoalveolar lavage diagnosis of bronchioloalveolar carcinoma. *Eur J Respir Dis* 1985;66(1):55–58.

NEUROENDOCRINE TUMORS

Aron M, Kapila K, Verma K. Carcinoid tumors of the lung: a diagnostic challenge in bronchial washings. *Diagn Cytopathol* 2004 Jan;30(1):62–66.

Nicholson SA, Ryan MR. A review of cytologic findings in neuroendocrine carcinomas including carcinoid tumors with histologic correlation. *Cancer* 2000 Jun 25;90(3):148–161.

Renshaw AA, Haja J, Lozano RL, Wilbur DC. Distinguishing carcinoid tumor from small cell carcinoma of the lung: correlating cytologic features and performance in the College of American Pathologists Non-Gynecologic Cytology Program. *Arch Pathol Lab Med* 2005May; 129(5):614–618.

LARGE CELL NEUROENDOCRINE CARCINOMA

Hiroshima K, Abe S, Ebihara Y, Ogura S, Kikui M, Kodama T, Komatsu H, Saito Y, Sagawa M, Sato M, Tagawa Y, Nakamura S, Nakayama T, Baba M, Hanzawa S, Hirano T, Horai T. Cytological characteristics of pulmonary large cell neuroendocrine carcinoma. *Lung Cancer.* 2005 Jun;48(3):331–337. Epub 2005 Apr 7.

Kakinuma H, Mikami T, Iwabuchi K, Yokoyama M, Hattori M, Ohno E, Kuramoto H, Jiang SX, Okayasu I. Diagnostic findings of bronchial brush cytology for pulmonary large cell neuroendocrine carcinomas: comparison with poorly differentiated adenocarcinomas, squamous cell carcinomas, and small cell carcinomas. *Cancer.* 2003 Aug 25;99(4):247–54.

Wiatrowska BA, Krol J, Zakowski MF. Large-cell neuroendocrine carcinoma of the lung: proposed criteria for cytologic diagnosis. *Diagn Cytopathol* 2001 Jan;24(1):58–64.

SMALL CELL CARCINOMA

Gephardt GN, Belovich DM. Cytology of pulmonary carcinoid tumors. *Acta Cytol* 1982;26(4):434–438.

Kyriakos M, Rockoff SD. Brush biopsy of bronchial carcinoid: A source of cytologic errors. *Acta Cytol* 1972;16(3):261–268.

Michael CW, Collins B, Flint A. The cytologic classification of pulmonary neuroendocrine tumors: how far can we go? *Acta Cytol* 2000;44(5):902.

Mitchell ML, Parker FP. Capillaries, a cytologic feature of pulmonary carcinoid tumors. *Acta Cytol* 1991;35(2):183–185.

Nicholson SA, Ryan MR. A review of cytologic findings in neuroendocrine carcinomas including carcinoid tumors with histologic correlation. *Cancer (Cancer Cytopathol)* 2000;90(3):148–161.

Nguyen GK. Cytopathology of pulmonary carcinoid tumors in sputum and bronchial brushings. *Acta Cytol* 1995;39(6):1152–1160.

Sturgis CD, Nassar DL, D'Antonio JA, Raab SS. Cytologic features useful for distinguishing small cell from non-small cell carcinoma in bronchial brush and wash specimens. *Am J Clin Pathol* 2000;114(2):197–202.

Travis WD, Shimosato BC, Brambilla E. *Histologic Typing of Lung and Pleural Tumors.* Berlin: Springer; 1999. pp. 21–47.

Travis WD, Rush W, Flieder DB, Falk R, Fleming MV, Gal AA, Koss MN. Survival analysis of 200 pulmonary neuroendocrine tumors with clarification of criteria for atypical carcinoid and its separation from typical carcinoid. *Am J Surg Pathol* 1998;22(8):934–944.

Travis WD, Linnoila RI, Tsokos MG, Hitchcock CL, Cutler GB Jr, Nieman L, Chrousos G, Pass H, Doppman J. Neuroendocrine tumors of the lung with proposed criteria for large-cell neuroendocrine carcinoma. An Ultrastructural, immunohistochemical, and flow cytometric study of 35 cases. *Am J Surg Pathol* 1991;15(6):529–553.

ANAPLASTIC LARGE CELL CARCINOMA (ALCC)

Broderick PA, Corvese NL, LaChance T, Allard J. Giant cell carcinoma of lung: a cytologic evaluation. *Acta Cytol* 1975;19(3):225–230.

Burns TR, Underwood RD, Greenberg SD, Teasdale TA, Cartwright J Jr. Cytomorphometry of large cell carcinoma of the lung. *Anal Quant Cytol Histol* 1989;11(1): 48–52.

Johansson L. Histopathologic classification of lung cancer: relevance of cytokeratin and TTF-1 immunophenotyping. *Ann Diagn Pathol* 2004;8(5):259–267.

HEMATOPOIETIC MALIGNANCIES (HPM)

Bardales RH, Powers CN, Frierson HF Jr, Suhrland MJ, Covell JL, Stanley MW. Exfoliative respiratory cytology in the diagnosis of leukemias and lymphomas in the lung. *Diagn. Cytopathol* 1996;14(2):108–113.

Keicho N, Oka T, Takeuchi K, Yamane A, Yazaki Y, Yotsumoto H. Detection of lymphomatous involvement of the lung by bronchoalveolar lavage. Application of immunophenotypic and gene rearrangement analysis. *Chest* 1994;105(2):458–462.

Lorenzetti E, Nardi F. Diagnostic value of bronchial washing in a case of primary pulmonary non-Hodgkin lymphoma. *App Pathol* 1984;2(5):277–281.

Michael CW, Richardson PH, Boudreaux CW. Pulmonary lymphoma of the mucosa-associated lymphoid tissue type: Report of a case with cytological, histological, immunophenotypical correlation, and review of the literature. *Ann Diagn Pathol* 2005;9(3):148–152.

Riazmontazer N, Bedayat G. Cytology of plasma cell myeloma in bronchial washing. *Acta Cytol.* 1989;33(4):519–522.

Stanley C, Wolf P, Haghighi P. Reed-Sternberg cells in sputum from a patient with the Hodgkin's disease. A case report. *Acta Cytol* 1993;37(1):90–92.

Zompi S, Couderc LJ, Cadranel J, Antoine M, Epardeau B, Fleury-Feith J, Popa N, Santoli F, Farcet JP, Delfau-Larue MH. Clonality analysis of alveolar B lymphocytes contributes to the diagnostic strategy in clinical suspicion of pulmonary lymphoma. *Blood* 2004;103(8):3208–3215.

MISCELLANEOUS RARE TUMORS

Attwood HD, Price CG, Riddell RJ. Primary diffuse tracheobronchial amyloidosis. *Thorax* 1972;27(5):620–624.

Michael C W, Naylor B. Amyloid in cytologic specimens: differential diagnosis and diagnostic pitfalls. *Acta Cytol* 1999;43(5):746–755.

SALIVARY GLAND ANALOGUE TUMORS

Radhika S, Dey P, Rajwanshi A, Guleria R, Bhusnurmath B. Adenoid cystic carcinoma in a bronchial washing: A case report. *Acta Cytol* 1993;37(1):97–99.

Nguyen GK. Cytology of bronchial gland carcinoma. *Acta Cytol* 1988;32(2):235–239.

3

Body Cavity Fluids

Mohammad M. Yousef, and Claire W. Michael

> Malignant mixed müllerian tumor (MMMT) (carcinosarcoma)
> Cervical carcinoma
> Gastrointestinal (GI) tumors
>   Esophageal carcinoma
>   Gastric adenocarcinoma
>   Colonic adenocarcinoma
>   Pancreatic adenocarcinoma
>   Pseudomyxoma peritonei
>   Hepatocellular carcinoma (HCC)
>   Bile duct (cholangiocarcinoma)
>   Hematopoietic neoplasms (lymphoma and leukemia)
>   Primary effusion lymphoma (PEL)
> Miscellaneous malignant tumors
>   Sarcoma
>   Germ cell tumors
>   Seminoma (dysgerminoma)
>   Embryonal carcinoma
>   Yolk sac tumor (endodermal sinus tumor)
>   Melanoma
>   Renal cell carcinoma (RCC)
>   Urothelial cell carcinoma (UCC)
>   Wilms tumor (nephroblastoma)

INTRODUCTION

- The body cavities include the pleural, pericardial, and peritoneal (abdominal) cavities.
- They are lined by a monolayer of mesothelial cells
- Under the mesothelial cell layer is a thin connective tissue that is rich in blood and lymphatic vessels
- All cavities are lined by two layers: the parietal (lines the cavity's wall) and visceral (lines the organ surface), with a potential space in-between
- Normally, a small amount of fluid is present between the parietal layer and the visceral layer for lubrication
- The fluid is continuously, being produced and reabsorbed
- Imbalance between production and reabsorption of fluid leads to accumulation of fluid within the cavity otherwise known as an effusion
- The presence of effusion is always pathologic

TYPES OF EFFUSIONS

- Effusions are divided based on the fluid content into transudate and exudate

Transudate Fluids
- Defined as plasma ultrafiltrate, due to change in the hydrostatic and osmotic pressure
- Clear fluid, hypocellular with low protein content
- Caused by systemic diseases such as congestive heart failure (CHF), chronic renal failure (CRF), and liver cirrhosis
- Do not require cytologic examination in most of the cases. However, malignant effusions can not be ruled out since 1–10% of malignant effusions present as transudate

Exudate Fluids
- Always need cytologic examination
- Fluid appearance is variable and includes: Bloody, milky, bilious, turbid, and chylous
- Hypercellular and rich in protein
- The presence of blood is indicative of either malignancy or an infarct

■ Malignant effusions are not always bloody

■ Etiology includes malignant and nonmalignant diseases

■ Non malignant exudates include infectious diseases, collagen vascular diseases, inflammatory diseases, trauma, infarcts, and chylous effusion

■ Malignant exudates include primary tumor (e.g., mesothelioma) and metastatic tumors (e.g., adenocarcinoma)

MESOTHELIAL CELLS: FROM NORMAL TO REACTIVE

QUIESCENT MESOTHELIAL CELLS

Clinical Features

■ Present in both benign and malignant effusions

■ Shed in few numbers in benign effusions

■ Can be manually retrieved in peritoneal and pelvic washes performed for staging during gynecologic surgery

Cytologic Features

■ Present as a monolayer of flattened sheets arranged in a cobblestone pattern when manually exfoliated (classic examples are sheets seen in pelvic washes)

■ Cells break off as single cells or in few small groups when naturally exfoliated

■ Round to oval cells, 15–20 μm in diameter

■ Cytoplasm is moderate in amount, translucent, and contains peripheral vacuoles containing glycogen

■ Long slender microvilli under light microscopy appear as a pale zone at the periphery causing a fuzzy or a brush-like appearance

■ The central portion of the cytoplasm is denser and darker due to the perinuclear intermediate filaments resulting in a two-tone or endoectoplasmic demarcation

■ Cells may be single or binucleated

■ Nuclei are monotonous, centrally located, and oval to round, with evenly distributed chromatin

■ Nucleoli are distinct

■ Occasional cells exhibit the characteristic "window" and "cellular clasping" appearance

■ Presence of collagen balls (collagen covered with mesothelial cells) in 2–6% of peritoneal washing specimens

■ Degenerated cells may have vacuolated cytoplasm, eccentric nucleus, and mimic histiocytes or signet ring cells

Special Stains and Immunohistochemistry

■ PAS without digestion will stain the small glycogen droplets and the periphery

■ Positive reaction with mesothelial specific markers (described below)

Modern Techniques for Diagnosis

■ Noncontributory

3-1. Benign mesothelial cells
(left). Sheet of benign mesothelial cells retrieved during a pelvic wash. The cells are arranged in a cobblestone pattern and are monotonous with centrally located nuclei, small nucleoli, and opened chromatin. (Papanicolaou stain)

3-2. Benign mesothelial cells
(middle). Benign mesothelial cell exhibiting two tone cytoplasm and peripheral submembranous vacuoles (glycogen droplets). The nucleus is centrally located and bland. (Papanicolaou stain)

3-3. Benign mesothelial cells
(right). Benign mesothelial cells showing articulation with window spaces between the cells. Notice how the cytoplasm touches at the periphery leaving a space in between the cells. (Papanicolaou stain)

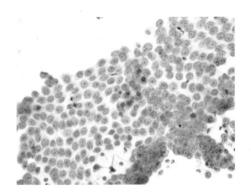
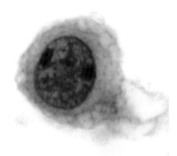
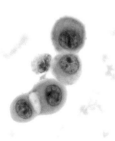

3-4A. Benign mesothelial cells. A row of benign mesothelial cells with clasp-like articulation. Notice how the cytoplasm of one cell extends to hug the other cell tightly. (Papanicolaou stain)

3-4B. Benign mesothelial cells. Two mesothelial cells with very tight articulation causing one cell to pinch the other and squeezing its cytoplasm in the opposite direction. (Papanicolaou stain)

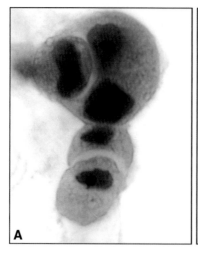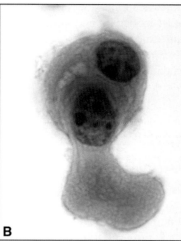

3-5. Benign mesothelial cells *(left)*. Mesothelial cells showing one cell within the other, a commonly seen feature. This is not cellular engulfment but simply one cell sitting on top of the other's cytoplasm similar to a plate and saucer. (Papanicolaou stain)

3-6. Benign mesothelial cells *(right)*. Multinucleated mesothelial cell. (Papanicolaou stain)

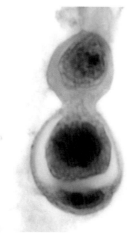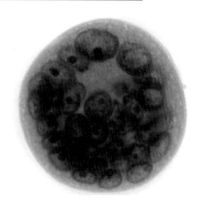

Differential Diagnosis

■ Macrophages
  ➤ Rounded cells with indistinct cell borders
  ➤ Pale vacuolated cytoplasm
  ➤ Peripherally located small folded nuclei
  ➤ Adjacent cells do not form "windows"
  ➤ Positive for CD68
■ Decidualized cells, squamous metaplasia, and epithelial cells
  ➤ Well-defined cell border
  ➤ No endoectoplasmic demarcation
  ➤ Absence of windows or cellular clasping between adjacent cells

REACTIVE MESOTHELIAL CELLS

Clinical Features

■ Hyperplastic/hypertrophied cells that may look atypical and may mimic malignant mesothelioma (MM) or adenocarcinoma
■ Underlying etiology include a list of benign factors:
  ➤ Heart failure
  ➤ Infection (pneumonia, lung abscess)
  ➤ Infarction (may shed in sheets)
  ➤ Liver disease such as hepatitis or cirrhosis (may cause pronounced hyperplasia)

➤ Collagen vascular disease
➤ Renal disease such as uremia or peritoneal dialysis
➤ Pancreatic disease
➤ Radiation
➤ Chemotherapy (bleomycin, cytoxan)
➤ Traumatic irritation (hemodialysis, surgery)
➤ Chronic inflammation (PID, pleuritis)
➤ Underlying mass causing irritation of the mesothelium (e.g., large ovarian cyst)
➤ Foreign substance (talc, asbestos)

Cytologic Features
▣ Shed as doublets and triplets, as well as small clusters with scalloped borders
▣ Few papillary groups may be formed
▣ Clasp-like articulations and intercellular windows are more obvious
▣ Cells are round to oval, 20–40 μm in diameter
▣ Abundant cytoplasm with endoectoplasmic demarcation and peripheral submembranous vacuoles
▣ Cytoplasmic protrusions distal to cellular clasping
▣ Nuclei are round to oval with some variation in size and chromatin distribution
▣ The cell size may vary slightly, however, within a small range and only few cells will appear out of proportion
▣ Nucleoli may become prominent
▣ Multinucleated cells increase
▣ Occasionally intranuclear inclusions are noted

Special Stains and Immunohistochemistry
▣ Some literature suggests that desmin and EMA could have a role in separating reactive from malignant mesothelial cells
    ➤ Reactive stains mostly positive to desmin and negative to EMA
    ➤ Malignant stains mostly negative to desmin and positive to EMA

Modern Techniques for Diagnosis
▣ Noncontributory

Differential Diagnosis
▣ Malignant mesothelioma
    ➤ Monotonous cell population with mild to moderate atypia
    ➤ Morules and numerous discohesive cells
    ➤ Numerous multinucleated giant mesothelial cells
    ➤ Markedly enlarged cells (5–10 times that of normal mesothelium)
    ➤ Background cells show a wide range of size
▣ Adenocarcinoma
    ➤ Pleomorphic population of cells with obvious atypia
    ➤ Little variation in size of cells
    ➤ Two-cell populations (background reactive mesothelium) may be detected
    ➤ Lack of two tone cytoplasm
    ➤ Cytoplasmic glycogen rarely seen (lung adenocarcinoma)
    ➤ True gland formation may be seen in some clusters

PEARLS

✶ Clinical history is not suspicious for malignancy
✶ Benign radiological findings
✶ Cells are not markedly enlarged

★ Variation in cellular size and shape is limited
★ Rare or few tight three-dimensional clusters

MACROPHAGES

Clinical features

▪ Present in both benign and malignant effusions
▪ Present in all serous fluid, especially in peritoneal fluid
▪ Seen in higher numbers when associated with hemorrhage, infarction, metabolic storage disease, infection, chronic inflammation, and as response to foreign body material

Cytologic Features

▪ Round to oval shape
▪ Vary in size from 20 to 25 μm up to 60–80 μm
▪ Eccentrically located small folded nuclei
▪ Indistinct nucleoli
▪ Ill-defined cell borders
▪ Pale (cyanophilic by Pap stain) usually vacuolated cytoplasm
▪ Can be seen singly or in loose groups
▪ Phagocytosed debris can be seen in the cytoplasm
▪ May exhibit slight atypia in patients presenting with effusions postsurgical manipulation

Special Stains and Immunohistochemistry

▪ Positive to CD68
▪ Negative to keratin

Modern Techniques for Diagnosis

▪ Noncontributory

Differential Diagnosis

▪ Degenerated mesothelial cells
  ➤ Round nuclei with distinct nucleoli
  ➤ Well-defined cell borders
  ➤ Dense two-tone cytoplasm
  ➤ Occasional cells exhibit the characteristic "window"
  ➤ Surface microvilli with brush-like appearance
▪ Signet ring adenocarcinoma
  ➤ Enlarged nuclei with hyperchromasia and more irregular nuclear membrane
  ➤ High nuclear to cytoplasmic ratio
  ➤ May exhibit intracellular mucin
  ➤ Positive reaction to epithelial markers

PEARLS

▪ Histiocytes may aggregate and present as sheets thus mimicking carcinomas
  ➤ There is usually no history of cancer
  ➤ There is no definite cellular atypia

HEMATOPOIETIC CELLS

▪ Benign lymphocytes are common
▪ Peripheral blood smear picture in cases with specimens contaminated by peripheral blood

■ The presence of megakaryocytes should raise a differential diagnosis of myelo-proliferative disorder, extramedullary hematopoiesis, metastatic carcinoma replacing the bone marrow, and pulmonary microvasculature bleeding into the pleural cavity

DETACHED CILIARY TUFTS (DCT)

■ DCTs are seen in peritoneal washing specimens
■ Result from detachment of the cilia lining the epithelium of the fallopian tubes
■ Motile on toluidine blue–stained wet preparations

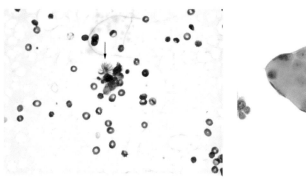 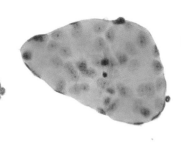

3-7. Detached ciliary tuft *(left)*. Detached ciliary tuft (arrow) in peritoneal fluid from a patient with recent abortion. (Papanicolaou stain)

3-8. Collagen ball *(right)*. Collagen ball seen in a pelvic wash. Notice the central collagen surrounded by flat mesothelium. (Papanicolaou stain)

EOSINOPHILIC EFFUSIONS

Clinical Features
■ Uncommon disorder
■ Most commonly seen in pleural effusions
■ Defined as the presence of high number of eosinophils (at least 10% of the total number of cells)
■ It is idiopathic in more than 30% of cases
■ Other disorders associated with eosinophilic effusions include collagen vascular diseases (most common), tuberculosis (TB), pneumonia, pneumothorax, pulmonary infarction, parasitic infections, allergic diseases, drugs reactions, and malignancies (e.g., Hodgkin's lymphoma)
■ High levels of vascular cell adhesion molecule-1 (VCAM-1) have been described in pleural fluids of patients with eosinophilic effusions
■ Resolve spontaneously in most of the cases

Cytologic Features
■ Cellular with high number of eosinophils (≥10% of total cells)
■ Reactive mesothelial cells
■ Charcot–Leyden crystals (most commonly seen in fluids stored more than twenty-four hours in refrigerator)
■ Mast cells have been described in some cases with no specific association

Special Stains and Immunohistochemistry
■ Noncontributory

Modern Techniques for Diagnosis
■ Noncontributory

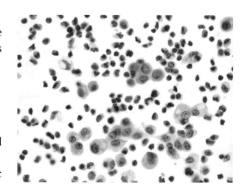

3-9. Eosinophilic effusion. Eosinophilic pleural fluid from a patient with pneumothorax. Notice the slightly reactive mesothelial cells shed in doublets and small clusters surrounded by numerous eosinophils. (Papanicolaou stain)

Differential Diagnosis

- Thoracic trauma (pneumothorax)
- Collagen vascular diseases
- Infections (TB, parasites)
- Allergy (drug)
- Malignancies
- Pulmonary infarction
- Peritoneal dialysis

PEARLS

- ✶ High number of eosinophils
- ✶ Usually in pleural fluids, rarely seen in peritoneal or pericardial fluids
- ✶ >30% of cases are idiopathic

RHEUMATOID PLEURITIS

Clinical Features

- Occur in less than 5% of patients with rheumatoid arthritis (RA)
- Rarely precedes the joint disease
- Usually unilateral, but can be bilateral or associated with pericardial effusion
- Long standing effusion (last days to years)
- Exudate effusion with low glucose and pH
- Pseudochylous effusions (rich in cholesterol) can be seen in long standing disease
- Rheumatoid factor (RF) is commonly present in pleural effusions
- Radiological studies and pleural biopsies reveal multiple rheumatoid nodules

Cytologic Features

- Consists predominantly of small and large clumps of necrotic granular debris (stain green, red, or orange by PAP stain)
- Round or spindle-shaped macrophages (may be present)
- Round or spindle-shaped multinucleated giant cells (up to 150 μm) with more than 20 nuclei (may be present)
- Rare to absent mesothelial cells
- Mixed inflammatory cells
- Nonspecific ragocytes or RA cells (granulocytes with small round cytoplasmic inclusions) may be identified
- Cholesterol crystals (nonspecific, seen in pseudochylous effusions)

Special Stains and Immunohistochemistry

- Noncontributory

Modern Techniques for Diagnosis

- Noncontributory

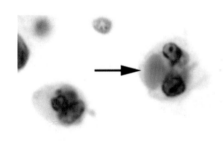

3-10. Rheumatoid pleuritis.
Pleural fluid with an LE cell from a patient with known lupus erythematosus. A neutrophil contains a green staining hematoxylin body (arrow). (Papanicolaou stain)

Differential Diagnosis

- Tuberculous effusion (TE)
  - ➤ Abundant T-cell lymphocytes
  - ➤ Rare giant cells
  - ➤ Histiocytes present in small numbers
- Bacterial infection
  - ➤ Abundant neutrophils
  - ➤ Absent giant cells
  - ➤ Reactive mesothelial cells

★ History of rheumatoid arthritis
★ Exudative pleural effusion with low pH and glucose
★ Necrotic granular material, round and spindle-shaped macrophages, and multinucleated giant cells are pathognomonic cytologic features of rheumatoid pleuritis

EFFUSIONS ASSOCIATED WITH SYSTEMIC LUPUS ERYTHEMATOSUS (SLE)

Clinical Features
▓ SLE is an autoimmune disorder that involves multisystem microvascular inflammation with the production of autoantibodies
▓ SLE occurs predominantly in women of childbearing age
▓ Effusions occur in one-third of patients with SLE
▓ Commonly affect pleural and pericardial cavities
▓ Rarely seen as the initial manifestation

Cytologic Features
▓ Presence of lupus erythematosus (LE) cells (characteristic but not pathognomonic)
　➤ Rarely seen in effusions of patients without SLE
　➤ LE cells are present in 27% of SLE-diagnosed patients with effusions
　➤ LE cells can be seen in effusions of patients with drug-induced lupus erythematosus
　➤ LE cell is a neutrophil or macrophage that contains cytoplasmic particle called hematoxylin body
　➤ The hematoxylin body stains green, blue, or purple with PAP stain
　➤ Presence of tart cells (same as LE cells but they ingest nuclei with visible chromatin instead of degenerated ones)
▓ Reactive mesothelial cells may range from mildly reactive to profound

Special Stains and Immunohistochemistry
▓ Noncontributory

Modern Techniques for Diagnosis
▓ Noncontributory

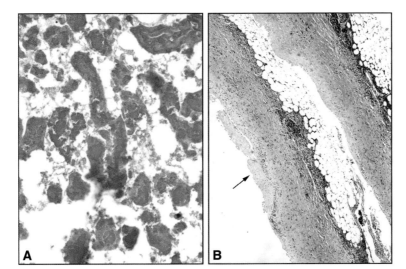

3-11A. Rheumatoid pleuritis. Pleural fluid from a patient with rheumatoid arthritis containing variable-sized clumps of granular necrotic material. (Papanicolaou stain)

3-11B. Rheumatoid pleuritis. Pleural biopsy showing small granulomas with opened surface (arrow) spilling the necrotic debris into the pleural space. (H&E stain)

Differential Diagnosis
■ Bacterial infection
➤ Abundant neutrophils
➤ Absent LE cells
➤ Reactive mesothelial cells
➤ Negative history for SLE

★ History of SLE
★ Positive antinuclear antibodies (ANAs) and anti double-stranded DNA (dsDNA) antibodies
★ Presence of LE cells

TUBERCULOUS EFFUSIONS

Clinical Features
■ May present as an acute (>60% of cases) or as a chronic illness
■ May occur without any obvious parenchymal involvement
■ Usually unilateral
■ The fluid is usually turbid, greenish in color
■ Typically, predominantly lymphocytic exudates
■ CD4:CD8 ratio is higher in pleural fluid than in the blood
■ The glucose may be low and adenosine deaminase (ADA) levels are usually elevated
■ ADA2 is the predominant isoform in the tuberculous pleural effusion (88% of total ADA activity)

Cytologic Features
■ They are characteristic but not specific
■ Highly cellular
■ Predominantly small lymphocytes
■ Lymphocytes are of T-cell origin (mainly helper cells CD4+)
■ Rare to absent mesothelial cells (in non-HIV patients)
■ Many reactive mesothelial cells in HIV patients

Special Stains and Immunohistochemistry
■ Acid-fast bacilli (AFB) stain
■ CD4+ and CD8+ lymphocytes

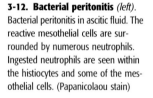

3-12. Bacterial peritonitis *(left).* Bacterial peritonitis in ascitic fluid. The reactive mesothelial cells are surrounded by numerous neutrophils. Ingested neutrophils are seen within the histiocytes and some of the mesothelial cells. (Papanicolaou stain)

3-13. Pneumonia *(right).* Pleural effusion from a patient with pneumonia showing reactive mesothelial cells appearing in clusters some with a central collagen core. The cells are single or binucleated with slightly enlarged nuclei and prominent nucleoli. The chromatin is vesicular and evenly distributed. Overall, the cells have a close size range. (Papanicolaou stain)

Modern Techniques for Diagnosis
■ Polymerase chain reaction (PCR) is more sensitive than AFB staining and culture for diagnosis, but with low specificity

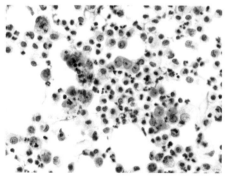

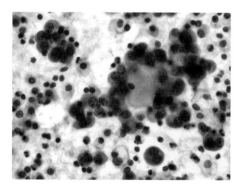

Differential Diagnosis
- Pneumonia
  - ➤ Polymorphous inflammatory cells
  - ➤ Reactive mesothelial cells
- Small lymphocytic lymphoma (SLL)/chronic lymphocytic leukemia (CLL)
  - ➤ Highly cellular
  - ➤ Absent or few background mesothelial cells
  - ➤ Small lymphocytes of B-cell origin
  - ➤ CD19+, CD20+, CD5+, and CD23+

PEARLS

- ✶ Elevated ADA levels
- ✶ Predominantly T-helper lymphocytes (CD4+)
- ✶ Presence of many mesothelial cells distinguishes HIV from non-HIV patients

BACTERIAL INFECTIONS

Clinical Features
- Causes acute pleuritis, pericarditis, and peritonitis
- Pleuritis usually associated with pneumonia
- Peritonitis is associated with bowel injury or inflammation
- The fluid is purulent (creamy yellow)
- Common organism include: streptococcus pneumonia (Gram-positive diplococci), staphylococcus (Gram-positive cocci in clusters)

FUNGAL/PARASITIC INFECTIONS

Cytologic Features
- Numerous neutrophils
- Reactive mesothelial cells

Special Stains and Immunohistochemistry
- Gram stain

Modern Techniques for Diagnosis
- Noncontributory

Differential Diagnosis
- Malignancy
  - ➤ High nuclear cytoplasmic (N:C) ratio
  - ➤ Three-dimensional clusters of atypical cells
  - ➤ Coarse chromatin

PEARLS

- ✶ Clinical history of infectious process
- ✶ Purulent fluid
- ✶ Positive Gram stain or culture
- ✶ Rule out metastatic malignancy causing a secondary infection

VIRAL INFECTIONS

Clinical Features
- Effusion is uncommon presentation
- Effusions can be from primary infection or secondary infection (pulmonary extension)
- Mostly seen in immunocompromised patients
- Common isolated viral infections include herpes simplex virus (HSV), cytomegalovirus (CMV), and herpes zoster virus (HZV)
- Cytopathic changes are rarely seen

Cytologic Features
- Usually lymphocytes in the background
- Atypical reactive mesothelial cells
- Challenging smear due to the difficulty in recognizing the cytopathic changes and the accompanying marked mesothelial atypia
- CMV changes include cell enlargement and large intranuclear inclusion
- HSV and HZV changes include multinucleation, molding, and ground-glass appearance of nuclei

Special Stains and Immunohistochemistry
- Antiviral antibodies on cell block material

Modern Techniques for Diagnosis
- Noncontributory

Differential Diagnosis
- Malignancy
  - High nuclear cytoplasmic (N:C) ratio
  - Three-dimensional clusters of atypical cells
  - Coarse chromatin
  - Negative antiviral antibodies

PEARLS
- Immunocompromised patient
- Viral inclusions
- Positive antiviral antibodies or culture
- Atypical reactive mesothelial cells mimicking malignancy

FUNGAL/PARASITIC INFECTIONS

Clinical Features
- Fungal infections are common in immunocompromised patients; however, identification of organisms in fluid is difficult
- Parasitic infections are rarely associated with effusions especially in Western countries and usually a history of traveling or immigration guide the identification of the organism
- Common isolated fungal infections include: *Cryptococcus neoformans*, *Histoplasmosis capsulatum*, mucormycosis, coccidioides immitis, aspergillus, candida, and blastomyces dermatitidis
- Some parasitic infections include: schistosoma (Japan, Egypt, South America), echinococcus granulosus (East Africa, Middle East), leishmania donovani (Mediterranean, Africa, South America, Asia), and wuchereria bancrofti (India, Asia, Pacific islands)
- *Pneumocystis jiroveci* has been reported in pleural and peritoneal effusions

Cytologic Features
- Usually mix inflammatory background
- Reactive mesothelial cells
- *P. jiroveci* cytology is similar to that seen in respiratory specimens (refer to "Respiratory" chapter)

Special Stains and Immunohistochemistry
- Grocott methenamine silver (GMS) stain on cell block material

Modern Techniques for Diagnosis
- Noncontributory

Differential Diagnosis
- Reactive mesothelium mimicking adenocarcinoma
  - High nuclear cytoplasmic (N:C) ratio
  - Three-dimensional clusters of atypical cells
  - Coarse chromatin
  - Negative GMS stain

PEARLS

- Immunocompromised patient
- Positive GMS stain
- Definitive diagnosis is established by culture

CIRRHOSIS

Clinical Features
- Effusions are the result of hypoalbuminemia and low osmotic pressure
- Usually transudate fluid
- Spontaneous bacterial peritonitis (SBP) can occur in longstanding peritoneal effusion, leading to an exudative fluid
- Spontaneous bacterial empyema (SBE) occur in patients with cirrhosis and pleural effusion
- SBE patients present with fever and dyspnea, but they may be asymptomatic

Cytologic Features
- Low cellularity (high cellularity seen in SBP)
- Usually mixed inflammatory background
- Abundant reactive/hyperplastic mesothelial cells in clusters may be seen in longstanding cirrhosis
- Longstanding unrefrigerated fluids can lead to nuclear hyperchromasia

Special Stains and Immunohistochemistry
- Positive reaction to mesothelial and negative to adenocarcinoma markers

Modern Techniques for Diagnosis
- Noncontributory

Differential Diagnosis
- Malignancy
  - Many single cells with high N:C ratio
  - Three-dimensional clusters of atypical cells
  - Coarse chromatin
  - Clinical history suspicious for malignancy

PEARLS

★ History of cirrhosis
★ Presence of numerous neutrophils should raise the suspicion of SBP

UREMIA

Clinical Features
▪ Seen in patients with chronic renal failure (CRF)
▪ Peritoneal dialysis
▪ Uremic pericarditis is the most common
▪ Usually the fluid is bloody

Cytologic Features
▪ Low cellularity
▪ Fragmented red blood cells (RBCs)
▪ Atypical reactive mesothelial cells
▪ Hyperplastic mesothelial groups with cytologic atypia may be seen in ascitic fluids from patients undergoing peritoneal dialysis

Special Stains and Immunohistochemistry
▪ Positive reaction to mesothelial markers
▪ Most cases will positively react to desmin

Modern Techniques for Diagnosis
▪ Noncontributory

Differential Diagnosis
▪ Adenocarcinoma
  ➤ High cellularity
  ➤ Many single cells with high N:C ratio
  ➤ Three-dimensional clusters of atypical cells
  ➤ Coarse chromatin
  ➤ Clinical history suspicious for malignancy
  ➤ Positive reaction to epithelial markers
▪ Malignant mesothelioma
  ➤ History of asbestos exposure in most cases
  ➤ Wide range of size of the mesothelial cells from benign appearing to giant cells and in-between
  ➤ Cytologic atypia more pronounced than in uremic fluid and with more prominent nucleoli
  ➤ Most cases will react positively to EMA and negatively to desmin

3-14. Chronic renal failure *(left)*. Peritoneal fluid from a patient with chronic renal failure and peritoneal dialysis showing reactive mesothelial cells in a background of broken red blood cells. (Papanicolaou stain)

3-15. Cirrhosis *(right)*. Ascitic fluid from a patient with liver cirrhosis. The reactive mesothelial cells are shed as single cells as well as clusters. Many of the cells are binucleated and multinucleated. (Papanicolaou stain)

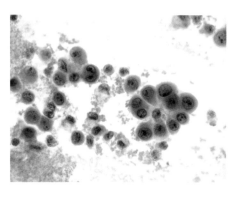
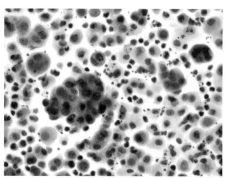

⋆ History of CRF
⋆ History of peritoneal dialysis
⋆ Bloody effusion with lysed RBCs

PANCREATITIS

Clinical Features
▢ Can cause chronic ascites and pleural effusion
▢ Bloody fluids
▢ Presence of high level of pancreatic enzymes is more sensitive than cytology for diagnosis

Cytologic Features
▢ Low cellularity
▢ Fragmented RBCs
▢ Presence of lymphocytes and eosinophils
▢ Reactive mesothelial cells

Special Stains and Immunohistochemistry
▢ Mesothelial markers separate reactive mesothelium from adenocarcinoma (see "Malignant Mesothelioma" section)

Modern Techniques for Diagnosis
▢ Noncontributory

Differential Diagnosis
▬ Malignancy
  ➤ Many single cells with high N:C ratio
  ➤ Three-dimensional clusters of atypical cells
  ➤ Coarse chromatin
  ➤ Clinical history suspicious for malignancy

History of pancreatitis
Presence of high levels of pancreatic enzymes

INFARCTION

Clinical Features
▢ Effusion is related to the hemorrhagic necrosis, caused by loss of blood supply, and associated inflammatory response
▢ Usually exudative fluid
▢ Can be associated with infection (e.g., bowel infarction)

Cytologic Features
▢ Usually cellular
▢ Usually mix inflammatory background with increased eosinophils
▢ Abundant atypical reactive mesothelial cells, some with degenerative changes
▢ Inflammatory cells vary with age of the infarct and the presence of superimposed infection

Special Stains and Immunohistochemistry
▫ Mesothelial markers separate the reactive cells from adenocarcinoma

Modern Techniques for Diagnosis
▫ Noncontributory

Differential Diagnosis
▪ Adenocarcinoma
  ➤ Many single cells with high N:C ratio
  ➤ Three-dimensional clusters of atypical cells
  ➤ Coarse chromatin and irregular nuclear membrane
  ➤ Prominent nucleoli
  ➤ Clinical history suspicious for malignancy
  ➤ Positive reaction to epithelial markers

PEARLS

★ History of infarction
★ Presence of numerous neutrophils should raise the suspicion of secondary infection

MALIGNANT MESOTHELIOMA (MM)

Clinical Features
▫ MM is a rare disease
▫ Approximately 2500–3000 cases are diagnosed per year in United States
▫ Extremely important to recognize it since mesothelioma has different therapeutic implications from other tumors and will spare the patients repeated procedures such as core biopsies that frequently carry the risk of seeding along the needle tract
▫ MM has no racial predilection
▫ Most patients develop MM in the fifth to seventh decade of life
▫ Some reported cases of MM were in childhood age (not related to asbestos exposure)
▫ More common in men, with a male- to -female ratio of 3:1
▫ Asbestos exposure is the most important factor associated with MM, including the duration and intensity of exposure
▫ More than 60% of cases are associated with asbestos exposure
▫ Usually occur thirty-five to forty-five years after asbestos exposure with a relative risk of 1000× compared to nonasbestos exposure
▫ Simian virus 40 (SV 40) has no direct role in developing MM, therefore, it has been suggested that it acts as possible co-carcinogen
▫ Most commonly seen in pleural cavities (right side > left side) followed by peritoneal cavity
▫ Primary pericardial MM is rarely seen
▫ Dyspnea and chest pain are the most common presenting symptoms
▫ Commonly the effusion is bloody
▫ Fluid or serum mesothelin-related protein (SMRP) levels are elevated in MM
▫ Early stage: appears as hundreds of tiny nodules on the serous membrane. Pleural thickening and plaques are noted when associated with asbestos exposure
▫ Late stage: nodules become confluent and the serosal membrane becomes thick and gradually the parietal and visceral membranes become fused together, with disappearance of any fluid
▫ Histologic types of MM include

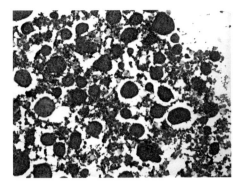
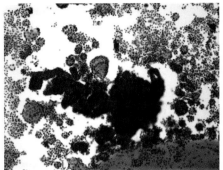
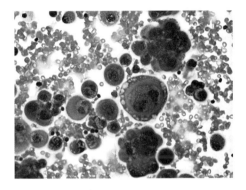
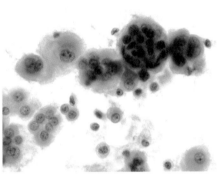
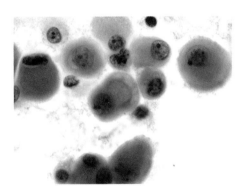
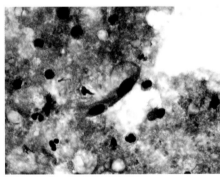

3-16. Malignant mesothelioma *(left)*. Malignant mesothelioma presenting predominantly as cellular spheres (morules) in a background of scattered single cells. (Papanicolaou stain)

3-17. Well differentiated tubulo-papillary mesothelioma *(right)*. Well-differentiated tubulopapillary mesothelioma presenting with complex papillary fragments and numerous spheres with collagen centers. (Papanicolaou stain)

3-18. Malignant mesothelioma *(left)*. Malignant mesothelioma presenting mainly as small clusters with scalloped borders and numerous single cells. The cells vary widely in size from small to gigantic and multinucleated. Notice the size of the central single cell almost approaching that of the adjacent clusters. (Modified gemsa stain)

3-19. Malignant mesothelioma *(right)*. Malignant mesothelioma showing similar features as the previous case. (Papanicolaou stain)

3-20. Malignant mesothelioma *(left)*. Malignant mesothelioma presenting predominantly as single cells. Notice the enlarged cells with abundant two-tone cytoplasm and rich glycogen droplets. (Papanicolaou stain)

3-21. Sarcomatoid mesothelioma *(right)*. Sarcomatoid mesothelioma with a sparsely cellular effusion containing rare yet highly atypical spindle cells. (Papanicolaou stain)

➤ Epithelioid (tubulopapillary, well-differentiated papillary, epithelioid, transitional, deciduoid, clear variant, microcystic, and small cell)
  • Most common type (particularly the first three patterns)
  • Very cellular
  • More commonly associated with effusion
  • Highest survival rate
➤ Sarcomatous
  • Uncommon
  • Hypocellular (difficult to diagnose)
  • Not commonly associated with effusion
  • Low survival rate
➤ Biphasic
  • Positive fluids will usually contain the epithelioid component and very rarely scarce sarcomatoid cells
➤ Anaplastic
  • The disease is fatal within four to eight months, if not treated
  • With treatment the survival increased to sixteen to nineteen months
  • Some patients have survived as long as five years

Cytologic Features

- Highly cellular smears (hypocellular in sarcomatoid variant)
- The increase in cell size is one of the most prominent features in mesothelioma (attain a gigantic size)
- All cells look alike, that is, no evidence of two-cell population
- Cellular spheres with smooth borders (morules)
- Tight and loose clusters with scalloped borders
- High number of cells within the clusters
- Individual cells show a wide variation in size and shape ranging from small to gigantic
- Large multinucleated cells with abundant cytoplasm, some of these cells approach the size of small morules
- Mesothelial cell features are easily recognized and exaggerated
- Yellow glycogen droplets are frequently detected
- Nuclei are usually bland or slightly atypical (nuclear irregularity, coarse chromatin and hyperchromasia)
- Very prominent nucleoli
- Background of numerous lymphocytes or abundant blood
- Thick extracellular matrix (hyaluronic acid) is frequently present causing a grossly recognized thick consistency described as "tar-like" or honey-like"
- This matrix can sometimes interfere with smear preparation particularly liquid-based preps
- Cell-in-cell engulfment
- EM is very accurate in diagnosing epithelioid mesothelioma
- Important features include
  - Cell surface: long, slender microvilli (length >15× diameter),
  - Cell junction: apical tight junctions and well as developed desmosomes
  - Cell cytoplasm: abundant tonofilaments around the nucleus, no secretory granules, and abundant glycogen

Special Stains and Immunohistochemistry

- Immunocytochemical results obtained with ThinPrep match those of cell block for most markers tested. However, cell block preparations are superior to ThinPrep for nuclear markers

POSITIVE MARKERS FOR MESOTHELIUM

- Calretinin
  - Regarded as the most sensitive and one of the most specific of the positive mesothelial markers
  - Frequently expressed in most histologic types of mesothelioma
  - The diagnosis of mesothelioma in the absence of staining with Calretinin should be considered cautiously
  - Staining pattern is strong and diffuse, and occurs in both the nuclei and cytoplasm (fried egg appearance)
  - Adenocarcinoma (ADC) staining has been reported between 0 and 38% but the staining is usually focal although occasionally strong and diffuse (lung 6–10%, ovary 31–38%, renal 0–4%). Squamous cell carcinoma could be immunoreactive in 23–39%.
- Wilms tumor 1 protein (WT-1)
  - Stains up to 93% of epithelioid mesotheliomas
  - It is also highly expressed in ovarian serous carcinoma
  - Lung ADC and squamous are reported to be negative or very minimal expression thus making WT-1 one of the best markers to distinguish between mesothelioma and lung ADC or squamous

- Keratins 5/6
  - Reported to stain 64–100% of mesotheliomas
  - Staining is cytoplasmic and can be very focal resulting in false negatives
  - Staining is positive and strong in most squamous cell carcinomas
  - Also could stain 22–35% of ovarian serous carcinoma and was reported to stain 0–19% of lung ADC
  - CK5/6 has no utility in distinguishing mesothelioma from squamous carcinoma
- Thrombomodulin
  - Reported to stain 34–100% of mesotheliomas (more around 75%), and between 5% and 77% of lung ADC (more around 14%)
  - Mesotheliomas tend to present with diffuse strong membranous pattern while adenocarcinoma showed focal week staining
  - Also expressed in angiosarcoma and squamous carcinoma
- D2-40
  - Antibody that reacts with oncofetal M2A antigen in fetal germ cells and germ cell tumors
  - Stains 86–96% of epithelioid component of mesothelioma with a membranous or luminal pattern
  - Also reported to stain about 15% of ovarian ADC but none of the other adenocarcinomas
- Podoplanin
  - This is a membrane mucoprotein detected on podocytes of glomerular epithelial cells. It has similar sensitivity and specificity as D2-40
- Mesothelin
  - Stains up to 100% of epithelioid mesotheliomas
  - Diffuse strong membranous staining
  - Positive staining also occur in a variety of adenocarcinomas (ovarian and pancreatic adenocarcinomas), though it may be cytoplasmic or focal
  - Despite the low specificity of this marker, a negative staining argues against the diagnosis of mesothelioma
- Keratin 7 and keratin 20
  - Keratin 7 is strongly expressed in epithelioid mesothelioma, lung ADC, and ovarian ADC
  - All the above are negative to keratin 20
  - Are not useful in the differential of mesothelioma from adenocarcinoma
  - Negative staining for both or strong staining to CK20 is evidence against mesothelioma
  - Rarely keratin 20 may be focally expressed in mesothelioma but these cases also show strong staining to keratin 7

NEGATIVE MARKERS FOR MESOTHELIUM

- MOC-31
  - Recognizes epithelial cell adhesion molecule
  - Currently considered to be the most sensitive and specific negative marker for mesothelioma although 5–10% are reported to show focal staining
  - Positive strong and diffuse cytoplasmic staining is reported in almost all adenocarcinomas of lung and ovary
  - Up to 50% of renal cell carcinomas are positive
- CD15 (Leu-M1)
  - Negative in mesothelioma
  - 70–75% of lung ADC and 30–60% of ovarian ADC are immunoreactive
  - Majority of renal cell carcinomas are also positive
  - It is also expressed in Reed–Sternberg (RS) cells of Hodgkin's disease

- BG-8
  - Recognizes Lewis blood group antigen
  - Expressed in up to 89% of adenocarcinomas of various origins with strong diffuse cytoplasmic staining
  - Positive reaction seen in 3–7% of epithelioid mesothelioma; however, the reaction is usually focal or scant
  - Renal cell carcinomas are usually negative
- Ber-EP4
  - Stain 86–96% of a variety of adenocarcinomas
  - Staining is usually strong and diffuse
  - Almost all lung and ovarian ADC are reactive
  - 35–50% of renal cell carcinomas are reactive
  - It may show positive focal reaction in up to 20% of mesotheliomas
  - Some propose that only lateral membranous staining should be regarded as truly positive and that focal staining is of limited value
- Carcinoemberyonic antigen (CEA)
  - Expressed in up to 80% of lung ADC
  - Can also be expressed in gastrointestinal ADC particularly colon
  - Expressed in a minority of ovarian carcinomas (mucinous type)
  - Not expressed in renal cell carcinoma
  - It is considered to be one of the best negative mesothelioma markers to distinguish between epithelioid mesothelioma and lung ADC
- B72.3
  - Reacts with a tumor-associated protein TAG-72
  - Expressed in up to 80% of ADC from a variety of organs
  - Expressed in up to 81% of lung ADC, up to 87% of ovarian ADC, and less than 3% of epithelioid mesotheliomas
  - Not expressed by renal cell carcinoma
- CA19-9
  - Related to Lewis blood antigen
  - Has low sensitivity
  - Commonly expressed in tumors of gastrointestinal origin, pancreas, ovary, and lung
  - Although not expressed in mesothelioma, it is not useful to separate it from lung ADC as it is only expressed in 39–53% of those adenocarcinomas

OTHER IMMUNOSTAINS

- E-cadherin and N-cadherin
  - Originally thought to be useful in the differentiation between adenocarcinoma and mesothelioma (E-cadherin in adenocarcinoma and N-cadherin in mesothelioma)
  - Now believed to have no utility in the differential
- Desmin and EMA
  - These two are usually used to separate MM from reactive mesothelium
  - Benign mesothelium preferentially expresses desmin and loses such expression with the malignant transformation
  - The majority of mesotheliomas, up to 80%, are believed to express EMA
  - There is some controversy regarding the utility of these stains
  - Occasionally EMA is expressed focally in few cells in reactive mesothelium
  - Few background reactive mesothelium may express desmin in cases of mesotheliomas
- E-cadherin and calretinin
  - They can be used to differentiate between MMs and reactive mesothelial cells

➢ Malignant mesothelioma cells positively stain with E-cadherin while reactive mesothelial cells will be negative

➢ Calretinin is used as a complement to differentiate mesothelial from non mesothelial cells

▣ Renal cell carcinoma marker (RCC Ma)

➢ Reported to stain up to 80% of renal cell carcinoma

➢ Also may stain in few metastatic breast ADC

➢ 8% of mesotheliomas were reported to show focal staining in few cells

▣ CD10

➢ Stains the majority of renal cell carcinoma

➢ Up to 48% of mesotheliomas may also have positive staining

Modern Techniques for Diagnosis

▣ Most MM cases have shown multiple chromosomal abnormalities

▣ Chromosomal losses are more common than gains (the opposite occur in lung cancer)

▣ Most frequent losses are at 1p, 3p, 6q, 9p, 13q, 14q, 15q, and 22q

▣ Most commonly gained regions are 5p, 7p, 7q, 8q, and 17q

▣ Deletion in 9p21 is considered the most common cytogenetic abnormality in MM, the locus of CDKN2A, a tumor suppressor gene (TSG)

▣ The deletion of CDKN2A is a negative prognostic factor in MM and can be used as a target in gene therapy, as well as marker of malignancy in body cavities effusions

▣ Platelet-derived growth factor (PDGF) is found to be an early response to asbestos, and high levels of PDGF are associated with increase tumor incidence and decrease latency period

▣ As in neurofibromatosis type 2 (NF2), loss of chromosome 22 is a recurrent cytogenetic abnormality in MM; therefore, NF2 patients' risk to develop MM is increased with exposure to asbestos

Differential Diagnosis

▣ Reactive mesothelium

➢ One cell population with monotonous appearance

➢ Atypia is not very pronounced

➢ Cellular clusters may be present but not as tight as spheres

➢ Little variation in size or shape of cells

▣ Adenocarcinoma

➢ Pleomorphic population of cells with obvious atypia

➢ Little variation in size of cells

➢ Two-cell population (background reactive mesothelium) may be detected

➢ Lack of two-tone cytoplasm

➢ Cytoplasmic glycogen rarely seen (lung adenocarcinoma)

➢ True gland formation may be seen in some clusters

▣ Poorly differentiated squamous cell carcinoma (please refer to SCC below)

➢ Third type cell with cyanophilic cytoplasm appearing singly or in large tight clusters (immature dysplastic cell shed in SCC particularly the poorly differentiated type. It was called third type cell simply as it was described after the "tadpole" and the "fiber/spindle" characteristic of invasive SCC)

➢ Cells show characteristic endoectoplasmic demarcation

PEARLS

✶ History of asbestos exposure, unexplained bloody effusion, and suggestive x-ray findings are highly suspicious for MM

✶ Not all malignant mesothelioma fluids are cellular

★ Although highly associated with asbestos exposure, one-third of the cases are not, and in many the history is not given to us
★ Mesothelioma effusions are large, unilateral, and recur fast and frequently
★ Although low cellularity on a repeated tap favors mesothelial hyperplasia, it can also occur in short interval taps and does not exclude mesothelioma

METASTATIC CARCINOMA

▥ Adenocarcinoma is the most common malignant type associated with body cavities effusions
▥ Metastatic lung carcinoma is the most common tumor associated with pleural effusions in male patients, while mammary carcinoma is the most common tumor present in female pleural effusions
▥ The most common tumor associated with peritoneal effusions in male patients is gastric carcinoma, while in peritoneal effusions of females; ovarian carcinoma is the most common
▥ The most common malignancies in pericardial effusions of adults are lung and breast

BREAST CARCINOMA

Clinical Features
▥ The most common metastatic tumor in pleural effusions in women
▥ It can be associated with peritoneal and pericardial effusions
▥ Most effusions present with a known clinical history of breast carcinoma
▥ Ductal carcinoma is the most common histologic type

Cytologic Features
▥ Highly cellular smears
▥ Many cells arranged in large three-dimensional clusters (cannon balls)
▥ Acinar or glandular groups (hollow spheres)

3-22. Metastatic breast carcinoma *(left)*. Pleural fluid from a patient with invasive ductal carcinoma of the breast. The fluid consists predominantly of cellular spheres very similar to those seen in mesothelioma. Notice, however, the irregular size and shape of these fragments compared to the regular spheres or morules seen in mesothelioma. (Papanicolaou stain)

3-23. Metastatic breast carcinoma *(right)*. Metastatic ductal breast carcinoma showing large fragments with geographic appearance and apparent cribriform pattern. (Papanicolaou stain)

3-24. Metastatic breast carcinoma *(left)*. Metastatic ductal breast carcinoma presenting mainly as highly atypical single cells with large nuclei and prominent nucleoli. (Papanicolaou stain)

3-25. Metastatic breast carcinoma *(right)*. Metastatic lobular breast carcinoma presenting as clusters, single cells, and cells arranged in a row. The cells have high nuclear to cytoplasmic ratio with eccentric nuclei and irregular nuclear membranes. (Papanicolaou stain)

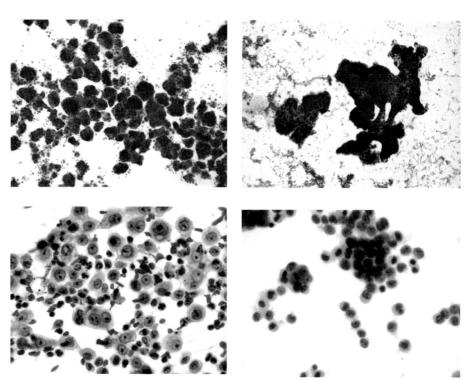

Small and large single cell pattern (occasionally mimic reactive mesothelial cells)

Linear arrangement of cells (very common in lobular carcinoma; however, it can also be seen in ductal type carcinoma)

Signet ring–like cells with eccentrically placed nuclei and mucin vacuoles (commonly seen in lobular carcinoma)

The cells are usually monotonous large (more common in ductal carcinoma) or small (lobular and ductal carcinomas)

The cytoplasm may be lacy or contains mucin vacuoles

High nuclear to cytoplasmic ratio

Nuclei with coarse chromatin and prominent nucleoli

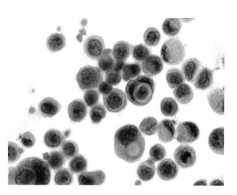

3-26. Metastatic breast carcinoma. Metastatic lobular breast carcinoma presenting as single cells with eccentric nuclei frequently indented by intracytoplasmic mucin droplets. Notice also the cell-within-cell appearance, a feature frequently seen in both ductal and lobular carcinoma. (Papanicolaou stain)

Special Stains and Immunohistochemistry
Positive markers in breast adenocarcinoma

CK7 (also, usually positive in lung, ovarian, pancreatic, urothelial, endometrial, and papillary renal cell carcinoma)

Estrogen receptor (ER) (nuclear stain. Also, positive in ovarian and endometrial carcinoma. Negative in endocervical carcinoma and clear cell carcinoma of the ovary)

Progesterone receptor (PR) (nuclear stain. Positive in endometrial and ovarian carcinomas. Negative in endocervical carcinoma)

Mammaglobin (cytoplasmic stain. Positive in 55% of effusion cytology specimens and in <87% of surgical resection specimens. Not expressed in effusion cytology specimens associated with metastatic carcinoma of the ovary, lung, uterus, gastrointestinal (GI), or genitourinary (GU)

CRxA-01 (membranous stain. Expressed in 69% of breast carcinoma, 48% of ovarian serous papillary carcinoma, and 28% of endometrial carcinoma of surgical resection specimens. In effusion cytology specimens, it has been expressed in 60% of breast carcinoma, 67% of ovarian carcinoma, and 50% of endometrial carcinoma

Mammaglobin and CRxA-01 together have higher sensitivity and specificity for the detection of breast carcinoma in effusion specimens (stain 80% of metastatic breast carcinoma)

Gross cystic disease fluid protein 15 (GCDFP-15) (cytoplasmic stain. Has very low sensitivity, but high specificity)

Negative markers in breast carcinoma
CK20 (negative in lung adenocarcinoma and ovarian carcinoma)

WT-1 (positive in ovarian carcinoma, and mesothelioma)

TTF-1 (positive in lung adenocarcinoma and thyroid carcinoma)

Modern Techniques for Diagnosis
Noncontributory

Differential Diagnosis
- Lung adenocarcinoma
  - ➤ Clinical history of lung cancer
  - ➤ Pleomorphic cells with high N:C ratio
  - ➤ No single cells filing
  - ➤ Rarely seen signet ring–like cells
  - ➤ Positive for TTF-1 and negative for mammaglobin
- Ovarian adenocarcinoma
  - ➤ Clinical history of ovarian cancer
  - ➤ Most commonly associated with ascites
  - ➤ Many psammoma bodies
  - ➤ Positive for WT-1, ER, and PR receptors and negative for mammaglobin

- Small cell carcinoma
  - Positive clinical history
  - Small cells with scant cytoplasm
  - Cell-in-cell engulfment
  - Short chain of single cells
  - Hyperchromatic nuclei
  - Absence of nucleoli
  - Positive for TTF-1, chromogranin, synaptophysin, and CD56, and negative for mammaglobin

PEARLS

★ Most of the cases are female patients with clinical history of treated mammary carcinoma
★ Long chains of monomorphic single cells are highly suggestive of breast carcinoma
★ Positivity for mammaglobin and CRxA-01 is very sensitive and specific for breast carcinoma, particularly with the absence of WT-1 and TTF-1 expressions

LUNG CARCINOMA

Clinical Features
- Most common cause of pleural effusions in men
- Most of the lung carcinoma patients (50%) develop pleural effusion later in their courses
- Small percentage (15%) of patients develops pleural effusion at the time of the lung cancer diagnosis
- Cytologic presentation depends on the histologic type of the tumor
- Adenocarcinoma (ADC) is the most common lung cancer type associated with effusion
- Squamous cell carcinoma (SCC) is less frequently associated with pleural effusion
- Small cell carcinoma (SmCC) is aggressive with widespread metastases at an early stage and infrequent pleural effusion

ADENOCARCINOMA (ADC)

Cytologic Features
- Cohesive three-dimensional clusters of cells
- Large single cells
- Acinar or glandular formation
- Bland-looking monomorphic cells mimicking mesothelial cells can be seen in well differentiated carcinoma
- Prominent nucleoli with surrounding chromatin clearing
- Psammoma bodies can be seen (rarely)

Special Stains and Immunohistochemistry
Positive markers in lung ADC
- CK7 (also, usually positive in breast, ovarian, pancreatic, urothelial, endometrial, and papillary renal cell carcinoma)
- TTF-1 (nuclear stain. Highly sensitive and specific marker for lung ADC)
- Napsin A (It is an aspartic proteinase, involved in the maturation of the surfactant protein B (SP-B), and is expressed in the cytoplasm of cells of lung and kidney. Very sensitive and specific for lung ADC with granular cytoplasmic reactivity
- CEA
- Ber-EP4
- MOC-31 (positive in almost all lung and ovarian carcinomas)

Negative markers in lung ADC
- CK20 (negative in breast and ovarian carcinoma)
- K903 (positive in SCC and MM)
- CK5/6 (positive in MM and SCC). Also recently reported to be occasionally positive in serous ovarian and endocervical adenocarcinomas
- WT-1 (usually negative in lung ADC. Positive in ovarian carcinoma, and mesothelioma)
- Mammaglobin (positive in breast carcinoma)

Modern Techniques for Diagnosis
- Noncontributory

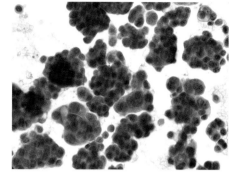

3-27. Metastatic lung adenocarcinoma. Metastatic lung adenocarcinoma presenting predominantly as cohesive clusters. (Papanicolaou stain)

Differential Diagnosis
- SCC (please see SCC below)
- MM
  - ➤ Clinical history of asbestos exposure
  - ➤ All cells look alike, that is, no evidence of two-cell population
  - ➤ Nuclei are usually bland or slightly atypical (nuclear irregularity, coarse chromatin, and hyperchromasia)
  - ➤ Large multinucleated cells with abundant cytoplasm: some of these cells approach the size of small morules
  - ➤ Positive for calretinin, CK5/6, WT-1, and negative for CEA, Ber-EP4, MOC-31, and TTF-1
- Ovarian ADC
  - ➤ Clinical history of ovarian cancer
  - ➤ Most commonly associated with ascites
  - ➤ Many psammoma bodies
  - ➤ Positive for WT-1, ER, and PR and negative for TTF-1 and napsin A
- Breast carcinoma
  - ➤ Positive clinical history
  - ➤ Linear arrangement of cells
  - ➤ Signet ring–like cells with eccentrically placed nuclei and mucin vacuoles
  - ➤ The cells are usually monotonous
  - ➤ Positive for mammaglobin, ER, PR, and CRxA-01 and negative for TTF-1 and napsin A

PEARLS

- ★ Most common malignant lung cancer associated with pleural effusion
- ★ Positivity for TTF-1 and napsin A is very sensitive and specific for lung ADC, particularly with the absence of WT-1, calretinin, and mammaglobin expression

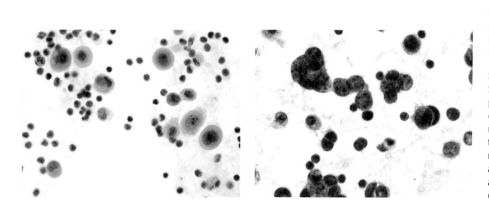

3-28. Metastatic lung adenocarcinoma *(left)*. Metastatic lung adenocarcinoma presenting mainly as single atypical cells in a background of mixed inflammatory cells. (Papanicolaou stain)

3-29. Small cell carcinoma *(right)*. Small cell carcinoma in a pleural fluid presenting as short cords and tight clusters. The cells have a very high nuclear to cytoplasmic ratio and tightly mold around each other. The nuclei are hyperchromatic with salt-and-pepper chromatin distribution and occasional chromocenters. (Papanicolaou stain)

SQUAMOUS CELL CARCINOMA (SCC)

Cytologic Features

▨ Well-differentiated SCC present with fragments and single cells with keratinizing cytoplasm (orangeophilic) and abnormal hyperchromatic nuclei

▨ Poorly differentiated SCC present mostly as third type cells with cyanophilic cytoplasm appearing singly or in large tight clusters and are difficult to distinguish from adenocarcinoma and mesothelioma (immature dysplastic cell shed in SCC particularly the poorly differentiated type. It was called third type cell simply as it was described after the "tadpole" and the "fiber/spindle" characteristic of invasive SCC)

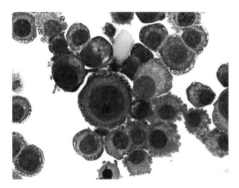

3-30. Poorly differentiated squamous cell carcinoma. Poorly differentiated squamous cell carcinoma in pleural fluid. The cells exhibit two tone cytoplasm very similar to that of mesothelioma. However, notice the well-defined cell borders and the high nuclear atypia in this case. Occasionally two adjacent cells with cell junctions oppose each other resembling window formation however there is no identified space between the cells. (modified Giemsa stain)

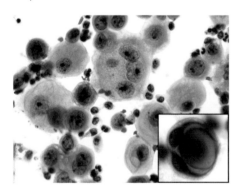

3-31. Squamous cell carcinoma. Squamous cell carcinoma presenting as large cells with two tone abundant cytoplasm. Notice the refractile ring in the middle corresponding the Herxheimer's spirals. The nuclei are highly atypical with very prominent nucleoli. Occasionally small clusters with cells wrapping around each other in an attempt to form pearls can be seen (inset). (Papanicolaou stain)

Cytologic Features of Poorly Differentiated SCC

▨ Cells with cyanophilic cytoplasm appearing singly or in large tight clusters

▨ Cells show characteristic endoectoplasmic demarcation

▨ Very dense and distinct cell border

▨ Significant nuclear atypia including hyperchromasia, irregular chromatin, and prominent nucleoli

▨ Dense periphery or hyaline in appearance (contrary to the fuzzy border of mesothelium) indicate attempt to keratinize

▨ Refractile rings indicative of abnormal keratinization (layers of hyaline as if successive zones of keratinization process is occurring)

▨ Endoectoplasmic demarcation (ectoplasm is dense while endoplasm is more textured) this is the result of keratinization from the periphery inwards

▨ Endoectoplasmic border can be ruffled or thrown into linear folds, and, if viewed in stretched cells, appear as "keratinizing fibrils" also known as "Herxheimer's spirals"

▨ Small clusters of cells arranged in whorls as they wrap around each other recapitulating a keratin pearl

▨ Positive for CK5/6, K903, and P16

Special Stains and Immunohistochemistry
Positive markers in lung SCC

▨ CK5/6 (also, usually positive in MM, and urothelial carcinoma)

▨ K903 (also, positive in MM)

▨ P16 (nuclear stain)

Negative markers in lung SCC

▨ TTF-1 (usually negative)

▨ MOC-31

▨ Calretinin and WT-1

▨ Ber-EP4 (may show focal membranous staining in some cases)

Modern Techniques for Diagnosis

▨ Noncontributory

Differential Diagnosis

▨ MM

➤ Clinical history of asbestos exposure

➤ Nuclei are usually bland or slightly atypical (nuclear irregularity, coarse chromatin, and hyperchromasia). This is the most significant difference

➤ Large multinucleated cells with abundant cytoplasm, some of these cells approach the size of small morules

> ➤ Single cells have a fuzzy cell border (microvilli)
> ➤ Positive for calretinin
- ADC
  > ➤ Pleomorphic population of cells with obvious atypia
  > ➤ Two cell population (background reactive mesothelium) may be detected
  > ➤ Lack of two-tone cytoplasm
  > ➤ True gland formation may be seen in some clusters
  > ➤ Negative for CK5/6, p16, and K903

PEARLS

★ Cells with cyanophilic cytoplasm appearing singly or in large tight clusters
★ Small clusters of cells arranged in whorls as they wrap around each other recapitulating a keratin pearl
★ Very dense and distinct cell border
★ Suspect SCC when both epithelial and mesothelial markers are negative in the work up of an effusion
★ Positive for CK5/6, K903, and P16 and negative for adenocarcinoma or mesothelial markers including WT-1 and calretinin
★ Ber-EP4 and MOC-31 and cellular adhesion markers and may positively react in 10-30% of SCC

SMALL CELL CARCINOMA (SMCC)

Cytologic Features
- Cytology is characteristic
- Cells tend to degenerate rapidly
- Tumor cells are about two times the size of resting lymphocytes, with scant cytoplasm and hyperchromatic nuclei
- Absence of nucleoli
- Small clusters of cells (may form larger clusters with an onion ring–like arrangement of nuclei)
- Short chains of single cells (characteristic)
- Cell-in-cell engulfment

Special Stains and Immunohistochemistry
Positive markers in lung SmCC
- TTF-1 (also, positive in lung ADC)
- Chromogranin A (granular cytoplasmic stain)
- Synaptophysin (granular cytoplasmic stain)
- CD56 (cytoplasmic stain)

Negative Markers In Lung SmCC
- CK20 (negative in breast adenocarcinoma)
- CD45 (positive in lymphoid neoplasm)
- Mammaglobin (positive in breast carcinoma)

Modern Techniques for Diagnosis
- Noncontributory

Differential Diagnosis
- Lymphoma
  > ➤ Cells are smaller in size

➤ Absence of cellular clusters or single filing
➤ Absence of nuclear hyperchromasia
➤ Lymphoglandular bodies (cytoplasmic fragments of lymphocytes) may be present
➤ Positive for CD45 and negative for TTF-1

■ Breast carcinoma
➤ Positive clinical history
➤ Linear arrangement of cells (long chains)
➤ Signet ring–like cells with eccentrically placed nuclei and mucin vacuoles
➤ Prominent nucleoli
➤ Positive for mammaglobin, ER, PR, and CRxA-01, and negative for TTF-1 and CD56

PEARLS

★ Short chains of cells with scant cytoplasm, hyperchromatic nuclei, and absent nucleoli are very characteristic for SmCC
★ Tight small clusters with onion skin appearance
★ Positive for CD56, TTF-1, synaptophysin, and chromogranin

OVARIAN CARCINOMA

Clinical Features
■ The most common malignant tumor associated with ascites
■ Most patients present in late stage
■ Epithelial ovarian tumors are the most common histologic type
■ Serous tumors are the most common epithelial neoplasm of the ovary and are divided into benign, borderline, and malignant categories
■ Borderline serous papillary (BSP) tumors account for 10–15% of all serous neoplasms and are associated with peritoneal implants in one-third of the cases
■ By definition, BSP tumors lack stromal invasion
■ Cytologic differentiation between primary peritoneal serous tumors and ovarian serous tumors is impossible, and the distinction is based on clinical history
■ BSP tumors have a better prognosis than serous papillary adenocarcinoma (SPADC)
■ By definition, SPADC is invasive tumor, and more commonly associated with peritoneal implants
■ Epithelial ovarian cancer metastasizes typically by intraperitoneal exfoliation and retroperitoneal lymphatic spread

OVARIAN SPADC

Cytologic Features
■ Highly cellular smears
■ Cells arranged in cohesive clusters (loose, noncohesive clusters seen in poorly differentiated [PD] SPADC)
■ Flat, branching or nonbranching papillary structures with common cell borders, frequently palisading at the periphery (in PDSPADC occasionally, not well-formed papillary structures seen with cells losing palisading at the periphery)
■ Large single cell pattern (more frequently seen in PDSPADC)
■ Marked variation in nuclear size
■ Vacuolated cytoplasm may be seen
■ High N:C ratio

- Nuclei with coarse chromatin, and prominent nucleoli
- Frequent mitoses
- Many psammoma bodies (less frequently seen in PDSPADC)

Special Stains and Immunohistochemistry
Positive markers in ovarian SPADC

- CK7
- Estrogen receptor (ER)
- Progesterone receptor (PR)
- WT-1
- Ber-EP4
- CA125 (membranous stain. Also, positive in 60% of lung ADC and 50% of breast ADC)

Negative markers in ovarian SPADC

- CK20
- Calretinin
- CK5/6
- TTF-1
- Mammaglobin
- CEA

Modern Techniques for Diagnosis
- Noncontributory

Differential Diagnosis
- Malignant mesothelioma
  - ➤ Can be differentiated based on cytology in most cases
  - ➤ Positive for calretinin and CK5/6 and negative for ER, PR, CEA, and Ber-EP4
  - ➤ Psammoma bodies are far less frequent
- Lung adenocarcinoma
  - ➤ Clinical history lung cancer
  - ➤ Most commonly associated with pleural effusion
  - ➤ Psammoma bodies rarely seen
  - ➤ Positive for TTF-1 and usually negative for WT-1
- Breast adenocarcinoma
  - ➤ Clinical history of breast cancer
  - ➤ Most commonly associated with pleural effusion
  - ➤ Chains of monomorphic single cells
  - ➤ Psammoma bodies may rarely be seen
  - ➤ Positive for mammaglobin and negative for WT-1

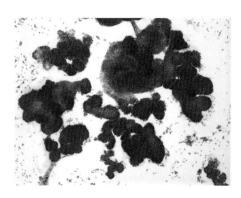

3-32. Well differentiated papillary serous carcinoma. Well-differentiated papillary serous carcinoma of the ovary presenting as complex papillary fragments. (Papanicolaou stain)

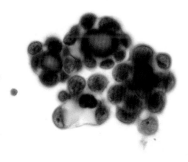

3-33. Papillary serous carcinoma. Papillary serous carcinoma of the ovary presenting as simple papillae with central psammoma bodies and obvious cellular atypia. (Papanicolaou stain)

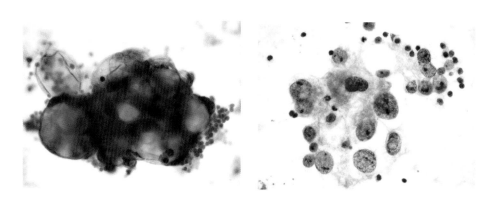

3-34. Mucinous carcinoma (left). Mucinous carcinoma of the ovary presenting as a tight cluster of highly vacuolated cells with eccentric nuclei. The nuclear membranes are irregularly indented by the distended cytoplasm, the chromatin is coarse, and the nucleoli are prominent. (Papanicolaou stain)

3-35. Clear cell carcinoma (right). Clear cell carcinoma of the ovary presenting as loose clusters of highly atypical cells. The nuclei are markedly enlarged with coarse chromatin and macronucleoli and occasional intranuclear inclusions. The cytoplasm is moderate to abundant and very fragile resulting in scattered bare nuclei. (Papanicolaou stain)

★ Most of the cases are postmenopausal female patients with clinical history of ovarian mass
★ Most common cause of ascites in women
★ Papillary structures with psammoma bodies
★ WT-1 is very helpful in differentiating ovarian SPADC from other lung and breast ADCs
★ ER, PR, and Ber-EP4 expressions with negative calretinin stain, support the diagnosis of ovarian SPADC and rule out papillary mesothelioma

OVARIAN BSP TUMOR

Cytologic Features
▪ Cellular smears
▪ Cells arranged in cohesive clusters
▪ Flat, large papillary structures with common cell borders, frequently palisading at the periphery
▪ Mild nuclear atypia
▪ Frequent psammoma bodies

Special Stains and Immunohistochemistry
Positive markers in ovarian BSP
▪ CK7
▪ Estrogen receptor (ER)
▪ Progesterone receptor (PR)
▪ WT-1
▪ Ber-EP4
▪ CA125 (membranous stain. Also positive in 60% of lung ADC and 50% of breast ADC)

Negative markers in ovarian BSP
▪ CK20
▪ Calretinin
▪ CK5/6
▪ TTF-1
▪ Mammaglobin
▪ CEA

Modern Techniques for Diagnosis
▪ Noncontributory

Differential Diagnosis
▪ Ovarian well-differentiated SPADC
  ➤ Differentiation is based on histology (presence of stromal invasion)
▪ Malignant mesothelioma
  ➤ Very hard to differentiate based on cytology only
  ➤ Mesotheliomas are positive for calretinin, CK5/6, and negative for ER, PR, CEA, and Ber-EP4

★ Most commonly associated with ascites
★ Papillary structures with psammoma bodies

⋆ ER, PR, and Ber-EP4 expressions with negative calretinin stain, support the diagnosis of ovarian BSP neoplasm and rule out papillary mesothelioma

OVARIAN MUCINOUS ADENOCARCINOMA (MADC)

Cytologic Features
▦ Cells occur in cohesive clusters
▦ Papillary structures may be seen (not as well formed as in SPADC)
▦ Vacuolated cytoplasm
▦ Mucin (intracellular and extracellular)
▦ High N:C ratio
▦ Nuclei (round to oval) with prominent nucleoli
▦ Psammoma bodies are absent

Special Stains and Immunohistochemistry
Positive markers in ovarian MADC
▦ CK7 and CK20 (positive in pancreatic and urothelial carcinomas)
▦ Muc2 (cytoplasmic stain. Positive in 70% of cases of ovarian MADC, and also, positive in colon cancers (>90%) and pancreatic cancers)
▦ Muc5AC (cytoplasmic stain. Expressed in almost all ovarian MADC, also positive in extramammary Paget disease, gastric carcinoma (90%), and pancreatic ADC)
▦ CEA
▦ Dpc4 (cytoplasmic stain. Positive in >90% of ovarian MADC and 90% of colonic ADC. It is only positive in 50% of pancreatic ADC)

Negative markers in ovarian MADC
▦ ER and PR (almost all MADC)
▦ Calretinin
▦ WT-1
▦ TTF-1
▦ CDX2 (usually negative, positive in 40%)

Modern Techniques for Diagnosis
▦ Noncontributory

Differential Diagnosis
▪ Gastrointestinal ADC
  ➤ Differentiation is based on history
  ➤ Present mostly as single cells or small clusters
  ➤ Colonic ADCs are negative for CK7 and villin, and negative for MUC5AC
  ➤ Pancreatic ADCs are usually negative for Dpc4
  ➤ CK20 and CDX2 may be helpful in distinguishing gastric ADC (usually CK20 negative and CDX2 positive) from Ovarian ADC
▪ Lung ADC
  ➤ Clinical history lung cancer
  ➤ Most commonly associated with pleural effusion
  ➤ Positive for TTF-1

PEARLS

⋆ Main differential is gastrointestinal ADC
⋆ Absence of psammoma bodies

UTERINE CARCINOMA

Clinical Features
- Uncommonly associated with effusion
- Endometrioid adenocarcinoma is the most common histologic type
- Mixed müllerian tumor (carcinosarcoma) is an aggressive uncommon histologic type, but usually associated with peritoneal effusion

ENDOMETROID ADENOCARCINOMA

Cytologic Features
- Cells occur in crowded cohesive groups with nuclear molding
- Ovoid nuclei with scant cytoplasm, coarse chromatin, and prominent nucleoli
- Cytoplasm may be vacuolated (secretory type)
- Positive fluids are usually not as cellular as those of PSADC

Special Stains and Immunohistochemistry
Positive markers in endometrial ADC (endometrioid type)
- CK7
- ER and PR
- CA125

Negative markers in endometrial ADC
- Calretinin
- WT-1
- TTF-1
- CK20

Modern Techniques for Diagnosis
- Noncontributory

Differential Diagnosis
- Lung ADC
  - ➤ Clinical history lung cancer
  - ➤ Most commonly associated with pleural effusion
  - ➤ Positive for TTF-1 and negative for ER and PR

PEARLS

★ Clusters of closely packed cells with nuclear molding

3-36. Endometrioid adenocarcinoma *(left)*. Endometrioid adenocarcinoma in a peritoneal washing presenting as clusters of malignant cells with no specific features. (Papanicolaou stain) Inset showing a higher magnification of one of the clusters

3-37. Borderline serous tumor *(right)*. Borderline serous tumor of the serosal surface with extensive psammoma body formation. The nuclei are mildly atypical with prominent nucleoli. (Papanicolaou stain)

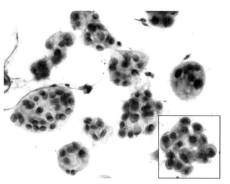
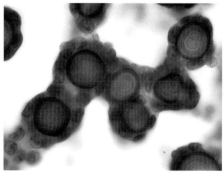

MALIGNANT MIXED MÜLLERIAN TUMOR (MMMT) (CARCINOSARCOMA)

Cytologic Features
▓ Epithelial cells are the most commonly seen
▓ Cells occur in discohesive clusters or as single bizarre cells
▓ Large pleomorphic nuclei with coarse chromatin and prominent nucleoli
▓ Scant cytoplasm with indistinct boarders
▓ Spindle cells with ill-defined cytoplasm and prominent nucleoli representing the sarcoma part

Special Stains and Immunohistochemistry
Positive markers in uterine MMMT
▓ Keratin (positive in the epithelial elements and focally in the mesenchymal elements)
▓ P53 (both elements have concordance positive or negative stains)
▓ The homologous stromal component reacts positively with vimentin. In heterologous stroma, depending on the type of mesenchymal differentiation it may express a differentiation antigen such as desmin or smooth muscle actin, etc.

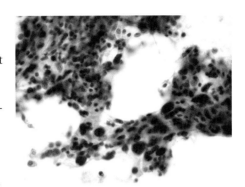

3-38. Malignant mixed müllerian tumor. Malignant mixed müllerian tumor unusually presenting as spindle highly atypical cells corresponding to the sarcomatous component. (Papanicolaou stain)

Negative markers in ovarian MMMT
▓ Calretinin
▓ WT-1
▓ TTF-1

Modern Techniques for Diagnosis
▓ Noncontributory

Differential Diagnosis
▓ Poorly differentiated ADCs
➤ Differentiation is based on history

PEARLS
★ MMMTs have poor prognosis and worse than poorly differentiated carcinoma of the endometrium
★ The overall prognosis is not related to the mesenchymal part

CERVICAL CARCINOMA
▓ Rarely associated with effusion
▓ Usually spread to the retroperitoneal space and later to the peritoneal cavity
▓ SCC is the most common histologic type and shares the cytologic and immunohistochemical features of other metastatic SCC of other organs
▓ The ADC type has no specific cytology

GASTROINTESTINAL (GI) TUMORS

Clinical Features
▓ Ranks as number 1 cause of malignant ascites in men and as a number 2 in women
▓ Commonly associated with malignant pleural effusions (usually second to lung cancers)

- Gastric cancers are the most common GI cancer associated with effusions
- Pancreatic ADCs are the second most common GI cancers associated with ascites
- The presence of positive fluid cytology is associated with poor outcome in patients with gastric carcinoma or pancreatic carcinoma. However, in cases of colonic carcinoma the positive cytology does not change prognosis
- Gastric and colonic ADCs are commonly associated with mucin production
- The cytologic features varies according to the histologic types (well differentiated, poorly differentiated, signet ring cell)
- Esophageal, hepatic, and small intestinal carcinomas are rarely associated with malignant effusions
- *Pseudomyxoma peritonei* (adenomucinosis and mucinous carcinomatosis) are most commonly associated with rupture appendiceal mucinous tumor
- Ruptured ovarian mucinous tumor is the second common cause of *Pseudomyxoma peritonei*

ESOPHAGEAL CARCINOMA

Clinical Features
- Rarely associated with effusion
- Esophageal ADC are usually associated with history of Barrett's mucosa

Cytologic Features
- SCC is the most common histologic type and shares the cytologic and immunohistochemical features of other metastatic SCC of other organs
- The ADC type is indistinguishable cytologically from gastric ADC

GASTRIC ADENOCARCINOMA

Clinical Features
- Gastric carcinoma is primarily in older patients and rarely seen below age 40
- History of atrophic gastritis or metaplasia
- Strong association between gastric ADC and *H. pylori* infection

Cytologic Features
- Large single cells (predominant feature)
- Cells of well differentiated (WD) ADC occur in small cohesive clusters (loose groups in PDADC)
- Round to ovoid nuclei with fine chromatin, moderate amount of cytoplasm, and small nucleoli are seen in WDADCs
- Large nuclei with high N:C ratio, coarse chromatin, and prominent nucleoli are in the PDADC type
- Vacuolated cytoplasm
- Signet-ring cells with eccentric crescent-like nuclei and vacuolated or granular cytoplasm
- Mucin (intracellular and extracellular)

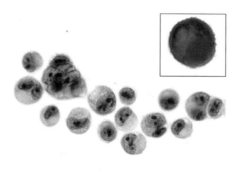

3-39. Metastatic gastric-esophageal adenocarcinoma. Ascitic fluid with metastatic gastro-esophageal adenocarcinoma. The signet ring cells have a very high nuclear to cytoplasmic ratio, eccentric nuclei, and prominent nucleoli. (Papanicolaou stain) Inset shows a high-power view of a positive mucicarmine stain

Special Stains and Immunohistochemistry
- The cytoplasmic vacuoles are mucicarmine and periodic acid–Shiff (PAS) stains positive

Positive markers in gastric ADC
- CK7 (71%)
- Muc2

▓ Muc5AC
▓ CEA

Negative markers in gastric ADC
▓ CK20 (positive in 40%)
▓ ER and PR
▓ Calretinin
▓ WT-1
▓ TTF-1

Modern Techniques for Diagnosis
▓ Noncontributory

Differential Diagnosis
■ Ovarian MADC
➤ Differentiation is based on history
➤ CK20 and CDX2 may be helpful in distinguishing gastric ADC (usually CK20 negative and CDX2 positive) from ovarian ADC
■ Colonic ADC
➤ Differentiation is based on history
➤ Colonic ADCs are positive for CK20 and villin
■ Lung ADC
➤ Clinical history lung cancer
➤ Most commonly associated with pleural effusion
➤ Positive for TTF-1

PEARLS

✶ The most common GI cancer associated with malignant ascites
✶ Large single cell pattern is a predominant feature
✶ Signet ring cells
✶ No specific immunostain
✶ PDADC presenting as signet rings may be difficult to detect and a mucin stain is recommended in cases with ADC history

COLONIC ADENOCARCINOMA

Clinical Features
▓ Known history of colonic mass in most cases
▓ Account for <5% of all primary tumors associated with malignant effusions
▓ Positive effusion cytology in patients who underwent curative resection has no prognostic value over the staging system

Cytologic Features
▓ Predominantly, cells are arranged in cohesive clusters (loose groups in PDADC)
▓ Ovoid to elongated nuclei (frequently, have parallel arrangement) with fine chromatin, moderate amount of cytoplasm and small nucleoli are seen in WDADCs
▓ Large nuclei with high N:C ratio, coarse chromatin, and prominent nucleoli are in the PDADC type
▓ Vacuolated cytoplasm
▓ Signet ring cells with eccentric crescent–like nuclei, and vacuolated or granular cytoplasm

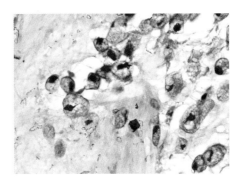

3-40. Metastatic signet ring adeno-carcinoma. Cell block of peritoneal fluid with metastatic signet ring adenocarcinoma of the colon with abundant mucin secretion in the background. (Hematoxylin and eosin stain)

- Mucin (intracellular and extracellular)
- Muciphage can be seen in mucinous cell–type carcinoma

Special Stains and Immunohistochemistry
- The cytoplasmic vacuoles are mucicarmine and periodic acid–Shiff stains positive with and without digestion

Positive markers in colonic ADC
- CK20
- Muc2
- CDX2
- Villin (98% express cytoplasmic stain)
- CEA
- Dpc4

Negative markers in colonic ADC
- CK7
- ER and PR
- Calretinin
- Muc5AC
- TTF-1

Modern Techniques for Diagnosis
- Noncontributory

Differential Diagnosis
- Ovarian MADC
  - ➤ Differentiation is based on history
  - ➤ Colonic ADC are positive for villin and negative for CK7 and Muc5AC
- Gastric ADC
  - ➤ Differentiation is based on history
  - ➤ Colonic ADCs are usually positive for CK20, villin
- Lung ADC
  - ➤ Clinical history lung cancer
  - ➤ Most commonly associated with pleural effusion
  - ➤ Positive for TTF-1

PEARLS

★ Tumor cells are positive for CK20, villin, CDX2, and negative for CK7
★ PDADC presenting as signet rings may be difficult to detect, and a mucin stain is recommended in effusions with history of colon ADC

PANCREATIC ADENOCARCINOMA

Clinical Features
- More common in men over age fifty years
- History of mass in the head of pancreas in about two-thirds of patients
- Patients may present with obstructive jaundice

Cytologic Features
- Cells are arranged in cohesive three-dimensional clusters or papillary structures
- Single cell pattern seen predominantly in PDADC

▒ Ovoid nuclei with wrinkled nuclear membrane, coarse chromatin, high N:C ratio, and prominent nucleoli
▒ Vacuolated cytoplasm may be seen
▒ Mucin may be seen
▒ Bizarre giant cells in undifferentiated carcinoma with osteoclast-like giant cell type

Special Stains and Immunohistochemistry
Positive markers in pancreatic ADC

▒ CK7 and CK20
▒ Muc2 and Muc5AC
▒ CEA
▒ CK19

Negative markers in pancreatic ADC

▒ ER and PR
▒ Calretinin
▒ Dpc4
▒ TTF-1

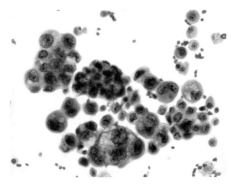

3-41. Pancreatic adenocarcinoma. Pancreatic adenocarcinoma presenting as loosely cohesive clusters and single cells with high degree of nuclear atypia. (Papanicolaou stain)

Modern Techniques for Diagnosis
▒ Noncontributory

Differential Diagnosis
▒ Ovarian MADC
  ➤ Differentiation is based on history
  ➤ Presents mostly as papillary groups
  ➤ Ovarian ADC are usually positive for Dpc4
▒ Gastric ADC
  ➤ Differentiation is based on history
  ➤ Frequently present with signet ring appearance
▒ Colonic ADC
  ➤ Differentiation is based on history
  ➤ Colonic ADC are positive for villin, Dpc4, and CDX2
▒ Lung ADC
  ➤ Clinical history lung cancer
  ➤ More commonly associated with pleural effusion
  ➤ Positive for TTF-1

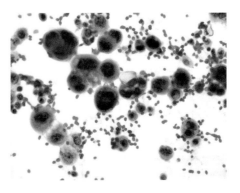

3-42. Pancreatic adenocarcinoma. Pancreatic adenocarcinoma presenting as single highly pleomorphic cells. (Papanicolaou stain)

PEARLS

★ Account for 5–10% of all primary tumors associated with malignant effusions
★ No specific immunostain

PSEUDOMYXOMA PERITONEI

Cytologic Features
▒ Peritoneal adenomucinosis (PAM)
  ➤ Viscous, thick mucin (purple or magenta color in modified Giemsa stain and orange reddish in PAP stain)
  ➤ Bland columnar cells in small clusters or palisading arrangement
  ➤ Tansparent cytoplasm with small nuclei
  ➤ Ascitic fluids with PAM are very difficult to aspitrate and usually a small volume is retreived

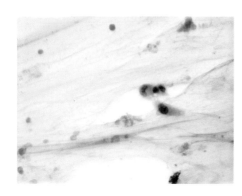

3-43. Pseudomyxoma peritonei.
Pseudomyxoma peritonei
(peritoneal adenomucinosis).
Background of thick mucin with few
floating columnar cells. (Papanicolaou stain)

➤ Peritoneal washings with PAM could present with impressive amount of extracellular thick mucin and variable number of cells
◼ Peritoneal mucinous (PM) ADC
➤ Viscous, thick mucin (purple or magenta color in DQ stain and orange reddish in PAP stain)
➤ Malignant cells in clusters
➤ Large nuclei with high N:C ratio, coarse chromatin, and prominent nucleoli

Special Stains and Immunohistochemistry
◼ Positive markers include Muc2, Muc5AC, and Muc5B

Modern Techniques for Diagnosis
◼ Noncontributory

Differential Diagnosis
◼ Ovarian MADC, gastric, colonic, and pancreatic ADCs
➤ Differentiation is based on history
➤ All are differential diagnosis of peritoneal mucinous ADC
➤ Absence of thick mucin

PEARLS

★ Appendiceal tumors are the most common cause
★ Poor prognosis due to infection, intestinal obstruction, peritonitis
★ PAM has better prognosis than PMADC
★ In the absence of epithelial cells, the presence of thick mucin alone is highly suggestive of pseudomyxoma peritonei

HEPATOCELLULAR CARCINOMA (HCC)

◼ Very rarely associated with effusion
◼ Cytologic features depend on the differentiation of the tumor
◼ In well-differentiated tumors the cells arrange in clusters with granular cytoplasm (occasionally bile stained), round nuclei, fine chromatin, and small nucleoli
◼ In poorly differentiated tumors, single large cell pattern predominate with large usually eccentric nuclei, moderate amount of granular cytoplasm, coarse chromatin, and prominent nucleoli
◼ Positive immunostains include: Hep Par-1 (cytoplasmic granular expression in 80–90%), polyclonal CEA (pCEA) in canalicular pattern (higher percentage in well-differentiated tumors), AFP (15–70%)
◼ Negative immunostains include: monoclonal CEA, EMA, CK7, CK20, K903, MOC31, Ber-EP4, and CD15

BILE DUCT CARCINOMA (CHOLANGIOCARCINOMA)

◼ Rarely associated with effusion
◼ Cytologic features are similar to the pancreatic ADC
◼ No specific immunostain
◼ CK19 positive

HEMATOPOIETIC NEOPLASMS (LYMPHOMA AND LEUKEMIA)

Clinical Features
- Lymphoma and leukemia patients commonly present with malignant effusions
- Most of the effusions occur later in the course of the disease
- Rarely effusions present as the initial manifestation of malignant hematologic disease
- More common in males
- Most commonly involve the pleura (account for 10% of pleural effusions)
- Lymphoma is ranked number 3 as a cause of pleural effusion
- Non-Hodgkin's lymphoma (NHL) is the most common lymphoma associated with pleural effusion
- On the other hand, malignant ascites is rarely associated with lymphoma

Cytologic Features
- NHL
    - Highly cellular smear
    - Monomorphic lymphoid population
    - Large, intermediate, or small single cell pattern
    - Nuclei are round or irregular with coarse chromatin and scant to moderate cytoplasm
    - Cleaved nuclei with scant cytoplasm seen in follicular lymphoma
    - Prominent nucleoli and numerous mitotic figures are seen in Burkitt and Burkitt-like lymphoma
    - Karyorrhexis is common
    - Absence of mesothelium
- Hodgkin's lymphoma (HL)
    - Presence of mononucleated or binucleated large cells with fine chromatin and prominent nucleoli (RS cells)
    - Background with mix inflammatory cells
- Leukemia
    - Immature large myeloid or monocytoid cells with large, round or irregular nuclei, scant cytoplasm, and multiple nucleoli
    - In chronic myelogenous leukemia (CML), it is difficult to differentiate from an inflammatory process
    - Chronic lymphocytic leukemia (CLL) show a high number of monomorphic small lymphocytes

Differential Diagnosis
- TB
    - Differentiation is based on history
    - Usually as a differential of SLL/CLL
    - Lymphocytes are of T-cell type (CD4+ and CD8+)
- Small cell carcinoma
    - Larger cells in clusters
    - Nuclei with salt and pepper chromatin
    - Absence of nucleoli
    - Positive for CD56, TTF-1, and chromogranin
- Small round blue cell tumors in children
    - Immunostain will vary depending on the type of tumor

PEARLS

- Most patients have history of treated lymphoma/leukemia

⋆ Combined flow cytometry and cytology have 100% sensitivity and 94% specificity in diagnosing lymphoma/leukemia

⋆ Presence of effusion is associated with poor prognosis

PRIMARY EFFUSION LYMPHOMA (PEL)

Clinical Features

▣ Rare high-grade large cell lymphoma almost always associated with effusion in the absence of tumor mass or lymphadenopathy

▣ Commonly associated with HHV-8 in advanced HIV or immunocompromised patients

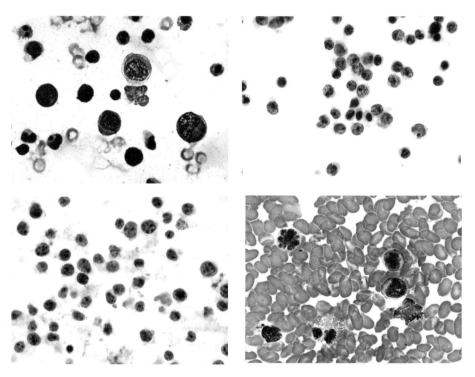

3-44. Primary effusion lymphoma *(left)*. Anaplastic large T-cell primary effusion lymphoma. Large hematopoietic cells with enlarged irregular nuclei, prominent nucleoli and scant to moderate cytoplasm. (modified Giemsa stain)

3-45. Follicular center cell lymphoma *(right)*. Follicular center cell lymphoma. A mixture of centrocytes (cleaved cells) and centroblasts (large noncleaved cells). (Papanicolaou stain)

3-46. Burkitt's lymphoma *(left)*. Burkitt's lymphoma. Medium-sized lymphocytes with rounded non cleaved nuclei and multiple nucleoli. (Papanicolaou stain)

3-47. Mycosis fungoides *(right)*. Peritoneal fluid from a patient with disseminated mycosis fungoides. The T cells are small in size (compare with background RBCs and eosinophil) with cribriform nuclei. (modified Giemsa stain)

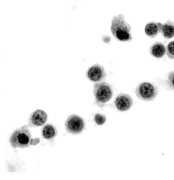

3-48. Multiple myeloma. Multiple myeloma in a pleural fluid. The cells have eccentric nuclei, clumped chromatin and moderate amount of cytoplasm. The cart wheel chromatin and perinuclear huff are not always visible and high-grade cells may easily mimic epithelial cells. (Papanicolaou stain)

▦ Usually associated with EBV

▦ Some isolated case reports about involvement of lymph node, tongue base, and intestine

▦ Also, it has been reported in HIV and HHV-8 negative patients with or without hepatitis C virus (HCV)

Cytologic Features

▦ Single pleomorphic large cells with moderate basophilic cytoplasm (DQ stain) range from immunoblastic to anaplastic in appearance

▦ Round or irregular nuclei with prominent nucleoli

Special Stains and Immunohistochemistry

▦ Tumor cells are positive for CD45, CD30, CD138, EMA, HHV8, EBV (usually), HLA-DR, and variable CD3

▦ Tumor cells are negative for CD19 and CD20

▦ Clonal rearrangements and somatic mutations of Ig heavy chain

▪ Main differential is anaplastic large cell lymphoma (ALCL) (HIV, EBV and HHV-8 negative, Alk-1+, CD3+, CD4+)

★ PEL is associated with poor prognosis (patients die within months)

MISCELLANEOUS MALIGNANT TUMORS

SARCOMA

Clinical Features
▪ Uncommonly associated with effusion (approximately 2–5% of malignant effusions)
▪ Most cases have effusions later in the course of the disease
▪ High-grade sarcomas are more frequently associated with effusion
▪ In general, the sarcoma cells lose their histologic features in tissue and tend to round up in fluids

Cytologic Features
▪ Cytologic patterns include
  ➤ Spindle (oval) cells, for example, leiomyosarcoma, malignant peripheral nerve sheath tumor (MPNST), synovial sarcoma
  ➤ Pleomorphic (bizarre) cells, for example, rhabdomyosarcoma, malignant fibrous histocytoma, high grade myxofibrosarcoma
  ➤ Small round cells, for example, Ewing's sarcoma, embryonal rhabdomyosarcoma

▪ Common cytologic features include
  ➤ Scant cellularity
  ➤ Single cell pattern
  ➤ Ill-defined cell borders
  ➤ Nuclei are oval or pleomorphic with coarse chromatin and prominent nucleoli
  ➤ Multinucleated cells can be seen
  ➤ Proteinaceous background

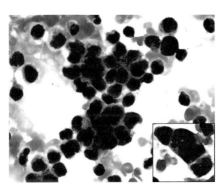

3-49. Metastatic embryonal rahbdomysarcoma in a peritoneal fluid. Cells appear in clusters or short cords (inset). The cells are small, round with eccentrically located nucleus and a rim of cytoplasm. (modified Giemsa stain)

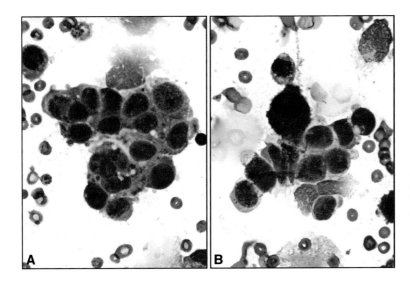

3-50A-B. Ewing sarcoma. Metastatic Ewing sarcoma in a pleural fluid. The cells appear in loose aggregates. The nuclei are rounded and mostly centrally located. The cytoplasm is moderate and occasionally bubbly due to its rich glycogen content. (modified Giemsa stain)

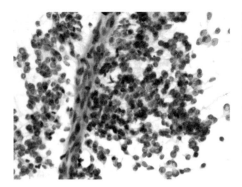

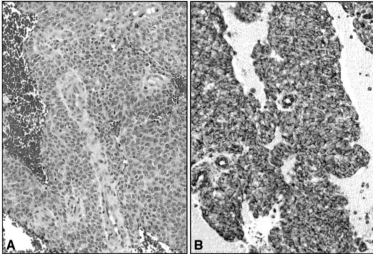

3-51. Fibrosarcoma *(above).*
Metastatic fibrosarcoma in peritoneal
fluid. Highly cellular fragments of
rounded to oval cells around a blood
vessel. (Papanicolaou stain)

3-52A. Fibrosarcoma *(middle).*
Cell block of the fibrosarcoma
showing similar features. (Hematoxylin and eosin stain)

3-52B. Fibrosarcoma *(right).*
Strongly positive vimentin stain. All
other stains were negative.

Special Stains and Immunohistochemistry

▪ Clinical history and immunohistochemical stains are very helpful in subclassifying sarcomas in most of the cases
▪ Leiomyosarcomas are positive for smooth muscle actin (SMA), and desmin
▪ Synovial sarcomas are positive for AE1/AE3, EMA, CD99, bcl-2
▪ MPNSTs and liposarcomas are positive for S-100
▪ Pleomorphic rhabdomyosarcomas are positive for myoglobin, desmin, skeletal muscle myogenin, and muscle-specific actin
▪ Angiosarcomas are positive for CD34

Modern Techniques for Diagnosis

▪ Synovial sarcomas have specific translocation, t(X;18)(p11.2; q11) – SYT-SSX1 genes, which can be detected in 90% of cases by PCR

GERM CELL TUMORS

▪ Rarely associated with effusion
▪ Effusion occurs late in the course of the disease

SEMINOMA (DYSGERMINOMA)

▪ Rarely associated with effusion
▪ Effusion occurs late in the course of the disease
▪ Uniform single cells with large round to oval nuclei, fine chromatin, and prominent nucleoli
▪ Multinucleated giant cells and lymphocytes
▪ Seminomas are positive for placental alkaline phosphatase (PLAP) and vimentin

EMBRYONAL CARCINOMA

▪ Pleomorphic large cells arrange in tight or loose clusters
▪ Round to oval nuclei with fine chromatin and prominent nucleoli
▪ Vacuolated cytoplasm may be seen with eccentric nuclei
▪ Tumor cells are positive for keratin and CD30

YOLK SAC TUMOR (ENDODERMAL SINUS TUMOR)

- Cells arrange in tight or loose clusters
- May form papillary structures
- Round to oval nuclei with fine chromatin and prominent nucleoli
- Vacuolated cytoplasm
- Tumor cells are positive for keratin and α-fetoprotein AFP

MELANOMA

- Rarely present with effusion without a known history of melanoma
- Malignant cells resemble mesothelial cells (usually single round cells with prominent nucleoli)
- Cytoplasmic brown pigmentation may be seen
- Bizarre pleomorphic cells can be seen
- Tumor cells are positive for S-100, HMB-45, and melan A

RENAL CELL CARCINOMA (RCC)

- Rarely associated with effusion
- More commonly associated with pleural effusions
- Clear cell type is the most common type
- Sarcomatoid RCC rarely show cells in fluids
- Cytologic features include: large single cells with abundant clear or granular cytoplasm, oval nuclei, and prominent nucleoli
- Cells may form loose clusters
- Papillary structures may be seen in papillary RCC
- Tumor cells are positive for keratin, EMA, RCC, and CD10

UROTHELIAL CELL CARCINOMA (UCC)

Clinical Features
- Rarely associated with effusion
- Effusion is more likely associated with high-grade UCC and disseminated disease

Cytologic Features
- Cellular groups with moderate dense cytoplasm, irregular nuclei, coarse chromatin, and prominent nucleoli
- Less-differentiated UCC may present as single cells morphologically mimicking SCC or ADC

Special stains and Immunohistochemistry
- Tumor cells are positive for CK7, CK20, high-molecular-weight cytokeratin (HMWCK)/34betaE12, CK5/6, and CEA

WILMS TUMOR (NEPHROBLASTOMA)

- Most common malignant kidney tumor in children
- One of the common causes of malignant effusions in children
- Cytologic features include round blue cells in clusters, with scant cytoplasm, round to oval hyperchromatic nuclei, and absent nucleoli
- The differential diagnosis includes all small blue cells tumors such as neuroblastoma, Ewing's sarcoma, and rhabdomyosarcoma
- Positive for WT-1, keratin, and EMA

3-53. Liposarcoma *(left)*. Liposarcoma in a peritoneal fluid. Highly vaculolated atypical cells are singly scattered against a background of mixed inflammatory cells (Papanicolaou stain) Inset showing a high magnification of a lipoblast

3-54. Endodermal sinus tumor *(right)*. Peritoneal fluid with endodermal sinus tumor (EST). The small cells are arranged in loose, elongated groups. The cells are small with rounded eccentric nuclei and a moderate amount of highly vacuolated cytoplasm. (Papanicolaou stain)

3-55. Endodermal sinus tumor *(left)*. Correlating histologic appearance of EST showing the reticular architecture and highly vacuolated cells. (Hematoxylin and eosin)

3-56. Clear cell sarcoma *(right)*. Peritoneal fluid with metastatic clear cell sarcoma (melanoma of soft tissue). Singly scattered medium-sized cells with prominent nucleoli and granular cytoplasm. (Papanicolaou stain) Inset showing positive reaction to HMB-45

3-57. Melanoma *(left)*. Metastatic melanotic melanoma. Single atypical cells, many obscured by abundant dark brown to black melanin pigment. (Papanicolaou stain)

3-58. Urothelial cell carcinoma *(right)*. Urothelial cell carcinoma in acitic fluid. The singly scattered abnormal cells have moderate to abundant cytoplasm, pleomorphic nuclei and occasional cell-within-cell appearance mimicking adenocarcinoma. (Papanicolaou stain)

3-59. Urothelial cell carcinoma *(left)*. Urothelial cell carcinoma in acitic fluid. The single cells have abundant two-tone cytoplasm and occasional cells exhibit articulation with windows mimicking mesothelioma. The nuclei, however, are obviously atypical. (modified Giemsa stain)

3-60. Urothelial cell carcinoma *(right)*. Metastatic high-grade renal cell carcinoma with clear cell features. The cells are markedly enlarged with pleomorphic features and abundant clear cytoplasm. The fragile cytoplasm breaks during manual smearing resulting in bare nuclei. (Papanicolaou stain)

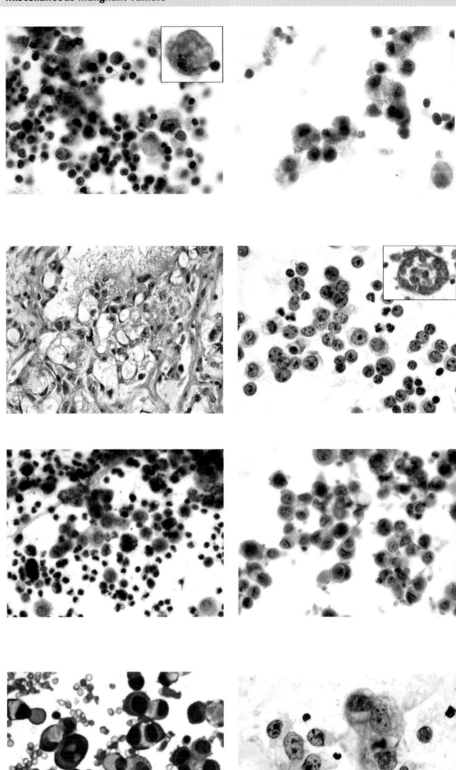

REFERENCES

TYPES OF EFFUSIONS

Carter D, True L, Otis CN. Serous membranes. In: Sternberg SS, editor. *Histology for Pathologists*, 2nd ed. Philadelphia: Lippincott-Raven, 1997, pp. 223–239.

Light RW, MacGregor MI, Lushsinger PC, Ball WC, Jr. Pleural effusions: the diagnostic separation of transudates and exudates. *Ann Intern Med* 1972; 77(4): 507–513.

Light RW. Management of pleural effusions. *J Formos Med Assoc* 2000; 99(7): 523–531.

Porcel JM, Alvarez M, Salud A, Vives M. Should a cytologic study be ordered in transudative pleural effusions? *Chest* 1999; 116:1836–7.

DETACHED CILIARY TUFTS (DCT)

Bedrossian CWM. Diagnostic problems in serous effusions. *Diagn Cytopathol.* 1998 Aug; 19(2):131–7.

Bedrossian CWM. *Malignant Effusions: A Multimodal Approach to Cytologic Diagnosis.* New York: Igaku-Shoin Medical Publishers Inc., 1994. pp. 26–51.

Bibbo M. *Comprehensive Cytopathology*, 2nd ed. Philadelphia: W. B. Saunders, 1997. pp. 551–621.

Domagala W, Koss LG. Surface configuration of mesothelial cells in effusions. A comparative light microscopic and scanning electron microscopic study. *Virchows Arch B Cell Pathol Incl Mol Pathol.* 1979 May 31; 30(2):231–43.

Koss L. Effusions in the absence of cancer. In: *Diagnostic Cytology and Its Histopathologic Bases*, 4th ed. Philadelphia: J.B. Lippincott, 1992, pp. 1082–1115.

McGowan L, Bunnang B. Morphology of mesothelial cells in peritoneal fluid from normal women. *Acta Cytol.* 1974 May–Jun; 18(3):205–9.

Radzum HJ, Dommes M, Henselmans M, Parwaresch MR. Resident human peritoneal macrophages: a monocytic cell line. *Acta Cytol.*1982; 26(3): 363–6.

Ryan GB, Groberty J, Majno G. Mesothelial injury and recovery. *Am J Pathol.* 1973 Apr; 71(1):93–112.

Vladutiu A, Brason FW, Alder RH. Differential diagnosis of pleural effusions. *Chest.* 1981; 79(3): 297–301.

Wojcik EM, Naylor B. Collagen balls in peritoneal washings: prevalence, morphology, origin and significance. *Acta Cytol.* 1992;36(4):446–70.

Zimmerman RL. Effusion cytology: Keeping researchers and journals in business for the past 20 years – and it is not over yet. *Curr Diagn Pathol.* 2005; 11: 194–202.

EOSINOPHILIC EFFUSIONS

Bertoli G, Anata CM, Agosti E. Mast cells in eosinophilic pleural effusions. *Acta Cytol.* 1981; 25(4):431–2.

Farah MG, Nassar VH, Shahid M. Marked eosinophilia and eosinophilic pleural effusion in Hodgkin's disease. Report of a case with review of the literature. *J Med Liban.* 1973; 26(5): 513–21.

Kalomenidis I, Mohamed KH, Lane KB, Peebles RS, Barnette R, Rodriguez RM, Light RW. Pleural fluid levels of vascular cell adhesion molecule-1 are elevated in eosinophilic pleural effusions. *Chest.* 2003; 124(1): 159–66.

Naylor B, Novak PM. Charcot-Leyden crystals in pleural fluids. *Acta Cytol.* 1985; 29(5): 781–4.

Veress JF, Koss LG, Schreiber K. Eosinophilic pleural effusions. *Acta Cytol.* 1979; 23(1): 40–44.

RHEUMATOID PLEURITIS

Bibbo M. Comprehensive Cytopathology, 2nd ed. Philadelphia: W.B. Saunders, 1997, p. 551–621.

Boddington MM, Sprigs AI, Morton JA, Mowat AG. Cytodiagnosis of rheumatoid pleural effusions. *J Clin Pathol.* 1971; 24(2): 95–106.

Fernandez-Muixi J, Vidal F, Razquin S, Torre L, Richart C. Pleural effusion as initial presentation of rheumatoid arthritis: cytological diagnosis. *Arch Bronconeumol.* 1996; 32(8): 427–9.

Montes S, Guarda LA. Cytology of pleural effusions in rheumatoid arthritis. *Diagn Cytopathol.* 1988; 4(1): 71–3.

Naylor B. The pathognomonic cytologic picture of rheumatoid pleuritis. *Acta Cytol.* 1990; 34(4): 465–73.

EFFUSIONS ASSOCIATED WITH SYSTEMIC LUPUS ERYTHEMATOSUS (SLE)

Chao T-Y, Huang SH, Chu CC. Lupus erythematosus cells in pleural effusions: diagnostic of systemic lupus erythematosus? *Acta Cytol.* 1997; 41(4): 1231–3.

Fazio J, Freidman HD, Swerdlow J, Michiel RR. Diagnosis of systemic lupus erythematosus in an elderly male by pericardial fluid cytology: a case report. *Diagn Cytopathol.* 1998; 18(5): 346–8.

Kaplan AI, Zakher F, Sabine S. Drug-induced lupus erythematosus with in vivo lupus erythematosus cells in pleural fluid. *Chest.* 1978; 73(6): 875–6.

Naylor B. Cytological aspects of pleural, peritoneal and pericardial fluids from patients with systemic lupus erythematosus. *Cytopathology.* 1992; 3(1):1–8.

Reda MG, Baigelman W. Pleural effusion in systemic lupus erythematosus. *Acta Cytol.* 1980; 24(6):553–7.

TUBERCULOUS EFFUSIONS

Ellison E, Lapuerta P, Martin SE. Cytologic features of mycobacterial pleuritis: logistic regression and statistical analysis of a blinded, case-controlled study. *Diagn Cytopathol.* 1998; 19(3):173–6.

Jones D, Lieb T, Narita M, Hollender ES, Pitchenik AE, Ashkin D. Mesothelial cells in tuberculous pleural effusion of HIV-infected patients. *Chest.* 2000; 117(1):289–91.

Kataria KP, Khurshid I. Adenosine deaminase in the diagnosis of tuberculous pleural effusion. *Chest,* 2001; 120(2):334–6.

Reechaipichitkul W, Lulitanond V, Sungkeeree S, Patjanasoontorn B. Rapid diagnosis of tuberculous pleural effusion using polymerase chain reaction. *Southeast Asian J Trop Med Public Health,* 2000; 31(3):509–14.

San Jose ME, Valdes L, Saavedra MJ, De Vega JM, Alvarez D, Vinuela J, Penela P, Valle JM, Seoane R. Lymphocyte populations in tuberculous pleural effusions. *Ann Clin Biochem.* 1999; 36(4):492–500.

Spieler P. The cytologic diagnosis of tuberculosis in pleural effusions. *Acta Cytol.* 1979; 23(5): 374–9.

Ungerer JP, Oosthuizen HM, Retief JH, Bissbort SH. Significance of adenosine, deaminase activity and its isoenzymes in tuberculous effusions. *Chest,* 1994; 106(1):33–37.

FUNGAL/PARASITIC INFECTIONS

Bedrossian CWM. *Malignant Effusions: A Multimodal Approach to Cytologic Diagnosis.* New York, NY: Igaku-Shoin Medical Publishers Inc., 1994. pp. 52–84.

Bibbo M. *Comprehensive Cytopathology,* 2nd ed. Philadelphia: W.B. Saunders, 1997, pp. 551–621.

Elwood LJ, Dobrzanski D, Feuerstein IM, Solomon D. Pneumocystis carinii in pleural fluid:the cytologic appearance. *Acta Cytol.* 1991; 35(6):761–4.

Goodman ZD, Gupta PK, Frost JK, Erozan YS. Cytodiagnosis of viral infections in body cavity fluids. *Acta Cytol.* 1979; 23(3):204–8.

INFARCTION

Anderson WJ, Skinner DB, Zuidema GD, Cameron JL. Chronic pancreatic pleural effusions. *Surg Gynecol Obstet.* 1973; 137(5): 827–30.

Bedrossian CWM. *Malignant Effusions: A Multimodal Approach to Cytologic Diagnosis.* New York: Igaku-Shoin Medical Publishers Inc., 1994, pp. 85–100.

Bibbo M. *Comprehensive Cytopathology,* 2nd ed. Philadelphia: W.B. Saunders; 1997, pp. 551–621.

Buja LM, Friedman CA, Roberts WC. Hemorrhagic pericarditis in uremia. Clinicopathologic studies in six patients. *Arch Pathol.* 1970; 90(4):325–330.

Craig R, Sparberg M, Ivanovich P, Rice L, Dordal E. Nephrogenic ascites. *Arch Intern Med.* 1974; 134(2):276–9.

Schindler SC, Schaefer JW, Hull D, Griffen WO, Jr. Chronic pancreatic ascites. *Gastroenterology.* 1970; 59(3):453–9.

Wilson JA, Suguitan EA, Cassidy WA, Parker RH, Chan CH. Characteristic of ascitic fluid in the alcoholic cirrhotic. *Dig Dis Sci.* 1979; 24(8): 645–8.

Xiol X, Castellote J, Baliellas C, Ariza J, Gimenez Roca A, Guardiola J, Casais L. Spontaneous bacterial empyema in cirrhotic patients: analysis of eleven cases. *Hepatology.* 1990; 11(3):365–70.

MALIGNANT MESOTHELIOMA (MM)

Attanoos RL, Griffin A, Gibbs AR. The use of immunohistochemistry in distinguishing reactive from neoplastic mesothelium. A novel use for desmin and comparative evaluation with epithelial membrane antigen, p53, platelet-derived growth factor-receptor, P-glycoprotein and Bcl-2. *Histopathology* 2003; 43(3):231–8.

Bedrossian CWM. *Malignant Effusions: A Multimodal Approach to Cytologic Diagnosis.* New York: Igaku-Shoin Medical Publishers Inc., 1994, pp. 101–119.

Bjorkqvist AM, Tammilehto L, Anttila S, Mattson K, Knuutila S. Recurrent DNA copy number changes in 1q, 4q, 6q, 9p, 13q, 14q and 22q detected by comparative genomic hybridization in malignant mesothelioma. *Br J Cancer* 1997; 75(4):523–7.

Carbone M, Kratzke RA, Testa JR. The pathogenesis of mesothelioma. *Semin Oncol.* 2002; 29(1):2–17.

Chu A, Litzky L, Pasha T, Acs G, and Zhang P. Utility of D2-40, a novel mesothelial marker, in the diagnosis of malignant mesothelioma. *Mod Pathol.* 2005; 18(1):105–110.

Cristaudo A, Foddis R, Vivaldi A, Buselli R, Gattini V, Guglielmi G, Cosentino F, Ottenga F, Ciancia E, Libener R, Filiberti R, Neri M, Betta P, Tognon M, Mutti L, Puntoni R. SV40 enhances the risk of malignant mesothelioma among people exposed to asbestos: a molecular epidemiologic case-control study. *Cancer Res.* 2005; 65(21):3049–52.

Flejter WL, Li FP, Antman KH, Testa JR. Recurring loss involving chromosomes 1, 3, and 22 in malignant mesothelioma: possible sites of tumor suppressor genes. *Genes Chromosomes Cancer* 1989; 1(2):148–54.

Gibas Z, Li FP, Antman KH, Bernal S, Stahel R, Sandberg AA. Chromosome changes in malignant mesothelioma. *Cancer Genet Cytogenet.* 1986;20(3-4):191–201.

Grundy GW, Miller RW. Malignant mesothelioma in childhood: report of 13 cases. *Cancer.* 1972; 30(5):1216–1218.

Hurlimann J. Desmin and neural marker expression in mesothelial cells and mesotheliomas. *Hum Pathol.* 1994; 25(8):753–7.

Illei PB, Ladanyi M, Rusch VW, Zakowski MF. The use of CDKN2A deletion as a diagnostic marker for malignant mesothelioma in body cavity effusions. *Cancer,* 2003; 99(1):51–6.

Kaneko C, Niimi H, Shinzato M, Shamoto M. Comparative studies of the same adenocarcinoma cells, macrophages, and mesothelial cells by light microscopy, scanning electron microscopy, and transmission electron microscopy. *Diagn Cytopathol.* 1994; 11(4):333–42.

Kimura N and Kimura I. Podoplanin as a marker for mesothelioma. *Pathol Int,* 2005; 55(2):83–86.

Kumar ND, Bhatia A, Misra K, Suri JC. Comparison of pleural fluid cytology and pleural biopsy in the evaluation of pleural effusion. *J Indian Med Assoc.* 1995; 93(8):307–309.

Ladanyi M. Implications of P16/CDKN2A deletion in pleural mesotheliomas. *Lung Cancer* 2005; 49(Suppl 1):S95–8.

Langerak AW, De Laat PA, Van Der Linden-Van Beurden CA, Delahaye M, Van Der Kwast TH, Hoogsteden HC, Benner R, Versnel MA. Expression of platelet-derived growth factor (PDGF) and PDGF receptors in human malignant mesothelioma in vitro and in vivo. *J Pathol.* 1996; 178(2):151–60.

Li Q, Bavikatty N, Michael CW. The role of immunohistochemistry in distinguishing squamous cell carcinoma from mesothelioma and adenocarcinoma in pleural effusion. *Semin Diagn Pathol.* 2006 Feb; 23(1):15–19.

Manfredi JJ, Dong J, Liu WJ, Resnick-Silverman L, Qiao R, Chahinian P, Saric M, Gibbs AR, Phillips JI, Murray J, Axten CW, Nolan RP, Aaronson SA: Evidence against a role for SV40 in human mesothelioma. *Cancer Res.* 2005; 65(7): 2602–9.

Ordoñez N. D2-40 and podoplanin are highly specific and sensitive immunohistochemical markers of epithelioid malignant mesothelioma. *Hum Pathol.* 2005; 36(4):372–80.

Ordoñez N. Immunohistochemical diagnosis of epithelioid mesothelioma: An update. *Arch Pathol Lab Med.* 2005; 129(11): 1407–14.

Ordoñez N. The diagnostic utility of immunohistochemistry in distinguishing between mesothelioma and renal cell carcinoma: A comparative study. *Hum Pathol.* 2004; 35(6): 697–710.

Ordoñez N. Value of E-cadherin and N-cadherin immunostaining in the diagnosis of mesothelioma. *Hum Pathol.* 2003; 34(8): 749–55.

Ordoñez N. Value of mesothelin immunostaining in the diagnosis of mesothelioma. *Mod Pathol.* 2003; 16(3):192–7.

Politi E, Kandaraki C, Apostolopoulou C, Kyritsi T, Koutselini H. Immunocytochemical panel for distinguishing between carcinoma and reactive mesothelial cells in body cavity fluids. *Diagn Cytopathol,* 2005 Mar; 32(3):151–5.

Prakash UB, Reiman HM. Comparison of needle biopsy with cytologic analysis for the evaluation of pleural effusion: analysis of 414 cases. *Mayo Clin Proc.* 1985; 60(3):158–164.

Prins JB, Williamson KA, Kamp MM, Van Hezik EJ, Van der Kwast TH, Hagemeijer A, Versnel MA. The gene for the cyclin-dependent- kinase-4 inhibitor, CDKN2A, is preferentially deleted in malignant mesothelioma. *Int J Cancer,* 1998; 75(4):649–53.

Puntoni R, Filiberti R, Cerrano PG, Neri M, Andreatta R, Bonassi S. Implementation of a molecular epidemiology approach to human pleural malignant mesothelioma. *Mutat Res.* 2003; 544(2–3):385–96.

Renshaw AA, Dean BR, Antman KH, Sugarbaker DJ, Cibas ES: The role of cytologic evaluation of pleural fluid in the diagnosis of malignant mesothelioma. *Chest,* 1997 Jan; 111(1):106–9.

Saad RS, Cho P, Liu Y, and Silverman JF. The value of epithelial membrane antigen expression in separating benign mesothelial proliferation from malignant mesothelioma: a comparative study. *Diagn Cytopathol.* 2005; 32(3):156–9.

Scherpereel A, Grigoriu B, Conti M, Gey T, Gregoire M, Copin MC, Devos P, Chahine B, Porte H, Lassalle P. Soluble mesothelin-related peptides in the diagnosis of malignant pleural mesothelioma. *Am J Respir Crit Care Med.* 2006; 173(10):1155–60.

Shivapurkar N, Virmani AK, Wistuba II, Milchgrub S, Mackay B, Minna JD, Gadzar AF. Deletions of chromosome 4 at multiple sites are frequent in malignant mesothelioma and small cell lung carcinoma. *Clin Cancer Res.* 1999; 5(1):17–23.

Sivertsen S, Berner A, Michael CW, Bedrossian C, Davidson B. Cadherin expression in ovarian carcinoma and malignant mesothelioma cell effusions. *Acta Cytol.* 2006 Nov–Dec; 50(6):603–7.

Taguchi T, Jhanwar SC, Siegfried JM, Keller SM, Testa JR. Recurrent deletions of specific chromosomal sites in 1p, 3p, 6q, and 9p in human malignant mesothelioma. *Cancer Res.* 1993; 53(18):4349–55.

Tao LC. Cytopathology of malignant effusions. In W.W. Johnston, editor. *ASCP Theory and Practice of Cytopathology 6,* American Society of Clinical Pathologists, 1996, pp. 203–29.

Wong L, Zhou J, Anderson D, Kratzke RA. Inactivation of p16INK4a expression in malignant mesothelioma by methylation. *Lung Cancer.* 2002; 38(2):131–6.

Yang CT, You L, Lin YC, Lin CL, McCormick F, Jablons DM. A comparison analysis of anti-tumor efficacy of adenoviral gene replacement therapy (p14ARF and p16INK4A) in human mesothelioma cells. *Anticancer Res.* 2003; 23(1A):331996, 8.

METASTATIC CARCINOMA

DeMay RM. *The Art and Science of Cytopathology.* Chicago, IL: ASCP Press, 1996, pp. 269–85.

Ehya H. Effusion cytology. *Clin Lab Med.* 1991; 11(2):443–67.

Galindo LM. Effusion cytopathology. In: Atkinson BF, Silverman JF, eds. *Atlas of Difficult Diagnoses in Cytopathology,* 1st ed. Philadelphia: WB Saunders, 1998, pp. 168–178.

Johnston WW. The malignant pleural effusion. A review of cytopathologic diagnoses of 584 specimens from 472 consecutive patients. *Cancer,* 1985; 56(4):905–9.

Naylor B. Pleural, peritoneal, and pericardial fluids. In: Bibbo M, ed. *Comprehensive Cytopathology,* 2nd ed. Philadelphia: WB Saunders, 1997, pp. 589–621.

Silverman JF. Effusion cytology of metastatic malignancy of unknown primary. *Pathol Case Rev.* 2001;6:154–160.

BREAST CARCINOMA

Bhargava R, Beriwal S, Dabbs DJ. Mammaglobin vs GCDFP-15: an immunohistologic validation survey for sensitivity and specificity. *Am J Clin Pathol.* 2007 Jan; 127(1):103–13.

Ciampa A, Fanger G, Khan A, Rock KL, Xu B. Mammaglobin and CRxA-01 in pleural effusion cytology: potential utility of distinguishing metastatic breast carcinomas from other cytokeratin 7-positive/cytokeratin 20-negative carcinomas. *Cancer (Cancer Cytopathol).* 2004; 102(6):368–72.

Lee BH, Hecht JL, Pinkus JL, Pinkus GS. WT1, estrogen receptor, and progesterone receptor as markers for breast or ovarian primary sites in metastatic adenocarcinoma to body fluids. *Am J Clin Pathol.* 2002 May; 117(5):745–50.

Staebler A, Sherman ME, Zaino RJ, Ronnett BM. Hormone receptor immunohistochemistry and human papillomavirus in situ hybridization are useful for distinguishing endocervical and endometrial adenocarcinomas. *Am J Surg Pathol.* 2002 Aug; 26(8):998–1006.

Tot T. Patterns of distribution of cytokeratins 20 and 7 in special types of invasive breast carcinoma: a study of 123 cases. *Ann Diagn Pathol.* 1999 Dec; 3(6):350–6.

Zhu W, Michael CW. WT1, monoclonal CEA, TTF1, and CA125 antibodies in the differential diagnosis of lung, breast, and ovarian adenocarcinomas in serous effusions. *Diagn Cytopathol.* 2007 Jun; 35(6):370–5.

ADENOCARCINOMA (ADC)

Chuman Y, Bergman A, Ueno T, Saito S, Sakaguchi K, Alaiya AA, Franzen B, Bergman T, Arnott D, Auer G, Appella E, Jornvall H, Linder S. Napsin A, a member of the aspartic protease family, is abundantly expressed in normal lung and kidney tissue and is expressed in lung adenocarcinomas. *FEBS Lett* 1999; 462(1–2):129–134.

Dejmek A, Naucler P, Smedjeback A, Kato H, Maeda M, Yashima K, Maeda J, Hirano T. Napsin A (TA02) is a useful alternative to thyroid transcription factor-1 (TTF-1) for the identification of pulmonary adenocarcinoma cells in pleural effusions. *Diagn Cytopathol.* 2007 Aug; 35(8):493–7.

Hirano T, Gong Y, Yoshida K, Kato Y, Yashima K, Maeda M, Nakagawa A, Fujioka K, Ohira T, Ikeda N, Ebihara Y, Auer G, Kato H. Usefulness of TA02 (napsin A) to distinguish primary lung adenocarcinoma from metastatic lung adenocarcinoma. *Lung Cancer,* 2003; 41(2):155–162.

Ng WK, Chow JC, Ng PK. Thyroid transcription factor-1 is highly sensitive and specific in differentiating metastatic pulmonary from extrapulmonary adenocarcinoma in effusion fluid cytology specimens. *Cancer.* 2002 Feb 25; 96(1):43–8.

Suzuki A, Shijubo N, Yamada G, Ichimiya S, Satoh M, Abe S, Sato N. Napsin A is useful to distinguish primary lung adenocarcinoma from adenocarcinomas of other organs. *Pathol Res Pract.* 2005; 201(8–9):579–586.

Ueno T, Linder S, Na CL, Rice WR, Johansson J, Weaver TE. Processing of pulmonary surfactant protein B by napsin and cathepsin H. *J Biol Chem.* 2004; 279(16):178–184.

SQUAMOUS CELL CARCINOMA (SCC)

Frost JK. The cell in health and disease: an evaluation of cellular morphologic expression of biologic behavior, In Wied GI, editor. *Monographs in Clinical Cytology*, 2nd ed. New York: Karger, 1986, pp. 165–186.

Li Q, Bavikatty N, Michael CW. The role of immunohistochemistry in distinguishing squamous cell carcinoma from mesothelioma and adenocarcinoma in pleural effusion. *Semin Diagn Pathol.* 2006 Feb; 23(1):15–19.

Ordóñez NG. The diagnostic utility of immunohistochemistry in distinguishing between epithelioid mesotheliomas and squamous carcinomas of the lung: a comparative study. *Mod Pathol.* 2006; 19(3): 417–28.

Smith-Purslow MJ, Kini SR and Naylor B. Cells of squamous cell carcinoma in pleural, peritoneal and pericardial fluids: Origin and morphology. *Acta Cytol.* 1989; 33(2): 245–53.

SMALL CELL CARCINOMA (SMCC)

Chhieng DC, Ko EC, Yee HT, Shultz JJ, Dorvault CC, Eltoum IAl. Malignant pleural effusions due to small-cell lung carcinoma: a cytologic and immunocytochemical study. *Diagn Cytopathol.* 2001; 25(6):356–60.

Kontogianni K, Nicholson AG, Butcher D, Sheppard MN. CD56: a useful tool for the diagnosis of small cell lung carcinomas on biopsies with extensive crush artifact. *J Clin Pathol.* 2005; 58(9):978–80.

Pereira TC, Saad RS, Liu Y, Silverman JF. The diagnosis of malignancy in effusion cytology: a pattern recognition approach. *Adv Anat Pathol.* 2006 Jul; 13(4):174–84.

Salhadin A, Nasiell M, Nasiell K, Silfversward C, Hjerpe A, Wadas AM, Enstad I. The unique cytologic picture of oat cell carcinoma in effusions. *Acta Cytol.* 1976; 20(4): 298–302.

Spieler P, Gloor F. Identification of types and primary sites of malignant tumors by examination of exfoliated tumor cells in serous fluids. Comparison with the diagnostic accuracy on small histologic biopsies. *Acta Cytol.* 1985; 29(5):753–767.

OVARIAN CARCINOMA

Creasman WT, Rutledge F. The prognostic value of peritoneal cytology in gynecologic malignant disease. *Am J Obstet Gynecol.* 1971; 110(6):773–781.

Keettel WC, Pixley EE, Buchsbaum HJ. Experience with peritoneal cytology in the management of gynecologic malignancies. *Am J Obstet Gynecol.* 1974; 120(2):174–82.

OVARIAN SPADC

Attanoos RL, Webb R, Dojcinov SD, Gibbs AR. Value of mesothelial and epithelial antibodies in distinguishing diffuse peritoneal mesothelioma in females from serous papillary carcinoma of the ovary and peritoneum. *Histopathology*, 2002 Mar; 40(3):237–44.

Barnetson RJ, Burnett RA, Downie I, Harper CM, Roberts F. Immunohistochemical analysis of peritoneal mesothelioma and primary and secondary serous carcinoma of the peritoneum: antibodies to estrogen and progesterone receptors are useful. *Am J Clin Pathol.* 2006 Jan; 125(1):67–76.

Covell JL, Carry JB, Feldman PS. Peritoneal washings in ovarian tumors. Potential sources of error in cytologic diagnosis. *Acta Cytol.* 1985; 29(3): 310–16.

Goldstein NS, Bassi D, Uzieblo A. WT1 is an integral component of an antibody panel to distinguish pancreaticobiliary and some ovarian epithelial neoplasms. *Am J Clin Pathol.* 2001 Aug; 116(2):246–52.

Ordóñez NG. Value of estrogen and progesterone receptor immunostaining in distinguishing between peritoneal mesotheliomas and serous carcinomas. *Hum Pathol.* 2005; 36(11):1163–7.

Zhu W, Michael CW. WT1, monoclonal CEA, TTF1, and CA125 antibodies in the differential diagnosis of lung, breast, and ovarian adenocarcinomas in serous effusions. *Diagn Cytopathol.* 2007 Jun; 35(6):370–5.

Ziselman EM, Harkavy SE, Hogan M, West W, Atkinson B. Peritoneal washing cytology. Uses and diagnostic criteria in gynecologic neoplasms. *Acta Cytol.* 1984; 28(2): 105–10.

OVARIAN BSP TUMOR

Gurley AM, Hidvegi DF, Cajulis RS, Bacus S. Morphologic and morphometric features of low grade serous tumours of the ovary. *Diagn Cytopathol.* 1994; 11(3):220–5.

Johnson TL, Kumur NB, Hopkins M, Hughes JD. Cytologic features of ovarian tumours of low malignant potential in peritoneal fluids. *Acta Cytol.* 1988; 32(4):513–8.

Pisharodi LR, Bedrossian CW. Cytopathology of serous neoplasia of the ovary and the peritoneum: differential diagnosis from mesothelial proliferations. *Diagn Cytopathol.* 1996; 15(4):292–5.

Stewart CJ, Kennedy JH. Peritoneal fluid cytology in serous borderline tumours of the ovary. *Cytopathology.* 1998; 9(1):38–45.

OVARIAN MUCINOUS ADENOCARCINOMA (MADC)

Albarracin CT, Jafri J, Montag AG, Hart J, Kuan SF. Differential expression of MUC2 and MUC5AC mucin genes in primary ovarian and metastatic colonic carcinoma. *Hum Pathol.* 2000 Jun; 31(6):672–7.

Groisman GM, Meir A, Sabo E. The value of Cdx2 immunostaining in differentiating primary ovarian carcinomas from colonic carcinomas metastatic to the ovaries. *Int J Gynecol Pathol.* 2004 Jan; 23(1):52–7.

Ji H, Isacson C, Seidman JD, Kurman RJ, Ronnett BM. Cytokeratins 7 and 20, Dpc4, and MUC5AC in the distinction of metastatic mucinous carcinomas in the ovary from primary ovarian mucinous tumors: Dpc4 assists in identifying metastatic pancreatic carcinomas. *Int J Gynecol Pathol.* 2002 Oct; 21(4):391–400.

Vang R, Gown AM, Barry TS, Wheeler DT, Ronnett BM. Immunohistochemistry for estrogen and progesterone receptors in the distinction of primary and metastatic mucinous tumors in the ovary: an analysis of 124 cases. *Mod Pathol.* 2006 Jan; 19(1):97–105.

Vang R, Gown AM, Wu LS, Barry TS, Wheeler DT, Yemelyanova A, Seidman JD, Ronnett BM. Immunohistochemical expression of CDX2 in primary ovarian mucinous tumors and metastatic mucinous carcinomas involving the ovary: comparison with CK20 and correlation with coordinate expression of CK7. *Mod Pathol.* 2006 Nov; 19(11):1421–8.

CERVICAL CARCINOMA

Covell JL, Carry JB, Feldman PS. Peritoneal washings in ovarian tumors. Potential sources of error in cytologic diagnosis. *Acta Cytol.* 1985; 29(3): 310–16.

Silverberg SG, Major FJ, Blessing JA, Fetter B, Askin FB, Liao SY, Miller A. Carcinosarcoma (malignant mixed mesodermal tumor) of the uterus. A Gynecologic Oncology Group pathologic study of 203 cases. *Int J Gynecol Pathol.* 1990; 9(1):1–19.

Ziselman EM, Harkavy SE, Hogan M, West W, Atkinson B. Peritoneal washing cytology. Uses and diagnostic criteria in gynecologic neoplasms. *Acta Cytol.* 1984; 28(2): 105–10.

GASTRIC ADENOCARCINOMA

Bedrossian CWM. *Malignant Effusions: A Multimodal Approach to Cytologic Diagnosis.* New York, NY: Igaku-Shoin Medical Publishers Inc., 1994, pp. 135–137.

Bonenkamp JJ, Songun I, Hermans J, van de Velde CJ. Prognostic value of positive cytology findings from abdominal washings in patients with gastric cancer. *Br J Surg,* 1996; 83(5):672–4.

Park SY, Kim HS, Hong EK, Kim WH. Expression of cytokeratins 7 and 20 in primary carcinomas of the stomach and colorectum and their value in the differential diagnosis of metastatic carcinomas to the ovary. *Hum Pathol.* 2002 Nov; 33(11):1078–85.

Tao LC. Cytopathology of malignant effusions. In W.W. Johnston, editor. *ASCP Theory and Practice of Cytopathology 6,* American Society of Clinical Pathologists, 1996, pp. 79–80.

COLONIC ADENOCARCINOMA

Bedrossian CWM. *Malignant Effusions: A Multimodal Approach to Cytologic Diagnosis.* New York: Igaku-Shoin Medical Publishers Inc., 1994, p. 137.

Gozalan U, Yasti AC, Yuksek YN, Reis E, Kama NA. Peritoneal cytology in colorectal cancer: incidence and prognostic value. *Am J Surg.* 2007 Jun; 193(6):672–5.

Park SY, Kim HS, Hong EK, Kim WH. Expression of cytokeratins 7 and 20 in primary carcinomas of the stomach and colorectum and their value in the differential diagnosis of metastatic carcinomas to the ovary. *Hum Pathol.* 2002 Nov; 33(11):1078–85.

Saad RS, Essig DL, Silverman JF, Liu Y. Diagnostic utility of CDX-2 expression in separating metastatic gastrointestinal adenocarcinoma from other metastatic adenocarcinoma in fine-needle aspiration cytology using cell blocks. *Cancer.* 2004; 102(3):168–173.

Suh N, Yang XJ, Tretiakova MS, Humphrey PA, Wang HL. Value of CDX2, villin, and alpha-methylacyl coenzyme A racemase immunostains in the distinction between primary adenocarcinoma of the bladder and secondary colorectal adenocarcinoma. *Mod Pathol.* 2005; 18(9):1217–22.

Tao LC. Cytopathology of malignant effusions. In W.W. Johnston, editor. *ASCP Theory and Practice of Cytopathology 6*, American Society of Clinical Pathologists, 1996, pp. 80–81.

Werling RW, Yaziji H, Bacchi CE, Gown AM. CDX2, a highly sensitive and specific marker of adenocarcinomas of intestinal origin: an immunohistochemical survey of 476 primary and metastatic carcinomas. *Am J Surg Pathol.* 2003 Mar; 27(3):303–10.

PANCREATIC ADENOCARCINOMA

Bedrossian CWM. *Malignant Effusions: A Multimodal Approach to Cytologic Diagnosis.* New York: Igaku-Shoin Medical Publishers Inc., 1994, pp. 137–9.

Lei S, Kini J, Kim K, Howard JM. Pancreatic cancer. Cytologic study of peritoneal washings. *Arch Surg.* 1994; 129(6):639–42.

Tao LC. Cytopathology of Malignant Effusions. In W.W. Johnston, editor. *ASCP Theory and Practice of Cytopathology 6*, American Society of Clinical Pathologists, 1996, p. 82.

Warsaw AL. Implications of peritoneal cytology for staging of early pancreatic cancer. *Am J Surg.* 1991; 169(1):26–34.

PSEUDOMYXOMA PERITONEI

Gu M, Zena RE. Columnar cells in smears from pseudomyxoma peritonei. Diagn Cytopathol. 1997 Feb;16(2):182–3.

Lee KR, Scully RE. Mucinous tumors of the ovary: a clinicopathologic study of 196 borderline tumors (of intestinal type) and carcinomas, including an evaluation of 11 cases with 'Pseudomyxoma peritonei'. *Am J Surg Pathol.* 2000 Nov; 24(11):1447–64.

Mall AS, Chirwa N, Govender D, Lotz Z, Tyler M, Rodrigues J, Kahn D, Goldberg P. MUC2, MUC5AC and MUC5B in the mucus of a patient with pseudomyxoma peritonei: biochemical and immunohistochemical study. *Pathol Int.* 2007 Aug; 57(8):537–47.

Ronnett BM, Zahn CM, Kurman RJ, Kass ME, Sugarbaker PH, Shmookler BM. Disseminated peritoneal adenomucinosis and peritoneal mucinous carcinomatosis. A clinicopathologic analysis of 109 cases with emphasis on distinguishing pathologic features, site of origin, prognosis, and relationship to "Pseudomyxoma peritonei". *Am J Surg Pathol.* 1995 Dec; 19(12):1390–408.

Yan H, Pestieau SR, Shmookler BM, Sugarbaker PH. Histopathologic analysis in 46 patients with *Pseudomyxoma peritonei* syndrome: failure versus success with a second-look operation. *Mod Pathol.* 2001 Mar;14(3):164–71.

HEPATOCELLULAR CARCINOMA (HCC)

Fan Z, van de Rijn M, Montgomery K, Rouse RV. Hep par 1 antibody stain for the differential diagnosis of hepatocellular carcinoma: 676 tumors tested using tissue microarrays and conventional tissue sections. *Mod Pathol.* 2003; 16(2):137–44.

Kakar S, Muir T, Murphy LM, Lloyd RV, Burgart LJ. Immunoreactivity of Hep Par 1 in hepatic and extrahepatic tumors and its correlation with albumin in situ hybridization in hepatocellular carcinoma. *Am J Clin Pathol.* 2003; 119(3):361–6.

Leong AS, Sormunen RT, Tsui WM, Liew CT. Hep Par 1 and selected antibodies in the immunohistological distinction of hepatocellular carcinoma from cholangiocarcinoma, combined tumours and metastatic carcinoma. *Histopathology.* 1998; 33(4):318–24.

Saad RS, Luckasevic TM, Noga CM, Johnson DR, Silverman JF, Liu YL. Diagnostic value of HepPar1, pCEA, CD10, and CD34 expression in separating hepatocellular carcinoma from metastatic carcinoma in fine-needle aspiration cytology. *Diagn Cytopathol.* 2004; 30(1):1–6.

PRIMARY EFFUSION LYMPHOMA (PEL)

Ansari MQ, Dawson DB, Nador R, Rutherford C, Schneider NR, Latimer MJ, Picker L, Knowles DM, McKenna RW. Primary body cavity-based AIDS-related lymphomas. *Am J Clin Pathol.* 1996; 105(2):221–9.

Ariad S, Benharroch D, Lupu L, Davidovici B, Dupin N, Boshoff C. Early peripheral lymph node involvement of human herpesvirus 8 associated body cavity-based lymphoma in a human immunodeficiency virus-negative patient. *Arch Pathol Lab Med.* 2000; 124(5): 753–5.

Banks PM, Warnke RA. Primary effusion lymphoma. In: Jaffe ES, Harris NL, Stein H, Vardiman JW, editors. *World Health Organization Classification of Tumours. Pathology and Genetics of Tumours of Haematopoietic and Lymphoid Tissues.* Lyon: IARC Press, 2001.

Das DK, Gupta SK, Ayyagari S, Bambery PK, Datta BN, Datta V. Pleural effusions in non-Hodgkin's lymphoma. A cytomorphologic, cytochemical and immunologic study. *Acta Cytol.* 1987; 31(2):119–24.

Dunphy CH. Combined cytomorphologic and immunophenotypic approach to evaluation of effusions for lymphomatous involvement. *Diagn Cytopathol.* 1996; 15(5):427–30.

Hallman JR, Geisinger KR. Cytology of fluids from pleural, peritoneal and pericardial cavities in children. A comprehensive study. *Acta Cytol.* 1994; 38(2):209–17.

Huang Q, Chang KL, Gaal K, Arber DA. Primary effusion lymphoma with subsequent development of a small bowel mass in an HIV-seropositive patient: a case report and literature review. *Am J Surg Pathol.* 2002; 26(10):1363–7.

Johnston WW. The malignant pleural effusion. A review of cytopathologic diagnoses of 584 specimens from 472 consecutive patients. *Cancer.* 1985; 56(4):905–9.

Mate JL, Navarro JT, Ariza A, Ribera JM, Castella E, Junca J, Tural C, Nomdedeu JF, Bellosillo B, Serrano S, Granada I, Milla F, Feliu E. Oral solid form of primary effusion lymphoma mimicking plasmablastic lymphoma. *Hum Pathol.* 2004; 35(5):632–5.

Morel P, Dupriez A, Plantier-Colcher J, Gosselin B, Declercq C, Pollet JP, Bauters F. Long-term outcome of follicular low-grade lymphoma. A report of 91 patients. *Ann Hematol.* 1993; 66(6):303–8.

Paner GP, Jensen J, Foreman KE, Reyes CV. HIV and HHV-8 negative primary effusion lymphoma in a patient with hepatitis C virus-related liver cirrhosis. *Leuk Lymphoma.* 2003; 44(10):1811–4.

Sahn SA. Malignant pleural effusion. In: Fishman AP, Elias JA, Fishman JA, Grippe MA, Kaiser LR, Senior RM, editors, *Fishman's Pulmonary Diseases and Disorders*, 3rd ed., New York: McGraw-Hill, 1998, pp. 1429–38.

Stonesifer KJ, Xiang JH, Wilkinson EJ, Bensen NA, Braylan RC. Flow cytometric analysis and cytopathology of body cavity fluids. *Acta Cytol.* 1987; 31(2):125–30.

Tanaka S, Katano H, Tsukamoto K, Jin M, Oikawa S, Nishihara H, Sawa H, Sawada K, Shimizu M, Sata T, Fujioka Y, Nagashima K. HHV8-negative primary effusion lymphoma of the peritoneal cavity presenting with a distinct immunohistochemical phenotype. *Pathol Int.* 2001 Apr; 51(4):293–300.

Vakar-Lopez F, Yang M. Peripheral T-cell lymphoma presenting as ascites: a case report and review of the literature. *Diagn Cytopathol.* 1999; 20(6):382–4.

MISCELLANEOUS MALIGNANT TUMORS

Abadi MA, Zakowski MF. Cytologic features of sarcomas in fluids. *Cancer.* 1998 Apr 25; 84(2):71–6.

Geisinger KR, Hajdu SI, Helson L. Exfoliative cytology of nonlymphoreticular neoplasms in children. *Acta Cytol.* 1984;28(1):16–28.

Kumar S, Perlman E, Harris CA, Raffeld M, Tsokos M. Myogenin is a specific marker for rhabdomyosarcoma: an immunohistochemical study in paraffin-embedded tissues. *Mod Pathol.* 2000 Sep; 13(9): 988–93.

YOLK SAC TUMOR (ENDODERMAL SINUS TUMOR)

Hajdu SI, Nolan MA. Exfoliative cytology of malignant germ cell tumor. *Acta Cytol.* 1975; 19(3): 255–60.

Kashimura M, Tsukamoto N, Matsuyama T, et al. Cytologic findings of ascites from patients with ovarian dysgerminoma. *Acta Cytol.* 1983;27:59–62.

Roncalli M, Gribaudi G, Simoncellu D, et al. Cytology of yolk-sac tumor of the ovary in ascetic fluid. *Acta Cytol.* 1988;31(1):113–6.

MELANOMA

Beaty M, Fetch PA, Wilder AM, et al. Effusion cytology of malignant melanoma. *Cancer Cytopathol.* 1997;81(1):57–63.

Walts AE. Malignant melanoma in effusions: a source of false-negative cytodiagnosis. *Diagn Cytopathol.* 1986; 2(2):150–3.

RENAL CELL CARCINOMA (RCC)

Ordoñez NG. The diagnostic utility of immunohistochemistry in distinguishing between mesothelioma and renal cell carcinoma: A comparative study. *Hum Pathol.* 2004; 35(6): 697–710.

Renshaw AA, Comiter CV, Nappi D, Granter SR. Effusion cytology of renal cell carcinoma. *Cancer.* 1998 Jun 25; 84(3):148–52.

UROTHELIAL CELL CARCINOMA (UCC)

Sears D, Hadju SI. The cytologic diagnosis of malignant neoplasms in pleural and peritoneal effusions. *Acta Cytol* 1987; 31(2):85–97.

WILMS TUMOR (NEPHROBLASTOMA)

Hajdu SI. Exfoliative cytology of primary and metastatic Wilms tumor. *Acta Cytol.* 1971; 15(4): 339–42.

4

Gastrointestinal Tract

Telma C. Pereira, Reda S. Saad, and Jan F. Silverman

ESOPHAGUS

CANDIDAL ESOPHAGITIS

Clinical Features
- Most frequent cause of infectious esophagitis
- Often in immunosuppressed patients
- Dysphagia, odynophagia, heart burn, or chest pain
- Endoscopic appearance: white plaques or fibrinopurulent exudate
- Brush cytology is superior to biopsy for diagnosis

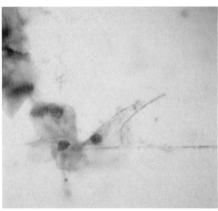

Cytopathologic Features
- Characteristic pseudohyphae or smaller budding yeast, both singly and in variably sized clusters in the smear as well as mixed directly with clusters of squamous cells, neutrophils, and necrotic material
- Neutrophilic infiltrate
- Degenerative changes of the epithelium

Special Stains and Immunohistochemistry
- Gomori methenamine silver (GMS) is usually not needed, but will be helpful in cases with few scattered organisms

Modern Techniques for Diagnosis
- Noncontributory

4-1. Candida esophagitis.
Eosinophilic pseudo-hyphae admixed with squamous cells (Papanicolaou stain)

Differential Diagnosis
- Rarely, other types of fungi, such as *Aspergillus:*
  - ➤ Immunocompromised patients, especially due to chemotherapy for lymphoproliferative disorders
  - ➤ Hyphae have true septation
  - ➤ Appear cyanophilic in Papanicolaou stain (in contrast to *candida*, which is eosinophilic)
- Primary bacterial infections
  - ➤ Can also have the neutrophilic and/or necrotic background
  - ➤ Frequent cause of esophagitis
  - ➤ Most cases due to saprophytes that involve individuals who are immunosuppressed or on long-term antibiotic therapy
  - ➤ Bacteria can usually be appreciated, although specific identification will require Gram stain and/or culture
  - ➤ Bacteria can also be seen in esophageal smears from individuals who have esophagitis due to other causes, and in this setting, either represent a contaminant or cocontributor

4-2A. Esophagitis *(left).* Marked acute inflammation in bacterial esophagitis (modified Gieimsa stain)

4-2B. Esophagitis *(right).* Reactive glandular cells in esophagitis. Arrow shows cluster of bacteria (modified Giemsa stain)

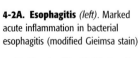
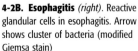
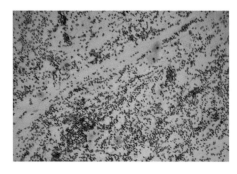
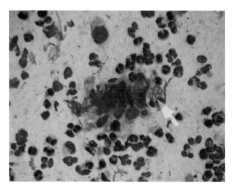

✴ In an esophageal brushing with neutrophils and granular debris, look carefully for fungus!

✴ Since *candida* is part of the normal flora of the GI tract, confirmation of infection requires identification of pseudohyphae (yeast alone might represent just colonization)

✴ If *candida* is seen without the background of inflammation and reactive/degenerative squamous cells, the possibility of an oral contaminant should be raised

✴ Coinfection of *candida* and other organisms is not uncommon, especially in immunocompromised patients

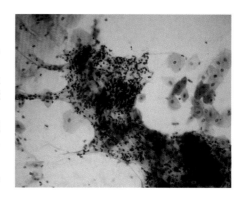

4-2C. Esophagitis. Squamous cells and marked acute inflammation in esophagitis (Papanicolaou stain)

HERPETIC ESOPHAGITIS

Clinical Features

▦ Most frequent type of viral esophagitis

▦ Dysphagia, odynophagia, heart burn, chest pain, or may be asymptomatic

▦ Patients usually have predisposing conditions: mucosal trauma (prior nasogastric intubation), malignancy (especially hematopoietic), prior chemotherapy and/or irradiation, immunosupression (AIDS, transplant)

▦ Occasionally occurs in otherwise healthy individuals

▦ Can resolve spontaneously, even in immunosuppressed patients

▦ Endoscopic appearance: multiple small, shallow ulcers with punched-out edges, mostly in the distal third of the organ

▦ The edge of the ulcer should be brushed (samples of the ulcer bed will be non-diagnostic)

Cytopathologic Features

▦ Viral cytopathic nuclear changes: the classic Cowdry type A viral inclusion or a pale basophilic homogeneous change to the chromatin

▦ Cowdry type A inclusions: eosinophilic, irregular, centrally positioned within the nucleus, separated from the thickened nuclear membrane by a distinct surrounding clear halo

▦ The more homogeneous type of viral inclusion body imparts a smooth pale basophilic refractile "ground-glass" appearance to the entire nucleus

▦ Virally infected squamous cells can become multinucleated with characteristic presence of nuclear molding and margination of the chromatin

▦ The infected squamous cells' cytoplasm is scanty, dense, and cyanophilic

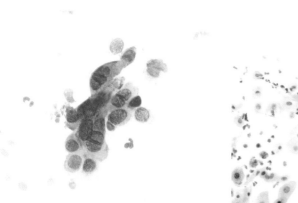

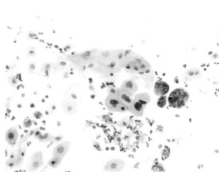

4-3A. Herpetic esophagitis *(left).* "3 M's" in herpetic esophagitis: multinucleation, molding and margination (modified Giemsa stain)

4-3B. Herpetic esophagitis *(right).* The multinucleated cells in the center have eosinophilic Cowdry type A intranuclear inclusions (Papanicolaou stain)

■ When the ulcer base is also sampled, necrotic debris and neutrophils are present
■ Background shows reactive epithelial cells with enlarged nuclei and prominent nucleoli, low N/C ratios, regular nuclear membrane, and "school of fish" cell arrangement of repair

Special Stains and Immunohistochemistry
■ Immunoperoxidase: If careful search with routine stains fail to disclose virocytes, then it is unlikely that immunoperoxidase will disclose anything further. However, it can be useful if routine cytology stains show cells that are suspicious but not diagnostic

Modern Techniques for Diagnosis
■ Noncontributory

Differential Diagnosis
■ Squamous cell carcinoma
  ➤ Chromatin is coarsely granular and hyperchromatic, in contrast to pale ground glass in herpes
  ➤ Potential pitfall is misinterpreting the viral inclusion bodies for huge macronucleoli of malignant cells. However, a perfectly clear halo is present around herpes viral inclusion, while in malignant cells, coarse chromatin granules are present in the nucleus
■ Small cell carcinoma
  ➤ Can show nuclear molding
  ➤ However, small cell carcinoma cells should have very little cytoplasm (almost imperceptible) and characteristic "salt-and-pepper" chromatin
■ Cytomegalovirus
  ➤ Single nucleus (very rarely binucleated)
  ➤ Cytoplasmic inclusions in addition to nuclear inclusions
■ Radiation esophagitis
  ➤ Radiated squamous cells can also have multiple nuclei and a degenerative chromatin that can simulate the homogeneous ground-glass virocytopathic change
  ➤ However, radiation esophagitis lacks the typical nuclear molding or viral inclusions

PEARLS

★ Infects squamous cells
★ 3 "Ms": multinucleation, margination (of chromatin), molding (of nuclei)

CYTOMEGALOVIRUS (CMV) ESOPHAGITIS

Clinical Features
■ Very rare in the general population, occurs with some frequency in patients with AIDS and other immunocompromised patients
■ The clinical features are nonspecific such as dysphagia and/or chest pain
■ Endoscopically, multiple well-circumscribed ulcers are seen
■ Biopsy is the modality of choice for identification of CMV, but it can occasionally be identified in brushings
■ The preferred site for brushing to retrieve CMV-infected cells is the ulcer bed, rather than the edge of the ulcer

Cytopathologic Features
■ Background of reactive epithelial cells, granulation tissue, and acute inflammation
■ Generally few CMV virocytes are present and are individually scattered cells with marked nuclear and cytoplasmic enlargement

■ The large viral inclusion bodies are surrounded by a large clear zone and a nuclear membrane that has a marginated appearance due to aggregation of chromatin along the inner border of the nuclear membrane causing contour irregularity

■ Small eosinophilic granular cytoplasmic inclusions can also be present

■ The alcohol-fixed, Papanicolaou-stained smears demonstrate the intranuclear inclusions to advantage, while air-dried modified Giemsa stained smears accentuate the cytoplasmic inclusions

Special Stains and Immunohistochemistry

■ Immunoperoxidase: If careful search with routine stains fail to disclose inclusions, then it is unlikely that immunoperoxidase will disclose anything further. However, it can be useful if routine cytology stains show cells that are suspicious but not diagnostic

Modern Techniques for Diagnosis

■ In situ hybridization can be useful if routine cytology stains show cells that are suspicious but not diagnostic

Differential Diagnosis

■ Herpes esophagitis

➤ Both herpes and CMV can have intranuclear inclusions, but herpes does not have cytoplasmic inclusions

➤ The cells in herpes infection show multinucleation, and in CMV infection the nucleus is usually single and very large

PEARLS

✶ Infects glandular cells, fibroblasts, and endothelial cells, not squamous cells

✶ The number of infected cells is frequently low, which often requires a very diligent search in order to identify the virocytes in the smears

RADIATION- AND CHEMOTHERAPY-RELATED ESOPHAGITIS

Clinical Features

■ Irradiation to chest and mediastinum and chemotherapy are a common cause of esophagitis

■ The effects of radiation and chemotherapy may potentiate each other by lowering the threshold for injury

■ Chemotherapy-associated atypia simulates cancer more closely than irradiation changes

■ Endoscopically, the esophagus is hyperemic, friable, and hemorrhagic

Cytopathologic Features

■ Significant nuclear and cytoplasmic enlargement, low nuclear to cytoplasmic ratios

■ Cells have a two-toned, blue and pink cytoplasm (bichromasia) with Papanicolaou staining

■ Degenerative nuclear and cytoplasmic vacuolization, karyolysis, and karyorrhexis

■ Nuclear membrane irregularity and multinucleation

■ Chromatin can have a finely granular appearance or smudged pattern

■ In chemotherapy-related esophagitis, nucleoli can be prominent, and the chromatin can be hyperchromatic and coarsely granular

Special Stains and Immunohistochemistry

■ Noncontributory

Modern Techniques for Diagnosis

■ Noncontributory

Differential Diagnosis

■ Herpes virus
➤ Nuclear molding
➤ Viral inclusions
■ Squamous cell carcinoma
➤ Definitive diagnosis of carcinoma should always be made with caution in patients with a known history of prior chemotherapy
➤ This diagnostic problem is further accentuated when the malignant cells also have superimposed treatment-related changes. However, malignant cells will also demonstrate high nuclear to cytoplasmic ratios, significant hyperchromasia with coarse chromatin, and nuclear irregularity in addition to the treatment-related change

PEARLS

★ Cells with atypia due to chemotherapy or radiation maintain a low N/C ratio

GASTROESOPHAGEAL REFLUX DISEASE (GERD)

Clinical Features

■ Most common cause of esophagitis
■ Endoscopically, an erythematous mucosa will be appreciated, with or without erosions, in the distal portion of the esophagus
■ Complications of reflux esophagitis include peptic ulcers, fibrosing strictures, and Barrett's esophagitis

Cytopathologic Features

■ Enlarged epithelial cells in flat cohesive sheets of varying sizes with well-defined cell border
■ Polarity is retained
■ "Streaming" effect: the cells and their nuclei all appear to be oriented in the same direction
■ Relative uniformity from cell to cell
■ Nuclei are large, round to oval, with smooth nuclear membrane
■ Chromatin is finely granular, uniformly distributed, and somewhat pale
■ Mitoses may be seen, but no atypical mitoses

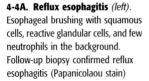

4-4A. Reflux esophagitis *(left).* Esophageal brushing with squamous cells, reactive glandular cells, and few neutrophils in the background. Follow-up biopsy confirmed reflux esophagitis (Papanicolaou stain)

4-4B. Reflux esophagitis *(right).* Reactive atypia in reflux esophagitis. The enlarged epithelial cells have prominent nucleoli, but maintain a low nuclear/cytoplasmic ratio (Papanicolaou stain)

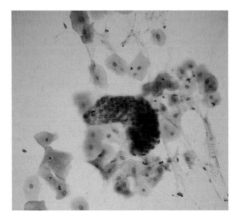
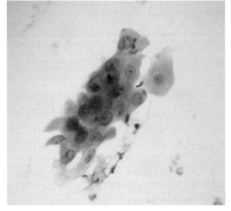

- Can have associated neutrophilic infiltration
- Lack of single atypical cells

Special Stains and Immunohistochemistry
- Noncontributory

Modern Techniques for Diagnosis
- Noncontributory

Differential Diagnosis
- Infectious esophagitis
  - Neutrophilic infiltrate, granulation tissue, and/or necrotic debris
  - Identification of infectious agent: fungus, bacteria, or viral inclusion
- Esophagitis following the ingestion of corrosive agents or lodging of pills in the esophagus
  - Clinical history is essential
- Barrett's
  - Goblet cells must be present for the diagnosis of Barrett's
  - Goblet cells have distended barrel-like contour secondary to abundant pale to clear mucinous cytoplasm and basally placed nuclei

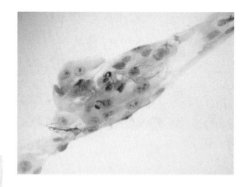

4-4C. Repair. Repair in esophageal brushing: Streaming effect, prominent eosinophilic nucleoli. The chromatin remains pale and delicate (Papanicolaou stain)

PEARLS

⭐ When diagnosing GERD, look for goblet cells to make sure there is no associated intestinal metaplasia (Barrett's esophagus)

BARRETT'S ESOPHAGUS

Clinical Features
- Complication of reflux esophagitis
- No specific clinical signs and symptoms in addition to the reflux symptoms
- Premalignant condition, can progress to low-grade dysplasia, to high-grade dysplasia, to adenocarcinoma

Cytopathologic Features
- Goblet cells:
  - Are required for diagnosis
  - Distended barrel-like contour due to abundant bluish gray mucinous cytoplasm

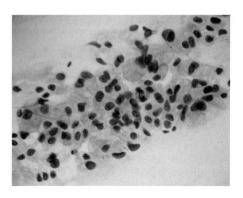 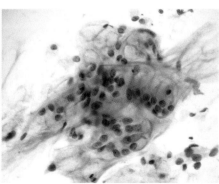

4-5A. Gastroesophageal reflux disease *(left)*. Intestinal metaplasia. The many goblet cells are distended with a large mucin vacuole that pushes the nucleus basally (Papanicolaou stain)

4-5B. Intestinal metaplasia *(right)*. Intestinal metaplasia. Group with numerous goblet cells with the characteristic "barrel-like contour" due to the large mucin vacuole that has a color distinctly different from the cytoplasm of the glandular cells in the same field (Papanicolaou stain)

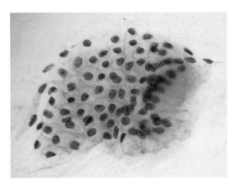

4-5C. Constipated glandular cells.
These foveolar cells are normal glandular cells from the cardia that can be present in an esophageal brushing. The cell distention due to an increased amount of cytoplasm can resemble goblet cells. These foveolar cells, however, have a pale cytoplasm that is similar in color to the neighboring glandular cells (Papanicolaou stain)

> The cytoplasm is about three times the size of the nucleus and pushes the nucleus basally
> Goblet cells are generally identified in cohesive groups of columnar cells
■ The columnar cells:
> Have uniform round to oval nuclei
> Delicate nuclear chromatin and smooth nuclear membranes.
> Are found in cohesive, flat cellular sheets arranged in a honeycomb or palisading pattern
> Can have reparative changes consisting of prominent nucleoli and a "streaming" pattern with all the nuclei flowing in the same direction and preserved polarity
> Occasionally groups of glandular cells (from the cardia or gastroesophageal junction) can look "constipated" with increased amount of cytoplasm and cell distention. They may be difficult to differentiate from true goblet cells. The cytoplasm, however, is pale and similar to the neighboring "non-constipated" glandular cells

Special Stains and Immunohistochemistry
■ Mucicarmine or PAS can highlight the goblet cells, but is seldom used in cytology
■ Goblet cells are Hep Par-1 positive

Modern Techniques for Diagnosis
■ Noncontributory

Differential Diagnosis
■ Low-grade dysplasia
> Predominance of cohesive glandular groups with more cell crowding and nuclear overlapping
> Nuclei are more elongated and hyperchromatic (as opposed to the oval vesicular nuclei of nondysplastic Barrett's esophagus)
> N/C ratio is slightly increased
> Occasional prominent nucleoli
■ High-grade dysplasia
> Greater degree of crowding, loss of polarity, and nuclear enlargement
> Changes overlap with changes of invasive adenocarcinoma (but there are no single atypical cells in dysplasia)

PEARLS

★ Presence of goblet cells is diagnostic of Barrett's esophagus
★ Once the diagnosis of Barrett's is made, the presence or absence of dysplasia should be noted in the report. Since brushing cytology is not sensitive for low-grade dysplasia, the presence or absence of high-grade dysplasia could be noted instead

DYSPLASIA IN BARRETT'S

Clinical Features
■ Dysplastic Barrett's epithelium is the precursor to invasive carcinoma
■ There are no specific signs or symptoms for dysplasia
■ Surveillance programs to monitor patients with Barrett's esophagus most often involve tissue biopsies, but a few protocols also include brushing cytology

■ Cytology is very sensitive to detect high-grade dysplasia in Barrett's esophagus, but has very poor sensitivity for low-grade dysplasia

Cytopathologic Features
■ Columnar-shaped glandular cells in three-dimensional groups with frayed margins
■ Lack of polarity, the cells are arranged haphazardly with overlapping nuclei
■ Nuclei are enlarged, oval to elongated, hyperchromatic, pleomorphic
■ Increased nuclear to cytoplasmic ratios
■ Can have large nucleoli
■ Delicate pale amphophilic cytoplasm with reduced mucin
■ Dysplasia may only have a few such cells in the cytology specimen
■ Low-grade dysplasia: the nuclei are more basally located
■ High-grade dysplasia: the nuclei approach the luminal glandular border, the nuclear membrane is irregular

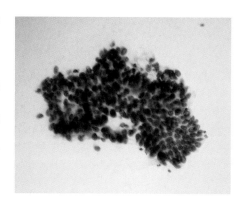

4-5D. Barrett's esophagus dysplasia. High-grade dysplasia in Barrett's esophagus. This three-dimensional group has frayed margins and loss of polarity, and the cells have high nuclear/cytoplasmic ratio and hyperchromatic nuclei (Papanicolaou stain)

Special Stains and Immunohistochemistry
■ Noncontributory

Modern Techniques for Diagnosis
■ Noncontributory

Differential Diagnosis
■ Well-differentiated adenocarcinoma
➤ Tumor diathesis and presence of many single atypical cells are features of adenocarcinoma
➤ However, in the absence of such features, high-grade dysplasia cannot be absolutely differentiated from a well-differentiated adenocarcinoma in the cytology smears

PEARLS
★ Dysplasia cannot be adequately graded by cytologic examination
★ Brush cytology is not a sensitive modality for the detection of low-grade dysplasia or differentiating it from reactive atypia
★ Dysplasia and well-differentiated adenocarcinoma can be impossible to distinguish by cytology
★ When in doubt, recommend a tissue biopsy!

SQUAMOUS CELL CARCINOMA

Clinical Features
■ Most common malignant neoplasm of the esophagus
■ Dysphagia: late symptom
■ Often causes considerable stenosis of the esophagus, being difficult or impossible to obtain tissue biopsies, so brushing cytology may be especially useful

Cytopathologic Features
■ Well-differentiated squamous cell carcinoma:
➤ Individually scattered cells and/or groups with intercellular cohesion relatively well maintained

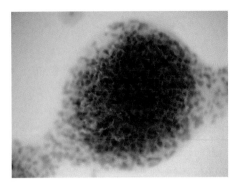

4-6A. Squamous cell carcinoma.
Squamous cell carcinoma in esophageal brushing. Three-dimensional cluster of cells with hyperchromatic nuclei, high nuclear/cytoplasmic ratio and cytoplasmic varying from orangeophilic to cyanophilic (Papanicolaou stain)

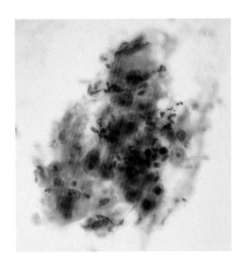

4-6B. Poorly differentiated squamous cell carcinoma. Malignant cells with hyperchromatic nucleus, prominent nucleoli, dense cytoplasm, and very sharply demarcated cytoplasmic edges (Papanicolaou stain)

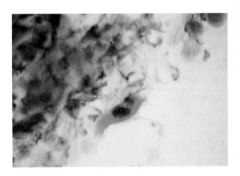

4-6C. Squamous cell carcinoma.
Individual irregularly shaped cell with bright orangeophilic cytoplasm and hyperchromatic angulated nucleus in esophageal squamous cell carcinoma (Papanicolaou stain)

➢ Variable–sized aggregates of large tumor cells having abundant dense cytoplasm
➢ Keratinization: bright orangeophilic cytoplasm with Papanicolaou stain
➢ Central nuclei, may have very sharply angulated contours
➢ Relatively low nuclear to cytoplasmic ratios
➢ Chromatin can vary from coarsely granular and hyperchromatic to almost pyknotic in appearance
➢ Keratin pearls can be appreciated, as well as individually scattered cells having bizarre shapes, including tadpole-like and spindle forms
➢ Numerous anucleated keratinized squamous and "parakeratotic" appearing cells may also be present
➢ "Dirty" necrosis and/or acute inflammation in the background

■ Poorly differentiated squamous cell carcinoma:
➢ Discohesion increases: numerous individually scattered malignant cells
➢ Dense cytoplasm more cyanophilic than orangeophilic (has less keratin than the well differentiated)
➢ Sharp cytoplasmic borders
➢ Higher N/C ratios
➢ Chromatin varies from finely to coarsely granular hyperchromatic
➢ Nucleoli are more apparent
➢ Dense pyknotic-like nuclei are infrequent
➢ "Dirty" necrosis and/or acute inflammation in the background

Special Stains and Immunohistochemistry
■ Noncontributory

Modern Techniques for Diagnosis
■ Noncontributory

Differential Diagnosis
■ Herpes
➢ Chromatin is ground glass
➢ Nuclear inclusions surrounded by clear halo
➢ Multinucleation with molding
■ Reactive changes of esophagitis
➢ Nucleoli can be seen both in repair/reactive changes and in poorly differentiated squamous cell carcinoma
➢ In repair, however, the cells have a uniform appearance, well-defined cell borders, preserved polarity, lower N/C ratios, fine chromatin, and there are no single atypical cells
■ Adenocarcinoma
➢ Adenocarcinoma has more open, vesicular chromatin
➢ Adenocarcinoma has more delicate cytoplasm in contrast to dense, opaque cytoplasm of squamous cell carcinoma
➢ Adenocarcinoma has more eccentric nuclei in contrast to more central nuclei of squamous cell carcinoma
➢ In poorly differentiated carcinomas, a careful search in the smears will demonstrate either focal mucin (in poorly differentiated adenocarcinomas) or focal keratin (in poorly differentiated squamous cell carcinomas)

★ Potential pitfall is misinterpreting herpes viral inclusion bodies for huge macro-nucleoli of malignant cells. However, a perfectly clear halo is present around herpes viral inclusion, while in malignant cells, coarse chromatin granules are present in the nucleus

ADENOCARCINOMA

Clinical Features

▨ Almost all adenocarcinomas arise in the background of preexisting Barrett's esophagus

▨ Adenocarcinomas almost always occur in the distal third of the esophagus and often involve the gastroesophageal junction

▨ Patients present with dysphagia, and endoscopically, have either large ulcers or fungating polypoid masses, which can significantly reduce the luminal diameter of the esophagus

Cytopathologic Features

▨ Cellular smears with many individually scattered abnormal cells and a small clusters in a three-dimensional arrangement

▨ Clusters smaller than in dysplasia

▨ Lack of polarity, and the cells are arranged haphazardly with overlapping abnormal nuclei

▨ The cells are columnar or cuboidal with increased N/C ratio

▨ Cytoplasm is clear, vacuolated, often with reduced cytoplasmic mucin

▨ Signet ring–type cells can also be seen

▨ Enlarged, hyperchromatic, pleomorphic nuclei with thick, irregular nuclear membranes

▨ Mitoses often seen

▨ One or more large irregular nucleoli present

▨ Tumor diathesis may be seen

Special Stains and Immunohistochemistry

▨ Noncontributory

Modern Techniques for Diagnosis

▨ Noncontributory

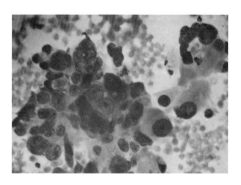

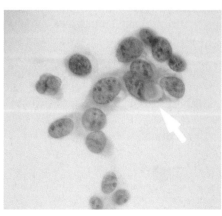

4-7A. Adenocarcinoma *(left)*. Adenocarcinoma in FNA of esophagus. Cluster of pleomorphic cells with overlapping nuclei and delicate cytoplasm (modified Giemsa stain)

4-7B. Adenocarcinoma *(right)*. Adenocarcinoma of esophagus. Arrow points to mucin vacuole (Papanicolaou stain)

Differential Diagnosis

■ Repair
  ➤ Cohesive, flat (two-dimensional) sheets of cells
  ➤ "Streaming" or "school-of-fish" appearance: the cells and their nuclei all appear to be oriented in the same direction, and appear somewhat stretched
  ➤ Polarity is preserved
  ➤ Cells have a uniform appearance, there is a homogeneity from cell to cell
  ➤ Sharp, well-defined cytoplasmic borders
  ➤ Enlarged nuclei, but N/C ratios remain low
  ➤ Uniform nuclei with round to oval nuclear contours
  ➤ Nuclear membrane is smooth, thin, and regular
  ➤ Cells have single prominent nucleolus that does not touch the nuclear membrane
  ➤ Nucleoli also have round smooth contours
  ➤ Finely granular, evenly distributed, pale chromatin
  ➤ Mitotic figures may be appreciated, but no atypical mitosis
  ➤ No diathesis
  ➤ Cellular cohesion is strictly maintained with absence of atypical single cells

■ Reactive stromal cells
  ➤ In brushings of ulcers, reactive stromal cells originating from the granulation tissue at the base of the ulcer may be present
  ➤ These cells are individually scattered or in loose clusters
  ➤ Spindle to stellate shapes
  ➤ Nuclei are oval to spindle
  ➤ Bland chromatin distribution and inconspicuous nucleoli

■ Radiation, chemotherapy, or laser atypia
  ➤ Nuclear and cytoplasmic enlargement, but maintain low N/C ratios
  ➤ The irradiated cells are often arranged in a repair pattern
  ➤ Cytoplasmic bichromasia (the cytoplasm stains with two different colors: cyanophilic and orangiophylic in the Papanicolaou stain)
  ➤ Vacuolization of nucleus and cytoplasm
  ➤ Degenerative chromatin (smudged)
  ➤ If the N/C ratio is significantly increased with nuclear membrane irregularity and many atypical intact single cells, consider the possibility of irradiated malignant cells

■ Melanoma (metastatic or primary)
  ➤ Can have a variety of different appearances
  ➤ Discohesive smear pattern with loosely cohesive clusters
  ➤ The size and shape of the tumor cells can vary significantly with polygonal, spindle to giant cell forms present
  ➤ Melanoma should be suspected when dispersed high-grade malignant cells with one or more large, eccentrically placed nuclei with thick nuclear membranes and huge nucleoli are identified
  ➤ Mirror image binucleated tumor cells are characteristic and the diagnosis is further supported when nuclear pseudoinclusions are found
  ➤ May have intracytoplasmic melanin pigment: dark brown, coarsely or finely granular pigment or the cytoplasm has a brownish dusky blush
  ➤ Positive for S-100, HMB-45, melan-A immunostains

■ Other primary or metastatic cancers
  ➤ Hematopoietic malignancies
  ➤ GIST and sarcomas
  ➤ Lymphoma
  ➤ Germ cell tumors

★ A definitive diagnosis of malignancy should never be made if only poorly preserved or degenerated cells are available for evaluation

SMALL CELL CARCINOMA

Clinical Features
- Neuroendocrine neoplasms of the esophagus are uncommon accounting for less than 5% of all esophageal tumors
- Small cell carcinoma is the most frequent neuroendocrine neoplasm in the esophagus
- Middle age or older individuals
- Middle or distal segment of the esophagus
- Nonspecific clinical symptom of dysphagia

Cytopathologic Features
- Population of small malignant cells both individually scattered and present within densely packed small groups, rosette-like structures, and chains
- Oval, round, or elongated nuclei
- Nucleoli should be absent or very small
- Chromatin is hyperchromatic, uniformly distributed, and finely to coarsely granular ("salt-and-pepper" quality)
- Exceedingly high nuclear to cytoplasmic ratios, the cytoplasm is barely visible
- Nuclear molding is a characteristic feature of this tumor
- Occasional mitoses can be seen

Special Stains and Immunohistochemistry
- Positive for low-molecular-weight cytokeratin (Cam5.2)
- Positive for neuroendocrine markers: synaptophysin, chromogranin, NSE, CD56, CD57, MAP-2
- Negative for, CD45, CD20, usually negative for TTF-1 (See below "Differential Diagnosis")

Modern Techniques for Diagnosis
- Noncontributory

Differential Diagnosis
- Metastasis from a small cell carcinoma, usually from the lung
  ➤ Esophageal small cell carcinomas are usually TTF-1 negative and CDX-2 positive, lung small cell carcinomas are the opposite
- Poorly differentiated squamous cell carcinoma
  ➤ A diligent search of the specimen will demonstrate at least some cells showing more obvious squamous differentiation
  ➤ Greater volumes of dense cytoplasm with sharp borders
  ➤ More hyperchromatic clumping chromatin
  ➤ Well-developed nucleoli
- Lymphoma
  ➤ Predominantly discohesive cell pattern
  ➤ Recognizable nucleoli
  ➤ Nuclear molding will not be appreciated in smears from lymphoma, although occasional clusters of lymphoid cells can show overlapping nuclei
  ➤ Lymphoglandular bodies (fragments of cytoplasm of lymphocytes, stain pale blue in modified Giemsa stain) in the background
  ➤ Positive for CD45 and negative for keratin and neuroendocrine markers

■ Benign chronic inflammation
> Lymphocytes also have fragile nuclei and can be artificially crushed, simulating the crush artifact of small cell carcinoma
> Lymphocytes have coarser chromatin
> Lymphoglandular bodies in the background
> A careful search of the smears will show intact cells where the morphology of lymphocytes can be appreciated

PEARLS

★ Relatively rare in the esophagus – important to exclude more common poorly differentiated squamous cell carcinoma – see above "Differential Diagnosis"
★ Even though the cells of small cell carcinoma are fragile and frequently have crush artifact, never make a definitive diagnosis without identifying some malignant cells with preserved, identifiable morphology

LEIOMYOMA AND OTHER MESENCHYMAL TUMORS

Clinical Features
■ Leiomyoma is the most common mesenchymal tumor of the esophagus
■ Sometimes present with dysphagia
■ Often incidentally found during endoscopic workup for other causes
■ Well-circumscribed, submucosal lesion arising from the muscular layer

Cytopathologic Features
■ Spindle cells in clusters with low to moderate cellularity
■ Cells haphazardly arranged in the clusters
■ Bland spindle-shaped cells that have cigar-shaped nuclei with minimal cytologic atypia

Special Stains and Immunohistochemistry
■ Leiomyoma: Positive for smooth muscle and muscle specific actins, negative for CD117, CD34, and S-100

Modern Techniques for Diagnosis
■ Noncontributory

Differential Diagnosis
■ GIST
> Groups of spindle cells are more cellular than in leiomyoma
> Positive for CD117, often positive for CD34, can be positive for actin
> Rare in the esophagus

4-8A. Leiomyoma and other mesenchymal tumors *(left)*. Endoscopic ultrasound-guided fine-needle aspiration cytology (EUS-FNA) of submucosal esophageal lesion. Hypercellular cluster of spindle cells can be found in mesenchymal tumors such as leiomyoma, leiomyosarcoma, and GIST (modified Giemsa stain)

4-8B. Leiomyoma and other mesenchymal tumors *(right)*. Same lesion of Figure 4-8A showing cluster of spindle cells in Papanicolaou stain

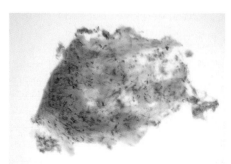

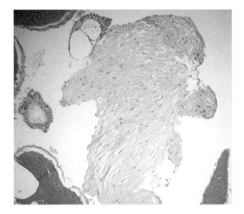
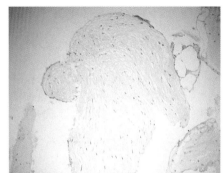
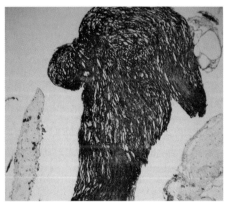
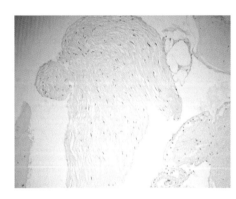

4-9. Leiomyoma of esophagus (same lesion of Figures 4-8A and 4-8B). (A) *(top, left)* Cell block with H&E stain, (B) *(top, right)* Negative immunostain for c-kit (CD117), (C) *(bottom, left)* Strongly positive smooth muscle actin, D: *(bottom, right)* negative S-100

- Leiomyosarcoma
  - ➤ Very rare in the esophagus
  - ➤ Cellular spindle cell lesion with marked cytologic and nuclear pleomorphism
  - ➤ Positive for smooth muscle actin and for muscle specific actin
  - ➤ Negative for CD34 and CD117
- Normal muscularis propria
  - ➤ Smaller cells, hypocellular fragments
  - ➤ Cells more evenly distributed in the fragments

PEARLS

★ Leiomyoma is the most common mesenchymal tumor of the esophagus, but keep the differential diagnosis in mind due to important treatment and prognostic implications!

STOMACH

GASTRITIS

Clinical Features
- May be due to a variety of etiologies
- Patients most commonly present with epigastric pain
- Acute gastritis is self-limited, so patients rarely undergo endoscopy
- *Helicobacter pylori* is the major cause of chronic gastritis

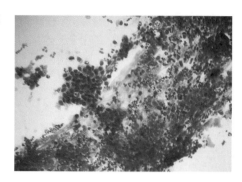
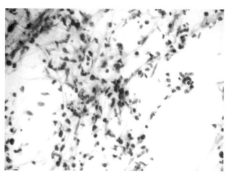

4-10A. Gastric ulcer *(left)*. Marked acute inflammation and reactive epithelium in FNA of gastric ulcer. Subsequent surgical resection proved it to be a benign ulcer (modified Giemsa stain)

4-10B. Gastric ulcer *(right)*. Reactive stromal cells admixed with acute inflammation and debris in gastric ulcer (Papanicolaou stain)

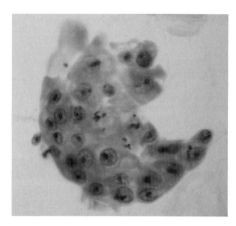

4-10C. Gastric repair. Enlarged cells with macro nucleoli maintain low nuclear/ cytoplasmic ratio and preserved polarity (papanicolaou stain)

Cytopathologic Features

▨ Chronic gastritis due to different etiologies share similar cytologic features

▨ Large cohesive flat honeycomb groups of glandular epithelial cells with preserved polarity

▨ The cells can show inflammatory atypia and/or reparative change with prominent nucleoli and enlarged nuclei, but the N/C ratios are preserved and the nuclear membrane is regular

▨ Background can have neutrophils and lymphocytes

▨ Cellular degeneration and necrotic debris may be present

▨ Occasionally goblet cells interspersed among the columnar cells (intestinal metaplasia)

▨ *Helicobacter*-associated gastritis also has numerous neutrophils and Helicobacter organisms can be seen

▨ *Helicobacter* organisms: 1–3 μm in length, curved or spiral configuration, closely associated with glandular cells or within clumps of extracellular mucus

▨ The long axis of the organism typically parallels the long axis of the mucous strands

Special Stains and Immunohistochemistry

▨ Helicobacter organisms are more easily identified in air-dried modified Giemsa stain or other Romanowsky-stained smears due to their larger size in these preparations

▨ Immunostain for *Helicobacter pylori* may also be helpful

Modern Techniques for Diagnosis

▨ Noncontributory

Differential Diagnosis

▨ Other organisms

➤ Cocci and rod-shaped bacteria may also be found in the smears and should be differentiated from the spiral-shaped *Helicobacter*

➤ Cytomegalovirus has been described in gastric smears, usually associated with systemic disease but most frequently in patients with AIDS and other immuno-compromised conditions

➤ Clusters of filamentous organisms have been described in both benign gastric brushings and associated with an underlying malignant tumor

PEARLS

✦ Cytologic features often nonspecific, it may be best to give a descriptive diagnosis

PEPTIC ULCER DISEASE

Clinical Features
■ Vast majority linked to *H. pylori* infection
■ Most frequently occurs in young to middle-aged adults, but can be seen in all ages
■ Burning epigastric pain occurring within an hour or so of eating
■ Endoscopic examination generally reveals a small ulcer usually measuring less than 3 cm in diameter, having round or ovoid and sharply delineated borders with the adjacent mucosa
■ Although characteristic, neither the radiologic nor endoscopic appearance can consistently and accurately distinguish benign from malignant ulcers

Cytopathologic Features
■ Brushing cytology smears will also contain numerous neutrophils and granular debris.
■ *H. pylori* may be appreciated also in the background or attached to some of the glandular cell surfaces
■ An admixture of bland-appearing glandular cells arranged in honeycomb clusters may be seen, along with other groupings showing inflammatory atypia and/or repair
■ Groups showing repair have enlarged nuclei with prominent nucleoli, but there is low N/C ratio, maintenance of polarity and relative preservation of cohesion with no atypical single cells (see detailed description of features of repair in the differential diagnosis of esophagus adenocarcinoma)

Special Stains and Immunohistochemistry
■ *Helicobacter* organisms are more easily identified in air-dried modified Giemsa Stain or other Romanowsky-stained smears due to their larger size in these preparations
■ Immunostain for *H. pylori* may also be helpful

Modern Techniques for Diagnosis
■ Noncontributory

Differential Diagnosis
■ Adenocarcinoma
  ➤ Loss of polarity
  ➤ Greater number of individually dispersed, intact abnormal-appearing single cells

PEARLS

★ The most important issue in the brushing cytology of a gastric ulcer is to exclude adenocarcinoma

DYSPLASIA

Clinical Features
■ Patients with atrophic gastritis have a statistically increased risk of developing adenocarcinoma, which is believed to evolve through glandular dysplasia

Cytopathologic Features
■ Background of atrophic gastritis: cohesive groups of benign glandular cells, which may include goblet cells, and mixed inflammatory cells including lymphocytes and plasma cells

▓ The dysplastic glandular epithelium recapitulates the cytologic findings of dysplasia in Barrett's mucosa
▓ The dysplastic aggregates vary from small to large and have irregular jagged edges
▓ The nuclei within the groups are crowded, overlapping, pseudostratified, and can demonstrate molding
▓ The dysplastic nuclei are larger than normal and are often elongated
▓ Nuclear contours vary from smooth to slightly irregular
▓ Finely to coarsely granular hyperchromatic chromatin
▓ One or more prominent nucleoli
▓ The nuclear to cytoplasmic ratios are increased
▓ Cytoplasmic mucin is reduced or not apparent

Special Stains and Immunohistochemistry
▓ Noncontributory

Modern Techniques for Diagnosis
▓ Noncontributory

Differential Diagnosis
▓ Benign repair
  ➤ Flat cohesive sheets of uniform cells with a "school-of-fish" arrangement
  ➤ Round to oval enlarged nuclei with smooth and regular nuclear membranes
  ➤ Fine chromatin and prominent nucleoli
  ➤ Low N/C ratios
  ➤ Absence of atypical single cells
  ➤ (See detailed description of features of repair in the section of differential diagnosis of esophagus adenocarcinoma)
▓ Adenocarcinoma
  ➤ Greater number of individually dispersed, intact abnormal-appearing single cells
  ➤ Syncytial arrangement
  ➤ Abnormal mitotic figures

PEARLS

★ Never diagnose adenocarcinoma without isolated (single) atypical cells

CHEMOTHERAPY-ASSOCIATED ATYPIA

Clinical Features
▓ In atypia associated with systemic chemotherapy the patients generally lack gastric symptoms
▓ Hepatic artery infusion chemotherapy has been associated with gastric ulcers because the hepatic artery also contributes a portion of the vascular supply to the stomach

Cytopathologic Features
▓ Marked cytologic atypia
▓ The atypical epithelial cells are arranged in large flat sheets, small clusters, and individually scattered
▓ Marked increase in cytoplasmic and nuclear volumes, but the nuclear to cytoplasmic ratios remains relatively low
▓ Although one or more prominent nucleoli are present and occasional mononucleated to multinucleated atypical cells can be seen, the nuclear contours remained relatively smooth and the chromatin was evenly distributed

Special Stains and Immunohistochemistry
- Noncontributory

Modern Techniques for Diagnosis
- Noncontributory

Differential Diagnosis
- Adenocarcinoma
  - ➤ Irregular nuclear contours
  - ➤ Coarse chromatin

PEARLS

★ The N/C ratio remains low

POLYPS

Clinical Features
- The two most frequent polyps to involve the gastric mucosa are hyperplastic polyps and adenomas
- Hyperplastic polyps have only a slightly increased risk of having an associated gastric carcinoma
- Gastric adenomas, in contrast, carry a markedly increased risk of adenocarcinoma of the stomach

Cytopathologic Features
- Hyperplastic polyps: reparative glandular epithelium with associated neutrophils and necrotic debris, cytologic features indistinguishable from those obtained from the edge of a gastric ulcer
- Gastric adenomas: the cells are indistinguishable from tubular adenomas of the lower GI tract, and dysplastic epithelium occurring in the setting of Barrett's esophagus or gastric-related diseases
  - ➤ The atypical glandular epithelium from an adenoma can occasionally show papillary-like fragments

Special Stains and Immunohistochemistry
- Noncontributory

Modern Techniques for Diagnosis
- Noncontributory

Differential Diagnosis
- Peptic ulcer
  - ➤ Clinical history of polypoid lesion is needed to differentiate gastric ulcer from hyperplastic polyp
- Gastric dysplasia
  - ➤ Clinical history of polypoid lesion is needed to differentiate gastric adenoma from gastric dysplasia

PEARLS

★ Knowledge of the endoscopic appearance of a polyp is essential

ADENOCARCINOMA

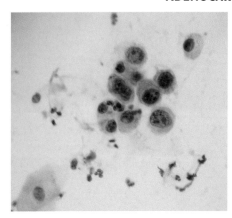

4-11A. Adenocarcinoma. Gastric adenocarcinoma, diffuse type. The overall cell size is not very large (compared to neutrophils in the bottom field), but the nuclear/cytoplasmic ratio is high and the chromatin is coarse (Papanicolaou stain)

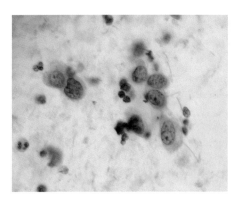

4-11B. Adenocarcinoma. Gastric adenocarcinoma with necrotic background and single malignant cells (Papanicolaou stain)

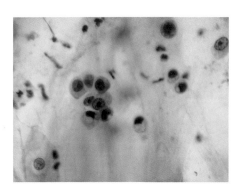

4-11C. Adenocarcinoma. Gastric adenocarcinoma, diffuse type with signet ring cells (Papanicolaou stain)

Clinical Features
- The overall incidence of gastric carcinoma is declining, although adenocarcinoma of the cardia region is increasing
- Middle age and older adults
- Nausea, heartburn, anorexia, weakness, and weight loss
- Patients with early gastric carcinoma are often asymptomatic

Cytopathologic Features
- Two major variants: intestinal gland-forming variant and diffuse form
- Intestinal form:
  - Highly cellular smears
  - Numerous 3-D aggregates of crowded cells with loss of polarity
  - Also numerous single (isolated) malignant cells throughout the smear
  - Marked pleomorphism, increased N/C ratios
  - Nuclei are large, round to oval, hyperchromatic, with irregular nuclear contours, thick nuclear membranes, abnormal nuclear chromatin, one to two prominent nucleoli
  - Cytoplasm is fragile, vacuolated to granular and amphophilic
  - Background contains granular necrotic debris and neutrophils
- Diffuse form (signet ring type):
  - Variable number of dispersed solitary tumor cells
  - Cells: single, round, with clear to foamy cytoplasm
  - Single eccentric nucleus
  - Sometimes low N/C ratio
  - Classic signet ring cell: large cytoplasmic mucin vacuole that displaces and distorts the nucleus producing a concave nuclear configuration with sharply pointed tips and angles
  - Nucleus can range from bland to obviously malignant

Special Stains and Immunohistochemistry
- Immunostain for keratins can be helpful to differentiate bland-looking signet ring cells from histiocytes filled with mucin (muciphages)

Modern Techniques for Diagnosis
- EUS-FNA may also increase the diagnostic accuracy for the diffuse type of adenocarcinomas, since this procedure is better suited to sample the involved wall of the stomach

Differential Diagnosis
- Repair (especially in the setting of benign gastric ulcers)
  - The aggregates are monolayered with preserved polarity and "school of fish" pattern
  - The cells are round, regular, and uniform
  - Fine chromatin and prominent nucleoli
  - Lack of single atypical cells
  - (See detailed description of features of repair in the section of differential diagnosis of esophagus adenocarcinoma)
- Dysplasia
  - No or few single atypical cells

■ Normal mucus-producing columnar (foveolar cells) and goblet cells or mucin containing histiocytes (vs. signet ring carcinoma)
➤ Lower nuclear to cytoplasmic ratios
➤ Histiocytes will have a characteristic bean-shaped nucleus that is not distorted by mucin vacuoles
➤ Individually scattered histiocytes and benign glandular cells lack the sharply pointed nuclear tips or flat, long surfaces of carcinoma
➤ Careful search of the smears in signet ring carcinoma will often demonstrate a few scattered cells with obvious malignant features
■ Gastric xanthoma
➤ Rare intramucosal lesions characterized by lipid-containing histiocytes (xanthoma cells)
➤ Can have xanthoma cells in clusters or isolated
➤ Typical xanthoma cells are large with abundant vacuolated cytoplasm and central nucleus with smooth chromatin, well-defined nuclear border, and no nucleoli
➤ Atypical xanthoma cells can be present and mimic signet ring cells
➤ Atypical xanthoma cells have eccentric nucleus with irregular nuclear border and prominent nucleolus, features probably due to degeneration
➤ Xanthoma cells are negative for PAS stain, positive for Oil red O
■ Metastasis
➤ Breast carcinoma (especially lobular)
➤ Bronchogenic carcinoma
➤ Malignant melanoma
➤ Ovarian cancer
➤ Pancreatic carcinoma
➤ Endometrial carcinoma
➤ Renal cell carcinoma

PEARLS

✴ Reparative change is a known pitfall for false-positive diagnosis of adenocarcinoma
✴ Never make an unequivocal diagnosis of malignancy without identifying at least a few isolated (single, not in a cluster), intact, obviously malignant cells
✴ The diagnosis of signet ring type adenocarcinoma can be challenging because the malignant cells can have a very bland appearance or there can be only few malignant cells that can be overlooked or easily confused with benign elements

CARCINOID TUMOR

Clinical Features
■ Adults who present with upper abdominal pain, GI bleeding, or the carcinoid syndrome
■ May arise in association with atrophy of the gastric body, or in patients who have Zollinger–Ellison syndrome with MEN syndrome
■ Endoscopic and gross appearance is that of a small submucosal lesion that may show overlying ulceration
■ EUS-FNA is better than brushings to sample submucosal nodules

Cytopathologic Features
■ Hypercellular smear with relatively clean background, although occasional granular background can be present due to spillage of intracytoplasmic neuroendocrine granules
■ Monotonous population of loosely cohesive small to moderately sized cells

4-12A. Carcinoid *(opposite, left).* Low power characteristic appearance of carcinoid: round, homogeneous cells singly and in small loosely cohesive clusters (modified Giemsa stain)

4-12B. Carcinoid *(opposite, right).* Gastric carcinoid. The cells are round, have mild variation in size, and a fair amount of cytoplasm (modified Giemsa stain)

4-12C. Carcinoid *(middle, left).* The neuroendocrine (salt-and-pepper) chromatin can be better appreciated in the Papanicolaou stain

4-12D. Carcinoid *(middle, right).* Cell block (H&E)

4-12E. Carcinoid *(bottom, left).* Synaptophysin strongly positive

4-12F. Carcinoid *(bottom, right).* Chromogranin strongly positive

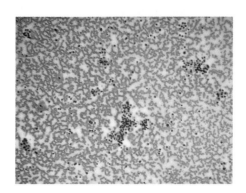
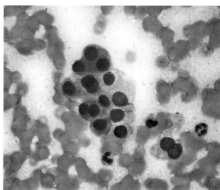
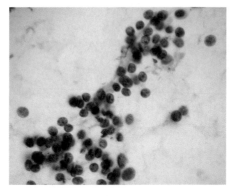
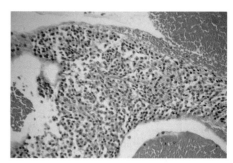
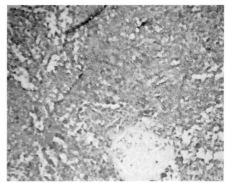
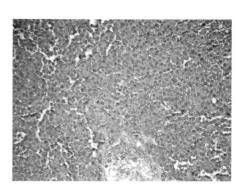

- Low-power architectural patterns: acini, rosettes, sheets, trabeculae, and dispersed single cells
- Round to polyhedral cells with moderate amount of delicate granular cytoplasm
- Round to ovoid nuclei, high N/C ratios, smooth nuclear borders
- Evenly dispersed, finely to moderately granular chromatin (salt and pepper)
- Small to inconspicuous nucleoli

Special Stains and Immunohistochemistry
- Positive for keratin and neuroendocrine markers (synaptophysin, chromogranin, NSE, MAP-2, CD56, CD57)
- Negative for CD45, CD20, CD117 (See below differential diagnosis)

Modern Techniques for Diagnosis
- Noncontributory

Differential Diagnosis
- Chronic inflammation
  - Discohesive cells
  - Polymorphic lymphocytes with variation in size and shape of nuclei
  - Negative for keratin and neuroendocrine markers
- Lymphoma
  - Usually no cohesion, scant cytoplasms
  - Nuclear contour might have clefts and indentations
  - Although the nuclear to cytoplasmic ratios can be high in cells from carcinoid tumor, they are higher in lymphoid lesions
  - The presence of nucleoli and nuclear irregularity would also favor lymphoma
  - Lymphoglandular bodies present, best seen in modified Giemsa stain, but also apparent in Papanicolaou stained smears
  - Negative for keratin and neuroendocrine markers
  - Positive for CD45, most are CD20-positive B-cell lymphomas
- Diffuse type of adenocarcinoma
  - Signet ring: coarse chromatin, sharp points in the nuclear contour, and a single dominant vacuole and moderate N/C ratios
  - The tumor cells show greater pleomorphism with prominent nucleoli and occasional cytoplasmic vacuoles
- Small cell carcinoma (primary and metastatic)
  - The cells from small cell carcinoma have more irregular, angulated nuclei with nuclear molding
  - Hyperchromatic chromatin
  - Extremely high N/C ratios
- Brunner's gland heterotopia:
  - Commonly small, rarely significant lesions
  - Always located in the gastric antrum
- Glomus tumor
  - Cohesive clusters of uniform round to polygonal cells
  - Scant cytoplasm and indistinct cell borders
  - Round hyperchromatic nuclei with homogeneous chromatin
  - Positive for smooth muscle actin and vimentin immunostains
- Heterotopic pancreas
  - Stomach and duodenum around the common bile duct are the most common sites for heterotopic pancreas
  - May present as an intramural nodule or a sessile polyp
  - Can be several centimeters in size
  - Characteristic endoscopic appearance: raised subepithelial mound with central umbilication in the prepyloric antrum
  - EUS-FNA shows a mixture of benign ductal and acinar cells
  - However, some lesions may be largely cystic or composed of ducts only (adenomyoma) and a cytologic diagnosis may not be possible
- Epithelioid GIST
  - Mainly single or small clusters of epithelioid cells with a moderate amount of granular to clear cytoplasm, small uniform nuclei with mild to marked nuclear envelope irregularities
  - Positive for CD117 (c-kit)
  - Negative for keratin and neuroendocrine markers

✶ Think about carcinoid in a loosely cohesive arrangement of bland epithelial cells in the smear
✶ Look for salt-and-pepper chromatin in carcinoid
✶ Keep the extensive differential diagnosis in mind and do immunostains if necessary

GASTROINTESTINAL STROMAL TUMOR (GIST)

Clinical Features
▓ The stomach is the most common organ of origin of GISTs (60–70%),
▓ Patients can present with nonspecific findings of upper GI bleeding and/or pain.
▓ The lesion is submucosal, and can cause a dome-shaped elevation in the mucosa with ulceration.
▓ EUS-FNA is the preferred method for cytology sample.
▓ It is best to avoid the term "benign" for any GIST, all GISTs should be considered potentially malignant.
▓ The relative risk of aggressive behavior can be defined into the following four different risk categories:
  ➤ Very low risk: size less than 2 cm, mitotic count less than 5/50 HPF
  ➤ Low risk: size between 2 and 5cm, mitotic count less than 5/50 HPF
  ➤ Intermediate risk: size less than 5 cm with 6–10 mitoses/50 HPF or size between 5 and 10 cm with mitotic count less than 5/50 HPF
  ➤ High risk: size more than 5 cm with mitotic count more than 5/50 HPF or size bigger than 10 cm with any mitotic rate or any size with a mitotic count of more than 10/50HPF
▓ Other prognostic factors for aggressive behavior include mucosal invasion and/or ulceration, and cystic or necrotic areas within the tumor
▓ Complete surgical resection is the treatment of choice
▓ For inoperable or metastatic tumors, tyrosine kinase inhibitors such as imatinib mesylate (Gleevec®) is the treatment of choice

Cytopathologic Features
▓ EUS-FNA cytology smears show variable numbers of cohesive sheets or clusters of spindle cells with occasional pleomorphism
▓ Variable numbers of single stripped nuclei are usually scattered in the smear background
▓ Relatively bland spindle or epithelioid cells
▓ Moderate cellularity
▓ High nuclear to cytoplasmic ratios
▓ Single elongated nuclei often with blunt ends
▓ Finely granular chromatin, evenly distributed
▓ Inconspicuous nucleoli
▓ Cytoplasm is cyanophilic with indistinct cell borders, causing the tumor cells to blend with each other or into the adjacent stromal matrix
▓ Mitosis, necrosis, and cell pleomorphism may be indicators of aggressive behavior

Special Stains and Immunohistochemistry
▓ Diffuse, strong staining for CD117 is confirmatory (and required for selecting patients for drug therapy)
▓ CD34 positive in 80% of the cases
▓ S-100 protein and smooth muscle actin can be positive or negative, but if CD117 is positive, the diagnosis should be GIST

Modern Techniques for Diagnosis
▨ PCR for c-kit mutations might be needed to diagnose the rare CD117-negative GISTs

Differential Diagnosis
▨ Epithelioid GISTs should be differentiated from:
  ➤ Carcinomas, neuroendocrine tumors, melanomas, glomus tumors, and other epithelioid mesenchymal neoplasms
  ➤ Smears of epithelioid GISTs show single or small clusters of epithelioid cells with a moderate amount of granular to clear cytoplasm, variable nuclear pleomorphism, binucleation, and intranuclear inclusions
▨ Schwannoma
  ➤ Moderately to highly cellular groups of haphazardly arranged bland spindle cells
  ➤ Delicate fibrillary cytoplasm
  ➤ Round to oval, wavy nuclei
  ➤ Positive for S-100, negative for CD117
▨ Leiomyoma
  ➤ Groups have low cellularity
  ➤ Negative for CD117, positive for actins
▨ Leiomyosarcoma
  ➤ Negative for CD117, positive for actins
▨ Granular cell tumors
  ➤ Sheets, clusters, and single cells with large round uniform eccentrically placed nuclei
  ➤ Cytoplasm: purple granular with modified Giemsa stain and cyanophilic with Papanicolaou stain
  ➤ Cell block: nests of cells with abundant granular eosinophilic cytoplasm and round nucleus
  ➤ Positive for S-100 protein
▨ Inflammatory fibroid polyp
  ➤ Negative for CD117, S-100 and actin
  ➤ Positive for CD34
▨ Normal muscularis propria
  ➤ Larger cell size and haphazardly arranged cell fascicles are clues in favor of GIST over normal bowel wall fragments that one might encounter in a routine transmural EUS-FNA

PEARLS

★ Good material for cell block should be obtained for immunostains
★ Although some studies have reported that EUS-FNA can predict behavior of GIST based on size (by imaging), mitotic figures and MIB-1–labeling index, we believe that not all the features can be adequately evaluated by EUS-FNA (such as necrosis and mitotic count), and that cytologic evaluation remains limited in its ability of predicting behavior of GISTs
★ CD117 can be at least focally positive in many tumors other than GIST (synovial sarcoma, malignant fibrous histiocytoma, dermatofibrosarcoma protuberans, fibromatosis, etc.) but fortunately, most do not occur in the GI tract

LYMPHOMA

Clinical Features
▨ Approximately 5% of all gastric cancers
▨ Adults who present with gastric ulcers, obstruction, and/or bleeding

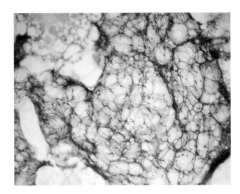

4-13A. Lipoma. Mature adipose cells in EUS-FNA of gastric submucosal lipoma (modified Giemsa stain)

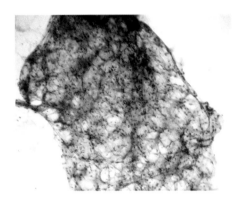

4-13B. Lipoma. Papanicolaou stain in same case as Figure 4-13A (gastric submucosal lipoma)

- Solitary mass having focal or diffuse involvement, can have the appearance of a mural nodule that is ulcerated, or massive rugal enlargement that may be indistinguishable from the more common adenocarcinoma
- Few cases present as multiple polypoid lesions
- Although a variety of different types of lymphoma can involve the stomach, diffuse large B-cell lymphoma and extranodal marginal zone lymphoma (mucosal-associated lymphoid tissue/MALT lymphoma) are the most common
- Intramural lesions might not be sampled by regular endoscopy
- EUS-FNA is a much better technique to obtain material for diagnosis of diffuse large B-cell lymphoma with the use of ancillary studies
- The diagnosis of extranodal marginal zone lymphoma may require the addition of an open biopsy for histomorphology

Cytopathologic Features
- Large numbers of individually scattered lymphoid cells with a uniformly atypical appearance
- Although tumor cells may appear to be crowded or clustered when entrapped in the mucoid exudate, there is no evidence of true cohesion
- Lymphoglandular bodies in the background (pale blue fragments of lymphocyte cytoplasm)
- In large cell lymphoma, the cells have a single nucleus with thick and sometimes irregularly shaped nuclear membranes, vesicular chromatin, and one or more conspicuous nucleoli with surrounding scanty cytoplasm, resulting in high nuclear-to-cytoplasmic ratios
- In MALT lymphoma, the atypical lymphoid cells are smaller with higher nuclear to cytoplasmic ratios, the chromatin is darker and nucleoli will be small
- Although a few neutrophils may be present, they do not make up a significant portion of the cellular infiltrate

Special Stains and Immunohistochemistry
- Most are CD20+ B-cell lymphomas
- Diffuse large B-cell lymphomas can be positive for CD10 and bcl-6
- MALT lymphomas are positive for CD20 and CD43, and negative for the markers for other small cell lymphomas: CD5, CD23, CD10, cyclin D-1, bcl-6

Modern Techniques for Diagnosis
- Flow cytometry, molecular diagnostics, cytogenetic studies

Differential Diagnosis
- Benign chronic inflammation (vs. low-grade lymphoma)
  - Inflammation should have a polymorphic population of lymphoid cells rather than the uniform population of atypical lymphoid cells in lymphoma
  - Tingible body macrophages and follicle center cell fragments may be present and are very helpful to support a reactive lymphoid processes
  - MALT lymphoma can have a prominent plasma cell component and admixed polymorphic population of cells. It can also show occasionally follicle center fragments and tingible body macrophages. Therefore, it may be impossible to diagnose MALT lymphoma by cytology and tissue biopsy remains the standard
- Diffuse form of gastric adenocarcinoma
  - Greater amount of cytoplasm and have eccentrically placed nuclei that are often displaced by an obvious mucin vacuole

➤ With careful searching of the smears, a few groups of truly cohesive epithelial cells will often be appreciated
➤ Positive for cytokeratin
■ Carcinoid tumors (vs. MALT lymphoma)
➤ There is some cohesion of cells
➤ The cells have more cytoplasm
➤ The nuclei are round, the chromatin is fine (salt and pepper)
➤ Lack prominent nucleoli
➤ Positive for cytokeratin, negative for CD45 and CD20
■ Stromal tumors
➤ Can also consist of individually scattered cells
➤ However, the cells tend to have a spindle or elongated configurations, with generally fine delicate chromatin and lack prominent nucleoli

PEARLS

★ It might not be possible to diagnose MALT lymphoma by cytology
★ If at the time of the on-site preliminary interpretation a lymphoma is suspected, specimens (additional passes) for flow cytometry and possibly other ancillary studies should be obtained

DUODENUM

INFECTIOUS AGENTS

Clinical Features
■ Nonspecific, often associated with concurrent or prior peptic ulcers
■ *Giardia lamblia*: more frequent in children, may be asymptomatic (carriers), or have severe diarrhea
■ In immunocompromised patients: Chronic diarrhea with fever: CMV, cryptosporidium, microsporidium, mycobacteria

Cytopathologic Features
■ Mixed inflammatory cell infiltrate, reparative changes, and gastric surface cell metaplasia can be present. Cytologic smears will resemble those obtained from *Helicobacter*-associated gastritis
■ For specific microorganism: see "differential diagnosis" below

Special Stains and Immunohistochemistry
■ Acid-fast stains for mycobacteria
■ Air-dried Romanowsky stain (modifed Giemsa Stain): is easier than Papanicolaou to see some microorganisms such as Giardia
■ Immunoperoxidase stain for CMV can be useful if routine cytology stains show cells that are suspicious but not diagnostic

Modern Techniques for Diagnosis
■ Transmucosal FNA cytology has been shown to be valuable in the diagnosis of mycobacterial infections

Differential Diagnosis
■ Giardia trophozoites
➤ Pear shaped, 12–15 μm
➤ When seen on edge: sickle-shaped configuration
➤ Two "mirror image nuclei"

- CMV
  - ➤ Cytoplasmic inclusions can also be seen
  - ➤ Nuclear and cytoplasmic enlargement (huge cells!)
  - ➤ Large basophilic nuclear inclusions surrounded by a halo
- Cryptosporidium
  - ➤ Cryptosporidium measuring 2–4 μm in diameter and having round to pyramidal shapes may be identified either lying freely or more characteristically, aligned along the luminal surface of the normal glandular cells
  - ➤ With the modified Giemsa–stained smear, the organisms have a basophilic stippled appearance
- Mycobacteria
  - ➤ Brushings are generally nondiagnostic
  - ➤ Necrotic debris, lymphocytes, and epithelioid histiocytes, sometimes granulomas
  - ➤ The smears from atypical mycobacteria can have pale macrophages having a striated pseudo-Gaucher appearance in the Papanicolaou-stained smears
  - ➤ With the use of air-dried or Wright-stained smears, the diagnostic negative images of the atypical mycobacterium comprising the *Mycobacterium avium* (MAI) complex can be identified

PEARLS

★ Look carefully for microorganisms if clinical history of immunosuppression

PEPTIC ULCER

Clinical Features
- Despite the fact that peptic ulcers are more common in the duodenum than in the stomach, histologic and cytologic exams are less often employed

Cytopathologic Features
- The cytologic findings recapitulate those seen in the gastric ulcers
- Flat sheets of benign glandular cells, including occasional groups showing reparative changes, as well as associated neutrophils and granular necrotic debris
- *Helicobacter*-type organisms may also be present (see description of *Helicobacter* organisms in the "Gastritis" section)

Special Stains and Immunohistochemistry
- Noncontributory

Modern Techniques for Diagnosis
- Noncontributory

Differential Diagnosis
- Ulcerations due to infections: mycobacteria, cytomegalovirus

PEARLS

★ In contrast to the stomach, almost all the duodenal ulcers are benign

ADENOCARCINOMA

Clinical Features
- Most common cancer involving the duodenum
- Jaundice, anemia, and/or obstructive symptoms

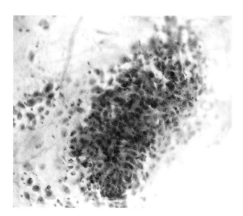

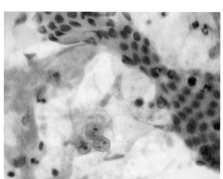

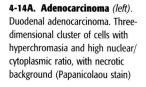

4-14A. Adenocarcinoma *(left).* Duodenal adenocarcinoma. Three-dimensional cluster of cells with hyperchromasia and high nuclear/cytoplasmic ratio, with necrotic background (Papanicolaou stain)

4-14B. Adenocarcinoma *(right).* Duodenal adenocarcinoma. As a cell-size reference, a cluster of benign epithelial cells is present on the top right. Compare with the much larger three malignant cells in the bottom center (Papanicolaou stain)

4-14C. Adenocarcinoma *(down).* Duodenal adenocarcinoma. Cells with prominent nucleoli and nuclear membrane irregularity resembling "bites" (Papanicolaou stain)

▨ In the duodenum, adenocarcinoma frequently involves the region of the ampulla of Vater, where it presents as an exophytic mass

▨ Less frequently, adenocarcinoma can involve the distal small bowel where it often presents as a napkin-ring growth causing obstruction

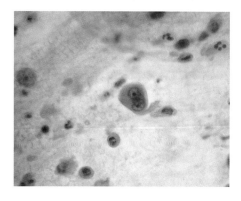

Cytopathologic Features
▨ The smears tend to be cellular with numerous malignant cells arranged in loose clusters, aggregates, and individually

Special Stains and Immunohistochemistry
▨ Noncontributory

Modern Techniques for Diagnosis
▨ Noncontributory

Differential Diagnosis
▨ Villous adenoma
➤ The presence of single cells favor adenocarcinoma, but it may not be possible to distinguish adenoma from adenocarcinoma in cytology
▨ Repair
➤ "School-of-fish" arrangement, uniform cells, fine chromatin, prominent nucleoli, low N/C ratios, lack of single atypical cells
➤ (See detailed description of features of repair in the section of differential diagnosis of esophagus adenocarcinoma)
▨ Metastatic malignancy
➤ Melanoma
➤ Carcinomas of the breast, ovary, and lung

PEARLS

★ Due to the extensive surgical treatment (Whipple), extreme caution is needed, be conservative and if in doubt recommend a biopsy

CARCINOID TUMOR

Clinical Features
▨ Can cause symptoms due to local infiltration: jaundice, pancreatitis, hemorrhage and intestinal obstruction
▨ Less frequently, can cause symptoms due to hormones produced

4-15A. Carcinoid *(top, left).*
Loosely cohesive round homogeneous cells (modified Giemsa stain)

4-15B. Carcinoid *(top, right).*
Nuclear detail can be better appreciated in Papanicolaou stain

4-15C. Carcinoid *(bottom, left).*
Cell block (H&E)

4-15D. Carcinoid *(bottom, right).*
Positive immunostain for synaptophysin

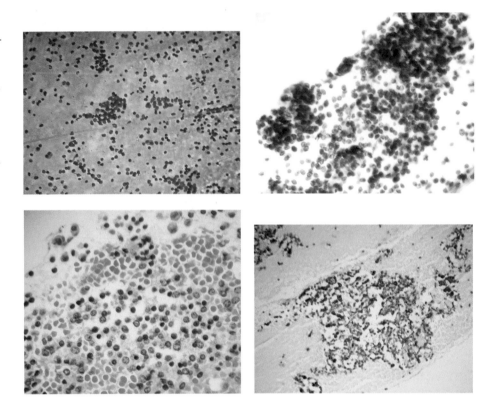

Cytopathologic Features
■ The cytologic features recapitulate those described for the stomach

Special Stains and Immunohistochemistry
■ Positive for keratin and neuroendocrine markers (synaptophysin, chromogranin, NSE, MAP-2, CD56, CD57)
■ Negative for CD45, CD20, CD117 (helpful in the differential diagnosis with lymphoma and GIST)

Modern Techniques for Diagnosis
■ Noncontributory

Differential Diagnosis
■ Brunner's gland hyperplasia
  ➤ Commonly found incidentally in the duodenum
  ➤ Presents as multiple small nodules at endoscopy
  ➤ Has no clinical significance
■ Brunner's gland hamartoma
  ➤ Located in the submucosa and muscularis propria
  ➤ Can be hyperechoic or cystic on EUS and ulcerated on endoscopy mimicking neoplasia
  ➤ Often composed of multiple tissue types, including pancreatic tissue, and is surrounded by a fibrous capsule
  ➤ Mucosal biopsies may be nondiagnostic
  ➤ EUS-FNA reveals glandular epithelium without atypia
■ Lymphoma, chronic inflammation, epithelioid GIST (see differential diagnosis of carcinoids in the stomach section)

★ (See detailed description of carcinoids in the stomach section)

GASTROINTESTINAL STROMAL TUMOR (GIST)

Clinical Features
▦ 20–30% of the GISTs occur in the small bowel
▦ The lesion is submucosal, EUS-FNA is the preferred method for cytology sample

Cytopathologic Features
▦ Similar to gastric GIST

Special Stains and Immunohistochemistry
▦ CD117 (c-kit) positive, CD34 positive in 80% of cases, variable staining for S-100 and actin

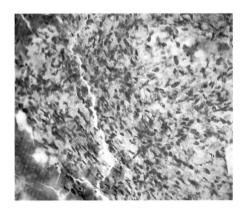
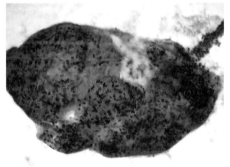

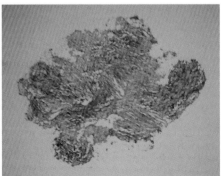
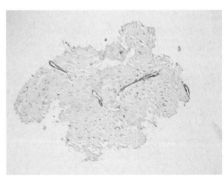

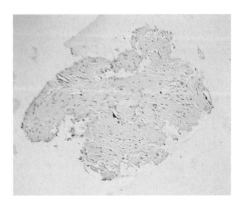
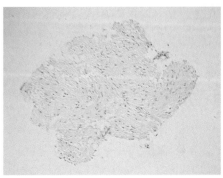

4-16A. Gastrointestinal stromal tumor *(top, left)*. GIST (Gastrointestinal stromal tumor) of duodenum. EUS-FNA shows hypercellular clusters of spindle cells (modified Giemsa stain)

4-16B. Gastrointestinal stromal tumor *(top, right)*. Papanicolaou stain in same case of Figure 4-16A (Duodenal GIST)

4-16C. Gastrointestinal stromal tumor *(middle, left)*. Immunostains performed on cell block of case of Figures 4-16A and 4-16B. Positive C-kit (CD117)

4-16D. Gastrointestinal stromal tumor *(middle, right)*. Negative CD34, showing an internal control staining in small vessels

4-16E. Gastrointestinal stromal tumor *(bottom, left)*. Negative smooth muscle actin

4-16F. Gastrointestinal stromal tumor *(bottom, right)* Negative S-100

Modern Techniques for Diagnosis
■ Genetic analysis for c-kit mutations might be needed to diagnose the rare CD117-negative GISTs

Differential Diagnosis
■ Epithelioid GISTs should be differentiated from carcinomas, neuroendocrine tumors, melanomas, glomus tumors, and other epithelioid mesenchymal neoplasms (see differential diagnosis of GISTs in the stomach section)
■ Spindle cell GISTs should be differentiated from normal muscularis propria, schwannomas, leiomyoma, leiomyosarcoma (see differential diagnosis of GISTs in the stomach section)

PEARLS

★ See detailed description of GISTs in the stomach section

LYMPHOMA

Clinical Features
■ Most lymphomas of the small intestine occur distal to the duodenum; therefore, there is infrequent sampling by endoscopic biopsies or brushings
■ Abdominal pain, obstruction, weight loss, diarrhea, and abdominal mass

Cytopathologic Features
■ Cytologic findings in duodenal lymphomas resemble those seen in the stomach
■ The majority of the non-Hodgkin's lymphoma is of B-cell type

Special Stains and Immunohistochemistry
■ Positive for CD45, CD20 and other lymphoma markers, negative for cytokeratin

Modern Techniques for Diagnosis
■ Flow cytometry, FISH, PCR for specific mutations

Differential Diagnosis
■ Carcinoid
  ➤ Loosely cohesive cells
  ➤ More cytoplasm
  ➤ Salt-and-pepper chromatin
  ➤ Positive for keratin and neuroendocrine markers
■ Small cell carcinoma
  ➤ True nuclear molding
  ➤ Homogeneous chromatin
  ➤ Rare in this location
  ➤ Positive for keratin and negative for CD45
■ Benign chronic inflammation
  ➤ Inflammation should have a polymorphic population of lymphoid cells rather than the uniform population of atypical lymphoid cells in lymphoma
  ➤ Tingible body macrophages and follicle center cell fragments (fragments of germinal centers) may be present and are very helpful to support a reactive lymphoid processes

★ If at the time of the on-site preliminary interpretation a lymphoma is suspected, specimens (additional passes) for flow cytometry and possibly other ancillary studies should be obtained

LARGE INTESTINE

INFLAMMATORY BOWEL DISEASE

Clinical Features
▦ Patients with idiopathic inflammatory bowel disease (especially ulcerative colitis) are at increased risk to develop colorectal adenocarcinoma

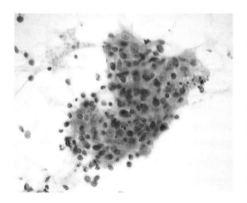
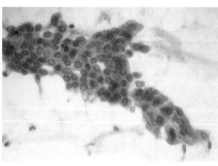

4-17A. Inflammatory bowel disease *(left)*. Colon brushing in inflammatory bowel disease shows reactive glandular epithelium admixed with acute inflammation (Papanicolaou stain)

4-17B. Inflammatory bowel disease *(right)*. Streaming effect (repair) in inflammatory bowel disease (Papanicolaou stain)

▦ Surveillance programs for dysplasia and early carcinomas include colonoscopies with biopsies
▦ Brushing cytology has been used in a few centers as a complimentary tool to biopsies
▦ Brushing is now seldom used and the main indication appears to be when a stricture does not allow advancement of the endoscope for visualization and biopsy

Cytopathologic Features – Inflammatory Bowel Disease without Dysplasia
▦ Reparative glandular epithelium and inflammation
▦ Cohesive groups of enlarged glandular epithelial cells
▦ Prominent nuclei with thick membranes and macronucleoli
▦ Marked neutrophilic inflammation in active disease
▦ Granulomas might be identified in patients with Crohn's disease
▦ Low-power arrangement: flat sheets with well-defined cell borders and preserved polarity
▦ The "streaming" nature of the cells is also a helpful feature
▦ Individually scattered intact atypical cells are nonexistent or very few in numbers

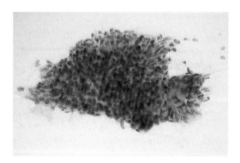

Special Stains and Immunohistochemistry
▦ Noncontributory

Modern Techniques for Diagnosis
▦ Noncontributory

4-17C. Dysplasia in inflammatory bowel disease. Rectal brushing with dysplasia showing aggregate of cells with loss of polarity and increased nuclear/cytoplasmic ratio (Papanicolaou stain)

Differential Diagnosis

■ Dysplasia

➤ Nuclei are larger than those seen in repair

➤ Chromatin is moderate to coarsely granular and hyperchromatic

➤ Nuclear membranes can be smooth or show some slight nuclear irregularity

➤ Nucleoli may be single or multiple and large

➤ Increased nuclear to cytoplasmic ratios

➤ The dysplastic cells are arranged in small aggregates with loss of polarity

➤ Abnormal nuclei can be crowded, overlapping, or show molding

➤ Syncytial pattern: groups of cells with merging of cytoplasmic borders and loss of polarity

■ Adenocarcinoma

➤ Individually scattered atypical cells

➤ However, reliably differentiating high-grade dysplasia from well-differentiated adenocarcinoma may not be possible in cytologic preparations

PEARLS

✭ Preserved polarity and "school of fish" are features of reactive/repair

✭ Crowded overlapping groups, syncytial groups and single atypical cells are features worrisome for dysplasia/adenocarcinoma

ADENOMAS AND ADENOCARCINOMA

Clinical Features

▦ Most often adults in the fifth and sixth decades

▦ Adenomas are precursors to adenocarcinoma

▦ Adenocarcinomas can be asymptomatic or present with rectal bleeding, anemia, obstruction, and/or change in bowel habits

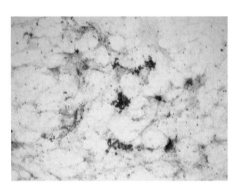

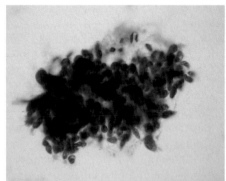

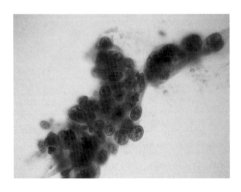

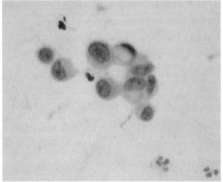

4-18A. Adenocarcinoma *(top, left).* Necrotic background in brushing of colonic carcinoma (Papanicolaou stain)

4-18B. Adenocarcinoma *(top, right).* Adenocarcinoma of colon. Three-dimensional aggregate of crowded cells with marked hyperchromasia and elongated pleomorphic nuclei (Papanicolaou stain)

4-18C. Adenocarcinoma *(bottom, left).* Marked pleomorphism and loss of polarity in colonic adenocarcinoma (Papanicolaou stain)

4-18D. Signet-ring cell adenocarcinoma *(bottom, right).* Signet ring cell in colonic adenocarcinoma (Papanicolaou stain)

■ Cytologic examination of colorectal adenomas have limited value since adenomas are often amenable to complete removal by polypectomy
■ The major use of brushing cytology is to sample colonic strictures when the biopsy forceps cannot pass the stricture site

Cytopathologic Features
■ Cellular smears with small to large three-dimensional groups of glandular cells
■ Villous adenomas: branched papillary patterns can be appreciated at low magnification
■ The nuclei can be crowded, overlapped, and stratified
■ The nuclei are elongated, cigar shaped, hyperchromatic, and pleomorphic
■ Cells have one or more nucleoli that vary in size from small to large
■ Individually dispersed abnormal cells favor a diagnosis of adenocarcinoma over adenoma
■ A necrotic background can be observed

Special Stains and Immunohistochemistry
■ Noncontributory

Modern Techniques for Diagnosis
■ Noncontributory

Differential Diagnosis
■ Repair
➤ Flat cohesive sheets of uniform cells with a "school-of-fish" arrangement
➤ Round to oval enlarged nuclei with smooth and regular nuclear membranes
➤ Fine chromatin and prominent nucleoli
➤ Low N/C ratios, absence of atypical single cells
➤ (See detailed description of features of repair in the section of differential diagnosis of esophagus adenocarcinoma)
■ Other primary and secondary cancers
➤ Lymphoma
➤ Melanoma
➤ GISTs
➤ Small cell carcinoma of the colon arising underneath a villous adenoma of colon and metastasizing to distant sites have also been reported
■ Endometriosis
➤ May rarely produce a colonic obstruction
➤ FNA will show sheets of tightly cohesive, three-dimensional groups of small glandular cells reminiscent of endometrial cells
➤ Hemosiderin-laden macrophages and stromal cells with elongated nuclei and little or no cytoplasm might be seen

PEARLS

★ Carcinomas cannot be cytologically differentiated from adenomas

ANUS

SQUAMOUS DYSPLASIA AND HPV

Clinical Features
■ Major risk factors: HPV infection, anoreceptive intercourse, and HIV infection

4-19A. Unsatisfactory specimen *(top, left)*. Anal brushing: A sample composed predominantly of anucleated squamous cells is unsatisfactory for evaluation (Papanicolaou stain)

4-19B. Ascus *(top, right)*. ASCUS (Atypical squamous cells of undetermined significance) in anal brushing (Papanicolaou stain)

4-19C. Low grade squamous intraepithelial lesion *(bottom, left)*. Anal brushing: Low-grade squamous intraepithelial lesion (LSIL) (Papanicolaou stain)

4-19D. Low grade intraepithelial lesion *(bottom, right)*. LSIL with HPV effect. Koilocyte with clear perinuclear zone and peripheral rim of dense cytoplasm (Papanicolaou stain)

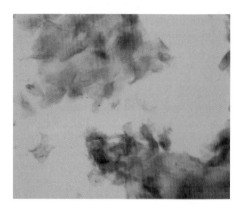
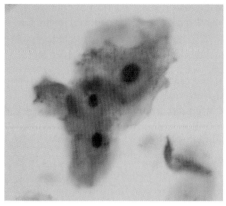
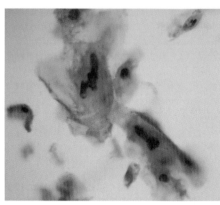
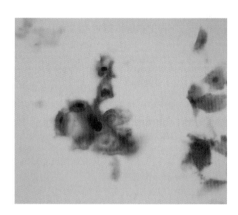

▦ HPV types 6 and 11 are most often associated with condyloma and low-grade dysplasia

▦ HPV types 16 and 18 have a greater association with high-grade dysplasia and carcinoma

▦ Anal–rectal brushing cytology has been used as a screening method for high-risk populations

Cytopathologic Features

▦ Diagnostic criteria and terminology are similar to cervical cytology
▦ Adequacy of the sample: the cellularity should approach that of a cervical sample
   ➤ Conventional smears: minimal cellularity 2000–3000 nucleated squamous cells
   ➤ Liquid-based Thinprep®: approximately one to two nucleated squamous cells per high-power field (40× objective)
   ➤ Liquid-based Surepath®: approximately three to six nucleated squamous cells per high-power field (40× objective)
   ➤ A sample composed predominantly of anucleated squames or mostly obscured by fecal material is unsatisfactory for evaluation
▦ The presence of anal transformation zone components (rectal columnar cells and/or squamous metaplastic cells) should be noted in the report
▦ An association between presence of columnar cells and anal intraepithelial lesion has been reported; however, a specimen without columnar cells should not be regarded unsatisfactory based on the current available data
▦ LSIL:
   ➤ Cells with all the following:
   ➤ "Mature," abundant well-defined cytoplasm
   ➤ Nuclear enlargement more than three times the area of normal intermediate nuclei

➤ Hyperchromasia, variation in size and shape of nuclei
➤ Cells can have either a single nucleus or be binucleated or multinucleated

▦ Koilocytes:
➤ Sharply delineated clear perinuclear zone and a peripheral rim of densely stained cytoplasm and large hyperchromatic dysplastic nuclei
➤ Less frequently present than in cervical cytology
➤ Helpful but not required for interpretation of LSIL

▦ ASC-US (Atypical squamous cells of undetermined significance):
➤ Nuclei 2 to 3× the area of the nucleus of a normal intermediate squamous cell nucleus
➤ Minimal nuclear hyperchromasia and irregularity in shape and chromatin distribution
➤ Slight increased N/C ratios
➤ Cells do not meet the criteria required for an interpretation of LSIL

▦ HSIL:
➤ N/C ratios are much higher than in LSIL
➤ Cytoplasm: "immature," metaplastic or orangeophilic (keratinization)
➤ Overall cell size is smaller than LSIL
➤ Nuclear membrane has irregular contour with indentations or grooves
➤ Nucleoli generally absent

Special Stains and Immunohistochemistry
▦ Noncontributory

Modern Techniques for Diagnosis
▦ Automated monolayer preparations (liquid-based cytology) enhance the diagnostic yield for anal dysplasia compared to conventional smears
▦ Reflex HPV testing by hybrid capture is helpful in triaging patients with a diagnosis of ASC-US

Differential Diagnosis
■ Herpes has also been diagnosed with brushing cytology:
➤ Multinucleated cells with molding nuclei, "ground-glass" chromatin with margination, and can have intranuclear inclusions
■ Squamous cell carcinoma
➤ Numerous pleomorphic cells, with irregular nuclear membranes, uneven chromatin distribution, hyperchromasia, often keratinized
➤ Prominent nucleoli
➤ Tumor diathesis may be present

PEARLS

✶ Criteria and terminology for HPV and dysplasia are similar to cervical/vaginal cytology

REFERENCES

CANDIDAL ESOPHAGITIS

Bronner MP, Geisinger KR. The esophagus. In Silverberg SG, DeLellis RA, Frable WJ, LiVolsi VA, and , Wick MR, editors. *Principles and Practice of Surgical Pathology and Cytopathology*, 4th ed. Philadelphia: Elsevier (Churchill Livingstone), 2006, pp. 1281–1319.

Geisinger KR, Stanley MW, Raab SS, Silverman JF, and , Abati A. *Modern Cytopathology*. Philadelphia: Churchill Livingstone, 2004, pp. 257–309.

Geisinger KR. Endoscopic biopsies and cytologic brushings of the esophagus are diagnostically complementary. *Am J Clin Pathol.* 1995;103:295–9.

Jhala N, and , Jhala D. Gastrointestinal tract cytology: advancing horizons. *Adv Anat Pathol.* 2003;10:261–77.

Wang HH, Jonasson JG, and , Ducatman BS. Brushing cytology of the upper gastrointestinal tract. Obsolete or not? *Acta Cytol.* 1991;35:195–8.

Wright RG, Augustine B, and , Whitfield A. *Candida* in gastroesophageal cytological and histological preparations: a comparative study. *Labmedica.* 1987;4:29–30.

Young JA, and , Elias E. Gastroesophageal candidiasis: diagnosis by brush cytology. *J Clin Pathol* 1985;38:293–6.

HERPETIC ESOPHAGITIS

Bronner MP, Geisinger KR. The esophagus. In Silverberg SG, DeLellis RA, Frable WJ, LiVolsi VA, and , Wick MR, editors. *Principles and Practice of Surgical Pathology and Cytopathology*, 4th ed. Philadelphia: Elsevier (Churchill Livingstone), 2006, pp. 1281–1319.

Geisinger KR, Stanley MW, Raab SS, Silverman JF, and , Abati A. *Modern Cytopathology.* Philadelphia: Churchill Livingstone, 2004, pp. 257–309.

Jhala N, and , Jhala D. Gastrointestinal tract cytology: advancing horizons. *Adv Anat Pathol.* 2003;10:261–77.

Lightdale CJ, Wolf DJ, Marcucci BA, and , Salyer WR. *Herpetic esophagitis in patients with cancer: antemortem diagnosis by brush cytology.* 1977;39:223–6.

Ramanathan J, Rammouni M, Baran Jr J, and , Khatib R. Herpes simplex virus esophagitis in the immunocompetent host: an overview. *Am J Gastroent.* 2000;95(9):2171–6.

Teot LA, Geisinger KR, and . Diagnostic esophageal cytology and its histologic basis. In Castell DO, editor. *The Esophagus*, 2nd ed. Boston: Little, Brown, 1995, pp. 179–204.

CYTOMEGALOVIRUS (CMV) ESOPHAGITIS

Bronner MP, Geisinger KR. The esophagus. In Silverberg SG, DeLellis RA, Frable WJ, LiVolsi VA, and , Wick MR, editors. *Principles and Practice of Surgical Pathology and Cytopathology*, 4th ed. Philadelphia: Elsevier (Churchill Livingstone), 2006, pp. 1281–1319.

Geisinger KR, Stanley MW, Raab SS, Silverman JF, and , Abati A. *Modern Cytopathology.* Philadelphia: Churchill Livingstone, 2004, pp. 257–309.

Geisinger KR. Endoscopic biopsies and cytologic brushings of the esophagus are diagnostically complementary. *Am J Clin Pathol.* 1995;103:295–9.

Jhala N, and , Jhala D. Gastrointestinal tract cytology: advancing horizons. *Adv Anat Pathol.* 2003;10:261–77.

Teot LA, Ducatman BS, and , Geisinger KR. Cytologic diagnosis for cytomegalovirus esophagitis: a report of three acquired immunodeficiency syndrome-related cases. *Acta Cytol.* 1993;37:93–96

Teot LA, Geisinger KR, and . Diagnostic esophageal cytology and its histologic basis. In Castell DO, editor. *The Esophagus*, 2nd ed. Boston: Little, Brown, 1995, pp. 179–204.

RADIATION- AND CHEMOTHERAPY-RELATED ESOPHAGITIS

Berthrong M, and , Fajardo LF. Radiation injury in surgical pathology II. Alimentary tract. *Am J Surg Pathol.* 1981;5:153–78.

Geisinger KR, Stanley MW, Raab SS, Silverman JF, and , Abati A. *Modern Cytopathology.* Philadelphia: Churchill Livingstone, 2004, pp. 257–309.

Geisinger KR, Wang HH, Ducatman BS, Teot LA, and . Gastrointestinal cytology. In Hajdu SI, editor. *Values and Limitations of Cytologic Examinations.* Vol. 11. Philadelphia: WB Saunders, 1991, pp. 403–441.

O'Morchoe PJ, Lee DC, and , Kozak CA. Esophageal cytology in patients receiving cytotoxic drug therapy. *Acta Cytol.* 1983;27:630–634.

Teot LA, Geisinger KR, and . Diagnostic esophageal cytology and its histologic basis. In Castell DO, editor. *The Esophagus*, 2nd ed. Boston: Little, Brown, 1995, pp. 179–204.

GASTROESOPHAGEAL REFLUX DISEASE (GERD)

Bronner MP, Geisinger KR. The esophagus. In Silverberg SG, DeLellis RA, Frable WJ, LiVolsi VA, and , Wick MR, editors. *Principles and Practice of Surgical Pathology and Cytopathology*, 4th ed. Philadelphia: Elsevier (Churchill Livingstone), 2006, pp. 1281–1319.

Geisinger KR, Stanley MW, Raab SS, Silverman JF, and , Abati A. *Modern Cytopathology.* Philadelphia: Churchill Livingstone, 2004, pp. 257–309.

Geisinger KR. Endoscopic biopsies and cytologic brushings of the esophagus are diagnostically complementary. *Am J Clin Pathol.* 1995;103:295–9.

Geisinger KR, and . Histopathology of human reflux esophagitis and experimental esophagitis in animals. In Castell DO, editor. *The Esophagus,* 2nd Ed. Boston: Little Brown, 1995, pp. 481–503.

Teot LA, Geisinger KR, and . Diagnostic esophageal cytology and its histologic basis. In Castell DO, editor. *The Esophagus,* 2nd ed. Boston: Little, Brown, 1995, pp. 179–204.

BARRETT'S ESOPHAGUS

Chu PG. Jiang Z., and Weiss LM. Hepatocyte antigen as a marker of intestinal metaplasia. *Am J Surg Pathol.* 2003;27(7):952–9.

Falk GW. Cytology in Barrett's esophagus. *Gastrointest Endosc Clin North Am.* 2003;13(2):335–48.

Geisinger KR, Teot LA, and , Richter JE. A comparative cytopathologic and histologic study of atypia, dysplasia and adenocarcinoma in Barrett's esophagus. *Cancer.* 1992;69:8–16.

Haggitt RC. Barrett's esophagus, dysplasia, and adenocarcinoma. *Hum Pathol.* 1994;25:982–993.

Jhala N, and , Jhala D. Gastrointestinal tract cytology: advancing horizons. *Adv Anat Pathol.* 2003;10:261–77.

Robey SS, Hamilton SR, Gupta PK, and , Erozan YS. Diagnostic value of cytopathology in Barrett's esophagus and associated carcinoma. *Am J Clin Pathol.* 1988;89:493–8.

Saad RS, Mahood LK, Clary KM, Liu Y, Silverman JF, and , Raab SS. Role of cytology in the diagnosis of Barrett's esophagus and associated neoplasia. *Diagn Cytopathol* 2003;29:130–5.

Wang HH, and , DrPH, Sovie S, et al. Value of cytology in detecting intestinal metaplasia and associated dysplasia at the gastroesophageal junction. *Hum Pathol.* 1997;28:465–71.

Wang HH, Ducatman BS, and , Thibault S. Cytologic features of premalignant glandular lesions in the upper gastrointestinal tract. *Acta Cytol.* 1991;35:199–203.

DYSPLASIA IN BARRETT'S

Geisinger KR, Teot LA, and , Richter JE. A comparative cytopathologic and histologic study of atypia, dysplasia and adenocarcinoma in Barrett's esophagus. *Cancer.* 1992;69:8–16.

Jhala N, and , Jhala D. Gastrointestinal tract cytology: advancing horizons. *Adv Anat Pathol.* 2003;10:261–77.

Robertson CS, Mayberry JF, and , Nicholson DA, et al. Value of endoscopic surveillance in the detection of neoplastic change in Barrett's esophagus. *Br J Surg.* 1988;75:760–3.

Robey SS, Hamilton SR, Gupta PK, and , Erozan YS. Diagnostic value of cytopathology in Barrett's esophagus and associated carcinoma. *Am J Clin Pathol.* 1988;89:493–8.

Saad RS, Mahood LK, Clary KM, Liu Y, Silverman JF, and , Raab SS. Role of cytology in the diagnosis of Barrett's esophagus and associated neoplasia. *Diagn Cytopathol.* 2003;29:130–5.

Wang HH, Doria MI, and , Purohit-Buch S, et al. Barrett's esophagus: the cytology of dysplasia in comparison to benign and malignant lesions. *Acta Cytol.* 1992;36:60–4.

Wang HH, and , DrPH, Sovie S, et al. Value of cytology in detecting intestinal metaplasia and associated dysplasia at the gastroesophageal junction. *Hum Pathol.* 1997;28:465–71.

Wang HH, Ducatman BS, and , Thibault S. Cytologic features of premalignant glandular lesions in the upper gastrointestinal tract. *Acta Cytol.* 1991;35:199–203.

SQUAMOUS CELL CARCINOMA

Bishop D, Lushpihan AR, and , Louis C. The cytology of carcinoma in situ and early invasive carcinoma of the esophagus. *Acta Cytol.* 1977;21:298–300.

Dawsey SM, Yu Y, and , Taylor PR, et al. Esophageal cytology and subsequent risk of cancer. A prospective follow-up study from Linxian, China. *Acta Cytol.* 1994;38:183–92.

Dowlatshahi K, Skinner DB, and , DeMeester TR, et al. Evaluation of brush cytology as an independent technique for detection of esophageal carcinoma. *J Thorac Cardiovasc Surg.* 1985;89:848–51.

Geisinger KR, Wang HH, Ducatman BS, Teot LA, and . Gastrointestinal cytology. In Hajdu SI, editor. *Values and Limitations of Cytologic Examinations.* Vol. 11. Philadelphia: WB Saunders, 1991, pp. 403–41.

Haddad NG, Fleischer DE, and . Neoplasms of the esophagus. In Castell DO, editor. *The Esophagus.* 2nd Ed. Boston: Little, Brown, 1995, pp. 269–91.

Jhala N, and , Jhala D. Gastrointestinal tract cytology: advancing horizons. *Adv Anat Pathol.* 2003;10:261–77.

Shen Q, Liu SF, and , Dawsey SM, et al. Cytologic screening for esophageal cancer: results from 12,877 subjects from a high-risk population in China. *Int J Cancer.* 1993;54:185–8.

Shu Y-J. Cytopathology of the esophagus. An overview of esophageal cytopathology in China. *Acta Cytol.* 1983;27:7–16.

Shu Y-J. *The Cytopathology of Esophageal Carcinoma. Precancerous Lesions and Early Cancer.* New York: Masson, 1985.

Teot LA, Geisinger KR, and . Diagnostic esophageal cytology and its histologic basis. In Castell DO, editor. *The Esophagus.* 2nd Ed. Boston: Little, Brown, 1995, pp. 179–204.

ADENOCARCINOMA

Belladonna JA, Hajdu SI, Bains MS, and , Winawer SJ. Adenocarcinoma in situ of Barrett's esophagus diagnosed by endoscopic cytology. *N Engl J Med.* 1974;291:895–6.

Caos A, Olson N, Willman C, and , Gogel HK. *Endoscopic "salvage" cytology in neoplasms metastatic to the upper gastrointestinal tract.* 1986;30:32–34.

Geisinger KR, Teot LA, and , Richter JE. A comparative cytopathologic and histologic study of atypia, dysplasia and adenocarcinoma in Barrett's esophagus. *Cancer.* 1992;69:8–16.

Hamilton SR, Smith RRL, and , Cameron JL. Prevalence and characteristics of Barrett's esophagus in patients with adenocarcinoma of the esophagus or esophagogastric junction. *Hum Pathol.* 1988;19:942–8.

Kadakia SC, Parker A, and , Canales L. Metastatic tumors to the upper gastrointestinal tract: endoscopic experience. *Am J Gastroenterol.* 1992;87:1418–1423.

Robey SS, Hamilton SR, Gupta PK, and , Erozan YS. Diagnostic value of cytopathology in Barrett's esophagus and associated carcinoma. *Am J Clin Pathol.* 1988;89:493–498.

Saad RS, Mahood LK, Clary KM, Liu Y, Silverman JF, and , Raab SS. Role of cytology in the diagnosis of Barrett's esophagus and associated neoplasia. *Diagn Cytopathol.* 2003;29:130–5.

Shurbaji MS, and , Erozan YS. The cytopathologic diagnosis of esophageal adenocarcinoma. *Acta Cytol.* 1991;35:189–94.

Sobel JM, Lai R, Mallery S, Levy MJ, Wiersema MJ, Greenwald BD, and , Gunaratnam NT. The utility of EUS-guided FNA in the diagnosis of metastatic breast cancer to the esophagus and the mediastinum. *Gastroint Endosc.* 2005;61(3):416–20.

SMALL CELL CARCINOMA

Briggs JC, and , Ibrahim NBN. Oat cell carcinoma of the esophagus: a clinicopathologic study of 23 cases. *Histopathology.* 1983;7:261–77.

Chen KT. Cytology of small cell carcinoma arising in Barrett's esophagus. *Diagn Cytopathol.* 2000;23(3):180–2.

De Lott LB, Morrison C, Suster S, Cohn DE, and , Frankel WL. CDX-2 is a useful marker of intestinal-type differentiation: A tissue microarray-based study of 629 tumors from various sites. *Arch Pathol Lab Med.* 2005;129(9):1100–5.

Geisinger KR, Stanley MW, Raab SS, Silverman JF, and , Abati A. *Modern Cytopathology.* Philadelphia: Churchill Livingstone, 2004, pp. 257–309.

Hoda SA, and , Hajdu SI. Small cell carcinoma of the esophagus. Cytology and immunohistology in four cases. *Acta Cytol.* 1992;36:113–20.

Jhala N, and , Jhala D. Gastrointestinal tract cytology: advancing horizons. *Adv Anat Pathol.* 2003;10:261–77.

Ordonez NG. Value of thyroid transcription factor-1 immunostaining in distinguishing small cell carcinomas from other small cell carcinomas. *Am J Surg Pathol.* 2000;24:1217–23.

Tenvall J, Johansson L, and , Albertson M. Small cell carcinoma of the esophagus: a clinical and immunohistopathologic review. *Eur J Surg Oncol.* 1990;16:109–15.

LEIOMYOMA AND OTHER MESENCHYMAL TUMORS

Bardales RH, Stelow EB, Mallery S, Lai R, and , Stanley MW. Review of endoscopic ultrasound-guided fine-needle aspiration cytology. *Diagn Cytopathol.* 2006;34:140–75.

Geisinger KR, Stanley MW, Raab SS, Silverman JF, and , Abati A. *Modern Cytopathology.* Philadelphia: Churchill Livingstone, 2004, pp. 257–309.

Hunt GC, Rader AE, and , Faigel DO. A comparison of EUS features between CD-117 positive GI stromal tumors and CD-117 negative GI spindle cell tumors. *Gastroint Endosc.* 2003;57(4):469–74.

Jhala N, and , Jhala D. Gastrointestinal tract cytology: advancing horizons. *Adv Anat Pathol.* 2003;10:261–77.

Stelow EB, Jones DR, and , Shami VM. Esophageal leiomyosarcoma diagnosed by endoscopic ultrasound-guided fine-needle aspiration. *Diagn Cytopathol.* 2007;35(3):167–70.

Stelow EB, Stanley MW, Mallery S, Lai R, Linzie BM, and , Bardales RH. Endoscopic ultrasound-guided fine-needle aspiration findings of gastrointestinal leiomyomas and gastrointestinal stromal tumors. *Am J Clin Pathol.* 2003;119(5):703–8.

GASTRITIS

Davenport RD. Cytologic diagnosis of Campylobacter pylori-associated gastritis. *Acta Cytol.* 1990;34:211–3.

Debongnie JC, Mairesse J, Donnay M, and , Dekoninck X. Touch cytology. A quick, simple, sensitive screening test in the diagnosis of infections of the gastrointestinal tract. *Arch Pathol Lab Med.* 1994;118:1115–8.

DeFrancesco F, Nicotina PA, and , Picciotto M, et al. Helicobacter pylori in gastroduodenal diseases: rapid identification by endoscopic brush cytology. *Diagn Cytopathol.* 1992;9:430–3.

Geisinger KR, Stanley MW, Raab SS, Silverman JF, and , Abati A. *Modern Cytopathology.* Philadelphia: Churchill Livingstone, 2004, pp. 257–309.

Rodriguez IN, de Santamaria SJ, and , Rubio Mdel MA, et al. Cytologic brushing as a simple and rapid method in the diagnosis of *Helicobacter pylori* infection. *Acta Cytol.* 1995;39:916–9.

Schnadig VJ, Bigio EH, and , Gourley WK, et al. Identification of *Campylobacter pylori* by endoscopic brush cytology. *Diagn Cytopathol.* 1990;6:227–34.

Strigle SM, Gal AA, and , Martin SE. Alimentary tract cytopathology in human immunodeficiency virus infection. A review of experience in Los Angeles. *Diagn Cytopathol.* 1990;6:409–20.

Trevisani L, Sartori S, and , Ruina M, et al. Touch cytology. A reliable and cost-effective method for diagnosis of *Helicobacter pylori* infection. *Dig Dis Sci.* 1997;42:2299–2303.

Walsh D, Immins E, and , Dutton J. Filamentous organisms in benign and malignant gastric cytology brushes. *Cytopathology.* 1997;8:63–9.

PEPTIC ULCER DISEASE

Dziura BR, Otis R, and , Hukill P, et al. Gastric brushing cytology: an analysis of cells from benign and malignant ulcers. *Acta Cytol.* 1997;21:187–190.

Geisinger KR, Stanley MW, Raab SS, Silverman JF, and , Abati A. *Modern Cytopathology.* Philadelphia: Churchill Livingstone, 2004, pp. 257–309.

Geisinger KR, Wang HH, Ducatman BS, Teot LA, and . Gastrointestinal cytology. In Hajdu SI, editor. *Values and Limitations of Cytologic Examinations*, Vol. 11. Philadelphia: WB Saunders, 1991, pp. 403–41.

Geisinger KR, and . Alimentary tract (esophagus, stomach, small intestine, colon, rectum, anus, biliary tract). In Bibbo M, editor. *Comprehensive Cytopathology*, 2nd ed. Philadelphia: WB Saunders, 1997, pp. 413–44.

Kiil J, Andersen D, and , Jensen M. Biopsy and brush cytology in the diagnosis of gastric cancer. *Scand J Gastroenterol.* 1979;14:189–91.

Qizilbash AH, Castelli M, Kowalski MA, and , Churly A. Endoscopic brush cytology and biopsy in the diagnosis of cancer of the upper gastrointestinal tract. *Acta Cytol.* 1980;24:313–8.

Schnadig VJ, Bigio EH, and , Gourley WK, et al. Identification of Campylobacter pylori by endoscopic brush cytology. *Diagn Cytopathol.* 1990;6:227–34.

Waldron R, Kerin M, and , Ali A, et al. Evaluation of the role of endoscopic biopsies and cytology in the detection of gastric malignancy. *Br J Surg.* 1990;77:62–3.

DYSPLASIA

Antonioli DA. Precursors of gastric carcinoma. A critical review with a brief description of early (curable) gastric cancer. *Hum Pathol.* 1994;25:994–1005.

Geisinger KR, Stanley MW, Raab SS, Silverman JF, and , Abati A. *Modern Cytopathology.* Philadelphia: Churchill Livingstone, 2004, pp. 257–309.

Hustin J, Lagneaux G, and . Donnay M.Debongnie J-C. Cytologic patterns of reparative processes, true dysplasia and carcinoma of the gastric mucosa. *Acta Cytol.* 1994;38:730–6.

Wang HH, Ducatman BS, and , Thibault S. Cytologic features of premalignant glandular lesions in the upper gastrointestinal tract. *Acta Cytol.* 1991;35:199–203.

CHEMOTHERAPY-ASSOCIATED ATYPIA

Becker SN, Sass MA, Petras RE, and , Hart WR. Bizarre atypia in gastric brushings associated with hepatic artery infusion chemotherapy. *Acta Cytol.* 1986;30:347–50.

Geisinger KR, Stanley MW, Raab SS, Silverman JF, and , Abati A. *Modern Cytopathology.* Philadelphia: Churchill Livingstone, 2004, pp. 257–309.

POLYPS

Geisinger KR, Stanley MW, Raab SS, Silverman JF, and , Abati A. *Modern Cytopathology*. Philadelphia: Churchill Livingstone, 2004, pp. 257–309.

ADENOCARCINOMA

Cook IJ, de Carle DJ, and , Haneman B, et al. The role of brushing cytology in the diagnosis of gastric malignancy. *Acta Cytol.* 1988;32:461–4.

Cusso X, Mones J, and , Ocana J, et al. Is endoscopic gastric cytology worthwhile? An evaluation of 903 cases of carcinoma. *J Clin Gastroenterol.* 1993;16:336–9.

Geisinger KR, Stanley MW, Raab SS, Silverman JF, and , Abati A. *Modern Cytopathology*. Philadelphia: Churchill Livingstone, 2004, pp. 257–309.

Kumar PV, Monabati A, Naini MA, Lankarani KB, Fattahi MR, and , Asadilari M. Gastric xanthoma: a diagnostic problem on brushing cytology smears. *Acta Cytol.* 2006: 50:74–9.

Mills AS, Contos MJ, Goel R. The Stomach. In Silverberg SG, DeLellis RA, Frable WJ, LiVolsi VA, and , Wick MR, editors. *Principles and Practice of Surgical Pathology and Cytopathology*, 4th Ed. Philadelphia: Elsevier (Churchill Livingstone), 2006, pp. 1321–1372.

Moreno-Otero R, Marron C, and , Cantero J, et al. Endoscopic biopsy and cytology in the diagnosis of malignant gastric ulcers. *Diagn Cytopathol.* 1989;5:366–370.

Sangha S, Gergeos F, Freter R, Paiva LL, and , Jacobson BC. Diagnosis of ovarian cancer metastatic to the stomach by EUS-guided FNA. *Gastrointest Endosc.* 2003;58(6):933–935. The diagnosis of lower digestive tract disease. *Endoscopy.* 2003; 35(11):966–9.

Sharma P, Misra V, and , Singh PA, et al. A correlative study of histology and imprint cytology in the diagnosis of gastrointestinal tract malignancies. *Indian J Pathol Microbiol.* 1997;40(2): 139–46.

Waldron R, Kerin M, and , Ali A, et al. Evaluation of the role of endoscopic biopsies and cytology in the detection of gastric malignancy. *Br J Surg.* 1990;77:62–3.

CARCINOID TUMOR

Bardales RH, Stelow EB, Mallery S, Lai R, and , Stanley MW. Review of endoscopic ultrasound-guided fine-needle aspiration cytology. *Diagn Cytopathol.* 2006;34:140–75.

Debol SM, Stanley MW, Mallery S, Sawinski E, and , Bardales RH. Glomus tumor of the stomach: cytologic diagnosis by endoscopic ultrasound-guided fine-needle aspiration. *Diagn Cytopathol.* 2003; 28(6):316–21.

Dong Q, McKee G, Pitman M, Geisinger K, and , Tambouret R. Epithelioid variant of gastrointestinal stromal tumor: diagnosis by fine needle aspiration. *Diagn Cytopathol.* 2003;29(2):55–60.

Geisinger KR, Stanley MW, Raab SS, Silverman JF, and , Abati A. *Modern Cytopathology*. Philadelphia: Churchill Livingstone, 2004, pp. 257–309.

Gu M, Nguyen PT, Cao S, and , Lin F. Diagnosis of gastric glomus tumor by endoscopic ultrasound-guided fine needle aspiration biopsy. A case report with cytologic, histologic and immunohistochemical studies. *Acta Cytol.* 2002;46(3):560–6.

Jhala N, and , Jhala D. Gastrointestinal tract cytology: advancing horizons. *Adv Anat Pathol.* 2003;10:261–77.

Lozowski W, Hajdu SI, and , Melamed MR. Cytomorphology of carcinoid tumors. *Acta Cytol.* 1979;23:360–5.

Mills AS, Contos MJ, Goel R. The stomach. In Silverberg SG, DeLellis RA, Frable WJ, LiVolsi VA, and , Wick MR, editors. *Principles and Practice of Surgical Pathology and Cytopathology*, 4th Ed. Philadelphia: Elsevier (Churchill Livingstone), 2006, pp. 1321–72.

Rodriguez FJ, Abraham SC, Allen MS, and , Sebo TJ. Fine-needle aspiration cytology findings from a case of pancreatic heterotopia at the gastroesophageal junction. *Diagn Cytopathol.* 2004;31(3):175–9.

GASTROINTESTINAL STROMAL TUMOR (GIST)

Ando N, Goto H, and , Niwa Y, et al. The diagnosis of GI stromal tumors with EUS-guided fine needle aspiration with immunohistochemical analysis. *Gastrointest Endosc.* 2002;55(1):37–43.

Bardales RH, Stelow EB, Mallery S, Lai R, and , Stanley MW. Review of endoscopic ultrasound-guided fine-needle aspiration cytology. *Diagn Cytopathol.* 2006;34:140–75.

Debol SM, Stanley MW, and , Mallery JS. Can fine needle aspiration cytology adequately diagnose and predict the behavior of gastrointestinal stromal tumors? *Adv Anat Pathol.* 2001;8(2):93–7.

Dong Q, McKee G, Pitman M, Geisinger K, and , Tambouret R. Epithelioid variant of gastrointestinal stromal tumor: diagnosis by fine needle aspiration. *Diagn Cytopathol.* 2003;29(2):55–60.

Elliott DD, Fanning CV, and , Caraway NP. The utility of fine-needle aspiration in the diagnosis of gastrointestinal stromal tumors: a cytomorphologic and immunohistochemical analysis with emphasis on malignant tumors. *Cancer*. 2006 Feb 25;108(1):49–55.

Fletcher CDM, Berman JJ, Corless C, Gorstein F, and , Lasota J, et al. Diagnosis of gastrointestinal stromal tumors: a consensus approach. *Hum Pathol*. 2002;33:459–65.

Fu K, Eloubeidi MA, Jhala NC, Jhala D, Chhieng DC, and , Eltoum IE. Diagnosis of gastrointestinal stromal tumor by endoscopic ultrasound-guided fine needle aspiration biopsy–a potential pitfall. *Ann Diagn Pathol*. 2002;6(5):294–301.

Li SQ, O'Leary TJ, Buchner SB, Przygodzki RM, Sobin LH, Erozan YS, and , Rosenthal DL. Fine needle aspiration of gastrointestinal stromal tumors. *Acta Cytol*. 2001;45(1):9–17.

Okubo K, Yamao K, and , Nakamura T, et al. Endoscopic ultrasound guided fine-needle aspiration biopsy for the diagnosis of gastrointestinal stromal tumors in the stomach. *J Gastroenterol*. 2004;39(8):747–53.

Rader AE, Avery A, Wait CL, McGreevey LS, Faigel D, and , Heinrich MC. Fine-needle aspiration biopsy diagnosis of gastrointestinal stromal tumors using morphology, immunocytochemistry, and mutational analysis of c-kit. *Cancer*. 2001;93(4):269–75.

Stelow EB, Stanley MW, Mallery S, Lai R, Linzie BM, and , Bardales RH. Endoscopic ultrasound-guided fine-needle aspiration findings of gastrointestinal leiomyomas and gastrointestinal stromal tumors. *Am J Clin Pathol*. 2003;119(5):703–8.

LYMPHOMA

Bardales RH, Stelow EB, Mallery S, Lai R, and , Stanley MW. Review of endoscopic ultrasound-guided fine-needle aspiration cytology. *Diagn Cytopathol*. 2006;34:140–75.

Geisinger KR, Stanley MW, Raab SS, Silverman JF, and , Abati A. *Modern Cytopathology*. Philadelphia: Churchill Livingstone, 2004, pp. 257–309.

Geisinger KR, Wang HH, Ducatman BS, Teot LA, and . Gastrointestinal cytology. In Hajdu SI, editor. *Values and Limitations of Cytologic Examinations*. Vol. 11. Philadelphia: WB Saunders, 1991, pp. 403–441.

Isaacson PG. Gastrointestinal lymphoma. *Hum Pathol*. 1994;25:1020–1209.

Jhala N, and , Jhala D. Gastrointestinal tract cytology: advancing horizons. *Adv Anat Pathol*. 2003;10:261–77.

Kolve ME, Fischbach W, and , Wilhelm M. Primary gastric non-Hodgkin's lymphoma: requirements for diagnosis and staging. *Recent Results Cancer Res*. 2000;156:63–68.

Layfield LJ, Reichman A, and , Weinstein WM. Endoscopically directed fine needle aspiration biopsy of gastric and esophageal lesions. *Acta Cytol*. 1992;36:69–74.

Sherman ME, Anderson C, and , Herman LM, et al. Utility of gastric brushing in the diagnosis of malignant lymphoma. *Acta Cytol*. 1994;38:169–174.

DUODENUM INFECTIOUS AGENTS

Clayton F, Heller T, and , Kotter DP. Variation in the enteric distribution of cryptosporidia in acquired immunodeficiency syndrome. *Am J Clin Pathol*. 1994;102:420 5.

Debongnie JC, Mairesse J, Donnay M, and , Dekoninck X. Touch cytology. A quick, simple, sensitive screening test in the diagnosis of infections of the gastrointestinal tract. *Arch Pathol Lab Med*. 1994;118:1115–8.

Geisinger KR, Stanley MW, Raab SS, Silverman JF, and , Abati A. *Modern Cytopathology*. Philadelphia: Churchill Livingstone, 2004, pp. 257–309.

Genta RM, Chapell CL, and , White AC Jr, et al. Duodenal morphology and intensity of infection in AIDS-related intestinal cryptosporidiosis. *Gastroenterology*. 1993;105:1769–75.

Guajardo RG, Quintana OB, and , Padilla PP. Negative images due to MAI infection detected in Papanicolaou-stained duodenal brushing cytology. *Diagn Cytopathol*. 1998;19:462–4.

Jhala N, and , Jhala D. Gastrointestinal tract cytology: advancing horizons. *Adv Anat Pathol*. 2003;10:261–77.

Marshall JB, Kelley DH, and , Vogele KA. Giardiasis: diagnosis by endoscopic brush cytology of the duodenum. *Am J Gastroenterol*. 1984;79:517–9.

Silverman JF, Levine J, and , Finley JL, et al. Small-intestinal brushing cytology in the diagnosis of cryptosporidiosis in AIDS. *Diagn Cytopathol*. 1990;6:193–6.

Strigle SM, Gal AA, and , Martin SE. Alimentary tract cytopathology in human immunodeficiency virus infection. A review of experience in Los Angeles. *Diagn Cytopathol*. 1990;6:409–20.

PEPTIC ULCER

Geisinger KR, Stanley MW, Raab SS, Silverman JF, and , Abati A. *Modern Cytopathology*. Philadelphia: Churchill Livingstone, 2004, pp. 257–309.

ADENOCARCINOMA

Abdul-Karim FW, O'Mailia JJ, and , Wang KP, et al. Transmucosal endoscopic needle aspiration: utility in the diagnosis of extrinsic malignant masses of the gastrointestinal tract. *Diagn Cytopathol.* 1991;7:92–94.

Bardales RH, Stelow EB, Mallery S, Lai R, and , Stanley MW. Review of endoscopic ultrasound-guided fine-needle aspiration cytology. *Diagn Cytopathol.* 2006;34:140–75.

Bardales RH. Stanley MW. Simpson DD. Baker SJ. Steele CT. Schaefer RF., and Powers CN. Diagnostic value of brush cytology in the diagnosis of duodenal, biliary, and ampullary neoplasms. *Am J Clin Pathol.* 1998;109(5):540–8.

Caos A, Olson N, Willman C, and , Gogel HK. *Endoscopic "salvage" cytology in neoplasms metastatic to the upper gastrointestinal tract.* 1986;30:32–34.

Geisinger KR, Stanley MW, Raab SS, Silverman JF, and , Abati A. *Modern Cytopathology.* Philadelphia: Churchill Livingstone; 2004, pp. 257–309.

CARCINOID TUMOR

Acs G, McGrath CM, and , Gupta PK. Duodenal carcinoid tumor: report of a case diagnosed by endoscopic ultrasound-guided fine-needle aspiration biopsy with immunocytochemical correlation. *Diagn Cytopathol.* 2000;23(3):183–6.

Bardales RH, Stelow EB, Mallery S, Lai R, and , Stanley MW. Review of endoscopic ultrasound-guided fine-needle aspiration cytology. *Diagn Cytopathol.* 2006;34:140–75.

Capella C, Solcia E, Sobin LH and Arnold R. Endocrine tumours of the small intestine. In Hamilton SR, and and Aaltonen LA, editors. *Health Organization Classification of Tumours. Pathology and Genetics of Tumours of the Digestive System.* Lyon, France: IARC Press. 2000, pp. 77–82.

Geisinger KR, Stanley MW, Raab SS, Silverman JF, and , Abati A. *Modern Cytopathology.* Philadelphia: Churchill Livingstone, 2004, pp. 257–309.

Stolpman DR, Hunt GC, Sheppard B, Huang H, and , Gopal DV. Brunner's gland hamartoma: a rare cause of gastrointestinal bleeding – case report and review of the literature. *Can J Gastroenterol.* 2002; 16(5):309–13.

GASTROINTESTINAL
STROMAL TUMOR (GIST)

Ando N, Goto H, and , Niwa Y, et al. The diagnosis of GI stromal tumors with EUS-guided fine needle aspiration with immunohistochemical analysis. *Gastrointest Endosc.* 2002;55(1):37–43.

Bardales RH, Stelow EB, Mallery S, Lai R, and , Stanley MW. Review of endoscopic ultrasound-guided fine-needle aspiration cytology. *Diagn Cytopathol.* 2006;34:140–75.

Elliott DD, Fanning CV, and , Caraway NP. The utility of fine-needle aspiration in the diagnosis of gastrointestinal stromal tumors: a cytomorphologic and immunohistochemical analysis with emphasis on malignant tumors. *Cancer.* 2006 Feb 25;108(1):49–55.

Fu K, Eloubeidi MA, Jhala NC, Jhala D, Chhieng DC, and , Eltoum IE. Diagnosis of gastrointestinal stromal tumor by endoscopic ultrasound-guided fine needle aspiration biopsy–a potential pitfall. *Ann Diagn Pathol.* 2002;6(5):294–301.

Fu K, Eloubeidi MA, Jhala NC, Jhala D, Chhieng DC, and , Eltoum IE. Diagnosis of gastrointestinal stromal tumor by endoscopic ultrasound- guided fine needle aspiration biopsy – a potential pitfall. *Ann Diagn Pathol.* 2002;6(5):294–301.

Laforga JB. Malignant epithelioid gastrointestinal stromal tumors: report of a case with cytologic and immunohistochemical studies. *Acta Cytol.* 2005;49:435–40.

Li SQ, O'Leary TJ, Buchner SB, Przygodzki RM, Sobin LH, Erozan YS, and , Rosenthal DL. Fine needle aspiration of gastrointestinal stromal tumors. *Acta Cytol.* 2001;45(1):9–17.

Stelow EB, Stanley MW, Mallery S, Lai R, Linzie BM, and , Bardales RH. Endoscopic ultrasound-guided fine-needle aspiration findings of gastrointestinal leiomyomas and gastrointestinal stromal tumors. *Am J Clin Pathol.* 2003;119(5):703–8.

LYMPHOMA

Abdul-Karim FW, O'Mailia JJ, and , Wang KP, et al. Transmucosal endoscopic needle aspiration: utility in the diagnosis of extrinsic malignant masses of the gastrointestinal tract. *Diagn Cytopathol.* 1991;7:92–4.

Bardales RH, Stelow EB, Mallery S, Lai R, and , Stanley MW. Review of endoscopic ultrasound-guided fine-needle aspiration cytology. *Diagn Cytopathol.* 2006;34:140–75.

Bardales RH. Stanley MW. Simpson DD. Baker SJ. Steele CT. Schaefer RF., and Powers CN. Diagnostic value of brush cytology in the diagnosis of duodenal, biliary, and ampullary neoplasms. *Am J Clin Pathol.* 1998;109(5):540–8.

Domizo P, Owen RA, and , Shepherd NA, et al. Primary lymphoma of the small intestine. A clinicopathological study of 119 cases. *Am J Surg Pathol.* 1993;17:429–42.

Geisinger KR, Stanley MW, Raab SS, Silverman JF, and , Abati A. *Modern Cytopathology.* Philadelphia: Churchill Livingstone, 2004, pp. 257–309.

Kadakia SC, Parker A, and , Canales L. Metastatic tumors to the upper gastrointestinal tract: endoscopic experience. *Am J Gastroenterol.* 1992;87:1418–1423.

LARGE INTESTINE

Festa VI, Hajdu SI, and , Winawer SJ. Colorectal cytology in chronic ulcerative colitis. *Acta Cytol.* 1985;29:262–8.

Galambos JT, Massey BW, Klayman MI, and , Kirsner JB. Exfoliative cytology in chronic ulcerative colitis. *Cancer.* 1959;9:152–9.

Geisinger KR, Stanley MW, Raab SS, Silverman JF, and , Abati A. *Modern Cytopathology.* Philadelphia: Churchill Livingstone, 2004, pp. 257–309.

Granqvist S, Granberg-Ohman I, and , Sundelin P. Colonoscopic biopsies and cytological examination in chronic ulcerative colitis. *Scand J Gastroenterol.* 1980;15:283–288.

Jhala N, and , Jhala D. Gastrointestinal tract cytology: advancing horizons. *Adv Anat Pathol.* 2003;10:261–77.

Melville DM, Richman PI, and , Shepherd NA, et al. Brush cytology of the colon and rectum in ulcerative colitis: an aid to cancer diagnosis. *J Clin Pathol.* 1988;41:1180–1186.

ADENOMAS AND ADENOCARCINOMA

Fehring A, and , Schmulewitz N. EUS-guided FNA diagnosis of recurrent follicular lymphoma in the transverse colon. *Gastroint Endosc.* 2006;64(4):652–3.

Geisinger KR, Stanley MW, Raab SS, Silverman JF, and , Abati A. *Modern Cytopathology.* Philadelphia: Churchill Livingstone, 2004, pp. 257–309.

Geramizadeh B, Hooshmand F, and , Kumar PV. Brush cytology of colorectal malignancies. *Acta Cytol.* 2003;47(3):431–4.

Jhala N, and , Jhala D. Gastrointestinal tract cytology: advancing horizons. *Adv Anat Pathol.* 2003;10:261–77.

Kannan V, and , Masters CB. Cytodiagnosis of colonic adenoma: morphology and clinical importance. *Diagn Cytopathol.* 1991;7:366–72.

Mortensen NJMcC, Eltringham WK, Mountford RA, and , Lever JV. *Direct vision brush cytology with colonoscopy: an aid to the accurate diagnosis of colonic strictures.* 1984;71:930–932.

Silverman JF, Baird DB, and , Teot LA, et al. Fine-needle aspiration cytology of metastatic small cell carcinoma of the colon: a report of three cases. *Diagn Cytopathol.* 1996;15:54–59.

Yu GH, Nayar R, and , Furth EE. Adenocarcinoma in colonic brushing cytology: High-grade dysplasia as a diagnostic pitfall. *Diagn Cytopathol.* 2001; 24:364–8.

Zargar SA, Khuroo MS, and , Mahajan R, et al. Endoscopic fine needle aspiration cytology in the diagnosis of gastroesophageal and colorectal malignancies. *Gut.* 1991;32:745–8.

ANUS

Bakotic WL, Willis D, Birdsong G, and , Tadros TS. Anal cytology in an HIV-positive population: a retrospective analysis. *Acta Cytol.* 2005;49:163–8.

Darragh TM, Birdsong GG, Luff RD and Davey DD. Anal–rectal cytology. In Solomon D, and , Nayar R, editors. *The Bethesda System for Reporting Cervical Cytology*, 2nd Ed. New York: Springer-Verlag, 2004, pp. 169–175.

de Ruiter A, Carter P, and , Katz DR, et al. A comparison between cytology and histology to detect anal intraepithelial neoplasia. *Genitourin Med.* 1994;70:22–5.

Maden C, Coates RJ, and , Sherman KJ, et al. Sexual practices, sexually transmitted diseases and the incidence of anal cancer. *N Engl J Med.* 1987;317:973–7.

Palefsky JM, Holly EA, and , Hogeboom CJ, et al. Anal cytology as a screening tool for anal squamous intraepithelial lesions. *J Acquired Immune Defic Syndr Human Retrovirol.* 1997;14:415–22.

Palefsky JM, Holly EA, and , Ralston ML. High incidence of anal high-grade squamous intraepithelial lesions among HIV-positive and HIV-negative homosexual and bisexual men. *AIDS.* 1998;12:495–503.

Scholefield JH, Johnson J, and , Hitchcock A. Guidelines for anal cytology – to make cytological diagnosis and follow up much more reliable. *Cytopathology*. 1998:9:15–22.

Sherman ME, Friedman HB, and , Busseniers AE, et al. Cytologic diagnosis of anal intraepithelial neoplasia using smears and Cytyc Thin-Preps. *Mod Pathol*. 1995;8:270–4.

Sonnex C, Scholefield JH, and , Kocjan G, et al. Anal human papillomavirus infection: a comparative study of cytology, colposcopy and DNA hybridization as methods of detection. *Genitourin Med*. 1991;67:21–5.

5

Urine Cytology

Güliz A. Barkan, Umesh Kapur, and Eva M. Wojcik

ELEMENTS OF NORMAL URINE

CELLS SEEN IN NORMAL URINE

▪ Urothelial cells – basal cells, intermediate cells, superficial (umbrella) cells
▪ Squamous cells – contaminant from the external genitalia, cells from trigone, squamous metaplasia

OTHER CELLS THAT COULD BE FOUND IN NORMAL URINE

▪ Glandular cells – prostatic, endometrial, cystitis glandularis, paraurethral glands
▪ Renal tubular cells – small cells with granular cytoplasm, small/pyknotic nuclei mostly with degenerative changes
▪ Leukocytes, lymphocytes, and RBCs
▪ Seminal vesicle cells – large cells with irregular hyperchromatic nuclei, prominent nucleoli, and yellowish brown cytoplasmic pigment
▪ Spermatozoa

NONCELLULAR ELEMENTS OF URINE

▪ Crystals – mostly form after the urine cools down from 37°C, and hence this finding has limited clinical importance. Most common cast seen is uric acid or amorphous urate crystals
▪ Casts – Cylindric structure formed in the renal tubules; red blood cell cast, white blood cell cast, epithelial cast, mixed cast, waxy cast, granular cast, and hyaline cast are different types
▪ Corpora Amylacea – eosinophilic concretions with laminations, derived from degenerate cells or thickened secretions
▪ Lubricant – clumps of dense, amorphous, basophilic material

5-1. Intermediate/Basal urothelial cells *(upper, left).* Columnar cells with homogenous dense cytoplasm, low N:C ratio, oval nucleus and smooth nuclear membrane. Columnar urothelial cells are seen in barbotage material. Three cells in the center are superficial (umbrella cells). (Papanicolaou stain)

5-2. Umbrella cell *(upper, right).* Large cell with abundant delicate, thin cytoplasm, multinucleation, and smooth chromatin (Papanicolaou stain)

5-3. Umbrella cell *(Lower, left).* Large cell with abundant thin cytoplasm, large round nucleus with hyperchromatic chromocenters. If this cell did not have abundant cytoplasm urothelial carcinoma would be in the differential diagnosis (Papanicolaou stain)

5-4. Squamous cells *(Lower, right).* Voided urine with squamous cells, some of which are anucleated. The squamous cells are larger than urothelial cells, have a denser cytoplasm and a small pyknotic nucleus. (Papanicolaou stain)

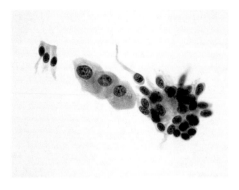
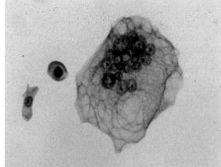
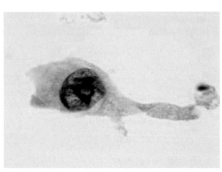
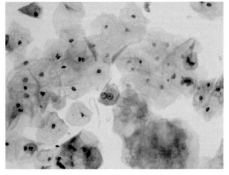

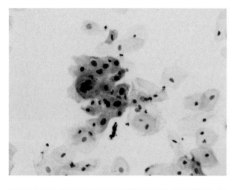

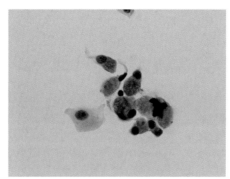

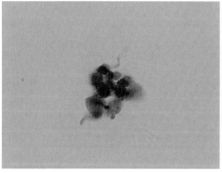

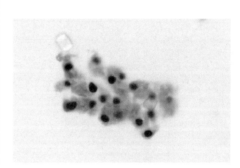

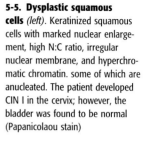

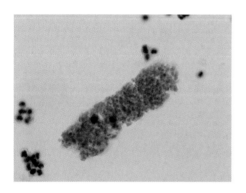

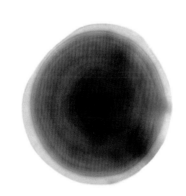

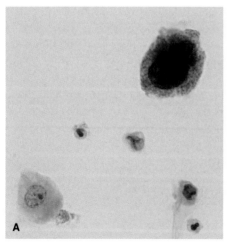

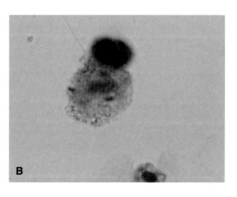

5-5. Dysplastic squamous cells *(left)*. Keratinized squamous cells with marked nuclear enlargement, high N:C ratio, irregular nuclear membrane, and hyperchromatic chromatin. some of which are anucleated. The patient developed CIN I in the cervix; however, the bladder was found to be normal (Papanicolaou stain)

5-6. Cystitis glandularis *(right)*. Columnar cells with mucin filled cytoplasm, low N:C ratio, eccentrically placed nucleus (Papanicolaou stain)

5-7. Cystitis glandularis *(opposite, left)*. Columnar cells with mucin filled cytoplasm staining pink with mucicarmine (Mucicarmine stain)

5-8. Renal tubular epithelial cells *(opposite, right)*. Polygonal cells with abundant granular cytoplasm, eccentrically placed round to oval nucleus (Papanicolaou stain)

5-9. Granular/Epithelial cast *(left)*. Mostly formed of coarse granular material and rare degenerated epithelial cells (Papanicolaou stain)

5-10. Corpora Amylacea *(right)*. Dense polychromatic, proteinaceous material with concentric laminations (Papanicolaou stain)

5-11A and B. Seminal Vesicle cells *(left and right)*. (A) A single cell with large, homogenous, hyperchromatic nucleus with faint focal yellow cytoplasmic pigment (Papanicolaou stain) (B) A Single cell with eccentrically placed hyperchromatic nucleus with abundant, yellow cytoplasmic pigment (Papanicolaou stain)

▦ Mucus – dense, thick basophilic amorphous substance
▦ Fecal material – vegetable cells with thick cell wall and degenerative changes, striated muscle cells
▦ Pollen – usually have a cell wall, and large central nucleus

5-12A and B. Spermatozoa *(left and right)*. (A) Aggregates of mature spermatozoa with round to fusiform nucleus and tails, accompanied by seminal vesicle cells (B) Corpora amylacea (Papanicolaou stain)

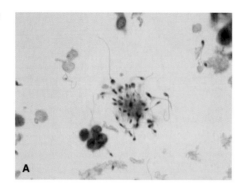

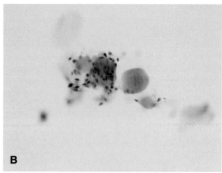

5-13. Crystals *(left)*. Yellow–brown uric acid crystals with various shapes (Papanicolaou stain)

5-14. Lubricant *(right)*. Dense amorphous basophilic material with sharp edges (Papanicolaou stain)

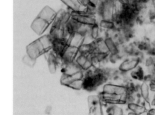

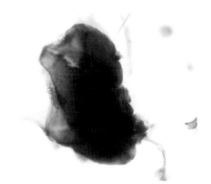

TYPES OF URINARY TRACT SPECIMENS

VOIDED URINE

- Most convenient and easily obtained
- Contamination from external genitalia and vagina
- Degenerated urothelial cells (eosinophilic inclusions, that is, Melamed–Wolinska bodies)

CATHETERIZED URINE

- Requires instrumentation
- Lack of contamination from external genitalia
- More cellular
- May have pseudopapillary urothelial fragments (DDX: low-grade urothelial carcinoma)

URINARY BLADDER WASHING/BARBOTAGE

- Requires instrumentation
- Lack of contamination from external genitalia
- More cellular
- Better preservation
- Monolayered sheets, pseudopapillary fragments, and single cells (DDX: low-grade urothelial carcinoma
- Columnar intermediate and deep cells

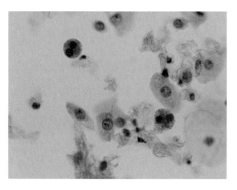

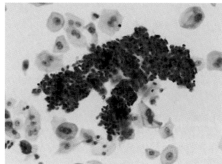

5-15. Voided urine *(left)*. Urothelial cells with degenerative changes. Two cells with cytoplasmic round eosinophilic inclusions "Melamed–Wolinska Bodies," which is in of the tell tale signs of degeneration (Papanicolaou stain)

5-16. Instrumented urine *(right)*. Highly cellular specimen with numerous cell clusters, and single umbrella cells and intermediate/basal cells (Papanicolaou stain)

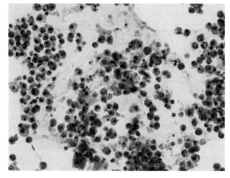

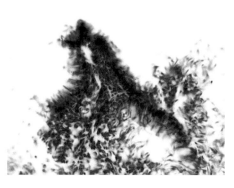

5-17A and B. Ileal conduit specimen *(left and right)*. A-B Very cellular specimen with mostly single cells and occasional clusters of degenerated glandular cells (Papanicolaou stain)

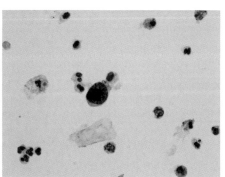

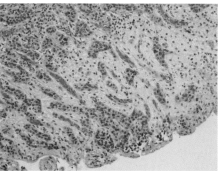

5-18A and B. Recurrent Urothelial carcinoma in ileal conduit specimen *(left and right)*. (A) In a background of degenerated urothelial cells and polymorphonuclear leukocytes there is a single cell with very high N:C ratio, and hyperchromatic nucleus (Papanicolaou stain) (B) Surgical biopsy showing nests of tumor cells in a desmoplastic stroma (recurrent urothelial carcinoma) in the ileal conduit (hematoxylin and eosin stain)

ILEAL CONDUIT

- Requires instrumentation
- Hypercellular
- Degenerated columnar/glandular cells of ileal epithelium in a dirty background of mucus and bacteria
- Degenerated urothelial cells with cytoplasmic inclusions
- Karyorrhexis

INFLAMMATORY CONDITIONS

NONINFECTIOUS

- Interstitial cystitis: Cytologic findings are nonspecific
- Eosinophilic cystitis: Eosinophils
- Hemorrhagic cystitis: Cytologic findings are nonspecific other than abundant RBC
- Could be an infectious or a noninfectious process: Etiology: *Escherichia coli;* adenoviruses, papovavirus; influenza A; cyclophosphamide, and radiation induced

Infectious

■ Viral: Polyoma virus

Clinical Features

■ A primary BK virus infection occurs during childhood and is usually subclinical
■ Over 90% of adults are seropositive for BK viral antibodies
■ The BK virus generally remains latent in the kidney, but intermittent viruria is demonstrable in 0.3% of healthy adults
■ The infection is reactivated in individuals with various degrees of immunological deficits

Cytologic Features

■ BK virus–infected cells are characterized by the presence of single, large, homogenous, basophilic inclusions occupying most of the enlarged nuclear area, and thickened nuclear membrane
■ The other type of cells commonly seen in BK infection are the "empty cells"
■ Urothelial cells affected by BK virus have an abnormal DNA content

Special stains and Immunohistochemistry

■ Immunohistochemical studies for JC/BK virus

Modern Techniques for Diagnosis

■ ELISA, RT-PCR, and electron microscopy

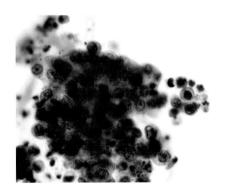

5-19. Acute bacterial cystitis.
Reactive urothelial cells with slightly enlarged N:C ratio, and prominent nucleoli and polymorphonuclear leukocytes (Papanicolaou stain)

Differential Diagnosis

■ Urothelial carcinoma
➤ Lacks basophilic nuclear inclusion
■ Cytomegalovirus
➤ Larger cell with perinuclear halo and both cytoplasmic and nuclear inclusions
■ Adenovirus
➤ Homogenous basophilic intranuclear inclusion, with multiple small irregular inclusions, and nuclear clearing
■ Herpes
➤ Multinucleation, margination of the chromatin, and molding of the nuclei

PEARLS

★ *Polyoma cells are also called "decoy cells,"* since they may be confused with urothelial carcinoma

INFECTIOUS

OTHER INFECTIOUS AGENTS

Viral

■ Herpes: usually seen in immunocompromised patients. Infected cells may be enlarged, showing the characteristic multinucleation, ground-glass nuclear inclusions, peripheral margination of the chromatin, and nuclear molding

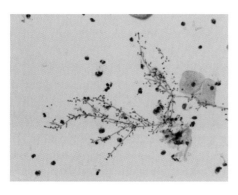

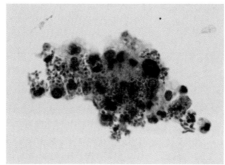

5-20A and B. Candida: (A-B). Pseudohyphae and yeast forms of candida in a background of acute inflammation and reactive urothelial cells (Papanicolaou stain)

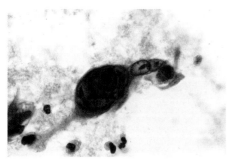

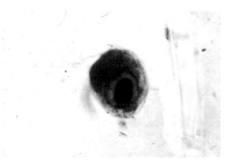

5-21. Herpes *(top, left)*. Large cell with multinucleation, nuclear margination and molding with a ground glass appearance and nuclear viral inclusion. (modified Giemya stain) *Picture courtesy of Dr. Bernard Naylor, emeritus professor, University of Michigan*

5-22. Cytomegalovirus *(top, right)*. Single large cell with both nuclear and cytoplasmic inclusions – "owl's eye." (modified Giemsa stain) *Picture courtesy of Dr. Bernard Naylor, emeritus professor, University of Michigan*

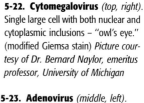

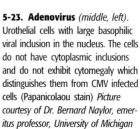

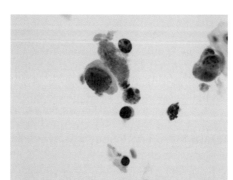

5-23. Adenovirus *(middle, left)*. Urothelial cells with large basophilic viral inclusion in the nucleus. The cells do not have cytoplasmic inclusions and do not exhibit cytomegaly which distinguishes them from CMV infected cells (Papanicolaou stain) *Picture courtesy of Dr. Bernard Naylor, emeritus professor, University of Michigan*

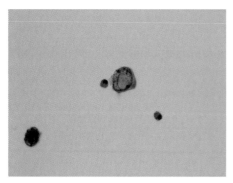

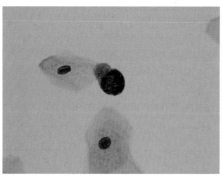

5-24A, B, and C. Polyoma virus (A) *(middle, right)*. Single cells with large, homogenous, basophilic inclusions occupying most of an enlarged nuclear area with an accentuated nuclear membrane. Since they it may be mistaken for urothelial carcinoma polyoma virus infected cells are also named as "decoy cell" (B) *(bottom left)*. the cells could also be hypochromatic hence the alias "empty cell" (C) *(bottom, right)*. and sometimes they may have a tail resembling a comet hence the other alias "comet cell" (Papanicolaou stain)

CMV

■ Most commonly seen in immuno-compromised patients showing large cells with perinuclear halo and both cytoplasmic and nuclear inclusions

Fungal

■ Candida is the most common fungal organism affecting the bladder. More common in immunosuppressive patients and diabetes. If seen accompanied by numerous squamous cells, bacterial organisms in women possibility of vaginal contamination should be raised

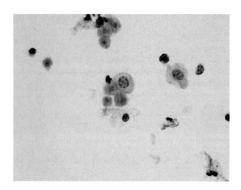

5-25. Trichomonas. Pear-shaped protozoan of 15–30 with a small, pale, eccentric nucleus, and eosinophilic cytoplasmic granules (Papanicolaou stain)

Parasitic
■ Trichomonas: rare sexually transmitted infection, frequently associated with genital coinfection. The organisms is a light gray, pear-shaped protozoan ranging in size between 15 and 50 μm, with cytoplasmic eosinophilic granules

Schistosoma
■ Endemic in Africa and some parts of Asia. The organisms are transmitted via fresh water snails. The eggs are oval, ranging between 100 and 150 μm, with a terminal (*S. hematobium*) or lateral (*S. mansoni*) spine

Bacterial
■ Fecal flora and malakoplakia (rarely blue targetoid calcospherules (Michaelis–Gutmann bodies)

UROLITHIASIS

Clinical Features
■ Pain with hematuria
■ Seen as a filling defect on IVP
■ Visualized on cystoscopy

Cytologic Features
■ Cellular and three-dimensional papillary fragments with smooth contours composed of cells with atypia
■ High N:C ratio, vacuolated cytoplasm, "cytoplasmic collar"

Special Stains and Immunohistochemistry
■ Noncontributory

Modern Techniques for diagnosis
■ Noncontributory

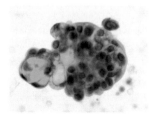

5-26A and B. Urolithiasis. (A) Three dimensional fragments, papillary clusters composed of cells exhibiting cytologic atypia, mild pleomorphism, and cytoplasmic vacuolization (B) There is a cytoplasmic collar and the nucleus is centrally placed with smooth nuclear borders and finely granular chromatin. (Papanicolaou stain)

Differential Diagnosis
■ Urothelial carcinoma
  ➤ Eccentrically placed nucleus, hyperchromasia, high nuclear cytoplasmic ratio, lack of cytoplasmic collar

PEARLS
★ Patients present with painful hematuria
★ Clinical history is crucial to avoid a false-positive diagnosis

TREATMENT-RELATED CHANGES

CYCLOPHOSPHAMIDE
■ High N/C ratio
■ Large nuclei
■ Hyperchromasia and degeneration
■ Granular and wispy cytoplasm

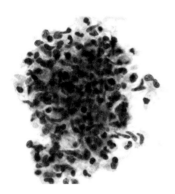

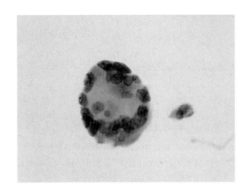

5-27A and B. BCG Effect *(left and right)*. (A) Granuloma composed of histiocytes and lymphocytes (B) Same case exhibiting a giant cell with peripherally located nuclei and rounded contours. (Papanicolaou stain)

MITOMYCIN AND THIOTEPA

- Umbrella cells mostly affected
- Marked nuclear enlargement
- Multinucleation
- Hyperchromatic, granular chromatin

RADIATION

- Cytomegaly
- Nucleomegaly
- Preserved N/C ratio
- Multinucleation
- Nuclear and cytoplasmic vacuoles

BCG

- Granulomas
- Inflammation
- Multinucleated giant cells

5-28. Chemotherapy effect. Urothelial cells showing marked enlargement, with vacuolated cytoplasm, hyperchromasia and prominent nucleoli. (Papanicolaou stain) *Picture courtesy of Dr. Bernard Naylor, emeritus professor, University of Michigan*

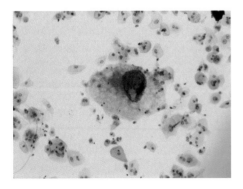

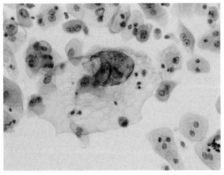

5-29A and B. Radiotherapy effect *(left and right)*. (A) Large urothelial cells with unchanged N:C ratio, cytoplasmic vacuolization and (B) polychromasia is evident. There is nuclear hyperchromasia. (Papanicolaou stain, stain)

UROTHELIAL CARCINOMA

Clinical Features
- Hematuria
- Dysuria
- Highest rate in North America, Western Europe
- Lowest rate in Japan

■ Male:Female – 3:1
■ Median age at Dx: sixty-five years

Cytologic Features
■ Low Grade
➤ Increased cellularity
➤ Presence of papillary, cohesive clusters
➤ Mild to moderate pleomorphism
➤ Eccentric, mildly enlarged nuclei
➤ Mild irregularity in nuclear membrane
➤ Granular, even chromatin
➤ Homogenous cytoplasm
➤ Inconspicuous nucleoli
➤ Low to moderate sensitivity and specificity

■ High Grade
➤ Increased cellularity
➤ Presence of loose clusters and single cells
➤ Moderate to marked pleomorphism
➤ Eccentric, enlarged, pleomorphic nuclei
➤ Irregular nuclear membrane
➤ Coarse chromatin
➤ ± Prominent nucleoli
➤ Squamous or glandular differentiation

CYTOLOGIC FEATURES OF UROTHELIAL PAPILLARY NEOPLASMS

	Papilloma	PUNLMP	Low grade	High grade
Nuclear size	Identical to normal	May be enlarged	Enlarged, variation in size	Enlarged, variation in size
Nuclear shape	Identical to normal	Elongated, round to oval, uniform	Round to oval, slight variation	Mod-marked pleomorphism
Chromatin	Fine	Fine	Mild hyperchromasia	Coarse, hyperchromatic
Nucleoli	Absent	Absent to inconspicuous	Usually inconspicuous	Multiple, prominent
Mitoses	Absent	Rare	Occasional	Usually frequent
Umbrella cells	Uniformly present	Present	Usually present	Mostly absent

Special Stains and Immunohistochemistry
■ CK20
■ CK5/6
■ E-cadherin
■ P63

Modern Techniques for Diagnosis
■ DNA ploidy
➤ Flow cytometry
➤ Static image analysis
➤ Laser scanning cytometry
■ Morphometry

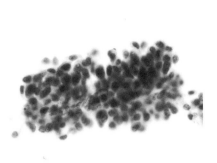 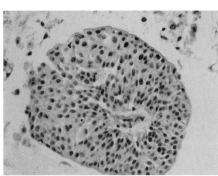

5-30A and B. Low-grade urothelial carcinoma *(left and right).* (A) Voided urine showing a papillary group with a thin fibrovascular core on ThinPrep (Papanicolaou stain) (B) Cell block sections (hematoxylin and eosin stain)

- Cytogenetic alterations and urothelial tumor markers
  - Microsatellite Instability Assays
  - FISH – Urovysion
  - Blood (ABO) group antigens and Lewis X
  - Urothelial tumor-associated monoclonal antibodies
  - CK20
  - E-cadherin
  - P53
  - The BARD bladder tumor antigen: BTA™
  - Nuclear matrix protein: NMP22™
  - Telomerase
  - Multiprobe FISH Assay: UroVision™
  - Cyfra 21-1
  - ImmunoCyte
  - Survivin

Differential Diagnosis
- Polyoma virus infection
  - Single, large, homogenous, basophilic inclusions occupying most of an enlarged nuclear area, "decoy cells"
  - Urothelial cells affected by BK virus have an abnormal DNA content
- Uroithiasis
  - Cellular and three-dimensional fragments composed of cells exhibiting significant pleomorphism may be seen
  - Clinical history is crucial to avoid a false-positive diagnosis
- Therapy
  - Details as above
- Seminal vesicle cells
  - Bizarre cells, with greatly enlarged nuclei and foamy, fragmented cytoplasm. The chromatin is hyperchromatic, degenerated and smudgy. In contrast, the chromatin of malignant cells is coarse
  - Golden-brown lipofuscin pigment and often, spermatozoa accompany seminal vesicle cells
  - These cells also have an abnormal DNA content
- Prostatic carcinoma
  - Cells with delicate cytoplasm and prominent nucleoli
  - Tumor cells are negative CK7 and CK20 and positive for PSA and PSAP
- Karyomegalic interstitial nephritis- a rare cause of progressive renal failure, which may be familial, and is frequently associated with a history of recurrent respiratory infections. The urine may contain large, pleomorphic cells, mimicking carcinoma

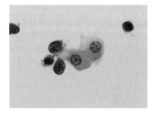

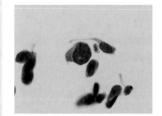

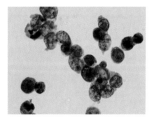

5-31A, B, and C. High-grade urothelial carcinoma *(top, middle, bottom).* (A–C) Urothelial cells with high N:C ratio, eccentrically located nucleus with irregular nuclear membrane and hyperchromasia. (Papanicolaou stain)

5-32. High-grade urothelial carcinoma *(left)*. Surgical biopsy of a patient with a positive barbotage showing disorganized markedly atypical, pleomorphic urothelial cells with high N:C ratio, prominent nucleoli and abundant mitotic figures (hematoxylin and eosin stain)

5-33. High-grade urothelial carcinoma with squamous differentiation *(right)*. Atypical squamoid cells with focal keratinization, high N:C ratio, and nuclear hyperchromasia. The follow up surgical biopsy showed an urothelial carcinoma with squamous differentiation (Papanicolaou stain)

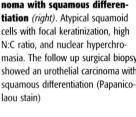
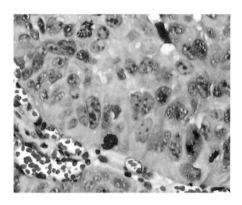
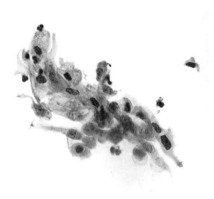

5-34A and B. High grade urothelial carcinoma with glandular differentiation *(left and right)*. (A) Atypical cells with focal cytoplasmic lumen formation, high N:C ratio, and nuclear hyperchromasia (Papanicolaou stain) (B) Mucicarmine stain shows pink stained intracytoplasmic mucin (Mucicarmine stain)

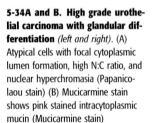
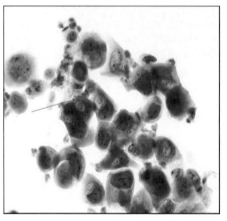
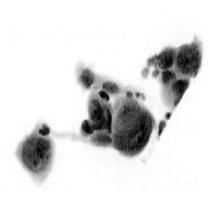

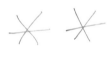
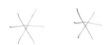

PEARLS

★ Although the morphologic features of papillary urothelial neoplasms are delineated above, the sensitivity and specificity of detecting lesions other that high-grade urothelial carcinoma has been shown to be very low and cannot be reliably diagnosed in urine cytology. The risk of progression to high-grade urothelial carcinoma is very low, and in such cases, usually a lesion is detected in cystoscopy and the surgical biopsy leads to the diagnosis. Therefore, for practical purposes, only high-grade urothelial carcinoma is diagnosed on cytology, and unless a true papillary fragment with a discernible fibrovascular core lined by slightly atypical urothelial cells is seen, a diagnosis of low-grade urothelial carcinoma should not be rendered

★ Stones can coexist with a neoplasm

★ Type of urine specimen (voided, instrumented, and ileal conduit) may influence the cellularity and the degree of preservation of the epithelial cells

★ In the presence of urothelial carcinoma if atypical squamous of glandular cells are identified a diagnosis of urothelial carcinoma with squamous or glandular differentiation could be rendered

★ Other epithelial cells including squamous (contaminant or metaplastic) and glandular cells – prostatic, endometrial, cystitis glandularis, paraurethral glands – may be seen

OTHER BLADDER NEOPLASMS

SQUAMOUS CELL CARCINOMA

Clinical Features

▪ Rare in the United States, accounting for less than 5% of all bladder carcinomas

▪ Associated with schistosomiasis, chronic inflammation, and urolithiasis

Cytologic Features
▨ Well-differentiated carcinoma; cells with dense cytoplasm, and orangophilia (if keratinizing), hyperchromatic small nuclei
▨ Poorly differentiated carcinoma; pleomorphic, hyperchromatic cells with high N:C ratio, prominent nucleoli, and necrotic background

Special Stains and Immunohistochemistry
▨ Noncontributory

Modern Techniques for Diagnosis
▨ Noncontributory

Differential Diagnosis
▧ Copresence of urothelial carcinoma and dysplastic squamous cells arising in the genital tract
  ➤ Cannot be reliably distinguished cytological from squamous cell carcinoma arising in the bladder
▧ Squamous cell carcinoma arising in the genital tract
  ➤ Cannot be distinguished cytological from squamous cell carcinoma arising in the bladder

★ In the presence of dysplastic squamous cells in the urine, a differential diagnosis of urothelial carcinoma with squamous differentiation, squamous cell carcinoma, and dysplastic cells arising in the genital tract should be raised

ADENOCARCINOMA

Clinical Features
▨ Rare, accounting for less than 2% of all bladder carcinomas
▨ May arise in the bladder or urachus

Cytologic Features
▨ Well-differentiated carcinoma; forming glandular structures, or isolated columnar cells with hyperchromatic nuclei and amphophilic, finely vacuolated cytoplasm
▨ Poorly differentiated carcinoma with signet ring cells or cells with high N:C ratio, and prominent nucleoli

Special Stains and Immunohistochemistry
▨ Cytokeratin 20 positive, cytokeratin 7–varying range of positivity 0–82%, beta-catenin negative
▨ In general, CDX-2 and villin are negative in adenocarcinoma arising in the bladder, however, there are reports stating otherwise as well

Modern Techniques for Diagnosis
▨ Noncontributory

Differential Diagnosis
▧ Metastatic adenocarcinoma
  ➤ Clinical history and above mentioned immunohistochemical studies will aid in the differential diagnosis
  ➤ Direct extension from the GI or GU tract – clinical history and above-mentioned immunohistochemical studies will aid in the differential diagnosis

■ Nephrogenic adenoma
  ➤ Although vacuolated cells could be seen, the N:C ratio is lower than that of adenocarcinoma and the nuclei are inconspicuous
■ Cystitis glandularis – glandular cells have bland cytologic features
  ➤ Instrumentation – cytoplasmic vacuolization and cytoplasmic collar formation around small groups of reactive appearing urothelial cells
■ Therapy-related changes
  ➤ See above for discussion on individual changes seen with different agents
■ Renal cell carcinoma
  ➤ Could be confused for clear cell carcinoma, history of a renal mass, lower N:C ratio with eccentrically placed nucleus, and immunohistochemical positivity for CD10 and RCC marker points toward a renal cell carcinoma

PEARLS

★ In general, low cellularity, low N:C ratio, bland nuclear features indicate of reactive conditions, whereas high N:C ratio, pleomorphism, and presence of necrosis indicate a neoplastic process

SMALL CELL CARCINOMA

Clinical Features
■ Highly aggressive malignancy, accounting for less than 1% of the bladder carcinomas
■ Majority of small cell carcinomas are seen in combination with urothelial carcinoma
■ Most common after sixth decade
■ Most common symptoms: hematuria, dysuria, and paraneoplastic syndromes

Cytologic Features
■ Identical to small cell carcinomas seen elsewhere; small round to oval cells, with high N:C ratio, scant cytoplasm, hyperchromatic nucleus with coarse "salt and pepper" chromatin, nuclear molding, and occasional mitotic figures

Special Stains and Immunohistochemistry
■ Chromogranin, synaptophysin, CD56: Positive

Modern Techniques for Diagnosis
■ Noncontributory

Differential Diagnosis
■ Metastatic small cell carcinoma
  ➤ Essentially impossible to differentiate from primary small cell carcinoma based on cytologic features alone
■ Hematopoietic malignancy (lymphoma/leukemia)
  ➤ More discohesive cells, positivity of hematopoietic markers such as CD45

PEARLS

★ Identification of small cell carcinoma is important because of the poor prognosis and therapeutic implications

SECONDARY MALIGNANCIES

- ~10% of bladder tumors
- Majority (~70%) – direct invasion from prostate, cervix, uterus, or GI tract
- Distant metastases – malignant melanoma, carcinomas of stomach, breast, kidney, and lung

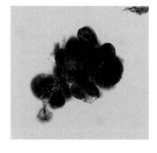

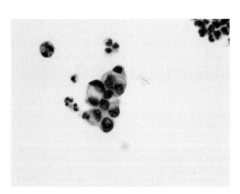

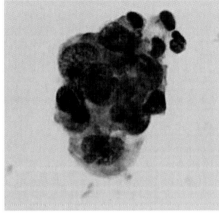

5-35. Prostatic adenocarcinoma *(above)*. Bladder barbotage specimen a small acinar cluster formed of cells with small scant cytoplasm and prominent nucleoli. Note the rare mitotic figure (Papanicolaou stain)

5-36A and B. Clear cell carcinoma *(left, right)*. (A) Bladder barbotage specimen showing small groups of pleomorphic cells with cytoplasmic vacuolization, nuclear hyperchromasia and prominent nucleoli. (B) A subsequent hysterectomy showed a clear cell carcinoma of the uterus (B) (Papanicolaou stain)

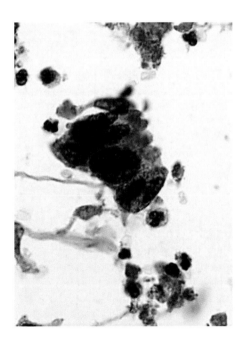

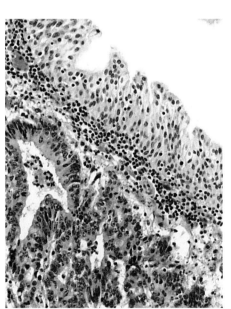

5-37. Colon carcinoma *(left, right)*. (A) Bladder barbotage specimen showing columnar cells with increased N:C ratio, irregular nuclear membranes and hyperchromasia in a background of acute inflammatory cells and necrosis (Papanicolaou stain) Surgical biopsy showing invasion of colon carcinoma into the bladder. (B) The colon carcinoma shows the classical features of columnar cells and central necrosis. (Hematoxylin and Eosin stain)

5-38A, B, and C. Mucinous adenocarcinoma *(below, left, middle, right)*. (A) Bladder barbotage specimen showing atypical glandular cells with nuclear hyperchromasia. (B) Background of abundant mucin (Papanicolaou stain). (C) The cell block sections showed signet ring cells with mucinous cytoplasm and nucleus pushed to one side (Hematoxylin and Eosin stain)

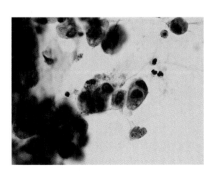

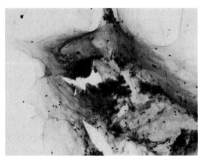

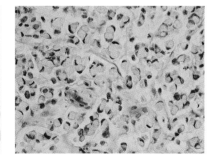

5-39A and B. Melanoma. (A) Bladder barbotage specimen showing single cells with nuclear hyperchromasia, prominent nucleoli and cytoplasmic pigmentation. (B) Rare cells are also binucleated (Papanicolaou stain)

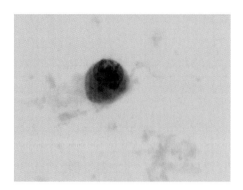
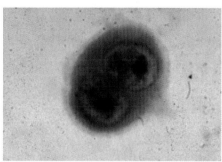

FINE-NEEDLE ASPIRATION OF UROTHELIAL CARCINOMA

Clinical Features: As Described Above
Cytologic Features
- Cellular aspirates
- Many single cells, true papillary structures with fibrovascular cores
- High N:C ratio, dense cytoplasm and eccentric nucleus
- Cells with bizarre shapes and prominent nucleoli in high-grade neoplasm
- Cells with blunt ended "tails," cercarial cells
- Rare cells with squamous or glandular differentiation

Special Stains and Immunohistochemistry
- Tumor cells are positive for CK7, CK20, and p63

Modern Techniques for Diagnosis
- Noncontributory

Differential Diagnosis
- Renal cell carcinoma
  - ➤ Clear cell carcinomas have abundant finely vacuolated cytoplasm with eccentrically placed nuclei and conspicuous nucleoli
  - ➤ Papillary carcinoma papillary clusters with fibrovascular cores covered with three to six layers epithelial cells, large groups of cells arranged in a spherical configuration – "cell ball's, and macrophages associated with the tumor cells, tumor cells could have intracytoplasmic hemosiderin
- Metastatic carcinoma
  - ➤ According to the primary site immunohistochemical studies may be helpful in distinguishing them from urothelial carcinoma (which is usually cytokeratin 7 and 20, and p63 positive)
- Lymphoma
  - ➤ Cohesive single cells, usually with scant cytoplasm; could be difficult to distinguish from a poorly differentiated urothelial carcinoma; positive for hematopoietic markers (CD45 etc.) and flow cytometric analysis

PEARLS

★ Urothelial carcinoma could mimic any malignancy, just like melanoma

REFERENCES

ELEMENTS OF NORMAL URINE

Coleman DV. The cytodiagnosis of human polyoma virus infection. *Acta Cytol.* 1975; 19: 93–96.

deVries CR, and , Freiha FS. Hemorrhagic cystitis: a review. *J Urol.* Jan 1990;143(1):1–9.

Droese M, and , Voeth C. Cytologic features of seminal vesicle epithelium in aspiration biopsy smears of the prostate. *Acta Cytol.* 1976; 20: 120–125.

Kahan AV, Coleman DV, and , Koss LG. Activation of human polyoma virus infection. Detection by cytologic techniques. *Am J Clin Pathol.* 1980; 74:326–332.

Koss LG, Sherman AB, and , Eppich E: Image analysis and DNA content of urothelial cells infected with human polyoma virus. *Anal Quant Cytol.* 1984; 6:89–94.

Koss LG, and . Cytologic manifestation of benign disorders affecting cells of the lower urinary tract. In: Koss LG, editor. *Diagnostic Cytology of the Urinary Tract: With Histopathologic and Clinical Correlation.* First edition. Philadelphia: Lippincott-Raven, 1996, pp. 52–55.

Koss LG, and . The urinary tract in the absence of cancer. In Koss LG, ed. *Diagnostic cytology Cytology and its Histopathologic Bases.*, Fifth edition. Koss LG. Philadelphia: JB Lippincott, 2006, pp. 739–776.

Lee HJ, Pyo JW, and , Choi EH, et al. Isolation of adenovirus type 7 from the urine of children with acute hemorrhagic cystitis. *Pediatr Infect Dis J.* Jul 1996;15(7):633–4.

Wojcik EM, Bassler TJ, and , Orozco R: DNA ploidy of seminal vesicle cells. A potential diagnostic pitfall in urine cytology. *Analyt Quant Cytol Histol.* 1999; 21: 29–34.

Wojcik EM, Miller MC, Wright BC, Veltri RW, and , O'Dowd GJ. Comparative analysis of DNA content in Polyoma Virus infected urothelial cells, urothelial dysplasia and transitional cell carcinoma. *Anal Quant Cytol Histol.* 1997;19: 430–436.

Yuste RS, Frías C, and , López A, Vallejo C Diagnostic value of JC/BK virus antibody immuno-histochemistry staining in urine samples from posttransplant immunosuppressed patients in relation to polyomavirus reactivation. *Acta Cytol.* 2008 Mar–Apr;52(2):191–5.

INFECTIOUS
OTHER INFECTIOUS AGENTS

Highman W, and , Wilson E. Urine cytology in patients with calculi. *J Clin Pathol.* 1982;35:350–6.

Rubben H, Hering F, Dahm HH, and , Lutzeyer W: Value of exfoliative urinary cytology for differentiation between uric acid stone and tumor of upper urinary tract. *Urol* 1982;22:571–3.

SECONDARY MALIGNANCIES

Bakhos R, Shankey TV, S. Fisher, Flanigan RC, and , Wojcik EM. Comparative analysis of DNA flow cytometry and cytology of urine barbotages – review of discordant cases. *Diagn Cytopathol.* 22: 65–69, 2000

Bassily NH, Vallorosi CJ, Akdas G, Montie J, and , Rubin MA. Coordinate expression of cytokeratins CK7 and CK 20 in prostate adenocarcinoma and bladder urothelial carcinoma. *Am J Clinical Pathol.* 2000; 113: 383–8.

Bastacky S, Ibrahim S, Wilczynski SP, and , Murphy WM. The accuracy of urinary cytology in daily practice. *Cancer.* 1999; 87: 118–28.

Brown FM: Urine cytology. It is still the gold standard for screening? *Urol Clin North Am.* 2000; 27: 25–37.

Curry JL, and , Wojcik EM: The effects of the current WHO/ISUP bladder neoplasm classification system on urine cytology results. *Cancer Cytopathol.* 2002; 96(3): 140–5.

Epstein JI, Amin MB, Reuter VR, and , Mostofi FK, Bladder Consensus Conference Committee: The World Health Organization/International Society of Urological Pathology Consensus Classification of urothelial (transitional cell) neoplasms of the urinary bladder. *Am J Surg Pathol.* 1998; 22: 1435–48.

Murphy WM: Current status of urinary cytology in the evaluation of bladder neoplasms. *Hum Pathol.* 1990;21: 886–96.

Palmer D, Lallu S, Matheson P, Bethwaite P, and , Tompson K.Karyomegalic interstitial nephritis: a pitfall in urine cytology. *Diagn Cytopathol.* 2007 Mar;35(3):179–82.

Pantanowitz L, and , Otis CN.Cystitis glandularis. *Diagn Cytopathol.* 2008 Mar;36(3):181–2.

Raab SS, Lenel JC, and , Cohen MB: Low grade transitional cell carcinoma of the bladder. Cytologic diagnosis by key features as identified by logistic regression analysis. *Cancer* 1994; 74: 1621–6.

Renshaw AA: Subclassifying atypical urinary cytology specimens. *Cancer Cytopathol* 2000; 90: 222–9.

Suh N, and , Yang XJ, et al. Value of CDX2, villin, and alpha-methylacyl coenzyme A racemase immunostains in the distinction between primary adenocarcinoma of the bladder and secondary colorectal adenocarcinoma. *Mod Pathol.* 2005 Sep;18(9):1217–22.

Watarai Y, Satoh H, and , Matubara M, et al.: Comparison of urine cytology between the ileal conduit and Indiana pouch. *Acta Cytol.* 2000; 44: 748–51.

Wojcik EM, Bassler TJ, and , Orozco R: DNA ploidy of seminal vesicle cells. A potential diagnostic pitfall in urine cytology. *Anal Quant Cytol Histol.* 1999; 21: 29–34.

Wojcik EM, Bridges VJ, Miller MC, and , O'Dowd GJ: The influence of season on the incidence of DNA hypodiploidy in urinary cytology. *Cytometry (Comm Clin Cytom).* 2000; 42: 218–20.

Wojcik EM, Brownlie RJ, Bassler TJ, and , Miller MC. Superficial urothelial cells (umbrella cells) – a potential cause of abnormal DNA ploidy results in urine specimens. *Analyt Quant Cytol Histol.* 2000; 22:411–5.

FINE-NEEDLE ASPIRATION OF UROTHELIAL CARCINOMA

Al-Agha OM, Khader SN, Cajigas A, Blank W, Grafstein N, and , Seymour AW. Fine needle aspiration of urethral recurrence of urothelial carcinoma after radical cystectomy presenting as a perineal mass: a case report. *Acta Cytol.* 2008 Jan–Feb;52(1):94–8.

Hida CA, and , Gupta PK. Cercariform cells: are they specific for transitional cell carcinoma? *Cancer.* 1999 Apr 25;87(2):69–74.

Renshaw AA, and , Madge R. Cercariform cells for helping distinguish transitional cell carcinoma from non-small cell lung carcinoma in fine needle aspirates. *Acta Cytol.* 1997 Jul–Aug;41(4):999–1007.

6

Cerebrospinal Fluid and Intraocular Cytology

Rosa M. Dávila

CEREBROSPINAL FLUID

BACTERIAL MENINGITIS

Clinical Features

- Patients usually have fever, neurologic symptoms, headache, neck stiffness, and photophobia
- Small children can have bulging fontanelle, convulsions, and lethargy
- A systemic infection like pneumonia and sinusitis usually precedes symptoms
- Bacteria reach the meninges via a hematogenous route
- Diagnosis is established by CSF analysis and culture
- The frequency of the type of bacteria varies according to the age group
  - *Escherichia coli* is more common in newborns
  - *Hemophillus influenzae* is more common in young children

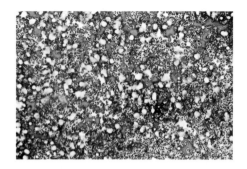

6-1. Bacterial meningitis. The presence of numerous neutrophils is typical of acute bacterial meningitis. Scattered macrophages and lymphocytes are also part of the cellular exudate (modified Giemsa stain)

➢ Neisseria meningitides is more common in adolescents
➢ *Streptococcus pneumonia* is more common in adults

Cytopathologic Features
■ Acute cases have leukocytosis with predominance of neutrophils (usually >90%)
■ Bacteria may be identified in Papanicolaou and Gram-stained slides
■ Subacute cases have increased number of lymphocytes, macrophages, and plasma cells

Special stains and Immunohistochemistry
■ Gram stain and culture of CSF are routinely used in diagnosing bacterial meningitis
■ Gram staining allows for identification of bacteria with a sensitivity of 60 – 90% and specificity of 97%

Modern Techniques for Diagnosis
■ Polymerase chain reaction (PCR) testing for specific bacteria provides higher sensitivity
■ Amplification of 16S rRNA gene by PCR
■ Ribosomal DNA assay

Differential Diagnosis
■ Distinction from viral meningitis, particularly when there is an abundant lymphocytic component, may be achieved with other laboratory data such as microbiologic culture and measurement of protein and glucose levels

PEARLS
★ Waterhouse–Friderichsen syndrome consists of septicemia, meningitis, and adrenal hemorrhagic infarction, petechial hemorrhages, and intravascular coagulopathy. It is usually associated with *N. meningococcus*
★ In patients with a brain abscess, the CSF is clear and colorless

VIRAL MENINGITIS

Clinical Features
■ It is the most common type of meningitis in the United States
■ Enterovirus is responsible for most cases of viral meningitis. It is transmitted via the oral–fecal route or respiratory droplets. It can occur in adults but it is more common in children during the summer. Prognosis is excellent in older children and adults but very poor in neonates
■ Usual signs and symptoms include fever, neck stiffness, headache, general malaise, and photophobia. It is often associated with gastrointestinal or respiratory problems such as diarrhea, vomits, and sore throat

Cytopathologic Features
■ CSF pleocytosis is observed. White blood count (WBC) is usually lower than in bacterial meningitis
■ Although a predominance of lymphocytes is considered a common finding in aseptic meningitis, predominance neutrophils can also be found
■ Atypical lymphocytes and plasma cells are part of the cellular milieu
■ Viral cytopathic changes are not usually present

Special Stains and Immunohistochemistry
▧ CSF Gram stain and bacterial cultures are negative. Sensitivity of viral cultures varies depending on the virus involved

Modern Techniques for Diagnosis
▧ PCR testing offers rapid identification of specific viruses

Differential Diagnosis
▪ Differentiation from bacterial or fungal meningitis is important
▪ Atypical lymphocytes need to be differentiated from malignant lymphoid cells

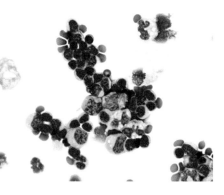

6-2. Viral meningitis. Although not unique of viral meningitis, a mixture of mature lymphocytes, reactive lymphocytes and monocytes is observed in the CSF (modified Giemsa stain)

PEARLS
★ The CSF glucose level is normal in viral meningitis

FUNGAL MENINGITIS

Clinical Features
▧ Cryptococcus, Coccidioides, and candida are the most common causes of fungal meningitis
▧ Fungi usually reach the leptomeninges via a hematogenous route. Therefore, fungal meningitis usually presents in patients with systemic mycosis
▧ Leptomeninges can be seeded via direct spread from adjacent paranasal or bone infections

Cytopathologic Features
▧ Variable cellularity
▧ Most cases have a predominance of mononuclear leukocytes
▧ Aspergillus, zygomycetes, and blastomyces can be associated with predominance of neutrophils
▧ Coccidiodes may be associated with the presence of eosinophils

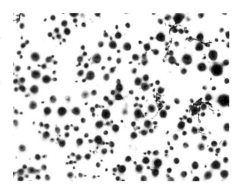

6-3. Viral meningitis. This air-dried, modified Giemsa stain CSF sample from an immunosuppressed patient reveals numerous yeast with narrow neck budding and a glassy outer layer that corresponds to the capsule. The morphologic features are consistent with cryptococcus (modified Giemsa stain)

Special Stains and Immunohistochemistry
▧ Fungal forms can be identified morphologically using histochemical stains such as Gomori methenamine silver and/or mucicarmine stains

Modern Techniques for Diagnosis
▧ Fungal cultures are necessary but are not very sensitive
▧ Antigen detection essays are useful

Differential Diagnosis
▪ Psammoma bodies
  ➤ May be confused with yeast forms but their concentric infrastructure and its large size allow for differentiation
▪ Contamination
  ➤ Always a concern and correlation with clinical and other laboratory findings is always advisable

PEARLS
★ Although fungal meningitis is more common in immunocompromised patients, it can also affect immunocompetent patients

PARASITIC INFECTIONS

Clinical Features
■ Helminths, particularly angiostrongyliasis, gnathostomiasis, and baylisascariasis, are worldwide responsible for most cases of eosinophilic meningitis, but they are not endemic in the United States
▥ Clinical symptoms vary according to the specific central nervous system (CNS) location of the lesions
▥ In the case of neurocystercosis, brain parenchymal involvement is more commonly encountered and it is usually asymptomatic
▥ Schistomomiasis can involve the CNS and can present with pseudotumor or myeloradiculopathy

6-4. Parasitic infections. Eosinophils are not normally present in the CSF. When present, they may represent the presence of a parasitic infection, foreign bodies such as shunts or intrathecal drug therapy (modified Giemsa stain)

Cytopathologic Features
▥ Cerebrospinal fluid (CSF) findings are not specific but a variable number of eosinophils are identified
▥ A 10% CSF eosinophils or ten or more eosinophils per microliter of CSF is required to make a diagnosis of eosinophilic meningitis

Special Stains and Immunohistochemistry
▥ Noncontributory

Modern Techniques for Diagnosis
▥ Detection of specific parasitic antigens can be achieved by various methods such as enzyme-linked immunosorbent assay
▥ Western blot can be used to detect serum antibodies directed to a specific parasite

Differential Diagnosis
The following are often associated with eosinophils in the CSF:
▥ Foreign material in central nervous system such as ventricular shunts
▥ Shunt infections
▥ Intraventricular drugs administration
▥ Malignant neoplasms such as eosinophilic leukemia
▥ Idiopathic hypereosinophilic syndrome
▥ Sarcoidosis
▥ Coccidioides immitis meningitis

PEARLS

★ Angiostrongyliasis cantonensis (rat lungworm) is considered the most common cause of eosinophilic meningitis in the world
★ Approximately 70% of *Coccidioides meningitis* cases have CSF eosinophilia
★ Eosinophils are not normally found in the CSF

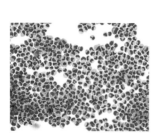

6-5. Leukemic meningitis. CSF involvement of this patient's acute promyelocytic leukemia is evident in this highly cellular sample (modified Giemsa stain)

LEUKEMIC/LYMPHOMATOUS MENINGITIS

Clinical Features
▥ Acute leukemia, predominantly acute lymphocytic leukemia (ALL) and non-Hodgkin's lymphoma are more prone to leptomeningeal involvement than chronic leukemia and Hodgkin's lymphoma
▥ Symptoms include headache, mental status changes, cranial nerve dysfunction, extremity weakness, and sensory loss
▥ When compared to patients with nonhematologic malignant meningitis, patients with leukemic/lymphomatous meningitis present more often with cranial nerve manifestations

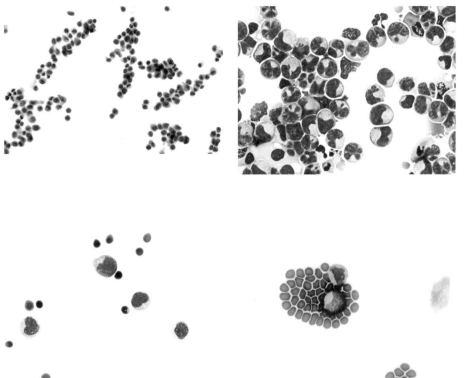

6-6. Leukemic meningitis *(left)*. When present in ethanol–fixed, Papanicolaou-stained slides, the cells may exhibit a loosely cohesive arrangement that should not be confused with that seen in epithelial cells (Papanicolaou stain)

6-7. Leukemic meningitis *(right)*. These AML blasts show a moderate amount of cytoplasm and a variable amount of chromatin clumping. Scattered cells have a prominent large nucleolus and a fine chromatin pattern (modified Giemsa stain)

6-8A. Leukemic meningitis *(left)*. This patient with a previous diagnosis of precursor B acute lymphoblastic leukemia (ALL) was found to have blasts in the CSF. The blasts are large, have round to irregular nuclear contours and scant cytoplasm (modified Giemsa stain)

6-8B. Leukemic meningitis *(right)*. These ALL blasts also have prominent nucleoli and a fine chromatin pattern (modified Giemsa stain)

■ In view of the success of prophylactic intrathecal chemotherapy in decreasing the incidence ALL CNS relapses, CSF samples from these patients are obtained early in their diagnosis and regularly during their treatment

Cytopathologic Features
■ Leukocytosis with variable number of blasts is seen in acute leukemia
■ Blasts are larger than normal lymphocytes, have higher nuclear:cytoplasmic ratio, prominent nucleoli, round to convoluted nucleus, and a fine chromatin pattern
■ Appearance of neoplastic cells varies according to the type of malignancy

Special Stains and Immunohistochemistry
■ Immunostains are helpful when the cellularity is low and differentiation between reactive and neoplastic lymphocytes is needed

Modern Techniques for Diagnosis
■ Flow cytometric analysis improves sensitivity by 75% but adequate cellularity is needed

Differential Diagnosis
■ Reactive immunoblasts
  ➤ Can be mistaken for leukemic blasts. Reactive immunoblasts usually have more cytoplasm and irregular chromatin pattern
■ Reactive lymphocytes
  ➤ Have coarsely clumped chromatin pattern and abundant cytoplasm
■ Blast-like cells
  ➤ Have been described in the CSF of neonates with hydrocephalus and are believed to originate in the germinal matrix

6-9. Lymphomatous meningitis. Large cell lymphoma will also have singly dispersed cells with large nuclei and large and prominent nucleoli. As in this example, the cells can be accompanied by degenerated cells and debris (Papanicolaou stain)

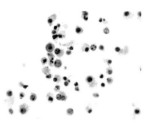

PEARLS

★ Patients with chronic leukemia who develop CSF leukocytosis are more likely to have an infectious process

★ Air-dried and Romanowski-stained preparations such as modified Giemsa stain facilitate evaluation of the lymphoid component

★ In the case of a bloody sample, it is difficult to determine if blasts originate from the CSF or the peripheral blood

LEPTOMENINGEAL CARCINOMATOSIS

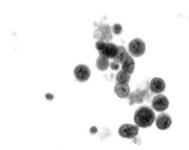

6-10. Leptomeningeal carcinomatosis. The "Indian file" arrangement of these cells is reminiscent of breast carcinoma (Papanicolaou stain)

Clinical Features

■ Found in up to 15% of patients with solid tumors

■ Adenocarcinoma is identified in most cases

■ Breast and lung are the most common sites of primary tumor

■ Most patients with leptomeningeal carcinomatosis have widely metastatic diseases

■ Presenting symptoms include, among other, headache, mental status changes, cranial nerve manifestations, and peripheral motor and sensory abnormalities

Cytopathologic Features

■ Morphologic identification of neoplastic cells is necessary to make the diagnosis

■ Morphologic findings vary according to the type of primary tumor

■ Malignant cells can be arranged in clusters or singly

■ The sensitivity of cytologic diagnosis is dependent on the extent of leptomeningeal involvement and on the number of CSF samples obtained. The sensitivity goes from 45% with one sample to 80% with two samples

Special Stains and Immunohistochemistry

■ Immunohistochemical staining for various antigens and tumor markers is helpful but limited by the number of cells available for evaluation

6-11. Leptomeningeal carcinomatosis. These cells can be readily classified as malignant. However, as in this case of breast ductal carcinoma, the malignant cells may not be cohesive enough to reveal their epithelial origin (Papanicolaou stain)

Differential Diagnosis

■ When the malignant cells are arranged singly, they may resemble reactive lymphocytes or macrophages

■ Choroidal/ependymal cell clusters have benign nuclear features and are usually seen in samples from patients with ventricular shunts

■ Meningothelial cell clusters also have benign nuclear features that allow differentiation form metastatic carcinoma

PEARLS

★ In the absence of a large intracranial mass it is unlikely that malignant cells in the CSF originate from a primary CNS tumor

6-12A. Leptomeningeal carcinomatosis *(left)*. As in other anatomic sites, metastatic adenocarcinoma can be easily diagnosed when the cells show significant nuclear abnormality and cytoplasmic vacuoles (modified Giemsa stain)

6-12B. Leptomeningeal carcinomatosis *(right)*. This higher magnification reveals the nuclear details of the malignant cells (modified Giemsa stain)

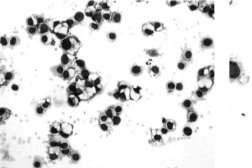
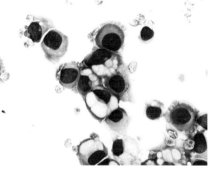

MEDULLOBLASTOMA

Clinical Features
▓ Most common malignant primary CNS tumor in childhood
▓ Most common CNS primary tumor involving the CSF during childhood
▓ Approximately 33% of patients have leptomeningeal seeding at initial presentation
▓ Usually presents with headache, vomiting and papilledema
▓ Median age at presentation nine years
▓ Most tumors (94%) are located in cerebellum, usually in the vermis
▓ Tumor recurrence is common during the two years after treatment

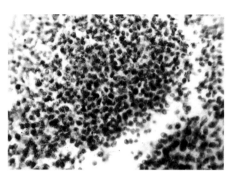

6-13. Medulloblastoma. This represents a recurrence of medulloblastoma in an eight-year-old boy. Since this is a fine-needle aspiration biopsy, numerous neoplastic cells are available for evaluation (Papanicolaou stain)

Cytopathologic Features
▓ Numerous neoplastic cells arranged singly or in clusters
▓ Neoplastic cells are slightly larger than lymphocytes, have scant cytoplasm, nuclear pleomorphism, and can show nuclear molding
▓ Rosette arrangement and small nucleoli are often seen
▓ Single cell necrosis and necrotic debris are common

Special Stains and Immunohistochemistry
▓ Due to the neuronal differentiation observed in medulloblastoma, synaptophysin, microtubule-associated protein 2, and neurofilament immunostains are usually positive
▓ Rare cases may show focal GFAP-positive immunostain

Modern Techniques for Diagnosis
▓ Most common structural genetic abnormality is isochromosome 17q
▓ Gene amplification of the MYC oncogenes is seen in large cell/anaplastic medulloblastomas

Differential Diagnosis
■ The presence of necrosis and history of intracranial mass help in distinction from ependymal or choroid plexus cells
■ Undifferentiated small cell carcinoma is more common in adults

PEARLS
★ Systemic spread occurs in about 7% of patients and bone is the most common site of systemic metastases

6-14A. Medulloblastoma *(left).* When medulloblastoma cells are detected in the CSF, they are often arranged in small groups such as this one (modified Giemsa stain)

6-14B. Medulloblastoma *(right).* In Papanicolaou-stained slides the cells are small, with scant cytoplasm and lack nucleoli (Papanicolaou stain)

GLIOBLASTOMA MULTIFORME

6-15A. Glioblastoma multiforme
(left). It is not common to
identify malignant cells in the CSF of
glioblastoma patients and when
present, they tend to be sparse
(modified Giemsa stain)

6-15B. Glioblastoma multiforme
(right). The cellular pleomorphism of
this tumor is reflected in the size and
shape of the neoplastic cells
encountered in the CSF (modified
Giemsa stain)

Clinical Features
- Most common primary CNS tumor that involves CSF in adults
- Median survival is twelve to fifteen months
- Belongs to the group of diffuse (infiltrating) astrocytomas
- Most tumors are supratentorial and solitary
- Symptoms are variable but headache, seizures, confusion, hemiplegia, and aphasia can be encountered

Cytopathologic Features
- Neoplastic cells are arranged singly or in small clusters
- High nuclear pleomorphism
- Irregular nuclear membranes
- Prominent nucleoli
- Coarse chromatin pattern
- Variable amount of cytoplasm

Special Stains and Immunohistochemistry
- GFAP positivity
- Immunopositivity has been observed for vimentin and epithelial markers such as AE1, AE3, and EMA

Modern Techniques for Diagnosis
- Trisomy/polysomy of chromosome 7, monosomy of chromosome 10, EGFR gene amplification and p53 deletion have been described in glioblastomas

Differential Diagnosis
- Metastatic carcinoma
  - ➤ can be considered in the differential diagnosis, particularly when positive immunostaining is observed with AE1/AE3 or EMA. Therefore, epithelial markers such as CK7 and CK20 may be helpful since they are absent in astrocytic tumors
- Melanoma
  - ➤ is the great imitator and should be considered in the differential diagnosis. Detection of melan A and HMB-45 will help in reaching the diagnosis of melanoma
- Pleomorphic sarcoma
  - ➤ can be excluded if GFAP positivity is detected

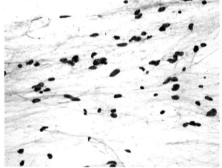

6-16. Glioblastoma multiforme.
As in the CSF sample, this
touch preparation from the resected
specimen shows the presence of
large spindle-shaped cells (H&E)

★ Can be associated with genetic syndromes such as Li–Fraumeni syndrome, neurofibromatosis type I, and Turcot's syndrome
★ Glioblastomas with p53 mutation usually arise from a previously existing lower grade astrocytoma and are referred to as secondary glioblastomas
★ Glioblastomas with EGFR amplification usually arise de novo

INTRAOCULAR CYTOLOGY

INTRAOCULAR HEMORRHAGE

Clinical Features

▪ Factors associated with intraocular hemorrhage: trauma, diabetes mellitus, coagulation disorders, anticoagulant therapy, systemic hypertension, sickle cell disease, and intraocular neoplasms
▪ Patients often develop a sudden, painless decreased visual acuity

Cytologic Features

▪ The cytologic findings may vary according to the chronicity and etiology of the hemorrhage
▪ Hemosiderin-laden macrophages and red blood cells are common
▪ Ghost erythrocytes are red blood cells that have lost their hemoglobin content
▪ Hemoglobin spherules are eosinophilic spheres of various sizes that correspond to hemoglobin
▪ When bleeding is related to fibrous membrane formation, microfragments of connective tissue can be seen
▪ In cases with neovacularization, capillary wall segments can be seen

6-17. Intraocular hemorrhage.
Patients with intraocular hemorrhage can undergo therapeutic vitrectomy as an attempt to improve visual acuity. We expect to see intact red blood cells and red blood cells that have lost their hemoglobin, also known as ghost erythrocytes (modified Giemsa stain)

Special Stains and Immunohistochemistry

▪ Iron stains such as Prussian Blue highlight the presence of iron in the cytoplasm of macrophages

Modern Techniques for Diagnosis

▪ Not contributory

Differential Diagnosis

▪ Tumor-related hemorrhage needs to be excluded in some patients and evaluation of the vitreous fluid will help in assessing the possibility
▪ Vitreous hemorrhage in young children should raise the possibility of shaken baby syndrome

★ Vitrectomy is therapeutic in these cases since the blood removal leads to improved visual acuity
★ Vitrectomy can also be diagnostic when the possibility of tumor-related bleeding is a consideration

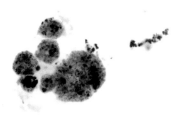

6-18. Intraocular hemorrhage.
Macrophages with hemosiderin cytoplasmic pigment are also seen (Papanicolaou stain)

ASTEROID HYALOSIS

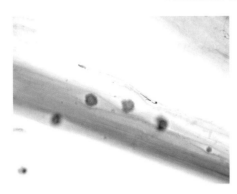

6-19A. Asteroid hyalosis. Identification of these acellular, spherical structures that vary in diameter is usually an incidental finding. This vitreous fluid is from a patient with chronic vitritis who was also known to have asteroid hyalosis (Papanicolaou stain)

Clinical Features
■ More common in men (up to 3:1)
■ Incidence increases with age (mean 67 years; range 9–97 years)
■ Unknown etiology
■ Usually asymptomatic
■ Usually unilateral (75% patients)
■ Association with diabetes, hypertension, hypercalcemia, hypercholesterolemia
■ Prevalence of 2% in autopsy studies
■ Ophthalmologic exam reveals small white or yellow-white spheres suspended in the vitreous fluid

Cytologic Features
■ Spherical structures ranging from 0.05 to 0.1 mm in diameter
■ Pink with bluish rim on Papanicolaou stain
■ Birefringence under polarized light

Special Stains and Immunohistochemistry
■ Spheres are colloidal iron and Alcian Blue positive
■ Weak posivity observed with Oil Red O

Modern Techniques for Diagnosis
■ Electron energy loss spectroscopy and energy-filtered transmission electron microscopy have demonstrated similarity between asteroids bodies and hydroxyapatite

Differential Diagnosis
■ Spheres may be confused with fungal structures by the inexperienced observer but the diameter of most spheres is greater than that seen in most yeast
■ Spheres may also be confused with a contaminant, however, clinical correlation will suggest the diagnosis

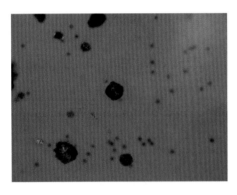

6-19B. Asteroid hyalosis. When the asteroid like structures are examined under polarized light, we can observe the presence of birefringent material (modified Giemsa stain)

PEARLS

★ Although patients with asteroid hyalosis are usually asymptomatic, abundance of the asteroid spheres may interfere with adequate ophthalmologic evaluation of patients that may have additional pathology

PHACOLYTIC GLAUCOMA

Clinical Features
■ Mean age at presentation is sixty-three years and is more common in women
■ This is an example of open angle glaucoma where patients have a milky anterior chamber (aqueous) fluid and a cataract
■ Lens material leaks into the aqueous fluid in the absence of a lens capsule rupture and elicits an inflammatory cellular response

Cytologic Features
■ Aqueous fluid contains macrophages and lens material is identified in their cytoplasm
■ Phacolytic cells are macrophages with ingested lens material

■ The lens material usually does not elicit a conspicuous lymphocytic response

Special Stains and Immunohistochemistry
■ Not contributory

Modern Techniques for Diagnosis
■ Not contributory

Differential Diagnosis
■ Inflammation due to other etiologies need to be excluded
■ Cataract extraction may result in retained lens fragments with the development of uveitis that require vitrectomy. Evaluation of such vitreous fluids may demonstrate lens material and macrophages. The number of macrophages can increase until approximately ninety days postop. In addition to macrophages, multinucleated giant cells and neutrophils can be also identified

6-20. Phacolytic granuloma. The presence of macrophages and lens fragments are supportive evidence for phacolytic glaucoma. These lens fragments should not be disregarded as a contaminant (Papanicolaou stain)

PEARLS

★ In the event of a lens capsule rupture, patients can develop phacoanaphylactic (phacoimmune) endophthalmitis characterized by a granulomatous inflammatory response containing granulation tissue, lymphocytes, plasma cells, scattered neutrophils, epitheliod histiocytes and multinucleated giant cells

BACTERIAL ENDOPHTHALMITIS

Clinical Features
■ Bacterial endophthalmitis can be endogenous or the result of bacterial seeding after surgery or ocular trauma
■ Patients with endogenous bacterial endophthalmitis usually have predisposing factors such as diabetes, intravenous catheters, hemodialysis, and immunosuppression
■ Gram-negative bacteria are responsible for approximately 60% of endogenous endophthalmitis. Klebsiella and *El coli* are the most commonly encountered bacteria
■ Gram-positive bacteria (coagulase negative *Staphylococcus*, *Staphylococcus aureus*, and *Streptococcus* species) are usually isolated in postsurgical endophthalmitis

Cytologic Features
■ When the causing agent is a virulent bacteria such as *S. aureus* and Gram-negative organisms, samples usually have numerous neutrophils with variable necrotic debris and macrophages

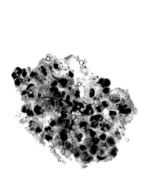 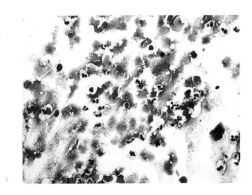

6-21. Bacterial endophthalmitis *(left)*. A mixture of macrophages and neutrophils in a vitreous fluid is very suggestive of a bacterial infectious process. The suspicion should be confirmed by microbiologic studies (Papanicolaou stain)

6-22. Bacterial endophthalmitis *(right)*. Staphylococcus aureus was isolated from this vitreous fluid containing neutrophils (modified Giemsa stain)

■ A chronic inflammatory exudate is present in less virulent bacteria such as *S. epidermidis* and *Proprionibacterium acnes*

Special Stains and Immunohistochemistry
■ Gram stain, anaerobe, and aerobe microbiologic cultures are routinely performed

Modern Techniques for Diagnosis
■ Molecular techniques such as PCR can be used in identification of specific micro-organisms

Differential Diagnosis
■ Bacterial endophthalmitis needs to be distinguished from other causes of endophthalmitis such as fungi

★ Microbiologic cultures remain the gold standard for bacterial endophthalmitis
★ Intraocular antibiotic treatment is preferred

FUNGAL ENDOPHTHALMITIS

Clinical Features
■ Candida causes most cases of exogenous and endogenous endophthalmitis
■ Patients complain of blurred vision, eye pain, and spots in the visual fields
■ Ophthalmoscopic exam reveals well circumscribed, whitish lesion in the choroid and retina and vitritis

Cytologic Features
■ Morphologic identification of the fungus can be made in direct smears stained with Gomori methenamine silver. Ethanol fixed, Papanicolaou stained smears may also show the fungi
■ A mixed inflammatory exudate of neutrophils, lymphocytes, and macrophages is also seen in vitreous samples

Special Stains and Immunohistochemistry
■ Gomori methenamine silver
■ When Crytococcus is suspected, mucicarmine or PAS stains are helpful

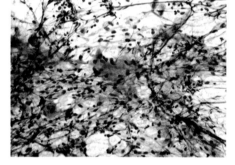

6-23. Fungal endophthalmitis.
The presence of a lymphocytic exudate and multinucleated histiocytes raised the possibility of a granulomatous inflammatory process associated with a fungal infection (Papanicolaou stain)

Modern Techniques for Diagnosis
■ PCR can detect and identify pathogenic fungi in a variety of ocular samples, including vitreous fluid

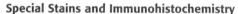

Differential Diagnosis
■ Other causes of endophthalmitis can have similar cytologic findings. Identification of the fungus is necessary to make the diagnosis

★ Endogenous fungal endophthalmitis is preceded by fungemia
★ Exogenous endophthalmitis is a result of trauma or surgery

VIRAL ENDOPHTHALMITIS

Clinical Features
- CMV and herpes viruses are the most common viruses causing endophthalmitis
- It can develop in immunocompetent and immunodeficient patients
- Incidence of viral retinopathy in HIV patients has decreased after highly active antiretroviral therapy was introduced

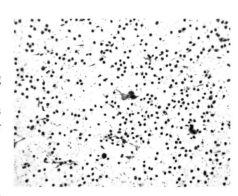

6-24. Viral endophthalmitis. Most cases of viral endophthalmitis will display a lymphocytic exudate with scattered macrophages (Papanicolaou stain)

Cytologic Features
- A mixture of macrophages and lymphocytes is seen in the vitreous fluid sample
- Viral cytopathic changes are rarely seen

Special Stains and Immunohistochemistry
- Documentation of the viral etiology is best documented by polymerase chain reaction (PCR)

Modern Techniques for Diagnosis
- PCR detection for viral antigens

Differential Diagnosis
- Malignant lymphoma and other infectious causes of uveitis need to be excluded

PEARLS
- ★ CMV persists in the retinal pigment epithelium

TOXOPLASMOSIS

Clinical Features
- Toxoplasmosis is caused by the protozoan *Toxoplasma gondii* and it presents as an acquired, postnatal infection or as a congenital infection
- The congenital form has bilateral ocular manifestations. Ophthalmoscopic evaluation reveals multiple macular inflammatory lesions
- The acquired disease occurs usually in young adults that are commonly asymptomatic. Patients can develop headaches, fever, malaise, myalgia, lymphadenitis, arthralgia and nigh sweats. The most common ophthalmologic finding is a focus of retinitis adjacent to a chorioretinal scar

Cytologic Features
- Cysts containing bradyzoites are rarely found in vitrectomy samples
- More commonly, evaluation of the vitreous fluid show a mixed inflammatory exudate with predominance of macrophages and lymphocytes

Special Stains and Immunohistochemistry
- GMS stain will highlight encysted bradyzoites

Modern Techniques for Diagnosis
- The diagnosis can be confirmed by PCR assays in ocular samples or by enzyme-linked immunosorbent assay of *T. gondii*–specific immunoglobulins

Differential Diagnosis

■ Since most vitreous fluids display a nonspecific inflammatory exudate, entities such as viral and idiopathic chronic endophthalmitis are included in the cytologic differential diagnosis

★ The disease is acquired by ingesting oocysts in contaminated food or water, cat feces present in soil or sand boxes, or ingestion of raw or undercooked meat

★ Toxoplasma can form tissue cysts that remain dormant until the patient develops problems of cellular immunity and the infection reactivates

TOXOCARA

Clinical Features

▓ Toxocariasis is caused by the nematodes *Toxocara canis* and *Toxocara catis*

▓ Visceral larva migrans (VLM) is the systemic disease with peripheral eosinophilia and various systemic manifestations reflecting inflammatory damage to specific organs

▓ Patients with ocular larva migrans (OLM) only have ocular manifestations

▓ It usually occurs in young children (five to ten years) that ingest eggs from contaminated soil

▓ The death of the larva elicits a delayed type and immediate type hypersensitivity response and eosinophilic granulomas are formed

▓ Children with OLM usually have unilateral decrease of visual acuity and strabismus

Cytologic Features

▓ Vitreous fluid reveals the presence of eosinophils accompanied by macrophages and lymphocytes

Special Stains and Immunohistochemistry

▓ Not contributory

Modern Techniques for Diagnosis

▓ Enzyme-linked immunosorbent assay for antigens secreted by the larva

▓ In OLM the ELISA is performed on vitreous or anterior chamber fluids and in VLM serum is used

Differential Diagnosis

▓ *Onchocerca volvulus* and *Tenia solium* are other helminthes that can cause ophthalmic disease

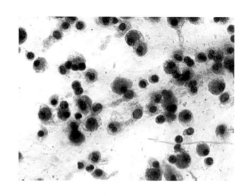

6-25. Toxocara. Identification of these protozoa is not expected in vitreous fluid. A mixed inflammatory exudate with eosinophils is typically seen. Since the eosinophil granules are not easy to identify in Papanicolaou stained slides, their identification relays on their bilobed nuclei (Papanicolaou stain)

★ Patients with OLM usually do not have clinical sign or symptoms of VLM and viceversa. Therefore, patients with OLM do not have peripheral eosinophilia and their stool examination for ova and parasite is usually negative

IDIOPATHIC CHRONIC UVEITIS

Clinical Features
▦ Uveitis refers to the presence of intraocular inflammation
▦ It usually affects patients in their third or fourth decade
▦ A vitreous sample is usually obtained in patients with chronic uveitis that persists after steroid treatment
▦ The vitreous sample is processed for cytologic evaluation, and various microbiologic studies as an attempt to identify a specific etiology

Cytologic Features
▦ Samples usually have a non specific inflammatory exudate with macrophages and lymphocytes

Special Stains and Immunohistochemistry
▦ The inflammatory process is T-cell mediated and the lymphoid component will express such differentiation by immunohistochemistry

Modern Techniques for Diagnosis
▦ Some authors advocate the use of PCR for evaluation of intraocular inflammatory mediators
▦ PCR has been used in evaluating the possibility of an infectious uveitis

Differential Diagnosis
▦ Malignant lymphoma is usually included in the clinical differential diagnosis of chronic uveitis
▦ Infectious causes of chronic uveitis can be identified in the clinical laboratory

6-26. Idiopathic chronic uveitis. The vitreous fluid from patients with idiopathic chronic uveitis usually has a mixture of benign lymphocytes and macrophages in the absence of necrosis (modified Giemsa stain)

PEARLS
★ Most cases of noninfectious uveitis are believed to be the result of autoimmunity

MALIGNANT MELANOMA

Clinical Features
▦ More common in the fifth decade and in Caucasian patients
▦ Usually unilateral
▦ Arises in the uveal tract

Cytologic Features
▦ Melanomas can be grouped into epitheliod or spindle melanomas

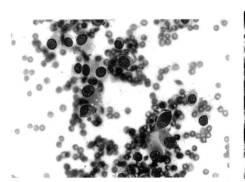
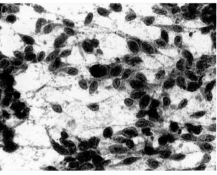

6-27A. Malignant melanoma, epithelioid type *(left)*. Fine-needle aspiration biopsies of epithelioid melanoma are usually richly cellular and the cells are not cohesive. The malignant cells have rounded nuclear profiles and large nucleoli (modified Giemsa stain)

6-27B. Malignant melanoma, epithelioid type *(right)*. Nuclear grooves and cytoplasmic pigment can be seen in epithelioid and spindle melanoma (Papanicolaou stain)

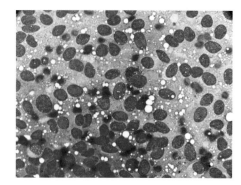

6-27C. Malignant melanoma, epithelioid type. The cytoplasmic melanin pigment is dark blue or black on modified Giemsa stained slides (modified Giemsa stain)

■ Epitheliod melanoma cells are large, and have rounded nuclear and cellular profiles. They exhibit high cellular and nuclear pleomorphism and multinucleated forms are seen. Large nucleoli, nuclear pseudoinclusion, and cytoplasmic pigment are also seen in this tumor type

■ Spindle melanoma cells have elongated cellular and nuclear profiles. The nuclei are smaller than those seen in epithelioid melanoma and nuclear grooves can be seen. They may also exhibit cytoplasmic pigment but lack significant nuclear pleomorphism and prominent nucleoli

Special Stains and Immunohistochemistry

■ Melan A and HMB-45 antibodies are used to confirm the melanocytic origin of the tumor

Modern Techniques for Diagnosis

■ Advances in molecular pathology have led to discover the role of various genetic alterations such as monosomy 3, cMyc and Bcl2, in prognosis

■ Gene expression profiling of RNA can also predict tumor behavior

Differential Diagnosis

■ Cutaneous malignant melanoma can metastasize to the eye and present as solitary or multiple masses

■ Amelanotic epitheliod melanoma and metastatic carcinoma need to be differentiated

■ Epitheliod melanoma and melanocytoma are distinguished based on the lack of significant nuclear atypia seen in the later

■ Cytologic features of spindle cell melanoma and spindle nevi overlap. The distinction between them is often based of the clinical behavior of the lesion

6-28A. Malignant melanoma, spindle cell type *(left).* Cells of spindle malignant melanoma have elongated cell profiles and oval to round nuclei. When nucleoli are identified, they are small (Papanicolaou stain)

6-28B. Malignant melanoma, spindle cell type *(right).* This example shows nuclear grooves and small nucleoli (Papanicolaou stain)

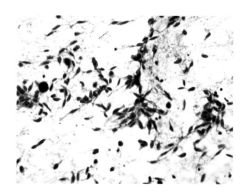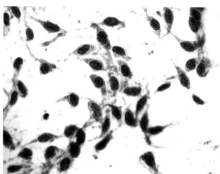

6-29a. Malignant melanoma *(left).* In some FNA samples, the melanoma cells can be arranged in tight clusters, raising the possibility of a carcinoma (Papanicolaou stain)

6-29b. Malignant melanoma *(right).* Immunostains for epithelial and melanocytic markers are helpful in distinguishing melanoma from carcinoma. In this example, the melanoma cells show strong immunostain for melan A

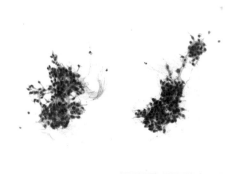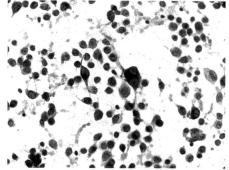

★ 90% of ocular melanomas arise in the choroid
★ Approximately 40% of patients are asymptomatic at the time of diagnosis
★ Ocular melanomas metastasize via hematogenous route, usually to the liver

PRIMARY INTRAOCULAR MALIGNANT LYMPHOMA

Clinical Features
▓ More common in fifth to seventh decades with a mean age of sixty-five years
▓ It is more common in immunosuppressed patients

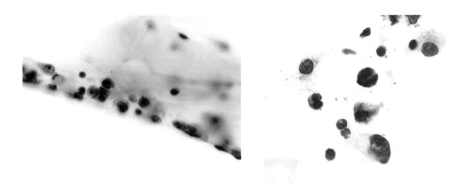

6-30A. Primary intraocular malignant lymphoma *(left)*. Vitreous samples from patients with intraocular lymphoma show a mixture of large neoplastic lymphoid cells, macrophages, and small lymphocytes (Papanicolaou stain)

6-30B. Primary intraocular malignant lymphoma *(right)*. The neoplastic lymphocytes are usually large, arranged singly, and display a large nucleolus and variable amount of cytoplasm (modified Giemsa stain)

▓ Most patients have bilateral disease and usually present with chronic posterior uveitis and vitritis
▓ Decreased visual acuity, eye pain, and floaters are common initial complaints
▓ Most patients will develop central nervous system involvement

Cytologic Features
▓ Vitreous fluid with primary ocular malignant lymphoma usually has abundant necrotic debris and a mixture of neoplastic lymphocytes and macrophages
▓ Since primary ocular malignant lymphoma is usually a large B-cell lymphoma, the neoplastic lymphocytes are large, with variable amount of cytoplasm, irregular nuclear contours and large nucleoli

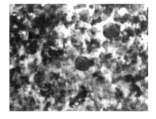

6-31. Primary intraocular malignant lymphoma. Most samples of primary intraocular malignant lymphoma have a necrotic background and sometimes the neoplastic cells are difficult to identify (modified Giemsa stain)

Special Stains and Immunohistochemistry
▓ Immunostains for B-and T-cell markers usually reveal a B-cell differentiation of tumor cells. If sufficient sample is available, kappa and lambda immunostains will demonstrate a monoclonal population

Modern Techniques for Diagnosis
▓ Flow cytometric analysis using lymphoid markers is also useful but the limited amount of vitreous fluid often does not have enough cells for flow cytometric analysis

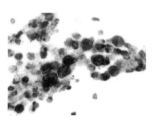

6-32. Primary intraocular malignant lymphoma. Since most primary ocular lymphomas are large B-cell type, immunostains for T-cell and B-cell markers are useful in confirming the diagnosis. This case shows strong CD20 immunostain in the large neoplastic cells. The presence of background staining is due to the accompanying necrotic debris

Differential Diagnosis
▓ Idiopathic chronic vitritis
▓ Primary ocular malignant lymphoma should be considered in any patient with chronic posterior uveitis and vitritis that persists after standard therapy

★ Lymphocytes involved in reactive/inflammatory processes of the vitreous fluid are usually T cells

RETINOBLASTOMA

Clinical Features
- Most common ocular malignant tumor in children
- Most common during the first three years of life
- It can be sporadic or familial. The familial form has a mutation of chromosome 13
- Preoperative biopsies are rarely performed. Older patients with unusual clinical presentation are the ones that may benefit from a preoperative biopsy
- Most familial cases are bilateral

Cytologic Features
- Abundant necrotic debris
- Viable tumor cells are rare
- Tumor cells are small, lack prominent nucleoli, and have scant or no cytoplasm

Special Stains and Immunohistochemistry
- Tumor cells are positive for neuroendocrine markers such as neuron specific enolase, S-100, and synaptophysin

Modern Techniques for Diagnosis
- Patients at risk of developing familial retinoblastoma can undergo DNA testing of the RB1 gene

Differential Diagnosis
- Other small round cell tumors such as lymphoma and neuroendocrine carcinomas

★ The typical clinical presentation described as a "white pupillary reflex," also known as leukocoria

METASTATIC CARCINOMA

Clinical Features
- Metastatic lesions are the most common malignant tumors of the eye
- Approximately 10% of patients with disseminated malignancy develop ocular metastases
- Most ocular metastases are carcinomas originating in the lung or breast in women and lung and gastrointestinal tract in men
- The choroid is the most common site of metastatic carcinoma

Cytologic Features
- The cytologic features of the tumor cells vary according to the histology of the primary tumor

▪ In general, the tumor cells will exhibit some degree of cohesion, revealing their epithelial nature

Special Stains and Immunohistochemistry
▪ Immunohistochemistry is very useful in documenting the epithelial differentiation of these lesions
▪ Since amelanotic melanoma is often considered in the clinical differential diagnosis of these tumors, melanocytic markers such as melan A can be applied

Modern Techniques for Diagnosis
▪ Not contributory

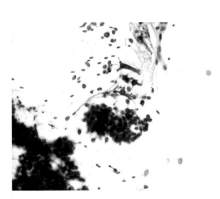

6-33. Metastatic carcinoma. The FNA from this ciliary body mass shows benign pigmented cells and cohesive clusters of small neoplastic cells (modified Giemsa stain)

Differential Diagnosis
▪ In the absence of a prior history of malignancy, primary ocular tumors need to be excluded
▪ Epithelioid melanoma can mimic carcinoma when it lacks cytoplasmic pigment and nuclear pseudoinclusions

PEARLS

★ Approximately one-third of patients with newly diagnosed metastatic carcinoma do not have prior history of cancer
★ Carcinoma associated retinopathy is a paraneoplastic retinal degeneration due to circulating antibodies to photoreceptors

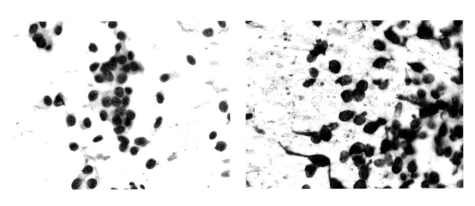

6-34A. Metastatic carcinoma *(left)*. In this case of breast ductal carcinoma metastatic to the eye the cells are arranged singly and in groups (Papanicolaou stain)

6-34B. Metastatic carcinoma *(right)*. In cases without previous history of carcinoma, immunostains for epithelial markers will help in confirming the epithelial differentiation of the tumor. A cytokeratin immunostain is shown in this case

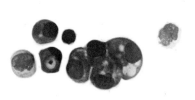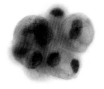

6-35A. Metastatic carcinoma *(left)*. This case of metastatic carcinoma to the eye was easily classified as an adenocarcinoma based on the presence of cytoplasmic vacuoles (modified Giemsa stain)

6-35B. Metastatic carcinoma *(right)*. The irregularity of the nuclear contours, prominent nucleoli and identification of these cells as foreign to the eye lead to a malignant diagnosis in this case (Papanicolaou stain)

REFERENCES

CEREBROSPINAL FLUID
BACTERIAL MENINGITIS

El Bashir H, Laundy M, Booy R. Diagnosis and treatment of bacterial meningitis. *Arch Dis Child.* 2003;88:615–20.

Overturf GD. Defining bacterial meningitis and other infections of the central nervous system. *Pediatr Crit Care Med.* 2005;6(3):S14–18.

Van de Beek D, de Gans J, Tunkel AR, Wijdicks EFM. Community-acquired bacterial meningitis in adults. *N Engl J Med.* 2006;354:44–53.

VIRAL MENINGITIS

Hashem M, Menegus MA. Molecular tools in the diagnosis and management of infectious diseases. *Pediatrics Rev.* 2005;26:15–21.

Negrini B, Kelleher KJ, Wald ER. Cerebrospinal fluid findings in aseptic versus bacterial meningitis. *Pediatrics.* 2000;105:316–9.

Redington JJ, Tyler KL. Viral infections of the nervous system, 2002. *Arch Neurol.* 2002;59: 712–8.

Rotbart HA. Viral meningitis. *Sem Neurol.* 2000;20:277–92.

FUNGAL MENINGITIS

Bicanic T, Harrison TS. Cryptococcal meningitis. *Br Med Bull.* 2004;72:99–118.

Gottfredsson M, Perfect JR. Fungal meningitis. *Sem Neurobiol.* 2000;20:307–22.

PARASITIC INFECTIONS

Lo Re V, Gluckman SJ. Eosinophilic meningitis. *Am J Med.* 2003;114:217–23.

Paz JA, Valente M, Casella EB, Marques-Dias MJ. Spinal cord schistosomiasis in children: analysis of seven cases. *Arquivos de Neuro-Psiquiatria.* 2002;60:224–30.

Vinshon M, Vallee L, Pirn L, Desreumaux P, Dhellemmes P. Cerebro-spinal fluid eosinophilia in shunt infections. *Neuropediatrics.* 1992;23:235–40.

LEUKEMIC/LYMPHOMATOUS MENINGITIS

Chamberlain MC, Nolan C, Abrey LE. Leukemic and lymphomatous meningitis: incidence, prognosis and treatment. *J Neuro-Oncol.* 2005;75:71–83.

Jaffey PB, Varma SK, DeMay RM, McLucas EJ, Campbell GA. Blast-like cells in the cerebrospinal fluid of young infants: further characterization of clinical setting, morphology and origin. *Am J Clin Pathol.* 1996;105(5):544–7.

Roma AA, Garcia A, Avagnina A, Rescia C, Elsner B. Lymphoid and myeloid neoplasms involving cerebrospinal fluid:comparison of morphologic examination and immunophenotyping by flow cytometry. *Diag Cytopathol.* 2002;27(5):271–5.

LEPTOMENINGEAL CARCINOMATOSIS

Chamberlain MC. Neoplastic meningitis. *Neurologist.* 2006;12:17987.

Grossman SA, Krabak MJ. Leptomeningeal carcinomatosis. *Cancer Treat Rev.* 1999;25:103–19.

Kolmel HW. Cytology of neoplastic meningiosis. *J Neuro-Oncol.* 1998;38:121–5.

MEDULLOBLASTOMA

Chhieng DC, Elgert P, Cohen JM, Jhala NC, Cangiarella JF. Cytology of primary central nervous system neoplasms in cerebrospinal fluid specimens. *Diagn Cytopathol.* 2002;26:209–12.

Ellison DW, Clifford SC, Gajjar A, Gilbertson RJ. What's new in neuron-oncology? Recent advances in medulloblastoma. *Eur J Paediatr Neurol.* 2003;7:53–66.

Koeller KK, Rushing EJ. From the Archives of the AFIP. Medulloblastoma: a comprehensive review with radiologic-pathologic correlation. *RadioGraphics.* 2003;23:1613–37.

Takei H, Bhattacharjee MB, Rivera A, Dancer Y, Powell SZ. New immunohistochemical markers in the evaluation of central nervous system tumors: a review of 7 selected adult and pediatric brain tumors. *Arch Pathol Lab Med.* 2007;131:234–41.

Urberuaga A, Navajas A, Burgos J, Pijoan JI. A review of clinical and histological features of Spanish paediatric medulloblastomas during the last 21 years. *Childs Nerv Syst.* 2006;22L: 466–74.

GLIOBLASTOMA MULTIFORME

Aldape KD, Okcu MF, Bondy ML. Molecular epidemiology of glioblastoma. *Cancer J.* 2003;9:99–106.

Chhieng DC, Elgert P, Cohen JM, Jhala NC, Cangiarella JF. Cytology of primary central nervous system neoplasms in cerebrospinal fluid specimens. *Diagn Cytopathol.* 2002;26: 209–12.

Necesalova, E. Vranova, V. Kuglik, P. Cejpek, P. Jarosova, M. Pesakova, M. Relichova, J. Veselska, R. Incidence of the main genetic markers in glioblastoma multiforme is independent of tumor topology. *Neoplasma.* 2007;54(3):212–8.

INTRAOCULAR HEMORRHAGE

Goff MJ, McDonald R, Johnson RN, Ai E, Jumper JM, Fu AD. Causes and treatment of vitreous hemorrhage. *Comp Ophthalmol Update.* 2006;7:97–111.

Zhai J, Harbour JW, Smith M, Dávila RM. Vitreous fluid cytology: A correlation study between benign cytomorphology and final clinical diagnosis. *Acta Cytol.* 2008;52(2):196–200.

ASTEROID HYALOSIS

Fawzi AA, Vo B, Kriwanek R, Ramkumar HL, Cha C, Carts A, Heckenlively JR, Foos RY, Glasgow BJ. Asteroid hyalosis in an autopsy population. The University of California at Los Angeles (UCLA) experience. *Arch Ophthalmol.* 2005;123:486–90.

Windler J, Lunsdorf H. Ultrastructure and composition of asteroid bodies. *Invest Ophthalmol Visual Sci.* 2001;42(5):902–7.

Zaharopoulos P, Schankig V. Vitreous cytology in asteroid hyalosis and observations on inter-pretation of cytologic findings in specimens of the posterior (vitreous) compartment of the eye. *Diagn Cytopathol.* 2003;28(2):88–91.

PHACOLYTIC GLAUCOMA

Kalogeropoulos CD, Malamou-Mitsi VD, Asproudis I, Psilas K. The contribution of aqueous humor cytology in the differential diagnosis of anterior uvea inflammations. *Ocular Immunol Inflammation.* 2004;12(3):215–25.

Venkatesh PV, Ramakrishnan R, Krishnadas R, Manoharan N. Lens induced glaucomas-visual results and risk factors for final visual acuity. *Indian J Ophthalmol.* 1996;44(3):149–55.

Wilkinson CP, Green WR. Vitrectomy for retained lens material after cataract extraction. The relationship between histopathologic findings and the time of vitreous surgery. *Ophthalmology.* 2001;108:1633–7.

BACTERIAL ENDOPHTHALMITIS

Callegan MC, Gilmore MS, Gregory M, Rmadan RT, Wiskur BJ, Moyer AL, Hunt JJ, Novosad BD. Bacterial endophthalmitis: therapeutic challenges and host pathogen interactions. *Prog Retin Eye Res.* 2007;26(2):189–203.

Josephberg RG. Endophthalmitis: the latest in current management. *J Retinal Vitreous Dis.* 2006;26(6):S47–50.

Smith SR, Kroll AJ, Lou PL, Ryan EA. Endogenous bacterial and fungal endophthalmitis. *Int Ophthalmol Clin.* 2007;47(2):173–83.

FUNGAL ENDOPHTHALMITIS

Ferrer C, Colom F, Frases S Mulet E, Abad JL, Alio JL. Detection and identification of fungal pathogens by PCR and by ITS2 5.8S ribosomal DNA typing of ocular infections. *J Clin Micro-biol.* 2001;39(8):2873–9.

Klotz SA, Penn CC, Negvesky GJ, Butrus SI. Fungal and parasitic infections of the eye. *Clin Microbiol Rev.* 2000;13(4):662–85.

VIRAL ENDOPHTHALMITIS

Fischler DF, Prayson RA. Cytologic specimens form the eye: a clinicopathologic study of 33 patients. *Diagn Cytopathol.* 1997;17(4):262–6.

Goldberg DE, Smithen LM, Angelilli A, Freeman WR. HIV-associated retinopathy in the HAART era. *Retina.* 2005;25:633–49.

Zhai J, Harbour JW, Smith ME, Dávila RM: Vitreous fluid cytology: A correlation study between benign cytomorphology and final clinical diagnosis. *Acta Cytol.* 2008;52(2):196–200.

TOXOPLASMOSIS

Cassaing S, Bessieres MH, Berry A, Berrebi A, Fabre R, Magnaval JF. Comparison between two amplification sets for molecular diagnosis of toxoplasmosis by real-time PCR. *J Clin Microbiol.* 2006;44(3):720–4.

Dodds EM. Toxoplasmosis. *Current Opin Ophthalomol.* 2006;17:557–61.

Garweg JG, Jacquier P, Boehnke M. Early aqueous humor analysis in patients with human ocular toxoplasmosis. *J Clin Microbiol.* 2000;38(3):996–1001.

Zhai J, Harbour JW, Smith ME, Dávila RM: Vitreous fluid cytology: a correlation study between benign cytomorphology and final clinical diagnosis. *Acta Cytol.* 2008;52(2):196–200.

TOXOCARA

Ament CS, Young LH. Ocular manifestations of helminthic infections: onchocersiases, cysticercosis, toxocariasis, and diffuse unilateral subacute neuroretinitis. *Int Ophthalmol Clin.* 2006;46(2):1–10.

Despommier D. Toxocariasis: clinical aspects, epidemiology, medical ecology and molecular aspects. *Clin Microbiol Rev.* 2003;16(2):265–72.

Sabrosa NA, de Souza EC. Nematode infections of the eye: toxocariasis and diffuse unilateral subacute neuroretinitis. *Curr Opin Ophthalmol.* 2001;12:450–4.

IDIOPATHIC CHRONIC UVEITIS

Chan CC, Shen D, Tuo J. Polymerase chain reaction in the diagnosis of uveitis. *Int Ophthalmol Clin.* 2005;45(2):41–55.

Manku H, McCluskey P. Diagnostic vitreous biopsy in patients with uveitis: a useful investigation? *Clin Exp Ophthalmol* 2005;33:604–10.

Zhai J, Harbour JW, Smith M, Dávila RM: Vitreous fluid cytology: A correlation study between benign cytomorphology and final clinical diagnosis. *Acta Cytologica.* 2008;52(2):196–200.

MALIGNANT MELANOMA

Ehlers JP Harbour JW. Molecular pathology of uveal melanoma. *Int Ophthalmol Clin.* 2006;46(1):167–8.

Faulkner-Jones BE, Foster WJ, Harbour JW, Smith ME, Dávila RM. Fine needle aspiration biopsy with adjunct immunohistochemistry in intraocular tumor management. *Acta Cytol.* 2005;49(3):297–308.

Onken MD, Worley LA, Davila RM, Char DH, Harbour JW. Prognostic testing in uveal melanoma by transcriptomic profiling of fine needle biopsy specimens. *J Molec Diagn.* 2006;8(5):567–73.

PRIMARY INTRAOCULAR MALIGNANT LYMPHOMA

Dávila RM, Miranda MC, Smith ME: The role of cytopathology in the diagnosis of ocular malignancies. *Acta Cytol.* 1998; 42:362–6.

Farkas T, Harbour JW, Dávila RM: Cytologic diagnosis of intraocular lymphoma in the vitreous aspirate. *Acta Cytol.* 2004;48:487–91.

Melcon MR, Mukai S. Intraocular lymphoma. *Int Ophthalmol Clin.* 2006;46(2):69–77.

RETINOBLASTOMA

Balmer A, Zografos L, Munier F. Diagnosis and current management of retinoblastoma. *Oncogene.* 2006;25:5341–9.

Davila RM, Miranda MC, Smith ME. Role of cytopathology in the diagnosis of ocular malignancies. *Acta Cytol.* 1998;42(2):362–6.

METASTATIC CARCINOMA

De Potter P, Disneur D, Levecq L, Snyers B. Ocular manifestations of cancer. *Journal Francais d Opthlmologie.* 2002;25(2):194–202.

Eliassi-Rad B, Albert DM, Green WR. Frequency of ocular metastases in patients dying of cancer in eye bank populations. *Br J Ophthalmol.* 1996;80(2):125–8.

Faulkner-Jones BE, Foster WJ, Harbour JW, Smith ME, Dávila RM: Fine needle aspiration biopsy with adjunct immunohistochemistry in intraocular tumor management. *Acta Cytol.* 2005;49(3):297–308.

Wickremansinghe S, Dansingani KK, Tranos P, Liyanage S, Jones a, Davey C. Ocular presentation of breast cancer. *Acta Ophthalmol Scand.* 2007;85:133–42.

7

Cytopathology of the Breast

Shahla Masood, and Marilin Rosa

> Myofibroblastoma
> Granular cell tumor
> Malignant mesenchymal tumors (sarcoma)
>
> Lymphomas
>
> Metastatic disease to the breast
>
> The male breast
>
> Prognostic/predictive factors
>
> Telomerase activity as a marker of breast carcinoma in cytology samples

SPECIMEN TYPES IN BREAST CYTOPATHOLOGY

FINE-NEEDLE ASPIRATION BIOPSY OF BREAST

Definition
- Fine-needle aspiration (FNA) is a technique for obtaining cellular material using a 21–25 gauge needle

Advantages
- Cost-effectiveness
- Minimal discomfort for the patient
- Rapid results and potential bedside diagnosis
- When compared to core needle biopsy in palpable breast lesions, FNA allows moving the needle in different directions, which permits better and more extensive sampling of the lesion

Accuracy
- Highly operator dependent
- Sensitivity for malignancy: 65–98%
- Specificity: 34–100%
- False-positive results: 0–2%
- False-negative results occur because of inaccurate sampling, interpretation, or both

Uses of FNA in Breast
- All palpable lesions
- Radiologically detected nonpalpable cystic lesions
- Therapeutic procedure for evacuation of cysts and abscesses
- Alternative procedure when surgical biopsy is not possible
- Tumor sampling for prognostic/ predictive factors and response to therapy

Complications
- Very low incidence of complications
- Occasionally, hematoma formation, bleeding, or infection and infarct of the lesion can occur

Techniques
- The triple test (physical examination, imaging studies, and cytological examination) should be used for diagnosis
- FNA of nonpalpable lesions are usually performed under ultrasound (US) or mammogram guidance
- The average number of passes recommended for adequate sampling of most palpable masses is two to four; however, more passes may be necessary in select cases

▦ Direct smearing is the preferred method of preparation of the slides

▦ Air-dried Romanowsky-type stains (modified Giemsa stain) and alcohol-fixed Papanicolaou (PAP) stains are optimal for diagnosis

▦ The cell block is prepared mainly when special stains and prognostic/predictive factors studies are anticipated. A separate pass can be dedicated for cell block preparation

▦ If the need for ancillary studies is expected, consult the laboratory for preferences in specimen preparation

Specimen adequacy

▦ There are no specific requirements for a minimum number of ductal cells

▦ A specimen is only considered adequate when it represents the lesion for which the biopsy has been performed

Diagnostic terminology

▦ Category system for reporting

   ➢ Benign: No evidence of malignancy

   ➢ Atypical/Indeterminate: Applied to adequate samples that represent entities difficult to diagnose by cytology, for example:

      ● Atypical ductal hyperplasia versus low grade ductal carcinoma in situ (DCIS)

      ● Papillary lesions: intraductal papilloma versus papillary carcinoma

      ● Fibroepithelial lesions: fibroadenoma versus benign phyllodes tumor

      ● Mucinous lesions: mucocele-like lesions versus mucinous carcinoma

   ➢ Suspicious: the findings are highly suggestive of malignancy, but other factors like preservation or the amount of cells fall short for the diagnosis

   ➢ Malignant: the cellular findings are diagnostic of malignancy

   ➢ Unsatisfactory/nondiagnostic: due to scant cellularity, artifacts, obscuring blood, etc.

Grading Breast Carcinomas in FNA

▦ Tumor/nuclear grading should be included in all cases if possible

▦ Several grading system exist, the simplest is dividing the lesion in low and high nuclear/histologic grades

Breast FNA Report

▦ The final report should include all the following if possible:

   ➢ Precise location of the lesion

   ➢ Specimen type

   ➢ Technique used

   ➢ Diagnosis

   ➢ Necessary comments

   ➢ Recommendations

DUCTAL LAVAGE

Definition

▦ Intraductal approach to breast tissue sampling for the detection of atypical and malignant breast ductal epithelial cells in women at high risk of developing breast cancer

Advantages

▦ Minimally invasive technique

▦ Superior to nipple aspirate in the detection of intraductal cellular abnormalities

▦ Allows the opportunity to study genetic alterations associated with breast cancer

Disadvantages
- Time-consuming procedure
- Factors that limit an adequate cellularity include old age, previous therapy, and anatomic abnormalities of the nipple
- Only retrieves cells from intraductal processes
- Unable to detect peripherally located lesions

Complications
- Rarely complications occur, including infection, ecchymoses, and breast engorgement

Accuracy
- The specificity and sensitivity of this procedure is still not defined
- The majority of lesions detected are representation of intraductal papillary lesions

Potential Uses of Ductal Lavage
- Selection of women for risk reduction intervention
- Diagnostic work-up of nipple discharge
- Early diagnosis of an occult cancer
- Study of the morphology and biology of breast cancer precursors

Technique
- A microcatheter is inserted into the ducts through the nipple surface orifices under local anesthesia
- The duct is infused with saline solution to retrieve cellular material for cytologic analysis
- May be prepared and stained by standard techniques using millipore filtration, cytospin, Thin Prep, and Papanicolaou staining

Specimen Adequacy
- There are not established criteria for adequacy in ductal lavage specimens. Some authors require the presence of ten epithelial cells to regard a specimen adequate

Diagnostic Terminology
- Diagnostic categories include
  - Benign
  - Mild changes
  - Marked changes
  - Malignant
  - Inadequate material for diagnosis
- The cytologic criteria for interpretation are similar to those of FNA

NIPPLE DISCHARGE CYTOLOGY

Definition
- Cytologic examination of the spontaneous nipple discharge in patients with no palpable abnormalities
- The majority of lesions causing bloody nipple discharge are of papillary origin

Advantages
- Noninvasive technique
- Low cost and discomfort for the patient
- Allows studying genetic alterations associated with breast cancer
- More useful in cases of unilateral discharge

Disadvantages
- It is not helpful as screening test
- Often insufficient material is retrieved for cytologic evaluation
- Only retrieves cells from intraductal processes
- Unable to detect peripherally located lesions
- Low sensitivity has been reported by some authors

Complications
- No complication has yet been reported

Accuracy
- The sensitivity for malignancy ranges from 41% to 60%

Uses of Nipple Discharge Cytology
- Selection of women for risk reduction intervention
- Diagnostic workup of nipple discharge
- Early diagnosis of an occult cancer

Technique
- Specimens are prepared by gently massaging the breast in the direction of the nipple
- A glass slide is used to touch the secreted drops
- The slides can be fixed by immersion in 95% ethyl alcohol for PAP-stained smears or air dried and stained with Romanowsky-type stains

Specimen Adequacy
- There are no specific requirements for a minimum number of ductal cells to be present and specimen adequacy is based in the operator and pathologist judgment

Cytologic Criteria
- The smears are usually sparsely cellular characterized by ductal cells in tight clusters, foam cells, inflammatory cells, and red blood cells
- Cytologic criteria of malignancy are similar to those of FNA and ductal lavage

THE NORMAL BREAST

Normal Histology
- The breast contains fifteen to twenty-five lactiferous ducts, which begin at the nipple, then branch into smaller ducts, and end in the terminal duct lobular unit (TDLU)
- All ducts and ductules are lined by an inner layer of cuboidal or columnar epithelial cells and an outer layer of myoepithelial cells
- The connective tissue within the lobule (intralobular stroma) is a mixture of fibroblasts, occasional lymphocytes, histiocytes, in a background of collagen and mucin
- The interlobular stroma is hypocellular and contains fibroadipose tissue

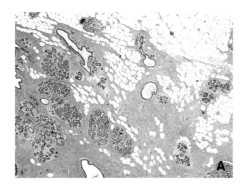
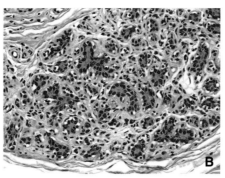

7-1. Histology of normal breast. (A) Ducts, lobules, interlobular stroma and adipose tissue. (B) High power view of normal breast lobule lined by an inner layer of cuboidal or columnar epithelial cells and an outer layer of myoepithelial cells (H&E)

7-2. Benign ductal epithelium
(left). A monolayer sheet without overlapping or atypia. The nuclei of benign ductal cells about one-and-half the size of a red blood cell (modified Giemsa)

7-3. Benign ductal cells intermixed with myoepithelial cells *(right)*. Myoepithelial cells can be also seen as naked, bipolar oval to elongated nuclei stripped of their cytoplasm in FNA (Papanicolaou stain)

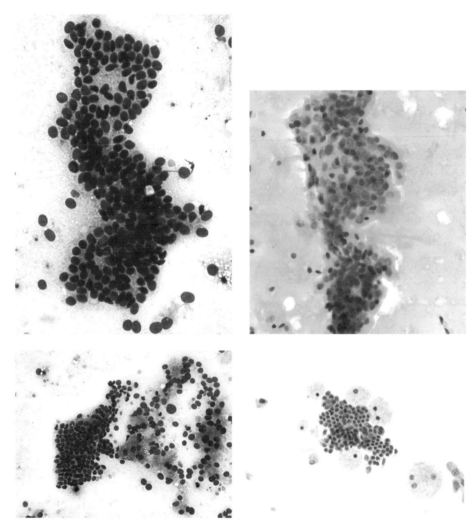

7-4. Contrast between benign and malignant ductal epithelium on FNA *(left)*. At the left of the picture: A group of benign ductal cells arranged in a monolayer sheet without overlapping or atypia. At the right of the picture: Malignant cells showing dyshesion, increased in nuclear size (as compared with the red blood cells seen in the background), lost of polarity and irregular chromatin with several nucleoli (modified Giemsa)

7-5. Foam cells *(right)*. Breast ductal lavage showing macrophages surrounding a group of benign ductal cells. The cytoplasm of macrophages is abundant and multivacuolated. The nuclei are bland (Papanicolaou stain)

Normal Components of Breast Cytology Samples

- Ductal cells
  - ➤ Highly cohesive, often two-dimensional flat sheets of small epithelial cells
  - ➤ Occasionally three-dimensional groups are aspirated (intact lobules). Few single epithelial cells are normally present
  - ➤ Cytologically ductal cells are uniform, with mild variability in cases of benign proliferative disease
  - ➤ The shape of the nuclei is round to oval and the size is about 1.5–2 times the diameter of a red blood cell (RBC)
  - ➤ The nuclear membrane is smooth and regular
  - ➤ The chromatin is fine, evenly distributed, and somewhat hyperchromatic

7-6. Apocrine cells. They form cohesive, regular sheets of cells with abundant, finely granular cytoplasm and uniform, eccentric nuclei with smooth nuclear membrane. A single, prominent nucleolus is present. Next to it, a sheet of benign ductal cells. Compare the characteristics of the cytoplasm. (A) PAP, (B) modified Giemsa

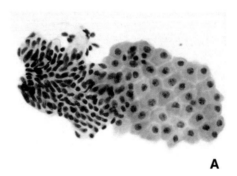

A

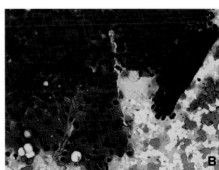

B

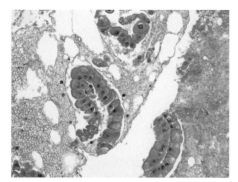

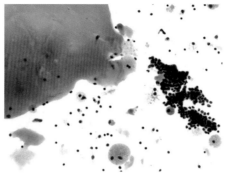

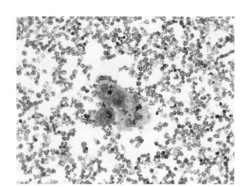

**7-7. Apocrine cells in a
cell block** *(top, left)*. The characteristics of
the cytoplasm and prominent nucleoli can be
clearly appreciated (H&E)

7-8. Ductal lavage *(top, right)*.
Ductal lavage showing a sheet of benign
ductal cells, macrophages, and proteinaceous
material in the background (Papanicolaou
stain)

7-9. Nipple discharge *(opposite)*.
Nipple discharge cytology characterized
by the presence of foam cells and abundant
blood in the background (Papanicolaou
stain)

- ➤ Nucleoli are normally inconspicuous and single
- ➤ The cytoplasm is usually scant and delicate, but may be more prominent and apocrine change is a common finding
- Myoepithelial cells
  - ➤ Their presence is a hallmark of a benign breast aspirate
  - ➤ Seen as naked, bipolar oval to elongated nuclei stripped of their cytoplasm in FNA
  - ➤ The length of the nuclei is about the diameter of a RBC
  - ➤ The chromatin is dark but bland without nucleoli
  - ➤ The nuclear outlines are fine and regular
- Foam cells
  - ➤ They could represent foamy ductal cells or histiocytes
  - ➤ Usually associated with benign lesions
  - ➤ They are found singly or in loose clusters
  - ➤ The cytoplasm is abundant, multivacuolated, and sometimes contains inclusions
  - ➤ The nuclei are bland and multinucleated cells are common
- Apocrine cells
  - ➤ Commonly found in benign breast aspirates associated with fibrocystic disease, fibroadenomas, papillary lesions, and cysts
  - ➤ They form cohesive, regular sheets of cells
  - ➤ The distinctive feature is the abundant, finely granular cytoplasm (due to the presence of abundant mitochondria), which stains blue–gray to purplish in modified Giemsa stain (DQ) and blue to orange in PAP stain
  - ➤ The nuclei are fairly uniform and eccentric and the nuclear membrane is smooth
  - ➤ The chromatin is finely granular
  - ➤ The nucleoli are single, round, and prominent
- Other components
  - ➤ Adipose tissue
  - ➤ Blood vessels

➤ Connective tissue fragments
➤ Lymphocytes or plasma cells: A few chronic inflammatory cells are acceptable
➤ Microcalcifications

PEARLS

★ The presence of a two-cell population (epithelial and myoepithelial) in a breast aspirate is the hallmark for benign disease; however, keep in mind that benign epithelial/myoepithelial cells can be seen admixed with malignant cells. This occurs during sampling of adjacent benign tissue

INFLAMMATORY BREAST LESIONS

MASTITIS

Clinical Features

▪ Acute mastitis: It is an inflammation of the breast that can occur as the result of lactation, infection or trauma
➤ Typically seen in the postpartum period
➤ Occurs in 1–3% of all lactating women
➤ The most common microorganisms implicated are staphylococci and streptococci
➤ If untreated can result in abscess formation
▪ Chronic mastitis: May evolve from an acute process or being associated with duct ectasia
➤ Plasma cell mastitis: A variant of chronic mastitis characterized by a prominent infiltrate of plasma cells
▪ Granulomatous mastitis: Its an inflammatory lesion of unknown etiology
➤ Usually occurs in patients in reproductive years
➤ It presents as a rapid growing mass that could mimic cancer

Cytologic Features

Mastitis	Cytomorphology
Acute mastitis	Abundant neutrophils Reactive ductal cells with enlarged nuclei and prominent nucleoli Foamy macrophages Cell debris in the background
Chronic mastitis	Abundant amorphus debris in the background Inflammatory infiltrate consistent of lymphocytes and plasma cells
Granulomatous mastitis	Multinucleated epithelioid histiocytes Multiple noncaseating granulomas Cellular aspirate Lymphocytes and plasma cells Ductal epithelial cells with reactive changes Cluster of fibroblasts

Special Stains and Immunohistochemistry

▪ Acute and chronic mastitis: With the appropriate clinical scenario no special studies are required
▪ Granulomatous mastitis: Since it is a diagnosis of exclusion, special stains for fungi, bacteria, and acid-fast organisms are mandatory

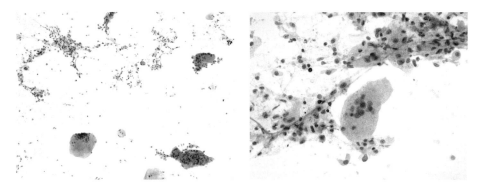

7-10 and 7-11. Granulomatous mastitis *(left and right)*. Reactive epithelial cells, macrophages, inflammatory cells, and multi-nucleated histiocytes (Papanicolaou stain)

▓ Occasionally the multinucleated histiocytes look atypical and need to be distinguished from neoplastic cells, requiring immunohistochemical staining to prove the histiocytic origin of the representative cells

Modern Techniques
▓ Noncontributory

Differential Diagnosis
▓ Granulomatous mastitis
➤ Duct ectasia: Characterized by the presence of plasma cells, granulomas and negative special stains
➤ Fat necrosis: Seen as a collection of lipophages, epithelioid and multi-nucleated giant cells
➤ Sarcoidosis: Granulomas without inflammation
➤ Tuberculosis: Background necrosis and positive acid-fast organisms
➤ Fungal infections: Can present as a palpable breast mass and special stains for fungal organisms (PAS and GMS) are necessary for the diagnosis, but only the culture is confirmatory regarding the classification of the organism
➤ Ruptured epidermal inclusion cyst: In addition to multinucleated giant cells, also keratinous material, anucleated squamous cells and inflammation are present
➤ Foreign body: Multinucleated foreign body giant cells containing ingested foreign material

PEARLS

★ It is recommended to be always cautious when making the diagnosis of malignancy in cases with marked inflammatory infiltrate

SUBAREOLAR ABSCESS

Clinical Features
▓ May be related to duct ectasia or to squamous metaplasia of the lactiferous ducts, with subsequent keratin plugging, dilatation, and rupture of the ducts
▓ Abscess formation is followed by sinus tract formation, chronic recurrent infections, and the development of fistula
▓ It is not related to lactation
▓ Occurs over a wide age range and can occur in men
▓ The treatment is surgical excision due to its propensity to recur after aspiration or drainage

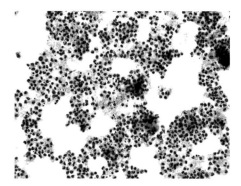

7-12. Acute mastitis. Dense acute inflammatory infiltrate composed of neutrophils and some macrophages (Papanicolaou stain)

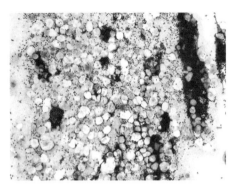

7-13. Subareolar abscess. Numerous anucleated squamous cells, neutrophils, histiocytes, multinucleated giant cells, and fat necrosis (modified Giemsa)

Cytologic Features
■ FNA yields a thick material containing numerous anucleated squamous cells, neutrophils, histiocytes, multinucleated giant cells, and fragments of granulation tissue
■ Occasionally groups of ductal cells with reactive changes can be aspirated

Special Stains and Immunohistochemistry
■ Noncontributory

Modern Techniques
■ Noncontributory

Differential Diagnosis
■ Malignancy: Subareolar abscess can mimic malignancy clinically and pathologically
➤ Clinically it can present as a mass, peau d'orange, and nipple inversion
➤ Cytologically the presence of reactive/atypical epithelium can be misleading to the diagnosis of malignancy
■ Other conditions affecting the nipple or areola such as
➤ Papillomas
➤ Lactational abscess
➤ Granulomas
➤ Fat necrosis
➤ Epidermal inclusion cysts

7-14. Subareolar abscess *(left)*. Numerous anucleated squamous cells, neutrophils, histiocytes, multinucleated giant cells, and fat necrosis (modified Giemsa)

7-15. Subareolar abscess (cell block) *(right)*. Abundant anucleated squamous cells and acute inflammation (H&E)

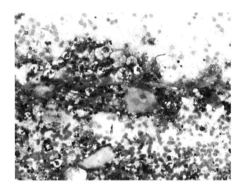 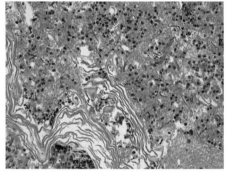

PEARLS

★ The cytologic hallmark of subareolar abscess is the presence of numerous anucleated squamous cells in a breast aspirate
★ Careful attention should be paid to the clinical presentation, the presence of inflammation and anucleated squamous cells in the background to avoid the diagnosis of malignancy when reactive atypia of the ductal epithelium is remarkable

FAT NECROSIS

Clinical Aspects
■ It occurs following trauma to the breast or previous surgical biopsy
■ It can mimic malignancy clinically and mammographically by presenting as a mass with skin retraction showing areas of calcifications

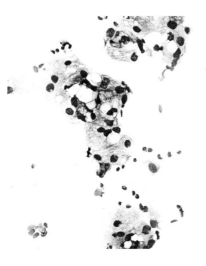

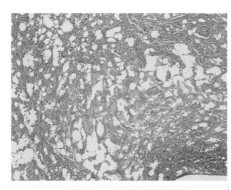

7-16. Fat necrosis *(left).* Histiocytes with vacuolated cytoplasm and inflammatory cells (modified Giemsa)

7-17. Fat necrosis histologic appearance *(right).* Necrosis of adipocytes and acute and chronic inflammatory infiltrate (H&E)

Cytologic Features
- Hypocellular smears
- Predominance of histiocytes with prominent cytoplasmic vacuoles or hemosiderin granules, kidney-shaped nuclei, and low nuclear to cytoplasmic ratio
- Multinucleated cells and fibroblasts
- Inflammatory and necrotic background
- Reactive epithelial cells
- Rare calcified particles

Special Stains and Immunohistochemistry
- Noncontributory

Modern Techniques
- Noncontributory

Differential Diagnosis
- Malignancy: Cytologically the reactive epithelial cells present in cohesive sheets without the degree of pleomorphism and discohesion seen in cancer
- Lactational adenoma: Can be rarely confused due to the vacuolated appearance of the cytoplasm of the histiocytes. Adequate clinical history helps in the differential diagnosis
- Silicone granuloma: The vacuoles seen in the cytoplasm of the histiocytes in reactions to ruptured silicone implant are larger and often have a signet ring appearance

PEARLS

⋆ Fat necrosis and cancer can occur together; for this reason the presence of fat necrosis does not completely exclude the possibility of malignancy

NONPROLIFERATIVE BREAST DISEASE

BREAST CYSTS

Clinical Features
- Cysts are the most common lesions of the female breast and are almost always benign
- They arise in the lobules (TDLU) and occur more often in premenopausal patients
- The cysts are classified as either Type I, containing a high level of potassium ions and a low level of sodium ions, or as Type II, with low potassium and high sodium ion concentrations

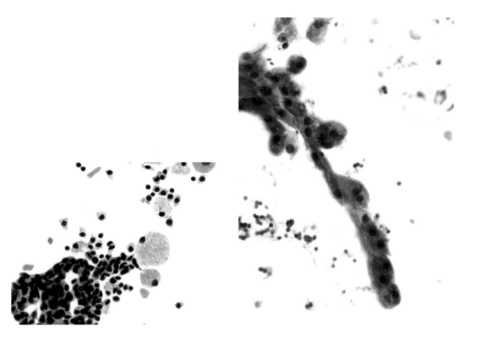

7-18. **Breast cyst** *(left)*. A sheet of benign ductal cells, foamy macrophages and few lymphocytes in the background (Papanicolaou stain)

7-19. **Breast cyst** *(right)*. A group of benign apocrine cells commonly seen in cyst aspirations (Papanicolaou stain)

▓ In some studies, women with Type I cysts are at increased risk for the development of breast cancer but more studies are necessary to reach a definitive conclusion

▓ FNA is mainly used as a therapeutic tool for evacuation of the cysts and the fluid aspirated is sent for cytological evaluation

▓ If a residual mass in the cyst wall persists after a cyst is aspirated, it should be re-aspirated and examined

▓ Epidermal inclusion cysts can also be found in breast

Cytologic Features
▓ Breast cyst
  ➤ The fluid appearance varies from clear to opaque to dark brown or bloody
  ➤ The aspirate contains mainly apocrine cells, foam cells and few ductal cells
  ➤ Benign apocrine cells are arranged in flat sheets or isolated cells, have abundant granular cytoplasm, and eccentric nuclei with prominent nucleoli
  ➤ Foam cells have abundant cytoplasm, which is vacuolated rather than granular
  ➤ Ductal cells could be arranged in sheets or tridimensional clusters.
▓ Epidermal inclusion cyst
  ➤ Contains anucleated squamous cells, debris, inflammatory cells, and multinucleated histiocytes
  ➤ They can rupture or become infected causing atypia of the squamous epithelium which can be worrisome for malignancy

Special Stains and Immunohistochemistry
▓ Noncontributory

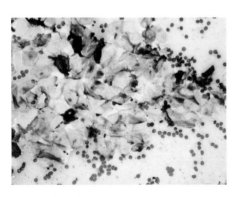

7-20. Epidermal inclusion cyst. Abundant anucleated squamous cells (modified Giemsa)

Modern Techniques
▓ Noncontributory

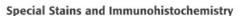

Differential Diagnosis
- Malignancy
  - ➤ Rarely medullary carcinomas become cystic. In those cases the fluid has a turbid appearance and the smear consists mostly of a mixture of inflammatory cells and tumor cells
- Papillary lesions
  - ➤ Most commonly produce a bloody aspirate or a residual mass is noted after aspiration
  - ➤ Cytologically papillary groups of ductal cells with variable degree of atypia are in more or less quantity present
- Apocrine carcinoma
  - ➤ This should be suspected when the specimen is hypercellular, marked atypia is present and there is striking cell dyshesion

PEARLS

★ If the fluid is clear and there is no residual mass after aspiration, the cyst is almost always benign

★ In general, the presence of apocrine cells support the diagnosis of a benign lesion, however they are frequently associated to papillary lesions, and in these cases the patient will require complete excision of the mass to exclude the possibility of a concomitant malignancy

COLLAGENOUS SPHERULOSIS

Clinical Features
- A benign lesion often associated with intraductal papilloma, sclerosing adenosis, or radial scar
- It is frequently an incidental finding and consists histologically of acellular, eosinophilic fibrillary structures formed by basal membrane collagen, surrounded by epithelial and myoepithelial cells
- Collagenous spherulosis is very rare, with an estimated incidence of less than 1% in excisional specimens and about 0.2% in cytology material
- It is important to correctly diagnose collagenous spherulosis not only because this lesion by itself is innocuous, but also because of its close resemblance on cytology to certain malignant entities of breast especially adenoid cystic carcinoma

Cytologic Features
- FNA is characterized by sparse to moderate cellularity
- Hyaline globules are surrounded by uniform ductal epithelial cells and attenuated myoepithelial cell layer
- The color of these spherules is pink in Giemsa-stained smears and green in Papanicolaou-stained smears

Special Stains and Immunohistochemistry
- The spherules are periodic acid–Schiff (PAS) positive

Modern Techniques
- Noncontributory

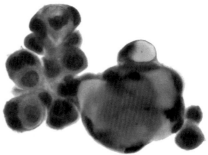

7-21. Collagenous spherulosis. Hyaline globules are surrounded by uniform ductal epithelial cells (Papanicolaou stain) Reproduced with permission from Masood S. Nipple fluid cytology. In: Masood S. Contemporary issues in Breast Cytopathology. Clin Lab Med. Saunders. Philadelphia. 25(4). 2005: 787–794

Differential Diagnosis

■ Adenoid cystic carcinoma
> ➤ Clinically it presents as a palpable mass whereas collagenous spherulosis is an incidental finding
> ➤ Cytologically the spherules in adenoid cystic carcinoma are surrounded by ductal cells with variable degree of atypia without myoepithelial cells

■ Signet ring carcinoma: The nuclei are eccentric and atypical. The spherules in signet ring carcinoma contain intracellular mucin

PEARLS

⋆ The presence of hyaline spherules in collagenous spherulosis can be troublesome and suggests the diagnosis of adenoid cystic carcinoma. It is important to be aware of this entity since no further treatment is required

MICROGLANDULAR ADENOSIS

Clinical Features

■ Microglandular adenosis is a benign proliferative lesion of the breast that can mimic adenocarcinoma

■ Presents as a localized mass in middle-aged women

■ Histologically characterized by being a poorly circumscribed, proliferation of glands with loose or fatty stroma

■ The glands are round, show regular size, and are composed of a single layer of cuboidal epithelium void of a myoepithelial layer

■ Rarely diagnosed in cytology, only two cases have been described in the literature

Cytologic Features

■ Sparse cellular smears
■ Monotonous population of epithelial cells with clear cytoplasm
■ Uniform nuclei with small nucleoli
■ Absence of myoepithelial cells in the background

Special Stains and Immunohistochemistry

■ Noncontributory

Modern Techniques

■ Noncontributory

Differential Diagnosis

All Breast lesions containing clear cells

■ Benign lesions
> ➤ Fibrocystic change: The presence of myoepithelial cells in the background helps in the differential diagnosis
> ➤ Fat necrosis and organized hematoma. The presence of necrosis or debris in the background arises the possibility of organized hematoma or fat necrosis.

■ Malignant lesions
> ➤ Secretory carcinoma: The presence of nuclear atypia, higher cellularity of the smears and abnormal cell architecture helps in the differential diagnosis of carcinoma.
> ➤ Colloid carcinoma: Abundant mucin is present in the background
> ➤ Lobular carcinoma: Lobular carcinomas have a typical single file arrangement and cells with intracellular lumens
> ➤ Metastatic renal cell carcinoma. The presence of cytologic atypia and the history of a renal mass are useful in the differential diagnosis

★ Microglandular adenosis is rarely diagnosed on cytology although the cytologic features can be easily recognized as benign

★ The absence of myoepithelial cells can be misleading, consequently in the absence of cytologic atypia it is advisable to refrain from rendering the diagnosis of malignancy and ask for excisional biopsy to further characterize these lesions

TUBULAR ADENOMA

Clinical Features

▓ Tubular adenoma is an uncommon benign tumor histologically sharply demarcated from adjacent breast tissue without a true capsule

▓ It is composed of uniform tubular structures lined by a single layer of epithelial cells and an attenuated layer of myoepithelial cells

▓ The intervening stroma is sparse and composed of a delicate fibrovascular network.

▓ Occurs most frequently in young nonpregnant women as a solitary well-defined mass

▓ Few cases have been described in the literature and confusion with fibroadenoma is a common diagnostic problem

Cytologic Features

▓ Very cellular smears

▓ Cells arranged as small, three-dimensional balls or clusters, tubules of different shapes, and less frequently as closely approximated acini

▓ Uniform cells with pale cytoplasm occasionally showing magenta granules in the Giemsa smears

▓ Opened tubules with myoepithelial cells

▓ Variable amount of stromal fragments

Special Stains and Immunohistochemistry

▓ The presence of myoepithelial cells around the tubules can be highlighted with myoepithelial cell markers, for example, calponin, p63, and smooth muscle myosin-heavy chain (SMM) among others

▓ The tubular luminal secretion is PAS positive

Modern Techniques

▓ Noncontributory

Differential Diagnosis

▓ Fibroadenoma

➤ They share several common features such as the presence of cohesive epithelial sheets some with staghorn pattern, bipolar naked nuclei in the background, and fragments of stroma

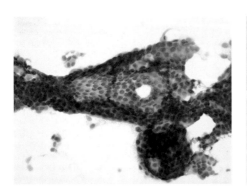

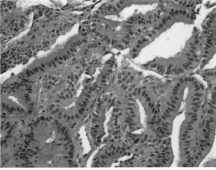

7-22. Tubular adenoma *(left).* Cells arranged in three-dimensional tubules of different shape with formation of lumina (Papanicolaou stain)

7-23. Tubular adenoma *(right).* Histology of the same case showing the presence of benign appearing back to back glands surrounded by myoepithelial cells (H&E)

> Straight tubules, closely approximated acini, and intracytoplasmic granules are not seen in aspirates from fibroadenomas
■ Tubular carcinoma
> The tubules in tubular adenomas always show myoepithelial cells, lack pleomorphism, and are more open than the angulated tubules of tubular carcinoma

PEARLS

★ The presence of conspicuous tubule formation in a smear that otherwise seems to be a fibroadenoma should alert the cytopathologist about the possibility of tubular adenoma

★ The use of combined cytologic criteria helps to make the correct diagnosis avoiding false-positive diagnosis and misclassification of this lesion

PREGNANCY AND LACTATIONAL CHANGES

Clinical Features
■ Characterized by increased acini per lobule and accumulation of secretory material in the lobular epithelial cells and lumina
■ When these changes occur as a discrete nodule it is called lactating adenoma
■ Pregnancy-associated changes can occur the novo or associated with previous lesions, for example, tubular adenomas and fibroadenomas
■ FNA is useful in distinguishing benign breast masses of pregnancy from those with marked cytologic atypia requiring surgical biopsy and may minimize the delayed diagnosis of carcinoma associated with pregnancy

Cytologic Features
■ Moderately cellular smears
■ Granular, proteinaceous background secondary to rupture of cells when smearing
■ Cells are single or in groups
■ Large epithelial cells with prominent nucleoli
■ The cytoplasm is finely vacuolated or granular
■ Foamy macrophages

Special Stains and Immunohistochemistry
■ Noncontributory

Modern Techniques
■ Noncontributory

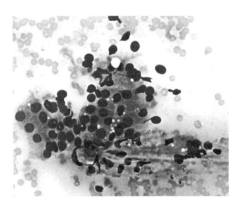
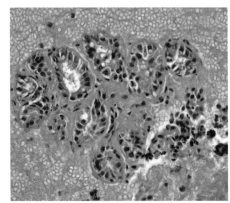

7-24. Lactational changes *(left).* Mildly enlarged epithelial cells with fine vacuoles in the cytoplasm (modified Giemsa)

7-25. Lactational changes *(right).* Cell block showing a cluster of ductal epithelium with vacuolated cytoplasm (H&E)

Differential Diagnosis

◼ Signet ring adenocarcinoma: The cytoplasmic vacuoles of signet ring cancer are single unlike several smaller vacuoles seen in lactational changes

◼ Galactocele

➤ Galactoceles are benign cystic lesions that generally occur during pregnancy and postpartum lactation

➤ Fine-needle aspiration yields milky/cloudy fluid and it is often both diagnostic and therapeutic

➤ Often the mass regresses immediately after aspiration

➤ The smear shows low to moderate cellularity with numerous foam cells

◼ Fibroadenoma with lactational changes: Clinically the presence of a smaller lesion before pregnancy substantiates the diagnosis

◼ Secretory breast carcinoma

➤ The presence of large, isolated cells with prominent nucleoli in lactational changes can rise the suspicious for a malignant lesion

➤ In malignant lesions more discohesion, loss of polarity, pleomorphism, and necrosis is present

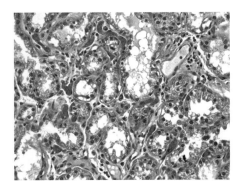

7-26. Lactational changes. Histology showing hyperplastic glandular epithelium with abundant secretion of ductal cells filling the glandular spaces (H&E)

PEARLS

★ Because breast cancer also occurs in pregnant women, it is important to distinguish between pregnancy-associated lesions and carcinoma of the lactating breast

★ Pregnancy-associated changes may present worrisome features; however, the clinical history of pregnancy and the distinct secretory changes in the epithelial cells are the clues to rendering an adequate diagnosis

TREATMENT-INDUCED CHANGES

Clinical Features

◼ Due to the increased use of breast conservative therapy combined with radiation, it is nowadays common to encounter breast biopsies where the distinction between recurrent carcinoma and radiation atypia is needed

◼ Clinically the patients present with thickening in the site of previous surgery or radiation therapy

◼ FNA biopsy has demonstrated a sensitivity of 86%, a specificity of 98%, a positive predictive value of 86%, a negative predictive value of 98%, and an efficiency of 97% in separating recurrent cancer versus radiation-induced changes

Cytologic Features

◼ Hypocellular aspirate

◼ Features of fat necrosis and granulation tissue

◼ Nuclear enlargement with preservation of low nuclear to cytoplasmic ratio (N/C ratio)

◼ Epithelial atypia characterized by hyperchromasia with prominent nucleoli

◼ Regular nuclear membrane and occasional multinucleation

■ Cytoplasmic vacuolization
■ Suture granuloma
■ Atypical squamous metaplastic cells (from the lining of seroma-type cavities following lumpectomy)

Special Stains and Immunohistochemistry
■ Noncontributory

Modern Techniques
■ Noncontributory

Differential Diagnosis
■ Recurrent malignancy
  ➤ The smears are usually more cellular with single malignant or atypical cells in a background of necrosis
  ➤ The nuclei show several nucleoli, anisonucleosis, and irregular membranes

PEARLS

★ The most important feature in the distinction of treatment-induced changes from malignancy is the cellularity of the specimen
★ Radiation-induced changes in breast tissue is a potential diagnostic pitfall, therefore when in doubt a tissue biopsy is recommended

PROLIFERATIVE BREAST DISEASE WITHOUT/WITH ATYPIA

Clinical Features
■ Comprise a group of lesions with features that range from physiologic alterations to approximately those seen in low grade in situ carcinomas
■ They vary in their severity and degree of atypia
■ It is further subdivided in two main groups
  ➤ Proliferative breast disease without atypia
  ➤ Proliferative breast disease with atypia
■ The categorization of these lesions is important in identifying women at increased risk for the subsequent development of breast cancer
  ➤ The risk is 1.5-2-fold in women with proliferative lesions without atypia, 4 to 5-fold in women with proliferative lesions with atypia

7-27. Proliferative breast disease without atypia *(left).* Cellular smear showing sheets of tight epithelial/ myoepithelial cells without pleomorphism or atypia (Papanicolaou stain)

7-28. Proliferative breast disease without atypia *(right).* Cellular smear showing sheets of tight epithelial/ myoepithelial cells without pleomorphism or atypia. Higher magnification (Papanicolaou stain)

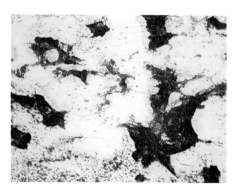
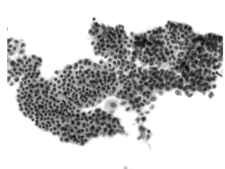

Cytologic Features

Group	Cytomorphology
Proliferative breast disease without atypia	Sheets of tight epithelial cells without nuclear overlapping Regular cellular spacing Nuclei with fine chromatin, regular nuclear outlines and lack of anisonucleosis Small inconspicuous nucleoli Myoepithelial cells are present
Proliferative breast disease with atypia	Sheets of tight epithelial cells with significant nuclear overlapping Irregular intercellular spacing that varies with the degree of atypia Small number of single cells Nuclei with coarser granular chromatin granular chromatin Prominent or multiple nucleoli Myoepithelial cells are present

Special Stains and Immunohistochemistry

▓ In proliferative breast disease the presence of myoepithelial cells can be highlighted using myoepithelial cell markers, for example, calponin, p63, and smooth muscle myosin heavy chain (SMM) among others

▓ Some pathologists use high-molecular-weight cytokeratins to differentiate between usual ductal hyperplasia and atypical ductal hyperplasia in histology; however, the authors have not found this approach helpful

Modern Techniques

▓ Noncontributory

Differential Diagnosis

▓ Papillary lesions

➤ Cytologically may be indistinguishable from proliferative breast disease. The presence of papillary fragment sometimes with visible fibrovascular cores aids in the differential diagnosis

➤ Clinically, papillary lesions present with nipple discharge or a subareolar mass

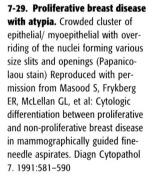

7-29. Proliferative breast disease with atypia. Crowded cluster of epithelial/ myoepithelial with overriding of the nuclei forming various size slits and openings (Papanicolaou stain) Reproduced with permission from Masood S, Frykberg ER, McLellan GL, et al: Cytologic differentiation between proliferative and non-proliferative breast disease in mammographically guided fine-needle aspirates. Diagn Cytopathol 7. 1991:581–590

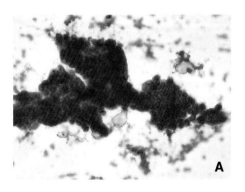
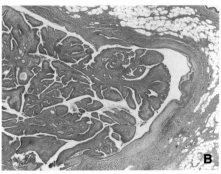

7-30. Papillary lesion. (A) Presence of three-dimensional papillary clusters without pleomorphism or nuclear atypia (PAP). (B) Surgical specimen of the same case showing a benign intraductal papilloma (H&E)

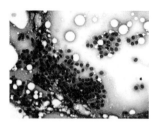

7-31. Papillary lesion with atypia. Presence of a papillary cluster conformed by a monomorphic population of plasmacytoid cells. The lack of a second cell type and discohesiveness are suspicious in this smear (modified Giemsa)

■ Fibroadenoma
  ➤ May be difficult to distinguish from proliferative breast disease; however, the presence of stromal fragments, a common feature of fibroadenomas, is less often seen in proliferative breast disease
  ➤ The presence of antler pattern in fibroadenoma is another clue to the diagnosis
■ Carcinoma
  ➤ The absence of cytologic atypia, pleomorphism, necrosis, and single malignant cells are the features that can distinguish proliferative breast disease with atypia from high grade breast carcinoma. However, there are limitations in the distinction between proliferative breast disease with atypia and low nuclear grade lesions, therefore follow-up surgical excision is required when the diagnosis of atypical hyperplasia is entertained in cytologic preparations

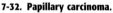

PEARLS

★ FNA can usually yield accurate diagnosis at either end of the spectrum; benign versus malignant, but a precise diagnosis of borderline lesions remain a challenge, even in tissue biopsies
★ In practice, the presence of myoepithelial cells within the cluster of atypical cells exclude the possibility of malignancy

7-32. Papillary carcinoma.
(A) Papillary cluster of atypical cells with fibrovascular core. Large atypical single cells and cuboidal to columnar cells (Papanicolaou stain).
(B) Histologic appearance of intracystic papillary carcinoma composed of fibrovascular cores lined by a monomorphic population of atypical cells without myoepithelial cells (H&E)

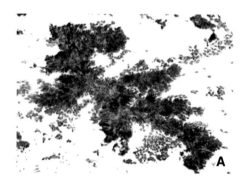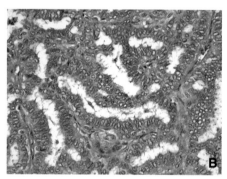

PAPILLARY LESIONS

Clinical Features
■ The assessment and categorization of papillary lesions remains one of the most challenging areas of breast pathology even in tissue sections
■ Nipple discharge cytology or FNA can be the method of evaluation
■ Papillomas are most common in women over fifty and can occur also in men
■ Papillary carcinomas
  ➤ Account for about 1–2% of breast cancers and are associated with good prognosis
  ➤ Defined as a malignant tumor with a predominantly frond-like pattern
  ➤ May be invasive or noninvasive, solid, or cystic
■ Both lesions present most commonly as nipple discharge, subareolar mass, or nipple retraction
■ All papillary lesions should be excised for histological evaluation

Cytologic Features

Lesion	Cytomorphology
Papilloma	Cellular aspirate Proteinaceous or bloody background Abundant foamy or hemosiderin-containing macrophages. Three-dimensional papillary clusters Presence of myoepithelial cells Cell balls Apocrine cells usually present
Papillary carcinoma	Highly cellular aspirate Often monomorphic population of cells Bloody background with hemosiderin-laden macrophages and necrotic debris Papillary clusters of atypical cells with fibrovascular cores Large atypical single cells and low to tall columnar cells Absence of myoepithelial cells

Special Stains and Immunohistochemistry

◼ In benign lesions, the presence of myoepithelial cells can be highlighted using myoepithelial cell markers, for example, calponin, p63, and smooth muscle myosin-heavy chain (SMM) among others

Modern Techniques
◼ Noncontributory

Differential Diagnosis
◼ Intraductal hyperplasia
➤ Clinically is rare for the patient to present with nipple discharge
➤ Characterized by two-dimensional arrangement of epithelial and myoepithelial cells
◼ Fibroadenoma
➤ Two-dimensional branching clusters often with folding, myoepithelial cells in groups and as naked nuclei in the background and fragments of stroma
◼ Papillary ductal carcinoma in situ: Often indistinguishable

PEARLS

★ Because the distinction between papilloma and papillary carcinoma is in cytology difficult, it is preferred to diagnose these cases as "papillary lesions"
★ Since about half of lesions showing papillary features on cytology prove to be malignant, all cases reported as papillary on cytology should be excised for histologic assessment

IN SITU LESIONS OF THE BREAST

DUCTAL CARCINOMA IN SITU (DCIS)

Clinical Features
◼ Marked increased risk of developing invasive breast cancer (8- to 10-fold)

Cytologic Features

- Cytologically DCIS should be graded as high nuclear grade or low nuclear grade
- Two groups: comedo and noncomedo
- Comedo carcinoma
  - Characterized by high nuclear pleomorphism and necrosis
  - Cytologically indistinguishable from infiltrating carcinoma
  - Highly cellular aspirates showing crowding and overlapping of epithelial cells
  - Pleomorphic population of neoplastic cells with necrotic background
  - Apoptosis and mitosis
  - Absence of myoepithelial cells
- Noncomedo DCIS
  - Cellularity varies
  - Monomorphic population of small to medium-sized cells
  - The clusters can be solid, papillary, or cribriform
  - Absence of myoepithelial cells

Special Stains and Immunohistochemistry

- Noncontributory

Modern Techniques

- Noncontributory

7-33. Atypical ductal hyperplasia vs. ductal carcinoma in situ. (A) Atypical ductal hyperplasia: Smear showing a monomorphic population of small-to medium-sized epithelial cells. Myoepithelial cells are admixed with the epithelial cells (PAP). (B) Ductal carcinoma in situ: Atypical population of epithelial cell without myoepithelial component forming glandular lumens (PAP)

7-34. Low grade ductal carcinoma in situ. (A) A monomorphic population of epithelial cells with minimal degree of atypia (Papanicolaou stain). (B) Histologic correlation of the case showing a low nuclear grade ductal carcinoma in situ with cribriform pattern and no necrosis (H&E)

7-35. High-grade ductal carcinoma in situ. (A) Smear of a high-grade ductal carcinoma in situ with necrosis. The epithelial cells show a high degree of pleomorphism and presence of several nucleoli. The background is necrotic (Papanicolaou stain). (B) Histologic correlation of the case showing comedo type ductal carcinoma in situ (H&E)

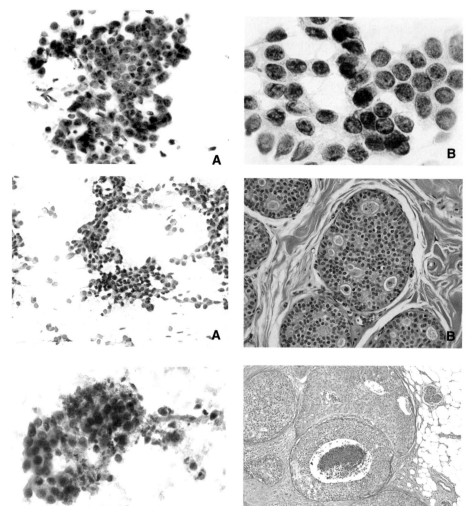
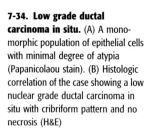
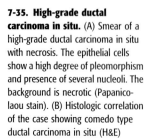

Differential Diagnosis

■ Proliferative breast disease with atypia (atypical ductal hyperplasia)
➤ The smear shows less number of atypical groups with less degree of atypia and disorganization
➤ The groups are cohesive and few single atypical cells are present
➤ Myoepithelial cells are present
➤ Benign elements can be seen
➤ The background is clean
■ Infiltrating carcinoma
➤ Comedo DCIS can be cytologically indistinguishable from infiltrating carcinoma; however, associated with clinical and imaging characteristics of the breast lesion, the combination of stromal infiltration, cribriform pattern, and necrosis in breast FNA are reliable predictors of the status of tumor invasion. Still in some cases, Histopathologic examination of the entire lesion may be necessary to confirm this diagnosis

PEARLS

✶ High-grade DCIS is easily identifiable on cytologic smears; however, distinction from invasive carcinoma may not be possible
✶ The cytologic diagnosis of low-grade DCIS is difficult. Recognition of cohesive cellular arrangements with crowding and punched-out spaces is crucial as single cells and prominent atypia are often lacking

LOBULAR NEOPLASIA

Clinical Features

■ The terminology lobular neoplasia (LN) encompasses the designations of atypical lobular hyperplasia (ALH) and lobular carcinoma in situ (LCIS)
■ Lobular neoplasia of the breast is a recognized marker for increased risk of invasive carcinoma and has well-established histologic criteria
■ The lesion is multicentric in up to 85% of cases and bilateral in 30–67% of patients
■ Close follow-up with regular mammography has been regarded as a possible management approach

Cytologic Features

■ Loosely cohesive cell groups
■ Uniform cells with eccentric regular nuclei and slight hyperchromasia
■ Presence of intracytoplasmic lumina
■ Small groups of cells similar to the acini of lobular neoplasia can be seen

Special Stains and Immunohistochemistry

■ Lobular neoplasia is typically E-cadherin and CK5 and CK6 negative and CK34BE12 positive. This pattern of staining is useful in the differential diagnosis with ductal lesions but does not help to differentiate LN from infiltrating lobular carcinoma
■ ALH and LCIS frequently resemble typical infiltrating lobular carcinoma with respect to expression of molecular markers, being ER and PR positive, and HER2-neu and p53 negative

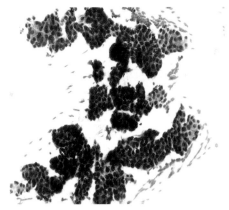

7-36. Lobular neoplasia.
A group of uniform small cells similar to the acini of lobular neoplasia is seen in this smear (Papanicolaou stain) Reproduced with permission from Masood S, Fibrocystic change, high risk, and premalignant breast disease. In: Johnston W. Cytopathology of the breast. ASCP press. 1996: 195

Modern Techniques

▪ The hallmark molecular feature of lobular malignancies, of both in situ and invasive forms, is loss or downregulation of E-cadherin, which can be tested by immuno-histochemistry

▪ Cytogenetic studies have shown that classic lobular carcinomas have relatively low numbers of changes, the most common being loss of 16q and gain of 1p

Differential Diagnosis

▪ Infiltrating lobular carcinoma
➤ FNA from infiltrating lobular carcinomas has some overlapping features with lobular neoplasia but is generally more cellular and has a higher proportion of noncohesive single cells with more nuclear atypia and pleomorphism
➤ The cells tend to present in small, indian-file groups, in cords or singly
➤ Occasionally, signet ring forms can be seen

PEARLS

★ FNA cannot reliably separate lobular neoplasia from infiltrating lobular carcinoma in many cases since this diagnosis is based on architectural features and basement membrane integrity that requires histologic study. However, since all these lesions require excisional biopsy, suggesting their presence (ex; lobular neoplasia) would be sufficient

PRIMARY BREAST CARCINOMA, COMMON TYPES

INFILTRATING DUCTAL CARCINOMA

Clinical Features

▪ It is the most common malignant tumor of the breast (65–80%)
▪ Occurs more commonly in women in their mid to late fifties, although can be also seen in younger patients
▪ It can be detected clinically or by mammography
▪ In advanced cases, the mass is associated with nipple retraction and skin changes

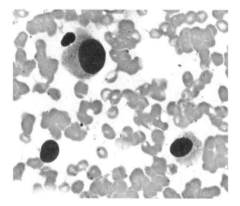

7-37. Malignant cells.
Isolated cells with excentric, enlarged nuclei with hyperchromatic coarse chromatin. The nuclear size is several times larger than that of the red blood cells seen in the background. Plasmacytoid cells are best appreciated in modified Giemsa stain

Cytologic Features

▪ Hypercellular smears
▪ Frequent isolated cells and poorly cohesive groups
▪ Dirty background
▪ Variable degree of pleomorphism
▪ Excentric, enlarged nuclei with hyperchromatic, fine or coarse granular chromatin
▪ Prominent nucleoli
▪ Occasionally plasmacytoid cells best appreciated in DQ stain

Special Stains and Immunohistochemistry

▪ Approximately 70–80% of infiltrating ductal carcinomas are ER positive and 15–30% are HER2/neu positive

Modern Techniques

▪ Genetic testing for inherited mutations in BRCA1 and BRCA2 has become integral to the care of women with a family history of breast or ovarian cancer and can assist in risk estimation for genetic counseling and breast cancer–screening programs

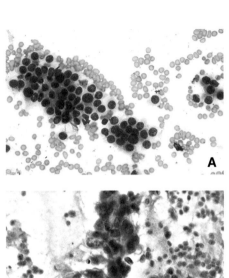
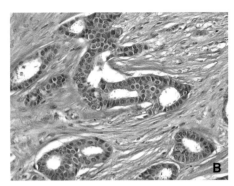

7-38. Low-grade ductal carcinoma. (A) Malignant epithelial group and absence of myoepithelial component. The malignant cells are arranged in clusters and isolated. Compare the nuclear size with the red blood cells seen in the background (modified Giemsa). (B) Histologic correlation of the case showing a well-differentiated infiltrating ductal carcinoma with prominent glandular formation (H&E)

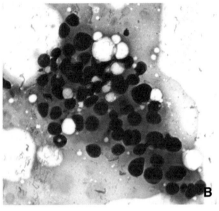
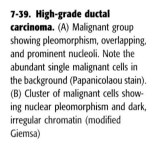

7-39. High-grade ductal carcinoma. (A) Malignant group showing pleomorphism, overlapping, and prominent nucleoli. Note the abundant single malignant cells in the background (Papanicolaou stain). (B) Cluster of malignant cells showing nuclear pleomorphism and dark, irregular chromatin (modified Giemsa)

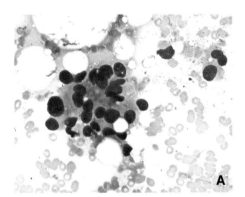
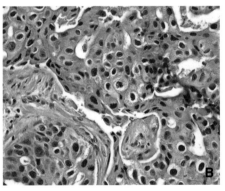

7-40. High-grade ductal carcinoma. (A) High power view of a malignant epithelial group with irregular, reddish chromatin. A few single malignant cells are also seen. Compare the nuclear size with the red blood cells are also seen in the background (modified Giemsa). (B) Histologic appearance of the tumor showing high nuclear grade and presence of mitosis (H&E)

Differential Diagnosis

■ Ductal carcinoma in situ
➤ Like invasive carcinoma, DCIS can present as a palpable mass or mammographic abnormality
➤ Cytologically there are no clear criteria to distinguish in situ from invasive carcinoma; however-the lack of cell cohesion and high cellularity of the specimen could be a diagnostic clue for an invasive process
➤ In most centers, the distinction between those two is not crucial since the management is similar; nevertheless, in cases that are amenable to preoperative chemotherapy this differentiation is fundamental and a confirmatory surgical biopsy is recommended
■ Fibroadenoma
➤ Stromal fragments and bipolar cells are more common in fibroadenomas
➤ Isolated cells with atypia are not commonly seen in fibroadenomas
■ Proliferative breast disease

> ➤ The presence of myoepithelial cells within the epithelial fragments and the absence of single atypical cells aid in the diagnosis
> ➤ The degree of cytologic atypia, pleomorphism, presence of necrosis, and single malignant cells are diagnostic of a malignant process
> ■ Pregnancy and lactational changes
> ➤ They can mimic malignancy due to the presence of single cells with prominent nucleoli
> ➤ The history of pregnancy and the absence of distinct cell membrane are clue to the correct diagnosis

PEARLS

★ Scirrhous carcinoma is characterized by dense fibrosis and can result in non-diagnostic FNA, in these cases a surgical biopsy is needed for diagnosis

★ In general, benign epithelial components are not seen in FNA smears of infiltrating ductal carcinoma, although sometimes benign breast tissue can be sampled in the way to the lesion

INFILTRATING LOBULAR CARCINOMA

Clinical Features

■ Accounts for 0.7–14% of all invasive breast carcinomas

■ The median age of occurrence is forty-five to fifty-seven years

■ Lobular carcinomas differ from duct carcinomas in the increased incidence of bilaterality and local recurrence after surgery, and the pattern of metastatic spread

■ Lobular carcinoma is difficult to identify as a malignant tumor on cytology due to the bland and relatively inconspicuous nuclear atypia

■ Clinically it does not produce a well-defined mass, which makes its detection difficult

Cytologic Features

■ Low to moderate cellularity

■ Presence of noncohesive single cells or small "balls" of slightly enlarged cells with some loss of cohesiveness

■ A single cell distribution and Indian-file pattern is characteristic

■ Uniform cells with mild atypia

■ Presence of small nucleoli

■ Occasional signet ring cells and intracytoplasmic vacuoles (targetoid mucin)

7-41. Lobular carcinoma. (A,B) Presence of noncohesive single cells. An Indian-file pattern is characteristic. Uniform cells with variable degree of atypia and prominent nucleoli. Occasional signet ring cells and intracytoplasmic vacuoles (targetoid mucin) are seen (Papanicolaou stain)

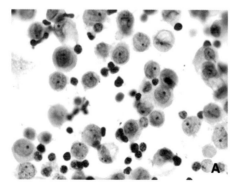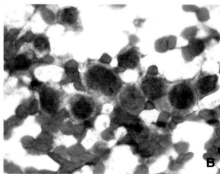

Special Stains and Immunohistochemistry

▦ Lobular carcinomas are E-cadherin and beta-catenin negative, helpful feature in the differential diagnosis with ductal carcinomas, which are positive for these markers

Modern Techniques

▦ The molecular profile of classic lobular neoplasms is distinctive, although not entirely unique. They are typically epidermal growth factor receptor 1 and HER2 negative, and the antibody 34BE12 (cytokeratins 1, 5, 10, and 14), ER and PR positive

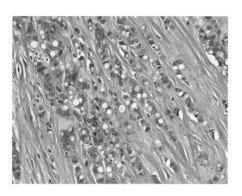

7-42. Infiltrating lobular carcinoma (histology). The presence of single cells with signet ring appearance is noted. The cells have an Indian-file infiltration pattern without glandular formation (H&E)

Differential Diagnosis

▦ Well-differentiated ductal carcinoma
➤ Usually more cellular and pleomorphic but can be confused with the pleomorphic variant of lobular carcinoma characterized by marked nuclear enlargement, hyperchromasia, and variation in cell size
▦ Lobular neoplasia (lobular carcinoma in situ)
➤ The distinction is crucial because lobular neoplasia is considered a risk factor for the subsequent development of breast cancer in either breast
➤ The smears in ILC are usually more cellular and have a higher proportion of noncohesive single cells with more nuclear atypia and pleomorphism
➤ The cells tend to present in small, indian-file groups, in cords or singly

PEARLS

✶ Identification of infiltrating lobular carcinoma showing classic features is possible, when in doubt, performance of immunostain for E-cadherin is helpful

PRIMARY BREAST CARCINOMA, SPECIAL TYPES

TUBULAR CARCINOMA

Clinical Features

▦ Tubular carcinoma of the breast is an invasive adenocarcinoma associated with an excellent prognosis and a low incidence of recurrence and metastases
▦ It represents only about 1% of all breast cancers
▦ It is a well-differentiated tumor with a specific microscopic pattern of branched angular tubules embedded in a loose fibrous stroma
▦ Diagnosis of tubular adenocarcinoma on aspiration biopsy can be difficult. An average of 11% of the cases described in the literature was given a benign diagnosis on FNA

Cytologic Features

▦ Smears are variable cellular
▦ Presence of angular glandular or tubular structures with sharp borders
▦ Oval cells perpendicularly arranged along the edges of the cellular clusters
▦ Regular, enlarged nuclei with occasional grooves
▦ Dispersed single epithelial cells with minimal atypia
▦ Cytoplasmic vacuoles
▦ Few bare oval nuclei in the background

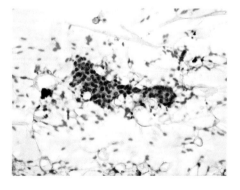

7-43. Tubular carcinoma. Presence of angular glandular or tubular structures with sharp borders and little cytologic atypia (Papanicolaou stain)

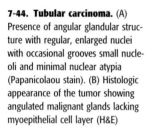

7-44. Tubular carcinoma. (A) Presence of angular glandular structure with regular, enlarged nuclei with occasional grooves small nucleoli and minimal nuclear atypia (Papanicolaou stain). (B) Histologic appearance of the tumor showing angulated malignant glands lacking myoepithelial cell layer (H&E)

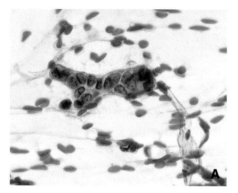

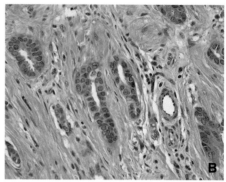

Special Stains and Immunohistochemistry

■ Myoepithelial cell markers, p63 and calponin, are helpful in the diagnosis of malignancy

Modern Techniques

■ Noncontributory

Differential Diagnosis

■ Fibroadenoma
  ➤ Tissue fragments are larger in size than those of tubular carcinoma
  ➤ Angulated glands are not seen in cases of fibroadenoma
■ Proliferative breast disease
  ➤ Atypical ductal hyperplasia may be confused with tubular adenocarcinoma on aspiration smears
  ➤ Features favoring atypical hyperplasia include cells arranged in sheets with distinct cell borders and the presence of myoepithelial cells in the background of the smears
■ Tubular adenoma
  ➤ May show tubular arrangements of uniform ductal epithelial cells, and these can be confused with tubular adenocarcinomas on aspiration smears
  ➤ Cytologically, tubular adenomas show sparse to moderately cellular smears with small spherical clusters of cells or tubular structures, both with abundant myoepithelial cells
  ➤ The tubules in tubular adenomas always contain myoepithelial cells and are more open than the angular tubules in tubular adenocarcinomas
■ Radial sclerosing lesions
  ➤ Angulated clusters have been described in radial scar. However, there is a higher prevalence of myoepithelial cells, a lower cellularity, and absence of nucleolus in radial scars
  ➤ Immunostains for myoepithelial markers can help in the differential diagnosis

PEARLS

★ The cytologic features of tubular carcinoma overlap with those of well-differentiated ductal carcinoma and lobular carcinoma. Because both can have a minor component of tubular carcinoma, in these cases a definitive diagnosis is rendered in surgical biopsy

MUCINOUS (COLLOID) CARCINOMA

Clinical Features
▦ It occurs in older patients.
▦ Pure colloid carcinoma is rare accounting for less than 4% of cases of breast carcinoma and more often is a component of ductal carcinoma
▦ It is a slow-growing cancer with a favorable prognosis,
▦ They are usually well circumscribed with soft gelatinous consistency

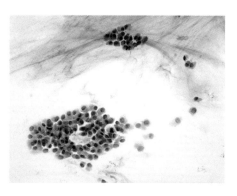

7-45. Mucinous carcinoma.
Clusters of bland tumor cells floating in a sea or whirlpool of mucin. The mucin is pale blue to pink in Papanicolaou stain-stained smears (Papanicolaou stain)

Cytologic Features
▦ Variable cellularity
▦ Clusters of bland tumor cells floating in a sea or whirlpool of mucin
▦ The mucin is pale blue to pink in PAP-stained smears and lightly metachromatic in DQ
▦ Single or clustered cells minimal cytologic atypia
▦ Fragments of stroma and branching capillaries
▦ Necrosis is not a feature

Special Stains and Immunohistochemistry
▦ A mucicarmine stain can be done to highlight the background, but this is not necessary for diagnostic purposes
▦ Myoepithelial cell markers can be helpful in the differentiation of mucocele-like lesions

Modern Techniques
▦ Noncontributory

Differential Diagnosis
▦ Mucocele-like lesion
➤ It is a rare benign condition that occurs more commonly in premenopausal women, in contrast to mucinous carcinoma that is a tumor of older patients
➤ Scant cellularity
➤ Presence of epithelial and myoepithelial cells embedded in the mucus whereas in mucinous carcinoma myoepithelial cells are absent
➤ Absence of nuclear atypia
➤ Mucinous carcinoma in general shows higher cellularity; abundant single, intact cells; three-dimensional cellular clusters in most cases; and variable nuclear atypia

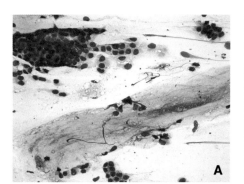
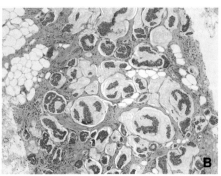

7-46. Mucinous carcinoma.
(A) Isolated or clustered epithelial cells with minimal cytologic atypia in a background of abundant mucin. The mucin is lightly metachromatic in modified Giemsa smears (modified Giemsa). (B) Histologic appearance of the tumor showing abundant mucin and papillary groups of malignant cells with mild cytologic atypia (H&E)

- Papillary carcinoma
  - ➤ Papillary formation can be seen in some cases of mucinous carcinoma and some papillary carcinomas can have mucinous background however, in general more cellularity, nuclear atypia, and less mucin is observed in papillary carcinomas
- Ductal carcinoma with mucinous differentiation
  - ➤ Cytologic features of both mucinous and ductal carcinoma should be present
  - ➤ Necrosis and scant amount of mucin favor ductal or mixed carcinoma
  - ➤ Abundant mucin in all smears, absence of pleomorphism and necrosis favor colloid carcinoma

PEARLS

☆ Because mucinous carcinomas are more commonly seen in postmenopausal women, extreme attention should be paid when considering this diagnosis in premenopausal women

☆ In cases that are not typical of either pure mucinous carcinoma or a mixed form, a diagnosis of "carcinoma with mucinous features" is preferred

☆ Excisional biopsy is advised for all hypocellular cases for further separation into benign and malignant mucinous lesions and to rule out the possibility of hypocellular mucinous carcinoma

MEDULLARY CARCINOMA

Clinical Features

- Medullary carcinoma of the breast is a rare variant of breast carcinoma, recognized to have good prognosis
- Accounts for 5–7% of breast tumors
- There is a higher incidence of medullary carcinomas in young patients, in particular in a *BRCA1* context

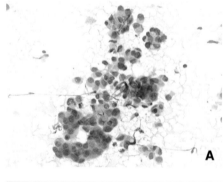
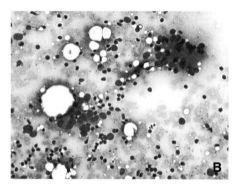

7-47. Medullary carcinoma. (A) Obviously malignant epithelial cells admixed with a few lymphocytes is shown here as "lymphoid tangles" as a consequence of smearing artefact (Papanicolaou stain). (B) Malignant epithelial cells, single and in groups, in a background of lymphocytes and plasma cells (modified Giemsa stain)

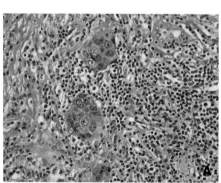
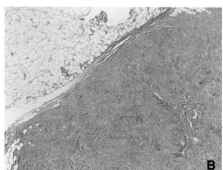

7-48. Medullary carcinoma (histology). (A) Syncytial groups of malignant epithelial cells surrounded by marked lymphoplasmacytic infiltrate. (B) Low power view of the same case showing the "pushing" border without infiltration of the surrounding breast tissue, an obligatory finding for the diagnosis (H&E)

▓ It shows aggressive pathological features but they are often associated with a more favorable outcome

▓ Histological diagnostic criteria include circumscription, intense lymphoplasma-cytic infiltrate, syncytial growth pattern, lack of tubule formation, high nuclear grade, and mitotic rate

Cytologic Features

▓ Very cellular smears

▓ Bizarre nuclei with macronucleoli, irregular nuclear membrane, and coarse chro-matin

▓ Predominance of single cells, naked atypical nuclei, or syncytial sheets of atypical cells

▓ Scarce to abundant cytoplasm with indistinct cell borders

▓ No gland formation and no mucin production

▓ Numerous mitosis

▓ Many lymphocytes and plasma cells in the background

▓ Lymphoglandular bodies can be seen

Special Stains and Immunohistochemistry

▓ Medullary carcinomas belong to the ER(−), PR(−), HER2/neu (−) group, harboring a basal-like immunophenotype with a higher rate of cytokeratins 5/6 positivity than basal-like carcinomas

Modern Techniques

▓ By fluorescence in situ hybridization (FISH) medullary carcinomas have genetic alterations in common with basal-like carcinomas, such as frequent *TP53* mutations, 8q gains or amplification, 1q gains or X amplicons. In addition, they are characterized by more frequent 10p, 9p, 3q and 16q gains, 4p losses, and 1q, 8p, 10p, and 12p amplicons

▓ A better knowledge of the heterogeneity of the basal-like tumor group should be useful in the near future for more appropriate patient management

Differential Diagnosis

▓ Poorly differentiated carcinoma with conspicuous chronic inflammatory infil-trate

▓ Metastasis of breast carcinoma to an intramammary lymph node

▓ Chronic mastitis

➤ Lacks the pleomorphic malignant cells seen in medullary carcinoma

▓ Intramammary lymph node

➤ Shows a polymorphic population of lymphoid cells without malignant epithe-lial cells typical of carcinomas

▓ Lymphoma

➤ The malignant cells seen in medullary carcinomas are larger and more pleo-morphic than those of large cell lymphoma

PEARLS

★ Medullary carcinoma is easily recognized as malignant in FNA, but although the diagnosis can be suspected, histologic evaluation of the resected specimen is nec-essary to exclude infiltrating margins. Such cases are better referred in FNA as Poorly differentiated carcinoma with prominent lymphoplasmacytic infiltrate and the diagnosis of medullary carcinoma can be suggested due to the prognostic impli-cations for the patient

METAPLASTIC CARCINOMA

Clinical Features

- Metaplastic carcinoma of the breast denotes tumors with epithelial and mesenchymal components, as well as mixed adenocarcinoma and squamous carcinoma
- It accounts for less than 1% of all invasive breast carcinomas
- The average age at presentation is fifty-five years
- Clinical presentation does not differ from that of ductal carcinomas in general
- It is associated with an unfavorable prognosis, especially if the mesenchymal component predominates

Cytologic Features

- Very cellular smears
- Malignant cells in a myxoid background
- The myxoid material can be fibrillar or metachromatic
- The mesenchymal cells are elongated, atypical, and pleomorphic
- Multinucleated forms of malignant or benign nature
- Single or clustered carcinoma cells
- Malignant cells show the same cytologic characteristics of any other malignant cells of adenocarcinoma or squamous cell carcinoma. (please refer to corresponding sections in the chapter)
- Presence of abnormal mitotic figures

Special Stains and Immunohistochemistry

- The squamous areas are in general negative for ER and PR and positive for broad-spectrum and high-molecular-weight cytokeratins (CK5/6 and CK34BE12)
- The spindle cell component may show positive reactivity for keratins, usually focally. Chondroid elements are frequently S-100 positive and may coexpress cytokeratins, but are negative for actin
- Even though the majority of the tumors are negative for ER/PR in both the adenocarcinoma and mesenchymal areas, the adenocarcinoma areas may be positive if they are well or moderately differentiated

Modern Techniques

- Noncontributory

Differential Diagnosis

- Subareolar abscess
  - ➤ A squamous component with background inflammation may suggest this diagnosis. The peripheral versus retroareolar position is a clue for the correct diagnosis
- Fibromatosis
  - ➤ The FNA contains microtissue fragments or single spindle cell with bland appearance

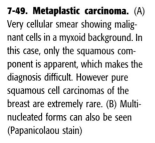

7-49. Metaplastic carcinoma. (A) Very cellular smear showing malignant cells in a myxoid background. In this case, only the squamous component is apparent, which makes the diagnosis difficult. However pure squamous cell carcinomas of the breast are extremely rare. (B) Multinucleated forms can also be seen (Papanicolaou stain)

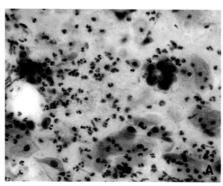
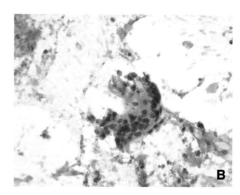

- Phyllodes tumor
  - ➤ In phyllodes tumor the mesenchymal element is usually arranged in stromal fragments rather than isolated cells. Also, the presence of benign epithelial component is conspicuous
- Primary breast sarcoma
  - ➤ It is cytologically indistinguishable from a pure sarcomatoid metaplastic carcinoma. The use of epithelial marker is useful in the differential diagnosis because metaplastic carcinomas will be at least focally positive for cytokeratins and EMA
- Adenocarcinoma
  - ➤ If only the glandular component is sampled, it is impossible to suspect the diagnosis of metaplastic carcinoma

PEARLS

★ The accurate diagnosis can only be made in the presence of both, epithelial and mesenchymal components, or adeno and squamous components

SQUAMOUS CELL CARCINOMA

Clinical Features
- Pure squamous cell carcinoma of the breast is an exceedingly rare form of primary breast tumor
- The incidence of this tumor is extremely low, estimated at less than 0.1% of all breast carcinomas
- The average age in the various published series varies between fifty-three and sixty-three years
- Squamous cell carcinoma of the breast tends to be larger (>4 cm) at presentation than other types of breast carcinomas, and more than 50% of these tumors are cystic

Cytologic Features
- Cellular smears
- Presence of syncytia and dissociated keratinized malignant squamous cells
- The nuclei are enlarged, hyperchromatic, and dense with angulated thickened nuclear membranes and coarse chromatin
- Rare prominent nucleoli
- Moderate pleomorphism, with occasional tadpole-shaped malignant squamous cells and rare cells with spindly configurations
- Bizarre nuclear forms can be seen
- Generally abundant cytoplasm, frequently glassy, eosinophilic, and keratinizing with sharp borders
- The background is usually necrotic with a moderate increase of inflammatory cells and keratin debris

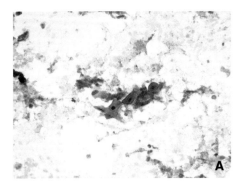 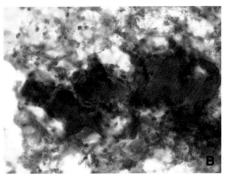

7-50. Squamous cell carcinoma. (A) Heavily keratinized atypical squamous cells. (B) Abundant keratin in a background of tumoral necrosis (Papanicolaou stain)

Special Stains and Immunohistochemistry
■ Squamous cell carcinomas are in general negative for ER and PR and positive for broad-spectrum and high-molecular-weight cytokeratins (CK5/6 and CK34BE12)

Modern Techniques
■ Noncontributory

Differential Diagnosis
■ Subareolar abscess
➤ Due to irritation and inflammation, the squamous cells can show variable degree of atypia and cause diagnostic problems. Also squamous cell carcinomas are often cystic. Clinical presentation of a subareolar versus intramammary mass can help in the differential diagnosis
■ Epidermal inclusion cyst
➤ Unless infected the squamous cells do not show cytologic atypia
■ Ductal carcinoma with squamous differentiation
➤ The presence of a malignant glandular population of cells completely rules out the diagnosis of pure squamous cell carcinoma
■ Metaplastic carcinoma
➤ The presence of any other malignant component (epithelial or mesenchymal) other than squamous cells, exclude the diagnosis of squamous cell carcinoma

PEARLS

★ The diagnosis of pure primary squamous cell carcinoma of the breast must fulfill three conditions
  • No other neoplastic elements, such as ductal or mesenchymal should be present in the tumor
  • The tumor is independent of adjacent cutaneous structures
  • No other primary squamous cell tumor exists in the patient, to exclude metastatic orgin

APOCRINE CARCINOMA

Clinical Features
■ It is an uncommon tumor, and the reported incidence ranges from 0.3% to 4% depending on the criteria used
■ It's defined as a carcinoma showing cytological and immunohistochemical features of apocrine cell in more than 90% of the tumor cells
■ Clinical, mammographical, and gross pathological presentation is the same as ductal carcinomas
■ Bilaterality is rare

7-51. Apocrine carcinoma.
(A) Loosely cohesive cluster of atypical apocrine cells with highly pleomorphic nuclei and prominent nucleoli. Abundant cytoplasm that stains gray with Papanicolaou stain. (B) Cell block of the same case showing the severe degree of cytologic atypia when comparing the single malignant cell with the residual benign apocrine lining on the right (H&E)

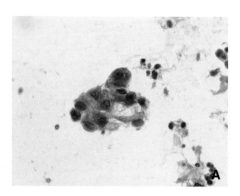
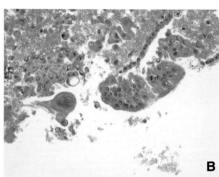

Cytologic Features
- Cellular smears
- Loose cohesive cluster of atypical apocrine cells
- Single neoplastic cells are often abundant
- Highly pleomorphic nuclei with prominent nucleoli
- Round to irregular nucleus usually eccentrically located with obvious malignant features
- Abundant and finely granular cytoplasm due to the presence of numerous mitochondria
- The cytoplasm stains variably pink or gray in PAP and gray–purple in DQ stain
- Occasional large, PAS-positive cytoplasmic inclusions
- Histiocytes and necrotic debris are often seen in the background

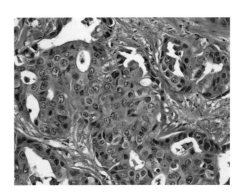

7-52. Apocrine carcinoma (histology): Infiltrating apocrine carcinoma showing abundant eosinophilic cytoplasm, high nuclear pleomorphism, and presence of mitosis (H&E)

Special Stains and Immunohistochemistry
- Apocrine carcinoma of the breast is typically, although not always, positive for gross cystic disease fluid protein-15 (GCDFP-15)
- They are also usually ER/PR negative and androgen receptor (AR) positive

Modern Techniques
- Malignant apocrine lesions, both in situ and invasive, commonly show gains of 1p, 1q, and 2q and losses of 1p, 12q, 16q, 17q, and 22q

Differential Diagnosis
- Benign and atypical apocrine change
  - ➤ Apocrine cancers are usually obviously malignant and often mixed with usual ductal carcinomas. The most useful characteristics are highly pleomorphic atypical nuclei, macronucleoli, and dyshesive pattern

PEARLS

★ Because apocrine cells can look very atypical and it is difficult to differentiate between atypia and malignancy even in histology, significant atypia must be observed before a diagnosis of apocrine carcinoma can be entertained

★ Cases diagnosed as atypical apocrine cells in cytology require excisional biopsy for further characterization of the lesion

FIBROEPITHELIAL TUMORS

FIBROADENOMA

Clinical Features
- Fibroadenoma is the most common tumor of the female breast
- Usually encountered in young age groups, especially those under thirty years of age
- It presents as a painless, solitary, firm, slowly growing, mobile, and well-defined nodule
- The development of cancer in fibroadenomas is quite rare (2.0–2.9%), usually of in situ or lobular type and this does not occur before the age of forty years
- They are associated with a slight increased risk of breast cancer, close to that of other benign proliferative lesions without atypical hyperplasia

Cytologic Features
- Cellularity varies
- Fibromyxoid stroma that stains bluish gray or green with the PAP stain and intensely red–purple with DQ

7-53. Fibroadenoma. (A) Low-power view showing a very cellular aspirate composed of large sheets of epithelial cells. (B) High-power view of the same case showing the finger-like clusters of ductal epithelial cells with sharply demarcated borders. The nuclei are small or round and regularly spaced. The chromatin is finely granular (Papanicolaou stain)

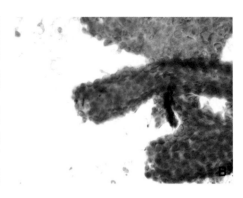

7-54. Fibroadenoma. (A) Three components of fibroadenoma; stromal fragments, epithelial groups, and bare myoepithelial cells in the background (modified Giemsa). (B) Histologic correlation of the tumor (H&E)

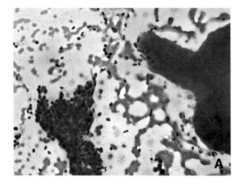
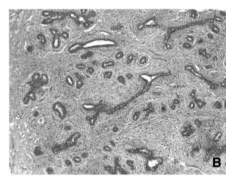

- Large honeycomb sheets
- Staghorn clusters of ductal epithelial cells
- Small or round nuclei with regular spacing
- Finely granular chromatin pattern
- Moderate to large number of bare bipolar nuclei

Special Stains and Immunohistochemistry
- Immunostains with myoepithelial markers can be used to identify myoepithelial cells in the smears

Modern Techniques
- Noncontributory

Differential Diagnosis
- Proliferative breast disease with or without atypia
  - Fibroadenomas presents as monolayer clusters with antler-horn pattern
  - Stromal fragments and papillary finger-like configurations are very uncommon in proliferative breast disease
- Phyllodes tumor
  - The distinction between benign phyllodes tumor and fibroadenomas is difficult
  - In phyllodes tumors the stromal fragments are more cellular
  - Stromal overgrowth, atypical stromal cells, and mitosis favor the diagnosis of malignant phyllodes tumor
  - Clinically, phyllodes tumor present in an older age group and as a larger, rapidly growing lesion

PEARLS

★ The cytological criteria for the diagnosis of fibroadenoma by FNA are reliable and when used in an appropriate setting (triple test) have high sensitivity and good reproducibility

PHYLLODES TUMOR

Clinical Features

▦ Phyllodes tumors represent a group of circumscribed biphasic tumors histologically characterized by a double layer of benign epithelial component arranged in clefts surrounded by an overgrowth of mesenchymal component forming leaf-like structures

▦ Accounts for less than 1% of all breast neoplasm and is more common in older patients

▦ It needs to be distinguished from fibroadenoma, which is about fifty times more common

▦ They are usually benign but recurrences are not uncommon

▦ In dependence of the characteristics of the mesenchymal component, they are histologically classified as benign, borderline, and malignant

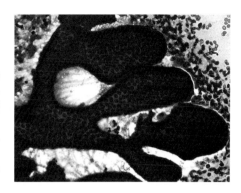

7-55. Phyllodes tumor. Large honeycomb sheets of uniform ductal epithelial cells with sharply demarcated borders (modified Giemsa stain)

Cytologic Features

▦ Cellular smears

▦ A dimorphic population of epithelial and stromal fragments

▦ Epithelial fragments indistinguishable from those of fibroadenoma

▦ The epithelial component is benign but can show cytologic atypia

▦ Stromal fragments cellularity varies with the grade of the tumor

▦ High stromal cellularity and stromal atypia help in the differentiation with fibroadenoma

▦ Bland or highly malignant stromal cells

▦ The presence of single, intact, spindle-shaped stromal cells is very helpful and can suggest a more aggressive lesion

▦ Myxoid, chondroid, or mucinous change may be seen in the stroma

Special Stains and Immunohistochemistry

▦ Stromal p53 protein expression is seen particularly in malignant phyllodes tumors

▦ Expression of c-kit (CD117) is also seen, particularly in malignant phyllodes tumors

▦ The stroma of all phyllodes tumors is vimentin positive and frequently positive for CD34, desmin, and actin

▦ The expression of ER and PR in phyllodes tumors is inversely related to the grade, suggesting interactions between the stroma and epithelium

Modern Techniques

▦ A recent study from the Curie Institut using combined comparative genomic hybridization (CGH) and FISH has found that borderline and malignant phyllodes

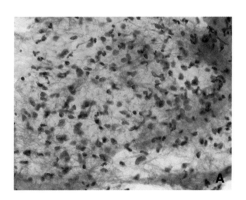
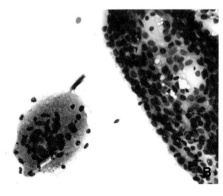

7-56. Phyllodes tumor. (A) High magnification of the stroma showing increased in cellularity but otherwise no cytologic atypia (PAP). (B) Epithelial component to the left and a stromal giant cell to the right (modified Giemsa stain)

tumors had significantly more chromosomal changes than benign phyllodes tumors. This suggests that there may be an important biological cut-off between borderline and benign phyllodes tumors. This may indicate that only two types of phyllodes tumors could be distinguished on a genomic basis: benign phyllodes tumors and malignant phyllodes tumors (which include the borderline and malignant pathologic categories)

■ In this study, 71% borderline and malignant phyllodes tumors and 11% of benign phyllodes tumors presented 1q gain and/or 13q loss

Differential Diagnosis

■ Fibroadenoma
  ➤ Fibroadenomas are often smaller than phyllodes tumors, however cytologically the distinction with phyllodes tumor is not based in the size but in the characteristics of the stroma
  ➤ The stromal fragments of phyllodes tumor are more cellular and contain more atypical cells than fibroadenoma

■ Borderline phyllodes tumor usually resembles fibromatosis or low-grade fibrosarcoma with occasional instances of chondroid, osseous, or lipomatous metaplasia

■ The stroma in malignant phyllodes tumor usually resembles fibrosarcoma or stromal sarcoma, with occasional cases showing heterologous elements such as angiosarcoma, liposarcoma, or myosarcoma

■ Ductal carcinoma
  ➤ In cases of great cytologic atypia some phyllodes tumor can be confused with ductal carcinoma
  ➤ The presence of stromal fragments and some benign ductal cells aid in the differential diagnosis

■ Mucinous carcinoma: When mucinous metaplasia is present
  ➤ Unlike mucinous carcinoma, phyllodes tumor shows a biphasic population of cells (stroma and epithelium)
  ➤ In the case of malignant phyllodes tumor with mucinous change, the absence of malignant epithelial component in the smears and the high cellularity of stromal fragments help to exclude mucinous carcinoma

■ Papillary lesions
  ➤ Large, folded sheets of epithelium that arise from the aspiration of the epithelium lining, the extremely elongated branching clefts can be confused with papillary fragments
  ➤ When combined with one or more stromal features of phyllodes tumor the cytologic diagnosis can be made

■ Metaplastic carcinoma: Can mimic phyllodes tumor because of the atypical spindle cell component, but in phyllodes tumor a benign epithelial component is also present

PEARLS

★ Although the accurate subclassification of phyllodes tumor is not always possible in FNA, the clinical features of the lesion (size, age of the patient, presentation) together with the cytological characteristics (stromal cellularity, mitosis and atypia) warrant a complete excision of the lesion for further classification

★ If only malignant stroma is present without epithelial component, the tumor is considered a stromal sarcoma. If stromal and epithelial components are present and both are malignant, the diagnosis is carcinosarcoma

MESENCHYMAL TUMORS

FIBROMATOSIS

Clinical Features
- It is a locally aggressive fibroblastic proliferation with variable amounts of collagen that may recur but lack metastatic potential
- Fibromatosis of the breast accounts for less than 0.2% of primary lesions in the breast
- Patients with mammary fibromatosis range in age from thirteen to eighty years at diagnosis, with a median age of twenty-five years in one series
- Fibromatosis has been associated with trauma, breast implants, and Gardner's syndrome
- The clinical impression is often suggestive of a carcinoma. If present, dimpling of the overlying skin reinforces the clinical impression of carcinoma. Mammography often reveals a spiculated tumor
- The frequency of local recurrence after local excision varies from 21% to 27%

Cytologic Features
- Moderately cellular aspirates
- Mixture of isolated spindle cells, stromal fragments, and inflammatory cells
- Background of amorphous proteinaceous material
- The spindle cells possess oval to elongated nuclei with fine chromatin and small distinct nucleoli
- The spindle cells vary in size and shape but marked nuclear pleomorphism is absent
- Mitotic activity is not present
- The cytoplasm is pale with tapered ends and ill-defined borders
- The stromal fragments are irregular in size and shape and composed of hyalinized collagen and scattered spindle cells
- The inflammatory cells consist of a heterogeneous population of small and large lymphocytes and a few plasma cells
- Benign groups of ductal epithelial cells can be present

Special Stains and Immunohistochemistry
- The spindle cells are vimentin positive and a small portion also smooth muscle actin (SMA) and desmin positive
- The spindle cells are negative for S-100, CD34, and keratins
- The cells are ER/PR and AR negative

Modern techniques
- Noncontributory

Differential Diagnosis
- Benign fibroepithelial tumors
  - ➤ The cytologic appearance of fibroepithelial neoplasms of the breast such as fibroadenoma and low-grade phyllodes tumour may resemble that of mammary fibromatosis
  - ➤ The presence of abundant ductal epithelial clusters, isolated bipolar naked nuclei in the aspirates and the clinical impression of a well-circumscribed mass are features against a diagnosis of mammary fibromatosis
- Metaplastic carcinoma
  - ➤ Because the fibroblastic proliferation tends to grow around preexisting epithelial structures, mammary ducts, and lobules become enclosed by the lesion. The presence of entrapped epithelial elements in the smears represents the major source of diagnostic problems

> ➤ Atypical hyperplastic changes of these ducts may be present, adding difficulties to the cytologic diagnosis of fibromatosis
> ■ Sarcomas (fibrosarcoma, malignant fibrous histiocytoma, and high-grade phyllodes tumour)
> ➤ The lack of pleomorphic, markedly atypical spindle cells and mitotic figures rules out high-grade sarcomas

☆ Due to the fact that clinically and mammographically fibromatosis is frequently confused with malignancy, preoperative recognition is essential since in many cases it would avoid unnecessary radical surgery

☆ Although the correct diagnosis by FNA is not always possible, the diagnosis of a benign lesion is sufficient preoperatively

LIPOMA AND SPINDLE CELL LIPOMA

Clinical Features

■ Lipoma presents as a solitary, well-circumscribed, soft, mobile mass microscopically composed of mature adipose tissue surrounded by a delicate capsule
■ The size ranges from small lesions to up to 10 cm
■ Spindle cell lipoma: Clinically is indistinguishable from lipoma and microscopically is composed of spindle-shaped fusiform and stellate cells with scant cytoplasm, mature adipocytes, mast cells and collagenous or myxoid stroma

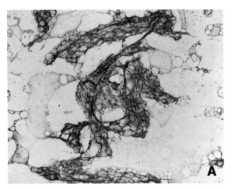

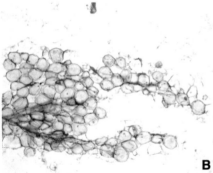

7-57. Lipoma. Mature adipose tissue fragments indistinguishable from the normal adipose tissue component of the breast. In these cases clinical presentation and absence of other breast elements in the smear are crucial for the diagnosis. (A) (modified Giemsa stain). (B) (Papanicolaou stain)

Cytologic features

■ Lipoma
   ➤ Mature adipose tissue fragments, small blood vessels, stromal cells, and few inflammatory cells
   ➤ Breast elements are not seen unless sampled unintentionally
■ Spindle cell lipoma
   ➤ Hypocellular aspirate
   ➤ Pleomorphic cells population, nuclear atypia, multinucleated giant cells
   ➤ Floret-like cells and absence of lipoblasts

Special Stains and Immunohistochemistry

■ Noncontributory

Modern Techniques

■ Noncontributory

Differential Diagnosis

■ Pleomorphic liposarcoma and benign spindle cell tumors
   ➤ Cytologically indistinguishable
   ➤ The clinical presentation is useful, but excisional biopsy is necessary to establish the definitive diagnosis

☆ Because mature adipose tissue is normal component of the breast, FNA findings should be correlated with the clinical presentation of the lesion

⋆ Awareness about the atypical cytologic characterists of spindle cell lipoma is important in order to avoid the diagnosis of malignancy

MYOFIBROBLASTOMA

Clinical Features
▨ Myofibroblastoma of the breast is an uncommon stromal tumor most often found in older men
▨ The mass ranges in size from 1 to 5 cm and presents as a nodular, round, slightly lobulated lesion
▨ It usually presents as a solitary well-circumscribed breast lesion, histologically consisting of slender bipolar spindle cells and broad bands of hyalinized collagen

Cytologic Features
▨ Moderate cellularity
▨ Spindle or round to polygonal cells
▨ Moderate cytoplasm
▨ Mildly pleomorphic nuclei
▨ Polygonal cells that may resemble epithelial cells
▨ Nuclei with occasional grooves and pseudoinclusion
▨ Single nucleolus
▨ No mitosis, significant nuclear atypia, or prominent nucleoli are present
▨ Numerous mast cells can be seen interspersed
▨ Myxoid-appearing matrix
▨ Absence of epithelial cells

Special Stains and Immunohistochemistry
▨ Immunohistochemistry reveal positivity for vimentin, desmin, SMA, and variable positivity for CD34 in the tumor cells
▨ Cytokeratin and S-100 are negative

Modern Techniques
▨ Noncontributory

Differential Diagnosis
▪ Fibroadenoma and phyllodes tumors
  ➤ Benign epithelial component in addition to a cellular stromal component
  ➤ Extremely uncommon in men
▪ Fibromatosis: Composed of monotonous slender spindle cells in fascicles
▪ Schwannoma
  ➤ Predominantly slender spindle cells
  ➤ S-100 positivity is useful
▪ Nodular fasciitis
  ➤ Myxoid background and pleomorphic cells admixed with leukocytes and histiocytes
  ➤ Mitotic figures are frequently seen
  ➤ Clinical presentation is a clue. In nodular fasciitis the swelling is of short duration and it rapidly grows over a few weeks
  ➤ Usually exceed 3 cm in diameter
▪ Malignancy
  ➤ Obvious nuclear atypia and malignant features
  ➤ Mammography can be a very useful adjunct in differentiating myofibroblastoma, which is a circumscribed lesion, from malignant neoplasm, which shows infiltrating margins

★ A cellular aspirate consistent of spindle to polygonal cells with ovoid mildly pleomorphic nuclei associated with extracellular matrix material and bands of hyalinized collagen should point to a diagnosis of myofibroblastoma, particularly in men in the appropriate clinical setting

GRANULAR CELL TUMOR

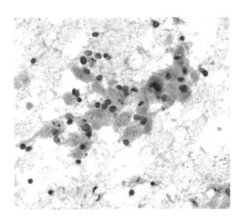

7-58. Granular cell tumor. Loosely cohesive cells with abundant granular blueish cytoplasm and ill-defined cell boundaries. The cytoplasm often appears to be disintegrating and falling apart, resulting in extracellular granular material (dirty background). The nuclei are irregular and central (Papanicolaou stain)

Clinical Features

■ Granular cell tumor is an uncommon neoplasm that has been described at many sites throughout the body, most commonly in the skin and the tongue

■ On the basis of its immunohistochemical and ultrastructural features, granular cell tumor is now considered to be of Schwann cell origin

■ About 8% of granular cell tumors occur in the breast

■ They are more common in middle-aged premenopausal patients especially African-American women

■ Granular cell tumor usually presents as a firm and painless mass, which may be fixed to the pectoral muscle or to the skin, thus mimicking a malignant lesion

■ Radiologic findings are also suggestive of malignancy

■ Mammography often reveals a stellate lesion without calcifications and ultrasonography usually shows a hypoechoic, ill-defined mass with posterior shadowing

Cytologic Features

■ Moderate cellular aspirates

■ Small and relatively large cohesive groups of cells

■ Small regular central nuclei

■ Occasional nucleoli

■ Abundant granular bluish cytoplasm in PAP stained smears

■ Cell boundaries are ill defined, resulting in a syncytial appearance

■ Single intact cells with granular cytoplasm can be also present

■ The cytoplasm of single cells often appears to be disintegrating and falling apart, resulting in extracellular granular material (dirty background)

Special Stains and Immunohistochemistry

■ The tumor cells are strongly immunoreactive to S-100 protein and also stain positively for CD68 and vimentin. There is no stain for cytokeratins, epithelial membrane antigen, and mucin

7-59. Granular cell tumor. (A) S-100 immunostain performed in the cell block showing positivity of the tumoral cells. (B) Histologic appearance of the tumor showing syncytial arrangement of the cells and abundant granular cytoplasm (H&E)

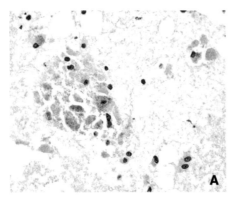

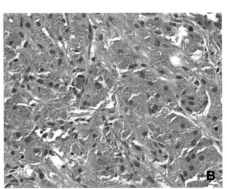

■ Cells are also negative for both estrogen and progesterone receptors

■ The cytoplasmic granularity can be highlighted by the PAS stain

Modern Rechniques

■ Noncontributory

Differential Diagnosis

■ Apocrine lesions

➤ The cytoplasm of apocrine cells is usually nongranular and, if granular, is generally pink in color with Romanowsky stains. This contrasts with the blue cytoplasmic granularity of granular cell tumor

➤ Apocrine cells tend to have well-defined boundaries in contrast to the cells of granular cell tumor where the cell membranes are ill defined

■ Histiocytes

➤ Histiocytes often contain indented nuclei and the cytoplasm tends to be foamy rather than granular and may contain pigment or cell debris

➤ If the cells are considered to be histiocytic, then the differential diagnosis may include fat necrosis, duct ectasia, or granulomatous mastitis

■ Malignancy

➤ The presence of "dirty" background may lead to a diagnosis of malignancy, but the absence of nuclear pleomorphism should aid in the diagnosis, since, typically, nuclei found in granular cell tumor are regular, ovoid to round with occasional small nucleoli

■ Malignant granular cell tumors: Very rare

➤ The following features suggest malignancy: a large tumor size (exceeding 5 cm), necrosis, cellular pleomorphism, prominent nucleoli, increased mitotic activity, and local recurrence

PEARLS

★ Granular cell tumor is a benign tumor often misdiagnosed as breast cancer both clinically and radiologically. Therefore, FNA biopsy plays an important role in the pre-operative diagnosis of these lesions. This emphasizes the significance of the triple test

MALIGNANT MESENCHYMAL TUMORS (SARCOMAS)

Clinical Features

■ Sarcomas of the breast are extremely rare and account for less than 1% of primary breast cancers

■ This group includes malignant fibrous histiocytoma (MFH), liposarcoma, osteosarcoma, chondrosarcoma, leiomyosarcoma, angiosarcoma, rhabdomyosarcoma, and so forth

■ These tumors are at high risk of recurrence and are known to have poor prognosis

■ Angiosarcoma arising in the irradiated breast after breast-conserving therapy is being reported with increasing frequency

Cytologic Features

■ Cellularity varies

■ Single spindle-shaped or rounded cells or highly discohesive cell population

■ Wispy, elongated cytoplasm

■ Hyperchromatic nuclei

■ Coarse granular chromatin

■ Prominent nucleoli

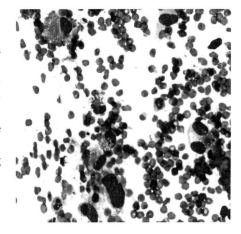

7-60. Sarcoma. Malignant fibrous histiocytoma: Highly pleomorphic single cells with wispy cytoplasm and overly malignant features that look "too malignant" to represent an epithelial tumor (modified Giemsa stain)

▪ The presence of mitosis, pleomorphism, and necrosis correlate with the tumor grade

▪ Tissue fragments with jagged, irregular borders and obvious vessels running through them at irregular angles. (This finding contrasts with the more rounded, less vascular clusters found in truly cohesive epithelial malignancies)

Special Stains and Immunohistochemistry

▪ A panel of immunostains is necessary for diagnostic purposes in the majority of the cases. This should include Keratins, CAM 5.2, 34betaE12, CK14, desmin, EMA, S-100, GFAP, SMA, CD34, and others according to the differential diagnosis

Modern Techniques

▪ During the last decade, molecular testing of mesenchymal tumors has become increasingly important, not only in the diagnostic approach of these lesions, but also regarding their prognosis and pathogenesis. A subset of sarcomas bears chromosomal abnormalities including reciprocal translocations, deletions, mutations, and amplifications. Besides their diagnostic value in sarcoma typing and subtyping, some of these abnormalities may also impact on treatment response and/or on prognosis

Differential Diagnosis

▪ Benign mesenchymal tumors
  ➤ The presence of cytologic atypia, pleomorphism, necrosis, and mitosis point to a malignant process
▪ Carcinoma
  ➤ At first glimpse, the tissue fragments seen in sarcomas may mimic a cohesive cell population as seen in carcinomas. On closer examination, however, these tissue fragments tend to have jagged, irregular borders with obvious vessels running through them at irregular angles
  ➤ High-grade sarcomas also can be confused with high-grade ductal carcinomas because of their pleomorphism and prominent nucleoli; however, sarcomas tend to have ill-defined, wispy cytoplasm in contrast to the well-defined, vacuolated cytoplasm of adenocarcinoma. It is important to say that vacuoles may occur in liposarcomas
  ➤ Spindle cell carcinoma: Spindle cell (sarcomatoid) carcinoma of the breast is a rare variant of breast cancer that has been classified under the broad group of metaplastic carcinoma

PEARLS

★ When confronted with a spindle cell neoplasm of the breast, a battery of keratins should be performed, including CK14, and 34betaE12, because spindle cell carcinomas of the breast are far more frequently encountered than primary spindle cell sarcomas of breast are

LYMPHOMAS

Clinical Features

▪ Lymphomas of the breast are rare and may mimic carcinoma clinically
▪ They can involve the breast either as primary neoplasm or as a systemic disease
▪ Breast lymphoma accounts for 1.7–2.2% of all extranodal lymphomas and 0.4–0.7% of all non-Hodgkin's lymphomas, with a roughly equal distribution between primary and secondary lesions
▪ The majority are of B-cell type, especially diffuse large B-cell lymphoma, follicular lymphoma, Burkitt lymphoma, and lymphoma of mucosa-associated lymphoid tissue

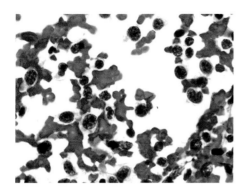 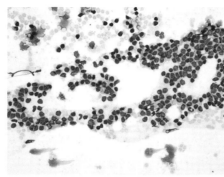

7-61. Non-Hodgkin's lymphomas *(left)*. Monomorphic population of single cells with atypia and prominent nucleoli. The nuclei outlines are irregular with indentations (Papanicolaou stain)

7-62. Intramammary lymph node *(right)*. Polymorphic population consistent of a mixture of small, medium, and large lymphocytes. Plasma cells are also present (modified Giemsa stain)

Cytologic Features

▨ The cytological features are the same of those lymphomas arising in the lymph nodes
▨ Single cell pattern with lymphoglandular bodies and frequently crushing artifact
▨ Monomorphic population of cells with variable degree of atypia and prominent nucleoli
▨ The size of the cell varies with the type of lymphoma

Special Stains and Immunohistochemistry

Groups by cell size	Lymphoma	Markers
Small cell group	Mantle cell lymphoma	CD20+, CD5+, CD23−, CD10−, cyclin D1+
	Marginal-zone lymphoma	CD5-, CD10-, CD23-, CD20+, CD43+, bcl-2 +/−
	Follicular lymphoma	CD20+, CD10+, CD5-, CD23+/-, bcl-2+
	Small lymphocytic lymphomas	CD5+, CD10-, CD23+, CD20+/-, CD43+
Intermediate cell group	Burkitt lymphoma	CD20+, CD10+, CD5-, bcl-2-, bcl-6+, Ki-67+, TdT-
	Small cell variant of anaplastic large cell lymphoma	CD45+, CD15-, CD20+/-, CD3+/-, CD30+, ALK+
Large cell group	Hodgkin's lymphoma	CD45-, CD30+, CD15+/-, CD20+/-, CD3,5-
	Anaplastic large cell lymphoma	CD45+, CD15-, CD20+/-, CD3+/-, CD30+, ALK+
	Follicular lymphoma Grade III	CD20+, CD10+, CD5-, CD23+/-, bcl-2+/-
	Large B-cell lymphoma	CD20+, CD45+

Modern Techniques

▨ Flow cytometric analysis and molecular studies are necessary for diagnosis and subclassification of lymphoproliferative disorders

Differential Diagnosis
▨ Reactive lymphoid proliferation and intramammary lymph node
  ➤ Polymorphic population consistent of a mixture of small, medium, and large cells
  ➤ Presence of tingible-body macrophages and lymphoglandular bodies
▨ Chronic mastitis
  ➤ Inflammatory infiltrate composed of lymphocytes and plasma cells

➤ The presence of granular debris and reactive epithelial fragments in chronic mastitis aids in the differential diagnosis
■ Amelanotic melanoma
   ➤ Highly cellular smears with mainly dispersed cells and occasional aggregates of round to polygonal cells
   ➤ Moderate to abundant amount of cytoplasm
   ➤ Eccentric nuclei, binucleation can be seen
   ➤ Prominent nucleoli
   ➤ Intranuclear inclusions are often seen
   ➤ Tumor cells are positive for S-100 and HMB-45
   ➤ The absence of a previous history of melanoma helps in the differential diagnosis
■ Small cell carcinoma
   ➤ Salt and pepper chromatin
   ➤ Inconspicuous nucleoli
   ➤ Cohesion and molding between the cells
   ➤ Small cell carcinomas are TTF-1(if lung primary), keratin, chromogranin, and synaptophysin positive and negative for lymphoid markers
   ➤ The presence of lymphoglandular bodies favors the diagnosis of lymphoma
■ Medullary carcinoma
   ➤ Its conspicuous lymphoplasmacytic component can be confused with lymphoma
   ➤ A careful search for a malignant epithelial component avoids making the wrong diagnosis

PEARLS

★ Because immunophenotyping is essential in the subclassification, when a diagnosis of lymphoma is suspected, more emphasis should be placed in obtaining satisfactory samples for flow cytometry
★ The fresh sample should be submitted in RPMI media. (RPMI was developed at **R**oswell **P**ark **M**emorial **I**nstitute, hence the acronym RPMI)

METASTATIC DISEASE OF THE BREAST

Clinical Features
■ Metastases from nonmammary malignant neoplasms to the breast are rare and represent 0.4–2% of all breast malignancies
■ The lesions are usually freely mobile, well defined, firm, and none of the skin changes often described in primary breast carcinomas are seen
■ Clinically and radiologically, metastatic neoplasms may mimic primary benign and malignant neoplasms of the breast
■ Hajdu et al. in their series of metastatic tumors to the breast reported eighteen carcinomas, sixteen lymphomas, fourteen melanomas, and three sarcomas
■ Among carcinomas, large-cell carcinoma of the lung, ovarian adenocarcinoma, squamous cell carcinoma of the cervix, endometrial adenocarcinoma, and gastric carcinoma are the most common
■ In men, metastases from prostatic carcinoma are commonest
■ Rhabdomyosarcoma and hematolymphoid tumors comprise the majority of malignant diagnoses in children

Cytologic Features
■ Aspirates are usually cellular
■ Classification is based on the pattern of cell distribution and individual cell morphology

- Adenocarcinomas, melanomas, Hodgkin's disease, large cell lymphoma, and pleomorphic sarcoma usually present as a pleomorphic large cell population
- Melanomas, leukemias, lymphomas, and carcinoid tumors have a dispersed cell pattern
- Sarcomatoid carcinoma, and true sarcomas have predominantly spindle cell morphology

Special Stains and Immunohistochemistry
- Depending on the cytological differential diagnosis, the panel of stain used include, keratins, thyroid transcription factor (TTF-1), epithelial membrane antigen (EMA), ER, PR, gross cystic disease fluid protein-15 (GCDFP-15), leukocyte common antigen (LCA), neuron specific enolase (NSE), S-100, HMB-45, muscle-specific antigen (MSA), desmin and vimentin
- A single positive immunostain is not enough to make a diagnosis

Modern Techniques
- Flow cytometry is very useful in this setting specially to diagnose lymphoproliferative disorders

Differential Diagnosis
- Cytologically the differential diagnosis between primary and metastatic disease is difficult because these tumors show the same or very similar characterists in both settings. The cytologic characterists of these tumors have been already discussed in other sections
- A suspicion of metastatic malignancy must come to mind if the tumor shows a pattern not matching the usual spectrum of a typical breast tumor. Past history and a review of biopsy material may be necessary for a correct diagnosis
- The clinical history combined with the use of immunohistochemistry help in the differential diagnosis

PEARLS

★ An accurate recognition of metastatic tumors to the breast results in prompt initiation of appropriate therapy and prevents unnecessary biopsy or mastectomy
★ Except for lymphomas and leukemias, the prognosis is usually poor, most patients die of disseminated metastases within a year of diagnosis

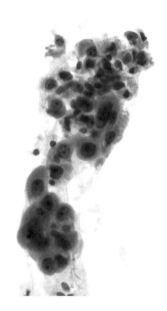

7-63. Metastatic lung adenocarcinoma to the breast. Cluster of malignant cells with high nuclear pleomorphism and macronucleoli difficult to differentiate from a poorly differentiated primary breast carcinoma on cytology only. The clinical history and use of appropriate immunostains aid in the diagnosis (Papanicolaou stain)

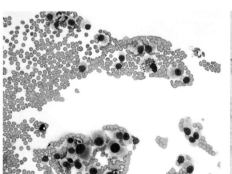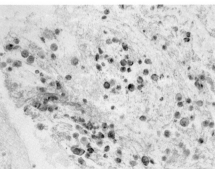

7-64. Metastatic malignant melanoma to the breast *(left).* Pleomorphic large cell and discohesive population. The malignant cells show finely vacuolated cytoplasm and excentric large nucleus. The presence of intracytoplasmic pigment in one of the cells is a clue for the diagnosis in this case (modified Giemsa stain)

7-65. Metastatic malignant melanoma to the breast *(right).* HMB-45 immunostain on the cell block showing positivity of the malignant cells

MALE BREAST

Clinical Features

▣ Male breast masses are uncommon pathologic findings. They are rarely aspirated, resulting in limited cytopathologic experience

▣ The majority of breast masses are the result of gynecomastia, a lesion that may pose some problems because under certain circumstances it can be confused with carcinoma

▣ Less than 1% of all breast cancers occur in men

▣ Cancer of the male breast is rare before three years of age, but the risk increases with age.

▣ There is no proven link between gynecomastia and breast cancer

▣ Metastatic tumors to the breast result in a large proportion of palpable breast masses in the males

Cytological Features

▣ Gynecomastia
  ➤ Variable cellular smears
  ➤ Large, tightly cohesive epithelial fragments often appearing as flat somewhat monolayered sheets
  ➤ Occasional finger-like projections reminiscent of a fibroadenoma
  ➤ Biphasic population of epithelial and stromal fragments
  ➤ Occasional naked bipolar to oval myoepithelial nuclei in the background
  ➤ Mild to marked epithelial atypia in the form of cellular crowding with nuclear overlap, nuclear hyperchromasia, high N/C ratio, loss of architecture, and some cellular discohesiveness

▣ Breast cancer
  ➤ Hypercellular smears with a predominant population of discohesive single malignant cells
  ➤ High N/C ratio, nuclear hyperchromasia with occasional prominent nucleoli
  ➤ Occasionally attempts of glandular formation
  ➤ Intracytoplasmic mucin vacuoles are also observed

▣ Metastatic tumors
  ➤ Suspect when cytologic findings are not usual for a primary breast malignancy
  ➤ The most common tumors are melanoma, lung adenocarcinoma, lymphoma, and prostate

Special Stains and Immunohistochemistry

▣ To distinguish between gynecomastia and adenocarcinoma, the presence of myoepithelial cells can be highlighted using myoepithelial cell markers. These studies should be interpreted with caution in cytologic samples

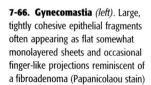

7-66. Gynecomastia *(left)*. Large, tightly cohesive epithelial fragments often appearing as flat somewhat monolayered sheets and occasional finger-like projections reminiscent of a fibroadenoma (Papanicolaou stain)

7-67. Gynecomastia *(right)*. Biphasic population of epithelial and stromal fragments. The epithelial component can show some degree of cytologic atypia, overlap, and hyperchromasia (modified Giemsa stain)

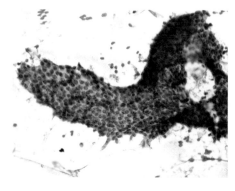

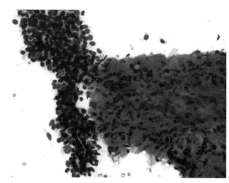

In the distinction between primary and metastatic malignancy a panel of immunostains is necessary. This includes prostate-specific antigen (PAS), prostatic acid phosphatase (PAP), CK7, CK20, TTF-1, S-100, ER, PR and others according to the morphologic characteristics of the tumor

Modern Techniques
- Noncontributory in gynecomastia
- For male breast cancer, same as in female breast cancer

Differential Diagnosis
- Fibroepithelial tumors
  - Fibroepithelial lesions are uncommon in the male breast. Most published reports describe phyllodes tumors
  - Fibroadenomas are extremely rare in the male breast
  - Gynecomastia has been known to coexist in both types of fibroepithelial lesions in men
  - Cytologically, fibroadenomas often show less degree of architectural disarray than gynecomastia
- Gynecomastia versus adenocarcinoma
  - In gynecomastia the typical cytological presentation is crowded epithelial sheets and stromal fragments with myoepithelial cells
  - Adenocarcinomas show higher degree of cytologic atypia, no stromal fragments and unlike gynecomastia the predominant cellular pattern almost always is that of cellular discohesiveness

PEARLS

★ Fine-needle aspiration is extremely useful in separating malignant breast lumps from the more common benign breast masses secondary to gynecomastia
★ Fine-needle aspiration is also useful in separating primary carcinomas of the male breast from metastatic malignancy. This distinction would result in appropriate and timely patient management
★ Gynecomastia associated with ductal hyperplasia with atypia may mimic adenocarcinoma, therefore necessitating a much higher threshold for carcinoma on cytopathologic evaluation

PROGNOSTIC/PREDICTIVE FACTORS IN BREAST CYTOLOGY

Definition
- Quantification of estrogen (ER), progesterone receptor (PR), HER2-neu, and marker of proliferation as Ki-67 in breast tumors is important in the clinical management of breast cancer patients. Their expression has been established as an independent prognostic factor and also to predict response to hormonal therapy

Advantages
- The material is obtained during FNA as a one step procedure
- Allows stratification of the patients that may benefit of neoadjuvant chemotherapy and could be of paramount importance for the preoperative planning of treatment
- Avoids unnecessary risk for those who will not benefit of an additional therapy
- The analysis can be repeated during preoperative therapy to see tumor response

Accuracy
- The accuracy is comparable to those of the histological evaluation

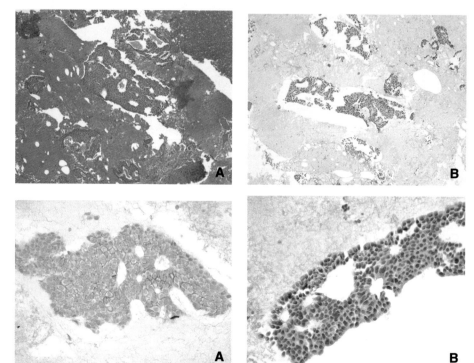

7-68. Prognostic/Predictive factors. (A) Cell block showing a cluster of malignant epithelial cells (H&E). (B) Immunostain for estrogen receptor showing strong nuclear staining of the cancer cells

7-69. Prognostic/Predictive factors. (A) Immunostain for HER2-neu oncoprotein showing positive stain of the cytoplasmic membranes (2+). (B) Immunostain for p53 showing scattered positive cells illustrated by their nuclear staining

Technique

■ Cell block preparations: During FNA, once the diagnosis has been reached on-site; an extra pass should be dedicated to obtain enough material for cell block preparation. The needle can be rinsed in CytoLyt (Cytyc) or Saccomanno solution
■ Cytospin preparation: It is also suitable for immunohistochemical studies
■ Thin-prep slides: The material is rinsed in CytoLyt for thin-prep preparation

Conclusions

■ Several studies have shown that quantification of prognostic/ predictive factors in cytologic samples is a reliable technique whenever surgical biopsy is not indicated and when this information is required at the time of the initial diagnosis

TELOMERASE ACTIVITY AS A MARKER OF BREAST CARCINOMA IN CYTOLOGY SAMPLES

Definition

■ Telomerase is normally inactivated in almost all somatic cells
■ With increasing age or cell divisions, the mean telomeric length of normal somatic cells gradually decreases

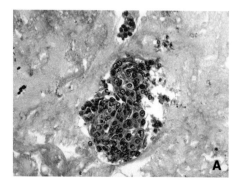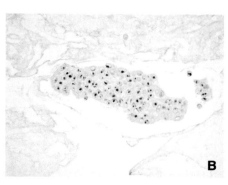

7-70. Telomerase. (A) Cell block showing a cluster of malignant epithelial cells (H&E). (B) Positive immunohistochemistry for telomerase

▦ Immortalized cell populations (cancer cells), by contrast, show an increased expression of telomerase that may lead to stabilization of telomeric length

Method
▦ An improved method for extraction and detection of telomerase activity, designated the telomeric repeat amplification protocol (TRAP), is capable of detection of telomerase activity from as few as a hundred cells
▦ With this method increased telomerase activity has been found in almost all breast carcinoma tissues, whereas it is not detected in most benign tumors

Advantages
▦ The application of molecular markers to increase the specificity and sensitivity of cytologic samples may lead to improved accuracy of diagnosis, prognosis, and clinical management
▦ Telomerase expression could be an ideal marker in cytologic samples, since the TRAP assay can detect activity of telomerase from malignant cells with a high level of sensitivity, even in the presence of a large background of normal cells
▦ It should not be used routinely on every breast fine-needle aspirate though it is valuable in the diagnosis of difficult cases

Disadvantages
▦ Possible reasons for the failure to detect telomerase in cytologically malignant samples (false negative results) could include poor specimen cellularity, specimen contamination by blood, degradation of telomerase activity, and failure of the tumor cells to express telomerase

Conclusions
▦ Several studies have shown that the use of the FNA-TRAP assay for telomerase detection is a highly sensitive and accurate method for the detection of telomerase activity in breast masses. Future application of these techniques should facilitate evaluation of telomerase as a tumor marker in the clinical management of breast and other solid malignancies

REFERENCES

SPECIMEN TYPES IN BREAST CYTOPATHOLOGY
Ducatman BS. Breast. In: Cibas ES, Ducatman BS, eds. *Cytology. Diagnostic Principles and Clinical Correlates*, 2nd ed. Philadelphia: Saunders, 2003, pp. 217–20.
Final Version: The uniform approach to breast fine-needle aspiration biopsy. *Breast J.* 1997 Jul; 3(4):149–68.
Guidelines of the Papanicolaou Society of Cytopathology for fine-needle aspiration procedure and reporting. The Papanicolaou Society of Cytopathology Task Force on Standards of Practice. *Diagn Cytopathol.* 1997 Oct;17(4):239–47.
Masood S. *Cytopathology of the Breast*. Chicago, IL: ASCP Press, 1995.
The uniform approach to breast fine-needle aspiration biopsy. NIH Consensus Development Conference. *Am J Surg.* 1997 Oct;174(4):371–85.

DUCTAL LAVAGE
Dooley WC, Ljung BM, Veronesi U, Cazzaniga M, Elledge RM, O'Shaughnessy JA, Kuerer HM, Hung DT, Khan SA, Phillips RF, Ganz PA, Euhus DM, Esserman LJ, Haffty BG, King BL, Kelley MC, Anderson MM, Schmit PJ, Clark RR, Kass FC, Anderson BO, Troyan SL, Arias RD, Quiring JN, Love SM, Page DL, King EB. Ductal lavage for detection of cellular atypia in women at high risk for breast cancer. *J Natl Cancer Inst.* 2001 Nov 7;93(21): 1624–32.
Dooley WC. Ductal lavage, nipple aspiration, and ductoscopy for breast cancer diagnosis. *Curr Oncol Rep.* 2003 Jan;5(1):63–5.

Krishnamurthy S, Sneige N, Thompson PA, Marcy SM, Singletary SE, Cristofanilli M, Hunt KK, Kuerer HM. Nipple aspirate fluid cytology in breast carcinoma. *Cancer.* 2003 Apr 25;99(2): 97–104.

Masood S, Khalbuss WE. Nipple fluid cytology. *Clin Lab Med.* 2005 Dec;25(4):787–94, vii–viii.

Masood S. Cytomorphology as a risk predictor: experience with fine needle aspiration biopsy, nipple fluid aspiration, and ductal lavage. *Clin Lab Med.* 2005 Dec;25(4):827–43.

NIPPLE DISCHARGE CYTOLOGY

Dooley WC. Ductal lavage, nipple aspiration, and ductoscopy for breast cancer diagnosis. *Curr Oncol Rep.* 2003 Jan;5(1):63–5.

Ducatman BS. Breast. In: Cibas ES, Ducatman BS, eds. *Cytology. Diagnostic Principles and Clinical Correlates,* 2nd ed. Philadelphia: Saunders, 2003, pp. 215–7.

Krishnamurthy S, Sneige N, Thompson PA, Marcy SM, Singletary SE, Cristofanilli M, Hunt KK, Kuerer HM. Nipple aspirate fluid cytology in breast carcinoma. *Cancer.* 2003 Apr 25;99(2): 97–104.

Masood S, Khalbuss WE. Nipple fluid cytology. *Clin Lab Med.* 2005 Dec;25(4):787–94, vii–viii.

Masood S. Cytomorphology as a risk predictor: experience with fine needle aspiration biopsy, nipple fluid aspiration, and ductal lavage. *Clin Lab Med.* 2005 Dec;25(4):827–43.

NORMAL COMPONENTS OF BREAST CYTOLOGY SAMPLES

Ducatman BS. Breast. In: Cibas ES, Ducatman BS, eds. *Cytology. Diagnostic Principles and Clinical Correlates,* 2nd ed. Philadelphia: Saunders, 2003, p. 220.

DeMay R. Breast. In DeMay R, ed. *The Art and Science of Cytopathology. Aspiration Cytology.* Chicago, IL: ASCP Press, 1996, pp. 854–6.

Masood S. *Cytopathology of the Breast.* Chicago, IL: ASCP Press, 1995, p. 51.

INFLAMMATORY BREAST LESIONS
MASTITIS

Ducatman BS. Breast. In: Cibas ES, Ducatman BS, eds. *Cytology. Diagnostic Principles and Clinical Correlates,* 2nd ed. Philadelphia: Saunders, 2003, pp. 227–8.

Masood S. *Cytopathology of the Breast.* Chicago, IL: ASCP Press, 1995, pp. 51–4.

Rosen PP. *Rosen's Breast Pathology.* 2nd ed. Philadelphia: LWW, 2001, pp. 33–9.

SUBAREOLAR ABSCESS

DeMay R. Breast. In DeMay R, ed. *The Art and Science of Cytopathology. Aspiration Cytology.* Chicago, IL: ASCP Press, 1996, pp. 856–57.

Ducatman BS. Breast. In: Cibas ES, Ducatman BS, eds. *Cytology. Diagnostic principles Principles and Clinical Correlates,* 2nd ed. Philadelphia: Saunders, 2003, p. 228.

Masood S. *Cytopathology of the Breast.* Chicago, IL: ASCP Press; 1995: pp. 52–3.

Silverman JF, Raso DS, Elsheikh TM, Lannin D. Fine-needle aspiration cytology of a subareolar abscess of the male breast. *Diagn Cytopathol.* 1998 Jun;18(6):441–4.

Versluijs-Ossewaarde FN, Roumen RM, Goris RJ. Subareolar breast abscesses: characteristics and results of surgical treatment. *Breast J.* 2005 May–Jun;11(3):179–82.

FAT NECROSIS

DeMay R. Breast. In DeMay R, ed. *The Art and Science of Cytopathology. Aspiration Cytology.* Chicago, IL: ASCP Press, 1996, pp. 858–9.

Ducatman BS. Breast. In: Cibas ES, Ducatman BS, eds. *Cytology. Diagnostic Principles and Clinical Correlates,* 2nd ed. Philadelphia: Saunders, 2003, pp. 226–7.

Masood S. *Cytopathology of the Breast.* Chicago, IL: ASCP Press, 1995, p. 55.

NONPROLIFERATIVE BREAST DISEASE
BREAST CYSTS

Bruzzi P, Dogliotti L, Naldoni C, Bucchi L, Costantini M, Cicognani A, Torta M, Buzzi GF, Angeli A. Cohort study of association of risk of breast cancer with cyst type in women with gross cystic disease of the breast. *BMJ.* 1997 Mar 29;314(7085):925–8.

DeMay R. Breast. In DeMay R, ed. *The Art and Science of Cytopathology. Aspiration Cytology.* Chicago, IL: ASCP Press, 1996, pp. 860–1.

Ducatman BS. Breast. In: Cibas ES, Ducatman BS, eds. *Cytology. Diagnostic Principles and Clinical Correlates,* 2nd ed. Philadelphia: Saunders, 2003, pp. 220–1.

Masood S. *Cytopathology of the Breast.* Chicago, IL: ASCP Press, 1995, pp. 77–8.

Parish DC, Ghilchik MW, Day JM, Eaton J, Purohit A, Reed MJ. Cytokines in human breast cyst fluid. *J Steroid Biochem Mol Biol.* 2007 May;104(3–5):241–5.

COLLAGENOUS SPHERULOSIS

Divani SN, Mavrogiannis L, Kostis J, Lioupis A. FNA cytology of collagenous spherulosis: recognizing a benign breast lesion. *J BUON.* 2003 Apr–Jun;8(2):171–2.

Gangane N, Joshi D, Anshu, Shivkumar VB. Cytological diagnosis of collagenous spherulosis of breast associated with fibroadenoma: report of a case with review of literature. *Diagn Cytopathol.* 2007 Jun;35(6):366–9.

Jain S, Kumar N, Sodhani P, Gupta S. Cytology of collagenous spherulosis of the breast: a diagnostic dilemma – report of three cases. *Cytopathology.* 2002 Apr;13(2):116–20.

Masood S. *Cytopathology of the Breast.* Chicago, IL: ASCP Press, 1995, pp. 92–3.

MICROGLANDULAR ADENOSIS

DeMay R. Breast. In DeMay R, ed. *The Art and Science of Cytopathology. Aspiration Cytology.* Chicago, IL: ASCP Press, 1996, p. 86.

Gherardi G, Bernardi C, Marveggio C. Microglandular adenosis of the breast: fine-needle aspiration biopsy of two cases. *Diagn Cytopathol.* 1993;9(1):72–6.

Masood S. *Cytopathology of the Breast.* Chicago, IL: ASCP Press, 1995, pp. 85–6.

TUBULAR ADENOMA

Kumar N, Kapila K, Verma K. Characterization of tubular adenoma of breast – diagnostic problem in fine needle aspirates (FNAs). *Cytopathology.* 1998 Oct;9(5):301–7.

Shet TM, Rege JD. Aspiration cytology of tubular adenomas of the breast. An analysis of eight cases. *Acta Cytol.* 1998 May–Jun;42(3):657–62.

PREGNANCY AND LACTATIONAL CHANGES

Ducatman BS. Breast. In: Cibas ES, Ducatman BS, eds. *Cytology. Diagnostic Principles and Clinical Correlates*, 2nd ed. Philadelphia: Saunders, 2003, pp. 225–6.

Masood S. *Cytopathology of the Breast.* Chicago, IL: ASCP Press, 1995, pp. 86–7.

Novotny DB, Maygarden SJ, Shermer RW, Frable WJ. Fine needle aspiration of benign and malignant breast masses associated with pregnancy. *Acta Cytol.* 1991 Nov–Dec;35(6):676–86.

Raso DS, Greene WB, Silverman JF. Crystallizing galactocele. A case report. *Acta Cytol.* 1997 May–Jun;41(3):863–70.

Vesoulis Z, Kashkari S. Fine needle aspiration of secretory breast carcinoma resembling lactational changes. A case report. *Acta Cytol.* 1998 Jul–Aug;42(4):1032–6.

TREATMENT-INDUCED CHANGES

Dornfeld JM, Thompson SK, Shurbaji MS. Radiation-induced changes in the breast: a potential diagnostic pitfall on fine-needle aspiration. *Diagn Cytopathol.* 1992;8(1):79–80.

Ducatman BS. Breast. In: Cibas ES, Ducatman BS, eds. *Cytology. Diagnostic Principles and Clinical Correlates*, 2nd ed. Philadelphia: Saunders, 2003, p. 227.

Filomena CA, Jordan AG, Ehya H. Needle aspiration cytology of the irradiated breast. *Diagn Cytopathol.* 1992;8(4):327–32.

Masood S. *Cytopathology of the Breast.* Chicago, IL: ASCP Press, 1995, pp. 88–9.

Saad RS, Silverman JF, Julian T, Clary KM, Sturgis CD. Atypical squamous metaplasia of seromas in breast needle aspirates from irradiated lumpectomy sites: a potential pitfall for false-positive diagnoses of carcinoma. *Diagn Cytopathol.* 2002 Feb;26(2):104–8.

PROLIFERATIVE BREAST DISEASE WITHOUT/WITH ATYPIA

Bottles K, Chan JS, Holly EA, Chiu SH, Miller TR. Cytologic criteria for fibroadenoma. A step-wise logistic regression analysis. *Am J Clin Pathol.* 1988 Jun;89(6):707–13.

DeMay R. Breast. In DeMay R, ed. *The Art and Science of Cytopathology. Aspiration Cytology.* Chicago, IL: ASCP Press, 1996, pp. 893–94.

Masood S. *Cytopathology of the Breast.* Chicago, IL: ASCP Press, 1995, pp. 169–171.

Masood S. Cytomorphology of fibrocystic change, high-risk proliferative breast disease, and premalignant breast lesions. *Clin Lab Med.* 2005; Dec;25(4):713–31, vi.

Sidawy MK, Stoler MH, Frable WJ, Frost AR, Masood S, Miller TR, Silverberg SG, Sneige N, Wang HH. Interobserver variability in the classification of proliferative breast lesions by fine-needle aspiration: results of the Papanicolaou Society of Cytopathology Study. *Diagn Cytopathol.* 1998; Feb;18(2):150–65.

PAPILLARY LESIONS

Collins LC, Schnitt SJ. Papillary lesions of the breast: selected diagnostic and management issues. *Histopathology*. 2008 Jan;52(1):20–9.

Ducatman BS. Breast. In: Cibas ES, Ducatman BS, eds. *Cytology. Diagnostic Principles and Clinical Correlates*. 2nd ed. Philadelphia: Saunders, 2003, pp. 228–30.

Jayaram G, Elsayed EM, Yaccob RB. Papillary breast lesions diagnosed on cytology. Profile of 65 cases. *Acta Cytol*. 2007 Jan–Feb;51(1):3–8

Masood S. *Cytopathology of the Breast*. Chicago, IL: ASCP Press, 1995, pp. 81–2, 209–10.

Nayar R, De Frias DV, Bourtsos EP, Sutton V, Bedrossian C. Cytologic differential diagnosis of papillary pattern in breast aspirates: correlation with histology. *Ann Diagn Pathol*. 2001 Feb;5(1):34–42.

IN SITU LESIONS OF THE BREAST
DUCTAL CARCINOMA IN SITU

Cangiarella J, Waisman J, Simsir A. Cytologic findings with histologic correlation in 43 cases of mammary intraductal adenocarcinoma diagnosed by aspiration biopsy. *Acta Cytol*. 2003 Nov–Dec;47(6):965–72.

DeMay R. Breast. In DeMay R, ed. *The Art and Science of Cytopathology. Aspiration Cytology*. Chicago, IL: ASCP Press, 1996, pp. 894–96.

Klijanienko J, Katsahian S, Vielh P, Masood S. Stromal infiltration as a predictor of tumor invasion in breast fine-needle aspiration biopsy. *Diagn Cytopathol*. 2004 Mar;30(3):182–6.

Masood S. *Cytopathology of the Breast*. Chicago, IL: ASCP Press, 1995, pp. 176–8.

Reis-Filho JS, Milanezi F, Amendoeira I, Albergaria A, Schmitt FC. p63 Staining of myoepithelial cells in breast fine needle aspirates: a study of its role in differentiating in situ from invasive ductal carcinomas of the breast. *J Clin Pathol*. 2002 Dec;55(12):936–9.

Sneige N, White VA, Katz RL, Troncoso P, Libshitz HI, Hortobagyi GN. Ductal carcinoma-in-situ of the breast: fine-needle aspiration cytology of 12 cases. *Diagn Cytopathol*. 1989;5(4):371–7.

Tavassoli FA, Hoefler H, Rosai J. Intraductal proliferative lesions. In: Tavassoli and Devilee, eds. *Tumours of the Breast and Female Genital Organs*. Lyon: IARC Press, 2003, pp. 63–72.

LOBULAR NEOPLASIA

Ayata G, Wang HH. Fine needle aspiration cytology of lobular carcinoma in situ on ThinPrep. *Diagn Cytopathol*. 2005 May;32(5):276–80.

Hanby AM, Hughes TA. In situ and invasive lobular neoplasia of the breast. *Histopathology*. 2008 Jan;52(1):58–66.

Salhany KE, Page DL. Fine-needle aspiration of mammary lobular carcinoma in situ and atypical lobular hyperplasia. *Am J Clin Pathol*. 1989 Jul;92(1):22–6.

Tavassoli FA, Hoefler H, Rosai J. Intraductal proliferative lesions. In: Tavassoliand Devilee, eds. *Tumours of the Breast and Female Genital Organs*. Lyon: IARCPress, 2003, pp. 60–62.

Ustün M, Berner A, Davidson B, Risberg B. Fine-needle aspiration cytology of lobular carcinoma in situ. *Diagn Cytopathol*. 2002 Jul;27(1):22–6.

PRIMARY BREAST CARCINOMA, COMMON TYPES
INFILTRATING DUCTAL CARCINOMA

Ducatman BS. Breast. In: Cibas ES, Ducatman BS, eds. *Cytology. Diagnostic principles Principles and Clinical Correlates*. , 2nd ed. Philadelphia: Saunders. 2003, pp. 23–233.

Ellis IO, Schnitt SJ, Sastre-Garau X, et al. Invasive breast carcinoma. In: Tavassoli and Devilee, eds. *Tumours of the Breast and Female Genital Organs*. Lyon: IARC Press, 2003, p. 19.

Masood S. *Cytopathology of the Breast*. Chicago, IL: ASCP Press, 1995, pp. 203–05.

Walsh T, Casadei S, Coats KH, Swisher E, Stray SM, Higgins J, Roach KC, Mandell J, Lee MK, Ciernikova S, Foretova L, Soucek P, King MC. Spectrum of mutations in BRCA1, BRCA2, CHEK2, and TP53 in families at high risk of breast cancer. *JAMA*. 2006 Mar 22;295(12):1379–88.

INFILTRATING LOBULAR CARCINOMA

Ducatman BS. Breast. In: Cibas ES, Ducatman BS, eds. Cytology. *Diagnostic Principles and Clinical Correlates*, 2nd ed. Philadelphia: Saunders, 2003, pp. 233–4.

Ellis IO, Schnitt SJ, Sastre-Garau X, et al. Invasive breast carcinoma. In: Tavassoliand Devilee, eds. *Tumours of the Breast and Female Genital Organs*. Lyon: IARC Press, 2003, p. 23.

Hanby AM, Hughes TA. In situ and invasive lobular neoplasia of the breast. *Histopathology*. 2008 Jan;52(1):58–66.

Joshi A, Kumar N, Verma K. Diagnostic challenge of lobular carcinoma on aspiration cytology. *Diagn Cytopathol*. 1998 Mar;18(3):179–83.

Masood S. *Cytopathology of the Breast*. Chicago, IL: ASCP Press. 1995, pp. 205–6.

PRIMARY BREAST CARCINOMA, SPECIAL TYPES
TUBULAR CARCINOMA

Bondeson L, Lindholm K. Aspiration cytology of tubular breast carcinoma. *Acta Cytol*. 1990;34:15–20.

Cangiarella J, Waisman J, Shapiro RL, Simsir A. Cytologic features of tubular adenocarcinoma of the breast by aspiration biopsy. *Diagn Cytopathol*. 2001 Nov;25(5):311–5.

Dawson AE, Logan-Young W, Mulford DK. Aspiration cytology of tubular carcinoma: diagnostic features with mammographic correlation. *Am J Clin Pathol*. 1994;101:488–92.

De la Torre M, Lindholm K, Lindgren A. Fine-needle aspiration cytology of tubular breast carcinoma and radial scar. *Acta Cytol*. 1994;38:884–90.

Ducatman BS.Breast. In: Cibas ES, Ducatman BS, eds. *Cytology. Diagnostic Principles and Clinical Correlates*, 2nd ed. Philadelphia: Saunders, 2003, pp. 236–7.

Gupta RK, Dowle CS. Fine-needle aspiration cytology of tubular carcinoma of the breast. *Acta Cytol*. 1997;41:1139–43.

Masood S. *Cytopathology of the Breast*. Chicago, IL: ASCP Press, 1995, pp. 207–8.

MUCINOUS (COLLOID) CARCINOMA

Cheng L, Lee WY, Chang TW. Benign mucocele-like lesion of the breast: how to differentiate from mucinous carcinoma before surgery. *Cytopathology*. 2004 Apr;15(2):104–8.

DeMay R. Breast. In DeMay R, ed. *The Art and Science of Cytopathology. Aspiration Cytology*. Chicago, IL: ASCP Press, 1996, pp. 877–8.

Haji BE, Das DK, Al-Ayadhy B, Pathan SK, George SG, Mallik MK, Abdeen SM. Fine-needle aspiration cytologic features of four special types of breast cancers: mucinous, medullary, apocrine, and papillary. *Diagn Cytopathol*. 2007 Jul;35(7):408–16.

Masood S. *Cytopathology of the Breast*. Chicago, IL: ASCP Press, 1995, pp. 210–3.

Stanley MW, Tani EM, Skoog L. Mucinous breast carcinoma and mixed mucinous-infiltrating ductal carcinoma: a comparative cytologic study. *Diagn Cytopathol*. 1989;5(2):134–8.

Wong NL, Wan SK. Comparative cytology of mucocelelike lesion and mucinous carcinoma of the breast in fine needle aspiration. *Acta Cytol*. 2000 Sep–Oct;44(5):765–70.

MEDULLARY CARCINOMA

DeMay R. Breast. In DeMay R, ed. *The Art and Science of Cytopathology. Aspiration Cytology*. Chicago, IL: ASCP Press, 1996, pp. 876–7.

Ducatman BS. Breast. In: Cibas ES, Ducatman BS, eds. *Cytology. Diagnostic Principles and Clinical Correlates*, 2nd ed. Philadelphia: Saunders, 2003, p. 235.

Haji BE, Das DK, Al-Ayadhy B, Pathan SK, George SG, Mallik MK, Abdeen SM. Fine-needle aspiration cytologic features of four special types of breast cancers: mucinous, medullary, apocrine, and papillary. *Diagn Cytopathol*. 2007 Jul;35(7):408–16.

Racz MM, Pommier RF, Troxell ML. Fine-needle aspiration cytology of medullary breast carcinoma: report of two cases and review of the literature with emphasis on differential diagnosis. *Diagn Cytopathol*. 2007 Jun;35(6):313–8.

Vincent-Salomon A, Gruel N, Lucchesi C, MacGrogan G, Dendale R, Sigal-Zafrani B, Longy M, Raynal V, Pierron G, de Mascarel I, Taris C, Stoppa-Lyonnet D, Pierga JY, Salmon R, Sastre-Garau X, Fourquet A, Delattre O, de Cremoux P, Aurias A. Identification of typical medullary breast carcinoma as a genomic sub-group of basal-like carcinomas, a heterogeneous new molecular entity. *Breast Cancer Res*. 2007;9(2):R24.

METAPLASTIC CARCINOMA

Ducatman BS. Breast. In: Cibas ES, Ducatman BS, eds. *Cytology. Diagnostic Principles and Clinical Correlates*, 2nd ed. Philadelphia, Saunders, 2003, pp. 237–8.

Ellis IO, Schnitt SJ, Sastre-Garau X, et al. Invasive breast carcinoma. In: Tavassoli and Devilee, eds. *Tumours of the Breast and Female Genital Organs*. Lyon: IARC Press, 2003, p. 37.

Johnson TL, Kini SR. Metaplastic breast carcinoma: a cytohistologic and clinical study of 10 cases. *Diagn Cytopathol*. 1996 May;14(3):226–32.

Lui PC, Tse GM, Tan PH, Jayaram G, Putti TC, Chaiwun B, Chan NH, Lau PP, Mak KL, Khin AT. Fine-needle aspiration cytology of metaplastic carcinoma of the breast. *J Clin Pathol*. 2007 May;60(5):529–33.

Masood S. *Cytopathology of the Breast.* Chicago, IL: ASCP Press, 1995, pp. 261–2.

Tse GM, Tan PH, Lui PC, Putti TC. Spindle cell lesions of the breast-the pathologic differential diagnosis. *Breast Cancer Res Treat.* 2007 Jul 18.

SQUAMOUS CELL CARCINOMA

Gupta RK, Dowle CS. Cytodiagnosis of pure primary squamous-cell carcinoma of the breast by fine-needle aspiration cytology. *Diagn Cytopathol.* 1997 Sep;17(3):197–9.

Pricolo R, Croce P, Voltolini F, Paties C, Schena C. Pure and primary squamous cell carcinoma of the breast. *Minerva Chir.* 1991;46:215–9.

Toikkanen S. Primary squamous cell carcinoma of the breast. *Cancer.* 1981;48:1629–32.

Vera-Alvarez J, García-Prats MD, Marigil-Gómez M, Abascal-Agorreta M, López-López JI, Ramón-Cajal JM. Primary pure squamous cell carcinoma of the breast diagnosed by fine-needle aspiration cytology: a case study using liquid-based cytology. *Diagn Cytopathol.* 2007 Jul;35(7):429–32.

APOCRINE CARCINOMA

DeMay R. Breast. In DeMay R, ed. *The Art and Science of Cytopathology. Aspiration Cytology.* Chicago, IL: ASCP Press, 1996, p. 879.

Ellis IO, Schnitt SJ, Sastre-Garau X, et al. Invasive breast carcinoma. In: Tavassoli and Devilee, eds. *Tumours of the Breast and Female Genital Organs.* Lyon: IARC Press, 2003, p. 36.

Gatalica Z. Immunohistochemical analysis of apocrine breast lesions. Consistent over-expression of androgen receptor accompanied by the loss of estrogen and progesterone receptors in apocrine metaplasia and apocrine carcinoma in situ. *Pathol Res Pract.* 1997;193(11–12):753–8.

Gupta RK, McHutchison AG, Simpson JS, Dowle CS. Fine needle aspiration cytodiagnosis of apocrine carcinoma of the breast. *Cytopathology.* 1992;3(5):321–6.

Haji BE, Das DK, Al-Ayadhy B, Pathan SK, George SG, Mallik MK, Abdeen SM. Fine-needle aspiration cytologic features of four special types of breast cancers: mucinous, medullary, apocrine, and papillary. *Diagn Cytopathol.* 2007 Jul;35(7):408–16.

Jones C, Damiani S, Wells D, Chaggar R, Lakhani SR, Eusebi V. Molecular cytogenetic comparison of apocrine hyperplasia and apocrine carcinoma of the breast. *Am J Pathol.* 2001 Jan;158(1):207–14.

Moinfar F, Okcu M, Tsybovskyy O, et al. Androgen receptors frequently are expressed in breast carcinomas: potential relevance to new therapeutic strategies. *Cancer.* 2003 Aug 15;98(4):703–11.

Unal E, Firat A, Gunes P, Kilicoglu G, Gulkilik A, Titiz I. Apocrine carcinoma of the breast: clinical, radiologic, and pathologic correlation. *Breast J.* 2007 Nov–Dec;13(6):617–8.

Yoshida K, Inoue M, Furuta S, Sakai R, Imai R, Hayakawa S, Fukatsu T, Nagasaka T, Nakashima N. Apocrine carcinoma vs. apocrine metaplasia with atypia of the breast. Use of aspiration biopsy cytology. *Acta Cytol.* 1996 Mar–Apr;40(2):247–51.

FIBROADENOMA

Bellocq JP, Magro G. Fibroepithelial tumors. In: Tavassoli and Devilee, eds. *Tumours of the Breast and Female Genital Organs.* Lyon: IARC Press, 2003, p. 99.

Dupont WD, Page DL, Parl FF, et al. Long-term risk of breast cancer in women with fibroadenoma. *N Engl J Med.* 1994;331:10–5.

Ducatman BS. Breast. In: Cibas ES, Ducatman BS, eds. *Cytology. Diagnostic Principles and Clinical Correlates,* 2nd ed. Philadelphia: Saunders, 2003, pp. 223–4.

Masood S. *Cytopathology of the Breast.* Chicago, IL: ASCP Press, 1995, pp. 79–80.

Kollur SM, El Hag IA. FNA of breast fibroadenoma: observer variability and review of cytomorphology with cytohistological correlation. *Cytopathology.* 2006 Oct;17(5):239–44.

Markopoulos C, Kouskos E, Mantas D, et al. Fibroadenomas of the breast: is there any association with breast cancer? *Eur J Gynaecol Oncol.* 2004;25:495–7.

PHYLLODES TUMOR

DeMay R. Breast. In DeMay R, ed. *The Art and Science of Cytopathology. Aspiration Cytology.* Chicago, IL: ASCP Press, 1996, pp. 865–6.

Ducatman BS. Breast. In: Cibas ES, Ducatman BS, eds. *Cytology. Diagnostic Principles and Clinical Correlates,* 2nd ed. Philadelphia: Saunders, 2003, pp 230–1.

Jayaram G, Sthaneshwar P. Fine-needle aspiration cytology of phyllodes tumors. *Diagn Cytopathol.* 2002 Apr;26(4):222–7.

Lae M, Vincent-Salomon A, Savignoni A, et al. Phyllodes tumors of the breast segregate in two groups according to genetic criteria. *Mod. Pathol.* 2007;20;435–444.

Lee AH. Recent developments in the histological diagnosis of spindle cell carcinoma, fibromatosis and phyllodes tumour of the breast. *Histopathology.* 2008 Jan;52(1):45–57.

Masood S. *Cytopathology of the Breast.* Chicago, IL: ASCP Press, 1995, pp. 79–80.

FIBROEPITHELIAL TUMORS
FIBROMATOSIS

Chhieng DC, Cangiarella JF, Waisman J, Fernandez G, Cohen JM. Fine-needle aspiration cytology of spindle cell lesions of the breast. *Cancer.* 1999 Dec 25; *Diagn Cytopathol.* 1997 Nov;17(5): 363–8. (6):359–71.

Chhieng DC, Cohen JM. Fine needle aspiration (FNA) cytology of mammary fibromatosis: a case report and review of literature. *Dign Cytopathol.* 1999 Oct;10(5):354–9.

López-Ferrer P, Jiménez-Heffernan JA, Vicandi B, Ortega L, Viguer JM.Fine-needle aspiration cytology of mammary fibromatosis: report of two cases. *Diagn Cytopathol.* 1997 Nov;17(5):363–8.

Nakano S, Ohtsuka M, Hasegawa T, Kudoh T, Ikebata K, Sakata H, Yamamoto M, Satake T. Fibromatosis of the breast: a case report. *Breast Cancer.* 2002;9(2):179–83.

Rosen PP, Ernsberger D. Mammary fibromatosis. A benign spindle cell tumor with significant risk for local recurrence. *Cancer* 1989;63:1363–9.

LIPOMA AND SPINDLE CELL LIPOMA

Drijkoningen M, Tavassoli FA, Magro G, et al. Mesenchymal tumors. In: Tavassoli and Devilee, eds. *Tumours of the Breast and Female Genital Organs.* Lyon: IARC Press, 2003, pp. 93–4.

Lew WY. Spindle cell lipoma of the breast: a case report and literature review. *Diagn Cytopathol.* 1993 Aug;9(4):434–7.

Masood S. *Cytopathology of the Breast.* Chicago, IL: ASCP Press, 1995, pp. 153–4.

MYOFIBROBLASTOMA

Formby MR, Hehir M. Myofibroblastoma of the breast. *Pathology.* 1997 Nov;29(4):431–3.

López-Ríos F, Burgos F, Madero S, Ballestín C, Martínez-González MA, de Agustín P. Fine needle aspiration of breast myofibroblastoma. A case report. *Acta Cytol.* 2001 May–Jun;45(3):381–4.

Masood S. *Cytopathology of the Breast.* Chicago, IL: ASCP Press, 1995, pp. 149–50.

GRANULAR CELL TUMOR

Akatsu T, Kobayashi H, Uematsu S, Tamagawa E, Shinozaki H, Kase K, Kobayashi K, Otsuka S, Mukai M, Kitajima M. Granular cell tumor of the breast preoperatively diagnosed by fine-needle aspiration cytology: report of a case. *Surg Today.* 2004;34(9):760–3.

El Aouni N, Laurent I, Terrier P, Mansouri D, Suciu V, Delaloge S, Vielh P. Granular cell tumor of the breast. *Diagn Cytopathol.* 2007 Nov;35(11):725–7.

Green DH, Clark AH. Case report: Granular cell myoblastoma of the breast: a rare benign tumor mimicking breast carcinoma. *Clin Radiol.* 1995;50:799.

McCluggage WG, Sloan S, Kenny BD, Alderdice JM, Kirk SJ, Anderson NH. Fine needle aspiration cytology (FNAC) of mammary granular cell tumour: a report of three cases. *Cytopathology.* 1999 Dec;10(6):383–9.

Ohnishi H, Nishihara K, Tamae K, Mitsuyama S, Abe R, Toyoshima S, Abe E. Granular cell tumors of the breast: a report of two cases. *Surg Today.* 1996;26(11):929–32.

MALIGNANT MESENCHYMAL TUMORS (SARCOMAS)

Carter MR, Hornick JL, Lester S, Fletcher CD. Spindle cell (sarcomatoid) carcinoma of the breast: a clinicopathologic and immunohistochemical analysis of 29 cases. *Am J Surg Pathol.* 2006 Mar;30(3):300–9.

Ducatman BS. Breast. In: Cibas ES, Ducatman BS, eds. *Cytology. Diagnostic Principles and Clinical Correlates,* 2nd ed. Philadelphia: Saunders, 2003, pp. 239–40.

Ewing CA, Miller MJ, Chhieng D, Lin O. Nonepithelial malignancies mimicking primary carcinoma of the breast. *Diagn Cytopathol.* 2004 Nov;31(5):352–7.

Hodgson NC, Bowen-Wells C, Moffat F, Franceschi D, Avisar E. Angiosarcomas of the breast: a review of 70 cases. *Am J Clin Oncol.* 2007 Dec;30(6):570–3.

Miettinen M. From morphological to molecular diagnosis of soft tissue tumors. *Adv Exp Med Biol.* 2006;587:99–113.

Pollard SG, Marks PV, Temple LN, Thompson HH. Breast sarcoma. A clinicopathologic review of 25 cases. *Cancer.* 1990;66:941–4.

LYMPHOMAS

Ducatman BS. Breast. In: Cibas ES, Ducatman BS, eds. *Cytology. Diagnostic Principles and Clinical Correlates,* 2nd ed. Philadelphia: Saunders, 2003, pp. 239–40.

Duncan VE, Reddy VV, Jhala NC, Chhieng DC, Jhala DN. Non-Hodgkin's lymphoma of the breast: a review of 18 primary and secondary cases. *Ann Diagn Pathol.* 2006 Jun;10(3):144–8.

Lamovec J, Wotherspoon A, Jacquemier J. Malignant lymphoma and metastatic tumors. In: Tavassoli and Devilee, eds. *Tumours of the Breast and Female Genital Organs.* Lyon: IARC Press, 2003, pp. 107–9.

Levine PH, Zamuco R, Yee HT. Role of fine-needle aspiration cytology in breast lymphoma. *Diagn Cytopathol.* 2004 May;30(5):332–40.

Shukla R, Pooja B, Radhika S, Nijhawan R, Rajwanshi A. Fine-needle aspiration cytology of extramammary neoplasms metastatic to the breast. *Diagn Cytopathol.* 2005 Apr;32(4):193–7.

Topalovski M, Crisan D, Mattson JC. Lymphoma of the breast. A clinicopathologic study of primary and secondary cases. *Arch Pathol Lab Med.* 1999;123:1208–18.

METASTATIC DISEASE OF THE BREAST

Domanski HA. Metastases to the breast from extramammary neoplasms. A report of six cases with diagnosis by fine needle aspiration cytology. *Acta Cytol.* 1996 Nov–Dec;40(6):1293–300.

Ferrara G, Nappi O. Metastatic neoplasms of the breast: fine-needle aspiration cytology of two cases. *Diagn Cytopathol.* 1996 Aug;15(2):139–43.

Hajdu, SI, Urban, JA. Cancers metastatic to the breast. *Cancer.* 1972;29:1691–6.

Masood S. *Cytopathology of the Breast.* Chicago, IL: ASCP Press; 1995, pp. 331–8.

Shukla R, Pooja B, Radhika S, Nijhawan R, Rajwanshi A. Fine-needle aspiration cytology of extramammary neoplasms metastatic to the breast. *Diagn Cytopathol.* 2005 Apr;32(4):193–7.

MALE BREAST

DeMay R. Breast. In DeMay R, ed. *The Art and Science of Cytopathology. Aspiration Cytology.* Chicago, IL: ASCP Press, 1996, pp. 890–1.

Lilleng R, Paksoy N, Vural G, Langmark F, Hagmar B. Assessment of fine needle aspiration cytology and histopathology for diagnosing male breast masses. *Acta Cytol.* 1995 Sep-Oct;39(5):877–81.

Shin SJ, Rosen PP. Bilateral presentation of fibroadenoma with digital fibroma-like inclusions in the male breast. *Arch Pathol Lab Med.* 2007 Jul;131(7):1126–9.

Siddiqui MT, Zakowski MF, Ashfaq R, Ali SZ. Breast masses in males: multi-institutional experience on fine-needle aspiration. *Diagn Cytopathol.* 2002 Feb;26(2):87–91.

Westenend PJ, Jobse C. Evaluation of fine-needle aspiration cytology of breast masses in males. *Cancer.* 2002 Apr 25;96(2):101–4.

PROGNOSTIC/ PREDICTIVE FACTORS IN BREAST CYTOLOGY

Konofaos P, Kontzoglou K, Georgoulakis J, Megalopoulou T, Zoumpouli C, Christoni Z, Papadopoulos O, Kouraklis G, Karakitsos P. The role of ThinPrep cytology in the evaluation of estrogen and progesterone receptor content of breast tumors. *Surg Oncol.* 2006 Dec;15(4):257–66.

Löfgren L, Skoog L, von Schoultz E, Tani E, Isaksson E, Fernstad R, Carlström K, von Schoultz B. Hormone receptor status in breast cancer – a comparison between surgical specimens and fine needle aspiration biopsies. *Cytopathology.* 2003 Jun;14(3):136–42.

Masood S. Prognostic/predictive factors in breast cancer. *Clin Lab Med.* 2005 Dec;25(4):809–25, viii

Nizzoli R, Bozzetti C, Savoldi L, Manotti L, Naldi N, Camisa R, Soresi AP, Guazzi A, Cocconi G. Immunocytochemical assay of estrogen and progesterone receptors in fine needle aspirates from breast cancer patients. *Acta Cytol.* 1994 Nov-Dec;38(6):933–8.

TELOMERASE ACTIVITY AS A MARKER OF BREAST CARCINOMA IN CYTOLOGY SAMPLES

Cunningham VJ, Markham N, Shroyer AL, Shroyer KR. Detection of telomerase expression in fine-needle aspirations and fluids. *Diagn Cytopathol.* 1998 Jun;18(6):431–6.

Fischer G, Tutuncuoglu O, Bakhshandeh M, Masood S. Diagnostic value of telomerase expression in breast fine-needle aspiration biopsies. *Diagn Cytopathol.* 2007 Oct;35(10):653–5.

Hiyama E, Saeki T, Hiyama K, Takashima S, Shay JW, Matsuura Y, Yokoyama T. Telomerase activity as a marker of breast carcinoma in fine-needle aspirated samples. *Cancer.* 2000 Aug 25;90(4):235–8.

Pearson AS, Gollahon LS, O'Neal NC, Saboorian H, Shay JW, Fahey TJ, 3rd. Detection of telomerase activity in breast masses by fine-needle aspiration. *Ann Surg Oncol.* 1998 Mar;5(2):186–93.

8

Fine-Needle Aspiration Cytology of Tumors of Unknown Origin

Tarik M. Elsheikh

INTRODUCTION

METASTATIC MALIGNANCIES OF UNKNOWN PRIMARY (MUP) SITE

- Eighth most common malignancy
- 5–10% of all noncutaneous malignancies
- Defined as biopsy-confirmed malignancy where a primary site is not found after rigorous, but limited initial clinical and radiographic evaluation, that is, careful history, physical examination, laboratory tests, x-rays, etc.
- Extensive radiological examinations and serum tumor markers are often unsuccessful in finding the primary site
- Decreased performance status, older age, and increased number of sites involved are associated with dismal prognosis
- Traditional treatment is cisplatin-based multiagent chemotherapy
- Poor prognosis; median survival approximately four to twelve months
- Recent literature indicates that optimal management may be organ specific, and rely on accurate determination of primary site

ROLE OF FINE-NEEDLE ASPIRATION (FNA) IN MUP

- FNA is essential in the initial evaluation
- Document/confirm diagnosis of metastasis
- Determine potential primary site
- Triage for ancillary studies such as immunohistochemistry, flow cytometry, and molecular studies

HISTOLOGIC TYPES OF MUP

HISTOLOGIC SUBSETS AND RESPONSE TO CHEMOTHERAPY

- Lymphoma, germ cell tumors, thyroid = good response
- Breast, ovary, prostate = fair response
- Gastrointestinal, urogenital = poor response

FAVORABLE CLINICAL SUBSETS OF MUP (MEDIAN SURVIVAL OF 23 MONTHS)

- Adenocarcinoma involving peritoneal surfaces in women
  - ➤ Treated as stage III ovarian or peritoneal carcinoma
- Adenocarcinoma metastatic to axillary nodes in women
  - ➤ Treated as stage II breast carcinoma
- Adenocarcinoma metastatic to skeleton and associated with elevated serum PSA in men
  - ➤ Treated as metastatic prostate carcinoma, with hormonal therapy for palliation
- Disseminated high-grade neuroendocrine carcinoma of nonpulmonary origin
  - ➤ 80% median response to chemotherapy
- Squamous carcinoma metastatic to cervical or inguinal lymph nodes
  - ➤ Treated as head and neck or anorectal/genital primary
  - ➤ Lymph node dissection and irradiation
- Poorly differentiated carcinoma involving mediastinum or retroperitoneum (especially in young men)
  - ➤ Treated as extragonadal germ cell tumor
  - ➤ Approximately 60% response to chemotherapy

MALIGNANCIES NOTORIOUS FOR LATE RECURRENCES AND LATE METASTASES

- Breast
- Renal cell carcinoma
- Thyroid
- Salivary gland
- Germ cell tumors
- Granulosa cell tumors

SPECIFIC HISTOLOGIC SUBTYPES OF MUP, I.E., MALIGNANCIES WITH RECOGNIZABLE CELL LINEAGE ON MICROSCOPY, AND THEIR RELATIVE FREQUENCIES

- Adenocarcinoma, well to moderately differentiated: 60%
- Poorly differentiated carcinoma: 30%
- Squamous cell carcinoma: 5%
- Undifferentiated malignancy: 5%
  - ➤ One-third to two-third are non-Hodgkin lymphoma
  - ➤ Sarcoma and melanoma < 15% of cases

ADENOCARCINOMA

- Most common MUP (60%)
- Well to moderately differentiated adenocarcinoma has worst prognosis than poorly differentiated adenocarcinoma (median survival is approximately three to six months)

▧ Lung and pancreas are most common primaries (40%), followed by gastrointestinal tract and liver
▧ May not be able to distinguish primary from metastasis by cytology alone
▧ Architectural patterns and immunohistochemistry are helpful in determining primary site

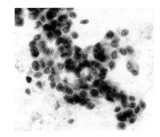

8-1. Adenocarcinoma. The neoplastic cells have delicate cytoplasm, round–oval nuclei, and prominent nucleoli. There is suggestion of gland formation (Papanicolaou stain)

SQUAMOUS CELL CARCINOMA

▧ Accounts for approximately 5% of MUP
▧ Presence of keratinization establishes the diagnosis
▧ Metastatic pattern is highly correlated with primary site
　➤ Upper cervical lymph node: head and neck
　➤ Lower cervical lymph node: lung
　➤ Inguinal lymph node: anorectal/genital
▧ Mixed glandular and squamous components may be appreciated
　➤ Adenosquamous carcinoma from various sites, usually high grade
　➤ Most commonly associated with lung and pancreatic primaries
　➤ Mucoepidermoid carcinoma of salivary glands and lung
　➤ Endometrioid carcinoma with squamous change

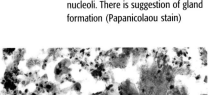

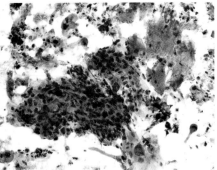

8-2. Squamous Carcinoma metastatic to kidney. The malignant cells show obvious keratinization and cytologic atypia (Papanicolaou stain)

LYMPHOMA

▧ Single-cell pattern
▧ Monomorphic population
▧ Lymphoglandular bodies
▧ Flow cytometry and/or immunohistochemistry is needed for confirmation

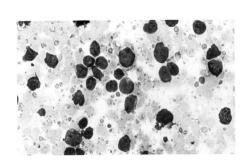

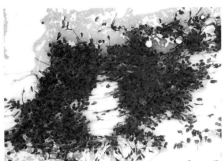

8-3. Large cell lymphoma *(left).* Note numerous lymphoglandular bodies in background (modified Giemsa stain)

8-4. Metastatic angiosarcoma to liver *(right).* (modified Giemsa stain)

SARCOMA

▧ Very unusual to present as MUP
▧ Primary site is often obvious
▧ Spindle, epithelioid, pleomorphic, small cell, and myxoid types
▧ Differential Diagnosis
　➤ Sarcomatoid carcinoma
　➤ Melanoma
　➤ Sclerosing lymphoma

8-5A. Classic presentation of melanoma. Large polygonal and pleomorphic cells with enlarged nuclei, prominent nucleoli, and scattered intranuclear inclusions. Note cytoplasmic pigmentation (Papanicolaou stain)

8-5B. Small cell variant of melanoma. Which must be distinguished from small cell carcinoma and lymphoma (modified Giemsa stain)

8-5C. Rhabdoid variant of melanoma. Huge pleomorphic cells with abundant dense cytoplasm, round eccentric nuclei, and prominent nucleoli (Papanicolaou stain)

8-5D. Plasmacytoid variant of melanoma. The cells show peripherally located nuclei and abundant cytoplasm, resembling plasma cells (modified Giemsa stain)

8-5E. Pleomorphic/giant cell variant of melanoma. (Papanicolaou stain)

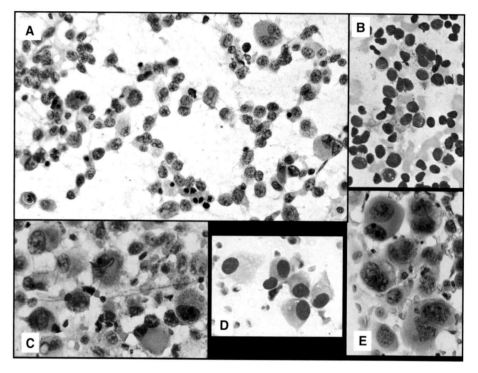

MALIGNANT MELANOMA

- Metastasis to unusual sites
- Primary may be occult or not apparent by history
- Often mimics the appearance of other malignancies
- Melanoma variants
  - Spindle
  - Signet ring
  - Myxoid
  - Desmoplastic
  - Small cell
  - Balloon cell
  - Rhabdoid

CYTOMORPHOLOGIC/ARCHITECTURAL PATTERNS

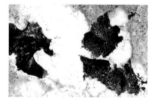

8-6. Columnar/ductal adenocarcinoma pattern. Low power shows cohesive clusters and geographic flat sheets (Papanicolaou stain)

MORPHOLOGIC PATTERNS OF METASTATIC MALIGNANCIES

- Columnar/ductal: low grade, and high grade
- Microacinar/microfollicular
- Mucinous
- Papillary
- Small cell, cohesive, and noncohesive
- Oncocytic/granular
- Clear cell
- Pleomorphic/giant cell
- Spindle cell
- Large cell polygonal, cohesive, and noncohesive

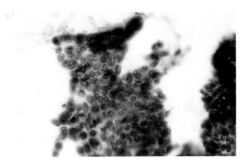 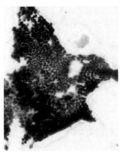 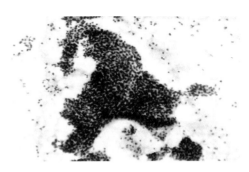

LOW-GRADE COLUMNAR/DUCTAL ADENOCARCINOMA

- Cohesive clusters and geographic flat sheets
- Uniform cell population with bland appearance, resembling benign ductal cells
- Sharp luminal borders are appreciated in some groups
- Round to elongated nuclei, low nuclear to cytoplasmic ratio
- Finely granular chromatin, small nucleoli
- Possible primary sites
  - Pancreas
  - Breast
  - Bile duct
  - Lung (bronchioalveolar carcinoma)
- Colon
  - Rarely presents with this morphology
- Carcinoid
  - Other features such as microacinar formation and salt-and-pepper chromatin should alert you to the diagnosis of carcinoid
  - Positive neuroendocrine markers such as chromogranin and synaptophysin

HIGH-GRADE COLUMNAR/DUCTAL ADENOCARCINOMA

- Cohesive clusters and flat sheets
- Marked nuclear overlapping, haphazard arrangement, significant pleomorphism
- Acinar formation may be focally seen
- Large vesicular nuclei with prominent nucleoli or elongated hyperchromatic nuclei
- Possible primary sites
  - Lung
  - Pancreas
  - Bile duct
    - Often indistinguishable from colon or pancreas
  - Prostate
  - Stomach
- Colon
  - Prominent nuclear elongation and palisading, dirty necrosis
- Endometrioid carcinoma (endometrium, ovary, cervix)

8-7A. Low grade columnar/ductal adenocarcinoma pattern (left). High power shows a uniform cell population. Note luminal border at 12:00 (Papanicolaou stain)

8-7B. Low grade columnar/ductal adenocarcinoma pattern (middle). Cholangiocarcinoma (Papanicolaou stain)

8-7C. Low grade columnar/ductal adenocarcinoma pattern (right). Carcinoid tumor (Papanicolaou stain)

8-8A. High grade columnar adenocarcinoma pattern (left). Metastatic lung adenocarcinoma to bone. There is significant nuclear overlapping and atypia (Papanicolaou stain)

8-8B. High grade columnar adenocarcinoma pattern (middle). Pancreatic adenocarcinoma metastatic to liver. The malignant cells have large vesicular nuclei with prominent nucleoli. Note prominent intracytoplasmic vacuoles (Papanicolaou stain)

8-8C. High grade columnar adenocarcinoma pattern (right). Colon adenocarcinoma metastatic to liver. The nuclei are elongated and hyperchromatic, and show palisading. This appearance is most commonly associated with colon carcinoma, but may also be seen in endometrioid carcinoma (Papanicolaou stain)

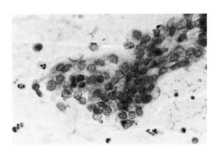 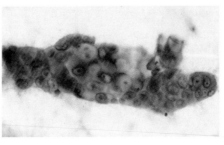 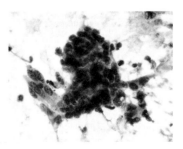

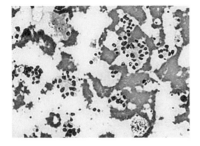
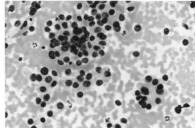
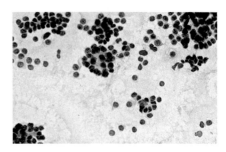

8-9A. Microacinar/microfollicular pattern *(left)*. Prostatic adenocarcinoma (modified Giemsa stain)

8-9B. Microacinar/microfollicular pattern *(middle)*. Follicular carcinoma of thyroid (modified Giemsa stain)

8-9C. Microacinar/microfollicular pattern *(right)*. Carcinoid tumor (Papanicolaou stain)

MICROACINAR/MICROFOLLICULAR COMPLEXES

- Predominant repetitive microacinar pattern
- Prostate is most common carcinoma to present with this appearance
    - Prostate-specific antigen+, prostate acid phosphatase+
- Thyroid follicular carcinoma and follicular variant of papillary carcinoma
    - Thyroglobulin+, TTF-1+
- Neuroendocrine tumors including carcinoid and small blue round cell tumors of childhood
- Granulosa cell tumor

MUCINOUS NEOPLASMS

- Prominent mucinous background
- Mucin often has a stringy appearance
- Neoplastic cells may or may not display significant atypia
- Possible primary sites
    - Colloid carcinomas from breast, gastrointestinal tract, pancreas, ovary, or lung (bronchioalveolar carcinoma)
    - Pseudomyxoma peritonei, usually of appendiceal origin
    - Salivary gland (mucoepidermoid carcinoma)
    - Myxoid sarcomas
- Chordoma
    - Proximal and distal axial skeleton
    - Physaliferous cells: vacuolated polygonal cells with displacement and scalloping of the nuclei
    - Extracellular myxoid material
    - Cytokeratin+, EMA+, S-100+

8-10A. Mucinous neoplasms *(left)*. Colloid carcinoma of breast. Note abundant stringy mucin in the background (Papanicolaou stain)

8-10B. Mucinous neoplasms *(right)*. Chordoma. Extracellular myxoid material and physaliferous cells with variable nuclear atypia (modified Giemsa stain)

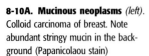
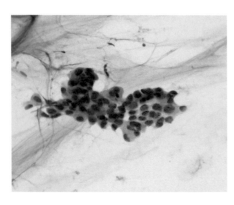
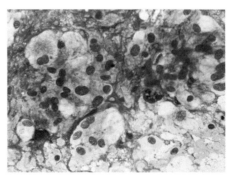

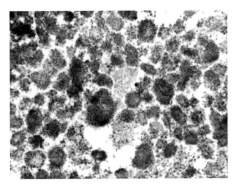

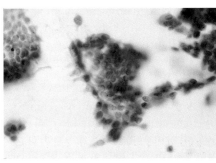

8-11A. Papillary configuration
(left). Papillary serous carcinoma of ovary (Papanicolaou stain)

8-11B. Papillary configuration
(right). Papillary thyroid carcinoma. Note characteristic nuclear features (Papanicolaou stain)

PAPILLARY CONFIGURATION

▥ Tightly cohesive clusters with three-dimensional configuration
▥ Clusters are of variable sizes and may show tufting
▥ Nuclear palisading may be appreciated at the periphery of some clusters
▥ Possible primary sites:
  ➤ Thyroid papillary carcinoma
    • Powdery chromatin, nuclear grooves, pseudo-inclusions
    • Thyroglobulin+, TTF-1+
  ➤ Ovary, endometrium
    • High-grade nuclear features
    • Prominent cytoplasmic vacuolization
  ➤ Kidney
  ➤ Breast
  ➤ Lung (bronchioalveolar carcinoma)

SMALL CELL, COHESIVE

▥ Small cells with minimal cytoplasm, presenting predominately as tight cohesive groups, and showing variable cytologic atypia
▥ Endometrioid carcinoma (ovary, endometrium, cervix)
▥ Basaloid squamous carcinoma
  ➤ Commonly presents as neck node metastases, so must distinguish from small cell carcinoma
  ➤ Cytokeratin 5/6+, p63+, TTF-1 negative
▥ Neuroendocrine carcinoma
  ➤ Low and intermediate grades (carcinoid and atypical carcinoid) show uniform cells with moderate amount of cytoplasm, eccentrically placed nuclei, salt-and-pepper chromatin, and mild to moderate atypia

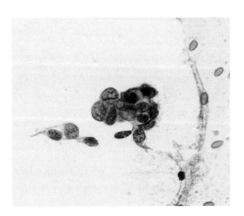

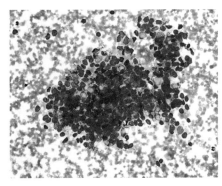

8-12A. Small cell cohesive pattern
(left). Endometrioid carcinoma from ovary (Papanicolaou stain)

8-12B. Small cell cohesive pattern
(right). Ewing's sarcoma (modified Giemsa stain)

➤ High-grade (small cell carcinoma) shows high nuclear/cytoplasmic ratio, nuclear irregularity and molding, and smearing artifact

➤ Cytokeratin 5/6 negative, p63 negative, TTF-1+(small cell carcinoma)

▪ Small blue round cell tumors of childhood

➤ Peripheral neuroectodermal tumor (PNET)/Ewing's sarcoma (ES)

➤ Wilms' tumor

➤ Neuroblastoma

➤ Embryonal rhabdomyosarcoma

➤ Uniform, small, round to oval cells with very high nuclear to cytoplasmic ratios

➤ Hyperchromatic nuclei, lack of prominent nucleoli

➤ Rosette formation can be occasionally appreciated in PNET and neuroblastoma

➤ Fine peripheral cytoplasmic vacuolization in PNET and ES

➤ Rhabdomyosarcoma can show a range of morphologic features with a greater degree of nuclear atypicality, including huge cells with large nuclei and prominent nucleoli

   • Ancillary studies, including immunohistochemistry for neuroectodermal markers, and molecular studies for fusion transcripts and chromosomal translocations

▪ Adenoid cystic carcinoma

➤ Hyaline globules

▪ Urothelial carcinoma

SMALL CELL, NONCOHESIVE

▪ Small cells with minimal cytoplasm, presenting mostly as a population of single cells. Occasional groups and clusters may be seen. There is variable cytologic atypia

▪ Major diagnostic considerations include neuroendocrine carcinoma, poorly differentiated carcinoma, and lymphoma

▪ Possible primary sites

➤ Neuroendocrine carcinoma including carcinoid tumor, Merkel cell carcinoma, and small cell carcinoma

   • Salt and pepper chromatin
   • Chromogranin+, synaptophysin+

➤ Small blue round cell tumors of childhood

➤ Lymphoma

   • Lymphoglandular bodies
   • Cytokeratin negative, CD45+
   • May be difficult to distinguish from reactive lymphoid hyperplasia, therefore, flow cytometry is needed for confirmation

➤ Lobular carcinoma

   • Estrogen/progesterone receptor+

➤ Signet ring carcinoma

   • Cytokeratin+, mucin+

➤ Melanoma

   • Cytokeratin negative, S-100+, HMB-45+, melan A+

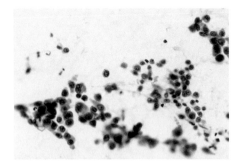

8-13. Small cell non-cohesive pattern. Lobular carcinoma of breast (Papanicolaou stain)

ONCOCYTIC/GRANULAR

▪ Large cells with abundant eosinophilic granular cytoplasm

▪ Cytoplasmic granularities can be due to increased numbers of mitochondria, smooth endoplasmic reticulum, lysosome-like bodies, secretory granules or neuroendocrine-type granules

▥ Thyroid, salivary gland, and kidney are most common primaries
▥ Immunohistochemistry and electron microscopy can help sort out these various neoplasms
▥ Possible primaries:
  ➤ Thyroid
    • Hürthle cell carcinoma
    • Medullary carcinoma: neuroendocrine markers +, calcitonin +
  ➤ Salivary glands
    • Oncocytic carcinoma
    • Acinic cell carcinoma
  ➤ Kidney
    • Oncocytic carcinoma
    • Granular cell carcinoma
  ➤ Hepatocellular carcinoma
    • Trabecular arrangement
    • Polyclonal CEA+ (canalicular pattern), Hep Par-1+
  ➤ Neuroendocrine tumors such as carcinoid and paraganglioma
  ➤ Apocrine carcinoma of breast
    • Gross cystic fluid protein-15+
  ➤ Adrenal cortical carcinoma
    • Often presents as a differential diagnosis of metastatic carcinoma
  ➤ Melanoma
  ➤ Soft tissue tumors
    • Granular cell tumor
    • Alveolar soft part sarcoma

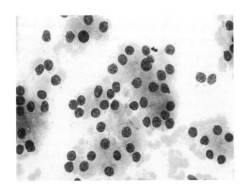 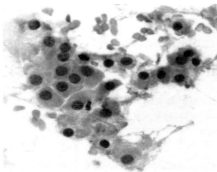

8-14A. Oncocytic/granular cell pattern *(left)*. Hepatocellular carcinoma (modified Giemsa stain)

8-14B. Oncocytic/granular cell pattern *(right)*. Medullary carcinoma of thyroid (Papanicolaou stain)

CLEAR CELL

▥ Abundant delicate cytoplasm with prominent microvacuolization
▥ Clear cell appearance may be due to intracytoplasmic glycogen or fat, paucity of organelles, and fixation or degeneration artifacts
▥ Possible primaries:
  ➤ Kidney
    • Most common malignancy with predominant clear cell features, therefore, must first be excluded
    • Prominent vascular background
  ➤ Gynecologic malignancies, especially ovary
  ➤ Lung
    • Often shows high-grade nuclear features
    • TTF-1+

8-15A. Clear cell pattern *(left).*
Renal cell carcinoma (modified
Giemsa stain)

8-15B. Clear cell pattern *(right).*
Seminoma. Large epithelioid cells
with abundant vacuolated cytoplasm,
coarse chromatin, and prominent
nucleoli. Few lymphocytes are seen
in the background (Papanicolaou
stain)

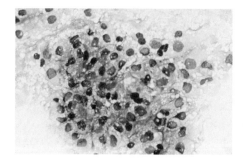
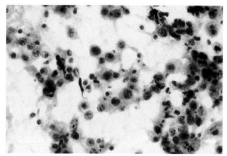

➤ Salivary gland
  • Clear cell carcinoma, epithelial–myoepithelial carcinoma
  • Mucoepidermoid and acinic cell carcinomas with clear cell change
➤ Germ cell tumors, such as seminoma
  • Large epithelioid cells with moderate-abundant fragile vacuolated cyto-
    plasm
  • Tigroid background on modified Giemsa stain
  • Large nuclei with coarse chromatin and prominent nucleoli
  • Variable number of lymphocytes in background
➤ Adrenal gland
➤ Thyroid
  • More conventional foci will often suggest the correct diagnosis
➤ Neuroendocrine tumors including paraganglioma
  • Zellballen pattern associated with a complex vasculature
➤ Chordoma

PLEOMORPHIC/GIANT CELL

▪ Huge cells with severe pleomorphism and variations in size and shape. Cells may
show binucleation and multinucleation
▪ Immunohistochemistry is necessary to exclude a nonepithelial malignancy
▪ Poorly differentiated carcinoma:
  ➤ Lung and pancreas
    • Most common primaries with this morphology
  ➤ Thyroid anaplastic carcinoma
  ➤ Hepatocellular carcinoma
    • Often mistaken for metastatic carcinoma, especially if multifocal in liver
▪ Lymphoma including anaplastic large cell lymphoma and Hodgkin disease
▪ Sarcoma including malignant fibrous histiocytoma and pleomorphic sarcoma

**8-16A. Pleomorphic/giant cell
pattern** *(left).* Giant cell carcinoma
of lung (Papanicolaou stain)

**8-16B. Pleomorphic/giant cell
pattern** *(right).* Pleomorphic
sarcoma/malignant fibrous histiocytoma (Papanicolaou stain)

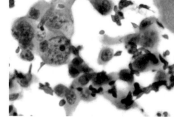
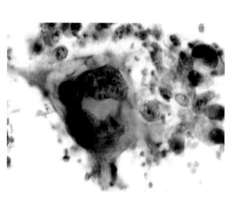

▧ Phaeochromocytoma
▧ Choriocarcinoma
▧ Melanoma

SPINDLE CELL

▧ Evaluation is greatly influenced by the site of involvement. A soft tissue lesion would most likely be a sarcoma, whereas an involved neck lymph node most likely represents a metastatic spindle carcinoma
▧ Lack of cell cohesion favors a sarcoma or melanoma
▧ Immunohistochemical markers are invaluable for the workup. A typical panel includes S-100 and HMB-45 for melanoma, cytokeratin for carcinoma, and specific soft tissue markers for a variety of sarcomas
▧ It is exceedingly unusual for spindle cell sarcoma to present as MUP. More likely, the malignancy represents a spindle cell carcinoma or melanoma
▧ Possible primaries:
  ➤ Spindle/sarcomatoid carcinoma
    • Sarcomatoid renal carcinoma
    • Metaplastic carcinoma of breast
    • Urinary bladder
    • Thyroid anaplastic carcinoma
    • Spindle squamous carcinoma
  ➤ Melanoma
    • Melanin pigment, prominent nucleoli, intranuclear inclusions
  ➤ Neuroendocrine carcinoma from variable sites including lung and medullary thyroid carcinoma
  ➤ Sarcoma including fibrosarcoma and leiomyosarcoma
  ➤ Mesothelioma
    • Cytokeratin 5/6+, calretinin+, WT-1+
  ➤ Lymphoma, sclerosing variant
    • Entrapped lymphoid cells within collagen can impart a cohesive spindle cell appearance
    • Single free lying cells will show hematopoietic appearance
    • CD45+, CD3 or CD20+, cytokeratin–, S-100–

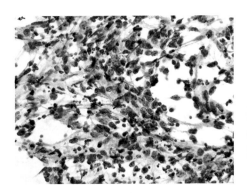
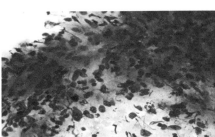

8-17A. Spindle cell pattern *(left).* Metastatic endometrial carcinosarcoma to spleen. The malignant cells showed a predominately spindle cell appearance (Papanicolaou stain)

8-17B. Spindle cell pattern *(right).* Sclerosing lymphoma (modified Giemsa stain)

LARGE CELL/POLYGONAL, COHESIVE

▧ Cohesive clusters of large round to polygonal cells with moderate to abundant cytoplasm and variable cytologic atypia

8-18A. Cohesive large cell/polygonal pattern *(left)*. Large cell carcinoma of lung (modified Giemsa stain)

8-18B. Cohesive large cell/polygonal pattern *(right)*. High-grade ductal carcinoma of breast (Papanicolaou stain)

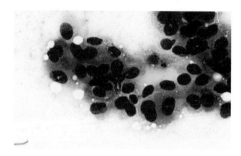
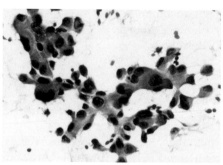

- Differential Diagnosis:
  - Poorly differentiated carcinoma, squamous or glandular
  - Neuroendocrine tumors including large cell neuroendocrine carcinoma and medullary carcinoma of thyroid
  - Melanoma
  - Anaplastic large cell lymphoma
    - May present as cohesive clusters mimicking carcinoma
    - CD30+, EMA+, CD45±, cytokeratin–

LARGE CELL/POLYGONAL, NONCOHESIVE

- Predominately single, round to polygonal cells with variable cytologic atypia. Occasional loosely cohesive groups
- Breast and stomach are most common adenocarcinomas to present as single cells
- May represent an undifferentiated carcinoma, not otherwise classified
- Immunohistochemistry is often needed to exclude a nonepithelial malignancy
- Possible primaries:
  - Signet ring carcinoma (stomach, pancreas, and colon)

8-19A. Non cohesive large cell/polygonal pattern *(top, left)*. Signet ring carcinoma from stomach (modified Giemsa stain)

8-19B. Non cohesive large cell/polygonal pattern *(top, right)*. Large cell lymphoma (Papanicolaou stain)

8-19C. Non cohesive large cell/polygonal pattern *(bottom, left)*. Medullary carcinoma of the thyroid. The neoplastic cells have a plasmacytoid appearance, that is, eccentrically placed nuclei with abundant dense cytoplasm (modified Giemsa stain)

8-19D. Non cohesive large cell/polygonal pattern *(bottom, right)*. Plasmacytoma. The patient presented with a lytic skull mass (modified Giemsa stain)

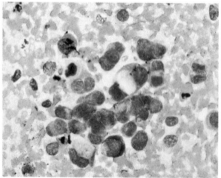

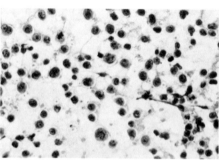
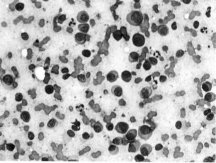

➤ Breast including pleomorphic lobular carcinoma and ductal carcinoma in the elderly
➤ Sarcoma
➤ Melanoma
➤ Lymphoma
➤ Neuroendocrine carcinoma
➤ Plasmacytoma
  • Other tumors with plasmacytoid appearance include carcinoid/islet cell tumor, melanoma, breast carcinoma

MISCELLANEOUS CYTOLOGIC FEATURES

INTRACYTOPLASMIC HYALINE GLOBULES

▩ Intracytoplasmic hyaline globules can be seen in a variety of carcinomas, sarcomas, lymphomas, germ cell tumors, and melanoma

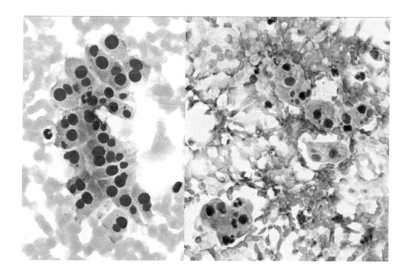

8-20. Intracytoplasmic hyaline globules. In renal oncocytic neoplasm (modified Giemsa stain and Papanicolaou stain)

▩ Possible primaries
➤ Hepatocellular carcinoma
➤ Renal cell carcinoma
➤ Germ cell tumors
➤ Ovarian carcinoma
➤ Malignancies with rhabdoid phenotype:
  • Intracytoplasmic globules are eosinophilic and prominent, and cells have large nuclei with prominent nucleoli
  • Malignancies are usually poorly differentiated and aggressive in behavior
  • Melanoma is one of the more common malignancies to show rhabdoid features

8-21. Intranuclear inclusions. Papillary thyroid carcinoma (Papanicolaou stain)

INTRANUCLEAR INCLUSIONS

▩ Papillary thyroid carcinoma
▩ Melanoma
▩ Hepatocellular carcinoma
▩ Bronchioalveolar carcinoma of lung
▩ Thyroid medullary carcinoma

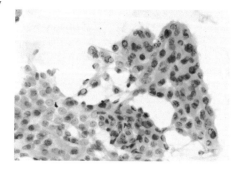

MALIGNANCIES ASSOCIATED WITH GRANULOMAS

- Squamous and adenosquamous carcinoma
- Nasopharyngeal carcinoma
- Seminoma
- Hodgkin disease
- T-cell lymphoma
- Epithelioid sarcoma
- Mesothelioma
- Papillary thyroid carcinoma
  - ➤ Associated with giant cells rather than true granulomas

IMMUNOHISTOCHEMISTRY

IMMUNOHISTOCHEMISTRY (IHC) APPROACH TO MUP

- Currently, immnohistochemistry is the main ancillary study utilized in determining the primary site or cell lineage of the malignancy
- If the malignancy is undifferentiated, then first determine the cell lineage, that is, carcinoma, lymphoma, melanoma, germ cell tumor, or sarcoma
- Diagnosis may be refined using different cytokeratins (CK) that are unique to certain tumor types, that is, CK7, CK20, and CK5/6
- Specific epithelial markers or hormonal receptor analysis, such as differential nonkeratins (CEA, EMA) and ER/PR receptors, may be added to the panel
- Organ specific and associated markers, such as PSA, TTF-1, and thyroglobulin can further narrow down the source of malignancy
- No single immunohistochemistry antibody can provide a definitive diagnosis, in most cases, so a panel of stains should always be utilized
- Interpretation of a panel of antibodies should be based on the pathologist's experience in own laboratory, as well as statistical analysis in the literature
- The antibodies chosen should be based on the morphologic and/or clinicopathologic features of the malignancies, in order for the evaluation to be meaningful

DIFFERENTIAL CYTOKERATINS

- CK7–/CK20+
  - ➤ *Colorectal carcinoma*
  - ➤ Merkel cell carcinoma

Table 8.1. Immunohistochemistry workup of undifferentiated malignancy

	AE-1/3	CD45	S-100	PLAP	Additional markers
Carcinoma	+	–	±	–[a]	Differential keratins, EMA, etc.
Melanoma	–	–	+	–	HMB-45, melan A, etc.
Lymphoma	–	+[b]	–	–	CD20, CD3, CD30, etc.
Germ cell tumor	–[c]	–	–	+	EMA, CD30, OCT-4

[a] Approximately 10% of nongerm cell carcinomas are PLAP+, but they are usually EMA+. Nonseminoma germ cell tumors are keratin+ and EMA–.

[b] CD45 is very specific, but misses approximately 10% of large cell lymphoma including anaplastic large cell lymphoma. May include CD30 if suspect lymphoma with negative initial panel.

[c] Seminoma and embryonal carcinoma are EMA–. Seminoma is CK–.

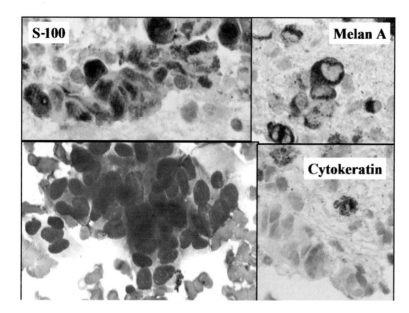

8-22. Immunohistochemistry workup of undifferentiated malignancy. This patient presented with a solitary lung mass. The staining pattern is consistent with metastatic malignant melanoma (modified Giemsa stain, S-100+, melan A+, cytokeratin–)

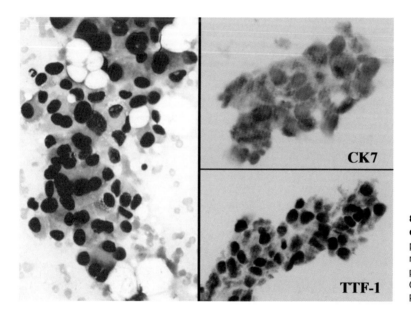

8-23. Metastatic adenocarcinoma consistent with lung primary. This patient presented with an osteolytic rib mass and a previous history of prostate carcinoma. (modified Giemsa stain, TTF1+, cytokeratin 7+, PSA– {not shown})

- CK7–/CK20–
  - Hepatocellular carcinoma
  - Prostate carcinoma
  - Renal cell carcinoma
  - Squamous cell carcinoma
  - Neuroendocrine carcinoma of lung
  - Adrenal cortical carcinoma
  - Germ cell malignancies
  - Thymoma
- CK7+/CK20–
  - Ovary (nonmucinous)
  - Endometrial carcinoma
  - Breast carcinoma (papillary and mucinous types can be CK20+)
  - Lung carcinoma (mucinous type can be CK20+)

➢ Mesothelioma (can also be CK20+)
➢ Salivary gland tumors
▪ CK7+/CK20+
  ➢ Urothelial carcinoma (can also be CK7+/CK20–)
  ➢ Pancreatic carcinoma
  ➢ Ovarian mucinous carcinoma
  ➢ Occasionally cholangiocarcinoma and gastric carcinoma
▪ CK5/6+
  ➢ Squamous cell carcinoma
  ➢ Urothelial carcinoma
  ➢ Mesothelioma
▪ CEA expression (monoclonal)
  ➢ Level of expression is proportional to degree of differentiation
  ➢ CEA positive:
    • Colorectal
    • Lung nonsmall cell carcinoma
    • Hepatocellular carcinoma (polyclonal CEA, canalicular pattern)
    • Mucinous carcinoma
  ➢ CEA negative:
    • Renal cell carcinoma
    • Prostate carcinoma
    • Endometrial carcinoma
    • Mesothelioma

EMA EXPRESSION

▪ EMA positive
  ➢ Adenocarcinoma
  ➢ Mesothelioma
  ➢ Plasmacytoma
  ➢ Anaplastic large cell lymphoma
▪ EMA negative
  ➢ Hepatocellular carcinoma
  ➢ Adrenocortical carcinoma
  ➢ Germ cell tumors (except occasional choriocarcinoma and teratoma)

ESTROGEN/PROGESTERONE RECEPTORS (1D5 CLONE, DAKO®)

▪ Sensitivity and specificity of ER receptor is dependent on the clone of antibody used
▪ ER/PR positive
  ➢ Breast carcinoma
  ➢ Ovarian, endometrial, cervical carcinoma
  ➢ Skin sweat gland (apocrine)
  ➢ Thyroid
  ➢ Neuroendocrine (Carcinoid)
▪ ER/PR negative
  ➢ Colorectal carcinoma
  ➢ Lung nonsmall cell carcinoma
  ➢ Hepatocellular carcinoma
  ➢ Gastric carcinoma
  ➢ Pancreatic carcinoma
  ➢ Thymoma
  ➢ Urothelial carcinoma

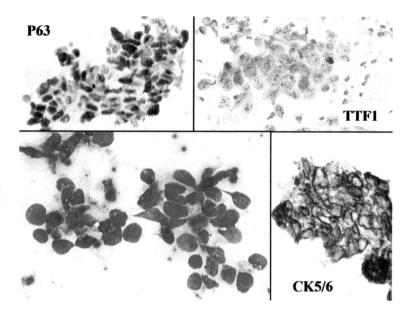

8-24. Metastatic basaloid squamous carcinoma. This patient presented with a left neck mass and no known primary. Cytologic differential diagnosis included small cell carcinoma and basaloid squamous carcinoma (modified Giemsa stain, cytokeratin 5/6+, p63+, TTF-1–, chromogranin and synaptophysin were negative [not shown])

Table 8.2. Tumor-specific markers

Marker	Staining pattern	Organ
TTF-1	Nuclear	Lung, thyroid, neuroendocrine carcinoma
CDX2	Nuclear	Colon, gastrointestinal (pancreas, stomach, bile duct), bladder adenocarcinoma, ovarian mucinous
Calretinin	Nuclear	Mesothelioma
WT-1	Nuclear	Serous ovarian, mesothelioma
MAP-2	Nuclear	Melanoma
Myogenin	Nuclear	Rhabdomyosarcoma
Prostate-specific antigen	Cytoplasmic	Prostate
Prostate acid phosphatase	Cytoplasmic	Prostate, carcinoid
Calcitonin	Cytoplasmic	Thyroid medullary carcinoma
Thyroglobulin	Cytoplasmic	Thyroid
GCFP-15	Cytoplasmic	Breast, salivary, sweat gland
Hep Par-1	Cytoplasmic	Hepatocellular carcinoma and hepatoid adenocarcinoma
Renal cell antigen	Membranous	Kidney
Uroplakin	Membranous	Urothelial carcinoma
Villin	Membranous	Colon, pancreas, bile duct, stomach, mucinous ovarian, bladder adenocarcinoma

CLINICAL PATTERNS OF METASTASES

COMMON SITES OF METASTASIS

- Lymph nodes
- Lung
- Large bones
- Liver
- Adrenal glands

UNUSUAL SITES OF METASTASIS

- Breast
- Thyroid
- Pancreas
- Kidney
- Small bones
- Eye
- Spleen

MOST COMMON PRIMARIES

- Lung
- Pancreas
- Gastrointestinal tract, including colon and stomach
- Liver
- Prostate
- Kidney

LYMPH NODES

- Most frequent site of metastasis
- Diagnostic accuracy for metastatic carcinoma is 82–99%
- Knowledge of exact location of involved lymph node is of prime importance

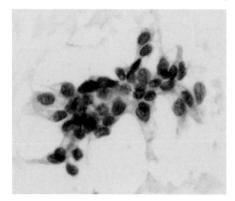

8-25. Metastatic urothelial carcinoma to left supraclavicular lymph node. The patient had a previous history of bladder carcinoma (Papanicolaou stain)

CERVICAL LYMPH NODES

- Head and neck squamous carcinoma and melanoma are most common primaries
- Adenocarcinoma from primaries arising in supraclavicular organs
  - Thyroid
  - Salivary glands
- Adenocarcinoma from primaries arising in infraclavicular organs
  - Lung
  - Gastrointestinal tract
  - Breast
  - Ovary
  - Prostate

SUPRACLAVICULAR LYMPH NODES (SCLN)

- Primary sites involving left SCLN *(Virchow's node)* are different from those involving right SCLN
- The majority of pelvic and abdominal malignancies preferentially metastasize to left SCLN

■ Thorax, breast, and head/neck malignancies show no difference in their metastatic pattern to left or right SCLN

■ Most common metastases to left SCLN are lung and breast > pelvis and testis > abdomen

■ Most common metastases to right SCLN are thorax and breast > lymphoma > pelvis and testis

AXILLARY LYMPH NODES

■ Most common primaries are breast, lung, skin of arm and regional trunk, and gastrointestinal tract

INGUINAL LYMPH NODES

■ Most common primaries are melanoma, skin of leg and trunk, cervix, vulva, anorectum, ovary, bladder, and prostate

Differential Diagnosis of Lymph Node Metastases

■ Large cell lymphoma may be difficult to distinguish from small cell carcinoma or from a poorly differentiated adenocarcinoma presenting in a predominantly discohesive pattern

■ Anaplastic large cell lymphoma may present in cohesive clusters and mimic metastatic carcinoma

■ Malignant melanoma should always be considered in the differential diagnosis of lymphoma and poorly differentiated carcinoma

■ Immunohistochemistry plays a pivotal role in establishing an accurate diagnosis

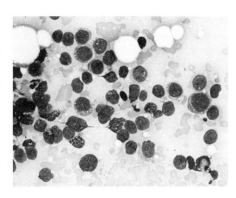

8-26. Metastatic large cell carcinoma from lung, involving cervical lymph node. The cytologic features may be confused with lymphoma, but notice the absence of lymphoglandular bodies (modified Giemsa stain)

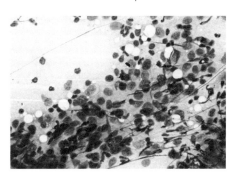

8-27. Anaplastic large cell lymphoma. The cohesive nature of this presentation can mimic carcinoma (modified Giemsa stain)

LARGE BONES

■ Radiologic findings in metastatic disease are seldom specific to allow for a definitive diagnosis

■ Bones with active hematopoietic marrow are more commonly involved by metastases
➤ Vertebral column
➤ Large bones
➤ Iliac bones
➤ Ribs
➤ Skull

■ Metastatic carcinoma is the most common malignancy of bone

■ Most frequent primaries
➤ Prostate
➤ Breast
➤ Kidney
➤ Lung
➤ Thyroid

■ Spindle cell malignancies in bone:
➤ Metastasis may have a spindle cell appearance, therefore mimicking a sarcoma
➤ Occasionally, metastasis may be associated with extensive osteoid formation or reactive osteoclastic proliferation simulating primary osteosarcoma or giant cell tumor of bone
➤ Metastatic spindle/sarcomatoid carcinoma (especially from kidney) and malignant melanoma must first be excluded

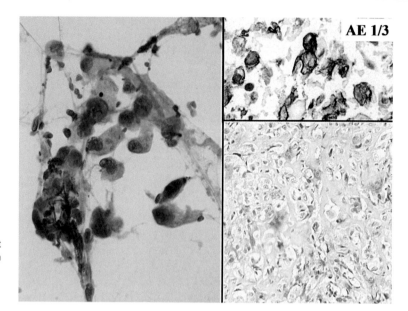

8-28. Spindle cell malignancy involving the bone. The cytokeratin staining is consistent with carcinoma. Follow-up revealed a primary sarcomatoid carcinoma of the kidney (Papanicolaou stain, H&E stain, cytokerain AE 1/3+)

LUNG

▦ Breast and gastrointestinal tract (colon, pancreas, stomach) are the most common primaries
▦ Any malignancy can metastasize to lung
▦ Multiple nodules is the most common presentation
▦ Metastasis may present as a single mass (3–9% of all solitary pulmonary nodules)
➤ Melanoma, breast, colon, kidney, sarcoma, germ cell tumor
▦ FNA of right lower lobe lung masses may inadvertently sample benign liver tissue, potentially leading to a false positive diagnosis of clear and/or granular cell carcinoma such as renal cell carcinoma
▦ Cavitation may be associated with metastatic malignancies arising in head and neck, cervix, colon, breast, bladder, and sarcoma

LIVER

▦ Metastases account for the great majority of liver malignancies
▦ Most common primary sites
➤ Gastrointestinal tract (pancreas, colon, stomach)
➤ Breast
➤ Lung
➤ Lymphoma
➤ Genitourinary
➤ Sarcoma
➤ Melanoma
▦ Most common histologic types
➤ Metastatic adenocarcinoma (40%)
➤ Hepatocellular carcinoma (24%)
➤ Neuroendocrine carcinoma (7%)
➤ Squamous cell carcinoma and lymphoma (4%)

Differential Diagnosis

■ Adenocarcinomas with small tubular or tubulopapillary architecture most likely arise from stomach, pancreas, or biliary tract

■ Light microscopy and immunohistochemistry will not distinguish cholangiocarcinoma from metastatic gastrointestinal carcinoma, in most instances

■ Metastatic colon adenocarcinoma often shows large well-formed glands, hyperchromatic cigar-shaped nuclei, and dirty necrosis in the background

■ Hepatocellular carcinoma
  ➤ Immunohistochemistry associated with elevated serum alpha-fetoprotein is helpful in confirming the diagnosis (pCEA+, Hep Par-1+, CK7−/CK20−)

■ Malignant melanoma
  ➤ Predominantly discohesive cell pattern
  ➤ S-100+, HMB-45+, melan A+, CK−

ADRENAL GLANDS

■ Metastases is found in up to 27–35% of patients with history of malignancy

■ Adenocarcinoma and squamous carcinoma are most frequent histologic types

■ Common primary sites
  ➤ Lung
  ➤ Breast
  ➤ Kidney
  ➤ Gastrointestinal tract (stomach, colon, pancreas)
  ➤ Liver
  ➤ Ovary
  ➤ Melanoma
  ➤ Lymphoma

■ Lung accounts for 50–70% of metastases, followed by breast

Differential Diagnosis

■ Metastatic adenocarcinoma
  ➤ CEA+, EMA+

■ Renal cell carcinoma
  ➤ CEA−, EMA±, CD10+, Renal cell antigen+

■ Benign adrenocortical nodule (BACN)
  ➤ CEA−, EMA−
  ➤ Verify that the tip of the sampling needle is within the adrenal nodule, since normal adrenal tissue is indistinguishable from BACN
  ➤ Benign liver tissue can occasionally mimic adrenal cortical tissue

■ Adrenocortical carcinoma may cytologically mimic BACN
  ➤ High-grade carcinoma shows significant atypia
  ➤ Distinguishing well-differentiated adrenocortical carcinoma from BACN remains problematic

■ Small blue round cell malignancy
  ➤ Neuroendocrine markers and TTF-1

SALIVARY GLANDS

■ Metastatic tumors account for approximately 10–16% of all salivary gland malignancies

■ Most commonly involve intraparotid or periparotid lymph nodes

■ Most frequent histologic types are squamous carcinoma and melanoma

■ Most common primary sites
  ➤ Head and neck
  ➤ Melanoma
  ➤ Lymphoma
  ➤ Lung
  ➤ Kidney

Differential Diagnosis

■ Squamous cell carcinoma versus primary high-grade mucoepidermoid carcinoma (MEC)
  ➤ Glandular differentiation and mucin positivity favors MEC
  ➤ Abundant keratinization favors metastatic squamous carcinoma
  ➤ Primary squamous cell carcinoma of the salivary gland is extremely rare
■ Branchial cleft cyst versus metastatic cystic squamous carcinoma
  ➤ In the absence of significant atypia, it is not possible to distinguish between them
  ➤ Diagnosis of squamous carcinoma should be rendered only in the presence of clusters and/or singly scattered highly atypical squamous cells
■ Clear cell carcinoma
  ➤ Must exclude metastatic renal cell carcinoma before considering primary salivary gland origin
■ Small cell carcinoma
  ➤ Must exclude pulmonary origin, before considering a primary salivary gland carcinoma
■ Poorly differentiated adenocarcinoma and undifferentiated carcinoma
  ➤ It is not possible to cytologically distinguish primary from metastatic cancer with this morphology
  ➤ Clinical correlation is needed

BREAST

■ Contralateral breast, melanoma, lung, lymphoma, and ovary are most common primaries
■ Other primaries include sarcoma, gastrointestinal tract, genitourinary
■ Extramammary malignancies account for 0.5–2% of breast malignancies
■ In men, most common primaries are prostate, lymphoma, lung, bladder
■ Often associated with disseminated disease
■ May present as the initial finding in up to 25–50% of patients
■ May present as a solitary mass (more common) or multiple nodules

Differential Diagnosis

■ Metastases should be suspected when cytology is unusual for a primary breast carcinoma, i.e.,
  ➤ Small cell carcinoma
  ➤ Melanoma
  ➤ Lymphoma
■ Distinguishing primary from metastatic malignancy is difficult when the metastasis has no distinctive cytologic features, that is,
  ➤ Poorly differentiated carcinoma
  ➤ Papillary carcinoma (ovarian vs. breast)
  ➤ Mucinous carcinoma (gastrointestinal vs. breast): immunohistochemistry is helpful
■ Differential diagnosis of spindle cell malignancy includes
  ➤ Metaplastic carcinoma of breast
  ➤ Sarcoma
  ➤ Melanoma

THYROID

- Rare site for metastases, approximately 1.3–25% of thyroid cancers
- May present as multiple nodules or a solitary tumor mass
- Kidney, lung, breast, and melanoma are most common primaries
- May be involved by direct extension from carcinoma of the upper aerodigestive tract
- Metastasis can be suspected when the cytology appears alien to the more common thyroid cancers such as papillary, follicular, and medullary carcinoma
- Immunohistochemistry is helpful, as thyroid cancers are usually positive for thyroglobulin and TTF-1

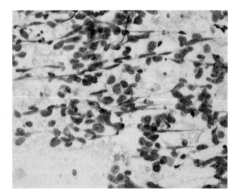

8-29. Metastatic renal cell carcinoma to the thyroid gland. The patient had a previous history of kidney cancer since fifteen years (Papanicolaou stain)

PANCREAS

- Metastases may be radiographically and clinically indistinguishable from primary neoplasms
- Make up approximately 10% of malignant pancreatic FNAs
- Lung, breast, kidney, lymphoma, liver, and melanoma are most common
- May be involved by direct extension from stomach, intestine, and biliary tract
- Cytology foreign to common primary pancreatic cancers is the most helpful clue to suspecting metastasis
- Small cell carcinoma is usually metastatic from lung, since primary small cell carcinoma is quite rare
- Squamous differentiation may occur in primary pancreatic carcinoma as part of adenosquamous carcinoma
- Pure squamous cell carcinoma is more suggestive of metastasis from pulmonary, esophageal or cervical origin

8-30. Metastatic small cell carcinoma to pancreas. The patient presented with obstructive jaundice and a mass in the head of pancreas (Papanicolaou stain)

KIDNEY

- Accounts for approximately 8–13% of renal tumors
- Current indications for kidney FNA:
  - ➤ Nonresectable tumor
  - ➤ Radiographically indeterminate lesions
  - ➤ High-risk surgical patients
  - ➤ Metastatic tumors
  - ➤ Drainage of benign cysts and abscesses
- Most common primaries include lung, breast, stomach, pancreas, contralateral kidney, and melanoma
- Most metastatic malignancies are easily distinguished cytologically from renal cell carcinoma
- It is difficult to distinguish occasional primary renal neoplasms such as collecting duct carcinoma from metastatic carcinoma

SMALL BONES

- Exceptionally rare, less than 0.3% of all bone metastasis
- Associated with an extremely poor prognosis
- Clinically, small bone metastases may mimic a variety of infectious and inflammatory skeletal diseases
- Lung, kidney, and breast are the most common to metastasize to small bones of the hand and feet

■ Gastrointestinal tract and melanoma may also involve small bones

■ In general, subdiaphragmatic malignancies metastasize to the feet, while malignancies arising above the diaphragm metastasize to the hand

ORBIT

■ FNA is not often used in the evaluation of intraocular neoplasms

■ Metastases in children are most often of embryonal or undifferentiated type

■ In adults, the most common metastatic epithelial malignancy is breast in women, and lung in men

■ Malignant melanoma is the most common nonepithelial metastasis

■ Uveal metastasis is second only to unveal melanoma as the most common diagnosis encountered in transocular FNAs

■ Other possible primaries include lymphoma, gastrointestinal tract, kidney, and prostate

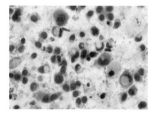

8-31. Metastatic signet ring carcinoma to spleen. A gastric primary was subsequently found (Papanicolaou stain)

SPLEEN

■ Splenic FNA is rarely utilized in the United States

■ Has been used mostly for diagnosis of lymphoma or nonneoplastic systemic disease (amyloidosis, sarcoidosis, infectious disease)

■ Lung, breast, and melanoma account for most metastases

■ May be involved by direct extension from pancreas and retroperitoneum

TUMOR TO TUMOR METASTASIS

■ Extremely rare

■ Both benign and malignant tumors can act as hosts to metastatic malignancies

■ Most common recipient benign tumors are thyroid adenoma, adrenal adenomas, and meningioma

■ Most common recipient malignancies are renal cell carcinoma, sarcoma, and lymphoma

■ Most common donor neoplasms are lung, prostate, and thyroid

■ Should be suspected when two distinctly different cytomorphologic features are seen in patients with known or suspected second malignancy

■ Immunohistochemistry is helpful in some metastatic cancers such as breast, prostate, thyroid papillary carcinoma and neuroendocrine carcinomas

SUMMARY

GENERAL PRINCIPLES TO BE CONSIDERED IN ANALYSIS OF SUSPECTED METASTASES

■ Pathologists should be familiar with cytology of common malignancies originating in a primary site

■ Unusual cytology for the site is the biggest clue to suspecting metastases

■ Knowledge of clinical patterns of metastases helps generate a short list of possible primary sites

■ Combination of cytomorphology and immunohistochemistry can then aid arriving to a more specific diagnosis

■ Inquire about a previous history of malignancy

■ Review and compare previous pathology material, when available

■ Recommend tissue confirmation in unresolved cases, before institution of definitive treatment

REFERENCES

INTRODUCTION

Abbruzzese JL, Lenzi R, Raber M. Carcinoma of unknown primary. In: Abeloff, Ed., *Clinical Oncology*, 2nd ed. Churchill Livingstone, Edinburgh, 2000.

Hainsworth JD, Erland JB, Kalman LA, et al. Carcinoma of unknown primary site: Treatment with 1-hour paclitaxel, carboplatin, and extended-schedule etoposide. *J Clin Oncol* 1997;5:2385–2393.

Haskell CM, Cochran AJ, Barsky SH, Steckel RJ. Metastasis of unknown origin. *Curr Probl Cancer* 1988;12(1):5–58.

Pasterz R, Savaraj N, Burgess M. Prognostic factors in metastatic carcinoma of unknown primary. *J Clin Oncol* 1986;4:1652.

Raber MN, Faintuch J, Abbruzzese JL, et al. Continuous infusion 5-flourouracil, etoposide and cisplatin in patients with metastatic carcinoma of unknown primary origin. *Ann Oncol* 1991;2:519–520.

Saghatchian M, Fizazi K, Borel C, et al. Carcinoma of an unknown primary site: A chemotherapy strategy based on histological differentiation – results of a prospective study. *Ann Oncol* 2001;12:535–540.

HISTOLOGIC TYPES OF MUP

DeMay RM. *The Art and Science of Cytopathology*. American Society of Clinical Pathologists Press, Chicago, IL, 1996.

Elsheikh TM, Silverman JF. Metastatic malignancies. In: Silverberg SG, Ed., *Principles and Practice of Surgical Pathology and Cytopathology*, 4th ed. Churchill Livingstone, Edinburgh, 2006.

Greco FA, Vaughn WK, Hainsworth JD. Advanced poorly differentiated carcinoma of unknown primary site: recognition of a treatable syndrome. *Ann Intern Med* 1986;104:547.

Gupta T, Bowden L, Berg JW. Malignant melanoma of unknown primary origin. *Surg Gynecol Obstet* 1963;117:341–345.

Haskell CM, Cochran AJ, Barsky SH, Steckel RJ. Metastasis of unknown origin. *Curr Probl Cancer* 1988;12(1):5–58.

Kambhu SA, Kelsen D, Fiore J, et al. Metastatic adenocarcinomas of unknown primary site. *Am J Clin Oncol* 1990;13:55.

Kirsten F, Chi HE, Leary JA, et al. Metastatic adeno- or undifferentiated carcinoma from an unknown primary site: Natural history and guidelines for identification of treatable subsets. *Quart J Med* 1987;62:143–161.

Lenzi R, Hess KR, Abbruzzese MC, et al. Poorly differentiated carcinoma and poorly differentiated adenocarcinoma of unknown origin: Favorable subsets of patients with unknown-primary carcinoma? *J Clin Oncol* 1997;15:2056–2066.

Newman KH, Nystrom JS. Metastatic cancer of unknown origin: non-squamous cell type. *Semin Oncol* 1982;9:427.

Sporn JR, Greenberg BR. Empiric chemotherapy in patients with carcinoma of unknown primary site. *Am J Med* 1990;88:49.

CYTOMORPHOLOGIC/ARCHITECTURAL PATTERNS

Bernacki EG. The cytologic faces of adenocarcinoma. *ASC Cytoteleconference*, February 1990.

Cerilli LA, Wick MR. Metastatic malignancies of unknown origin: a histologic and cytologic approach to diagnosis. *Pathology Case Rev* 2001;6(4):137–145.

DeMay RM. *The Art and Science of Cytopathology*. American Society of Clinical Pathologists Press, Chicago, IL, 1996.

Elsheikh TM, Silverman JF. Metastatic malignancies. In: Silverberg SG, Ed., *Principles and Practice of Surgical Pathology and Cytopathology*, 4th ed. Churchill Livingstone, Edinburgh, 2006.

Geisinger K, Silverman J, Wakely, Jr. P. Pediatric cytopathology. In: *ASCP Theory and Practice of Cytopathology 4*. American Society of Clinical Pathologists, Chicago, IL, 1994, pp. 265–353.

Sidawy MK, Bosman FT, Orenstein JM and Silverberg SG. Differential diagnosis of metastatic tumors. In: *Principles and Practice of Surgical Pathology and Cytopathology*, 3rd ed. Churchill Livingstone, New York, 1997.

Steckel AJ, Kagan AA. Metastatic tumors of unknown origin. *Cancer* 1991;67:1242–1244.

MISCELLANEOUS CYTOLOGIC FEATURES

DeMay RM. *The Art and Science of Cytopathology*. American Society of Clinical Pathologists Press, Chicago, IL, 1996.

Greco FA, Vaughn WK, Hainsworth JD. Advanced poorly differentiated carcinoma of unknown primary site: recognition of a treatable syndrome. *Ann Intern Med* 1986;104:547.

Karsell PA, Sheedy PF, O'Connell MJ. Computed tomography in search of cancer of unknown origin. *JAMA* 1982;248:340–343.

Kline TS. *Handbook of Fine Needle Aspiration Biopsy Cytology*, 2nd ed. Churchill Livingstone, New York, 1988, pp. 495–465.

IMMUNOHISTOCHEMISTRY

Anwar F, Schmidt RA. Thyroid transcription factor-1 (TTF-1) distinguishes mesothelioma from pulmonary adenocarcinoma. *Lab Invest* 1997;79:181A.

Brown RW, Campagna LB, Dunn JK, et al. Immunohistochemical identification of tumor markers in metastatic adenocarcinoma: a diagnostic adjunct in the determination of primary site. *Am J Clin Pathol* 1997;107:12–19.

Busam KJ, Jungbluth AA. Melan-A, a new melanocytic differentiation marker. *Adv Anat Pathol* 1996;6:12–18.

Dabbs DJ. Immunohistology of metastatic carcinomas of unknown primary. In: *Diagnostic Immunohistochemistry*, 2nd ed. Churchill Livingstone, Philadelphia, PA, 2006.

Dabbs DJ and Silverman JF. Immunohistochemical workup of metastatic carcinoma of unknown primary. *Pathology Case Rev* 2001;July/August:146–153.

Dabbs DJ, Landreneau RJ, Liu Y, Raab SS, Maley RH, Tung MY, Silverman JF. Detection of estrogen receptor by immunohistochemistry in pulmonary adenocarcinoma. *Ann Thorac Surg* 2002;73:403–406.

DeYoung BR, Wick MR. Immunohistologic evaluation of metastatic carcinomas of unknown origin: an algorithmic approach. *Semin Diagn Pathol* 2000;17(3):184–193.

Kaufmann O, Deidesheimer T, Muehlenberg M, et al. Immunohistochemical differentiation of metastatic breast carcinomas from metastatic adenocarcinomas of other common primary sites. *Histopathology* 1996;29:233–240.

Kovacs CS, Mase RM, Kovacs K, et al. Thyroid medullary carcinoma with thyroglobulin immunoreactivity in sporadic multiple endocrine neoplasia type 2-B. *Cancer* 1994;74:928–932.

Mazoujian G, Haagensen DE Jr. The immunopathology of gross cystic disease fluid proteins. *Ann N Y Acad Sci* 1990;586:188–197.

Niehans GA, Manivel JC, Copland GT, et al. Immunohistochemistry of germ cell and trophoblastic neoplasms. *Cancer* 1988;62:1113–1123.

Sidaway. Jiang C, Tan Y, Li E. Histopathological and immunohistochemical studies on medullary thyroid carcinoma. *Chung Hua Ping Li Hsueh Tsa Chih* 1996;25:332–335.

Wick MR, Swanson PE, Manivel JC. Placental-like alkaline phosphatase reactivity in human tumors: an immunohistochemical study of 520 cases. *Hum Pathol* 1987;18:946–954.

Wick MR, Lillemoe TJ, Copland GT, et al. Gross cystic disease fluid protein-15 as a marker for breast carcinoma. *Hum Pathol* 1989;20:281–287.

COMMON SITES OF METASTASIS

Abrams HL, Spira R, Goldstein N. Metastases in carcinoma: analysis of 1000 autopsied cases. *Cancer* 1950:74–85.

Allard P, Yankaskas BC, Fletcher RH, Parker LA, Halvorsen RA Jr. Sensitivity and specificity of computed tomography for the detection of adrenal metastatic lesions among 91 autopsied lung cancer patients. *Cancer* 1990;66:457–462.

Brage ME, Simon MA. Evaluation, prognosis, and medical treatment considerations of metastatic bone tumors. *Orthopedics* 1992;15(5):589–596.

Centeno BA. Pathology of liver metastases. *Cancer Control* 2006;13(1):13–26.

Cervin JR, Silverman JF, Loggie BW, Geisinger KR. Virchow's node revisited analysis with clinicopathologic correlation of 152 fine-needle aspiration biopsies of supraclavicular lymph nodes. *Arch Pathol Lab Med* 1995;119:727–730.

DeMay RM. *The Art and Science of Cytopathology*. American Society of Clinical Pathologists Press, Chicago, IL, 1996.

Dodd GD, Boyle JJ. Excavating pulmonary metastases. *Am J Roentgenol* 1961;85:277–293.

Elsheikh TM, Silverman JF. Fine needle aspiration cytology of metastasis to common and unusual sites. *Pathology Case Rev* 2001;6(4):161–172.

Elsheikh TM, Silverman JF. Metastatic malignancies. In: Silverberg SG, Ed. *Principles and Practice of Surgical Pathology and Cytopathology*, 4th ed. Churchill Livingstone, Edinburgh, 2006.

Filderman AE, Coppage L, Shaw C, Matthay RA. Pulmonary and pleural manifestations of extrathoracic malignancies. *Clin Chest Med* 1989;10:747–887.

Hertz G, Reddy VB, Freen L, Spitz D, Massarani-Wafai R, Selvaggi SM, Kluskens L, Gattuso P. Fine-needle aspiration biopsy of the liver: a multicenter study of 602 radiologically guided FNA. *Diagn Cytopathol* 2000;23:326–328.

Ishak KG, Goodman ZD, Stocker JT. Tumors of the liver and intrahepatic bile ducts. *Atlas of Tumor Pathology*, Third Series, Fascicle 31. Armed Forces Institute of Pathology, Washington, DC, 2001.

Jorda M, Luis R, Hanly A, Ganjei-Azar P. Fine-needle aspiration cytology of bone accuracy and pitfalls of cytodiagnosis. *Cancer (Cancer Cytopathol)* 2000;90:47–54.

Katz RL, Shirkhoda A. Diagnostic approach to incidental adrenal nodules in the cancer patient. *Cancer* 1985;55:1995–2000.

Lee JE, Evans DB, Hickey RC, Sherman SI, Gagel RF, Abbruzzese MC, Abbruzzese JL. Unknown primary cancer presenting as an adrenal mass: frequency and implications for diagnostic evaluation of adrenal incidentalomas. *Surgery* 1998;124:1115–11122.

Lioe TF, Elliott H, Allen DC, Spence RAJ. The role of fine needle aspiration cytology (FNAC) in the investigation of superficial lymphadenopathy; uses and limitations of the technique. *Cytopathology* 1999;10:291–297.

McCluggage WG, Anderson N, Herron B, Caughley L. Fine needle aspiration cytology, histology and immunohistochemistry of anaplastic large cell ki-1-positive lymphoma a report of three cases. *Acta Cytologica* 1996;40:779–785.

Min KW, Song J, Boesenberg M, Acebey J. Adrenal cortical nodule mimicking small round cell malignancy on fine needle aspiration. *Acta Cytol* 1988;32:543–546.

Mitchell ML, Ryan FP, Shermer RW. Pulmonary adenocarcinoma metastatic to the adrenal gland mimicking normal adrenal cortical epithelium on fine needle aspiration. *Acta Cytol* 1985;29:994–998.

Molinari R, Cantu G, Chiesa F, Podreccca S, Milani F, Del Vecchio M. A statistical approach to detection of the primary cancer based on the site of neck lymph node metastases. *Tumori* 1977;63:267–282.

Nasuti JF, Yu G, Boudousquie, Gupta P. Diagnostic value of lymph node fine needle aspiration cytology: an institutional experience of 387 cases observed over a 5-year period. *Cytopathology* 2000;11:18–31.

Poigenfurst J, Marcove RC, Miller TR. Surgical treatment of fractures through metastases in the proximal femur. *J Bone Joint Surg [Br]* 1968;50:743–756.

Powell JM. Metastatic carcinoid of bone. Report of two cases and review of the literature. *Clin Orthop* 1988;230:266–272.

Prasad RRA, Narasimhan R, Sankaran V, Veliath AJ. Fine needle aspiration cytology in the diagnosis of superficial lymphadenopathy: an analysis of 2,418 cases. *Diagn Cytopath* 1996;15:382–386.

Sasano H, Shizawa S, Nagura H. Adrenocortical cytopathology. *Am J Clin Pathol* 1995;104:161–166.

Toomes H, Delphendahl A, Manke HG, Vogt-Moykopf I. The coin lesion of the lung. A review of 955 resected coin lesions. *Cancer* 1983;51:534–537.

Unni KK. *Dahlin's bone tumors. General aspects and data on 11,087 cases.* Lippincott-Raven, Philadelphia, PA, 1996.

Vieco Pr, Azouz EM, Roeffel JC. Metastases to bone in medulloblastoma. A report of five cases. *Skeletal Radiol* 1989;18:445–449.

Wu HH, Cramer HM, Kho J, Elsheikh TM. Fine needle aspiration cytology of benign adrenal cortical nodules. A comparison of cytologic findings with those of primary and metastatic adrenal malignancies. *Acta Cytol* 1998;42:1352–1358.

UNUSUAL SITES OF METASTASIS

Alexander HR, Turnbull AD, Rosen PP. Isolated breast metastasis from gastrointestinal tract carcinoma. *J Surg Oncol* 1989;42:264–266.

Baloch ZW, LiVolsi VA. Pathology of the thyroid gland. In: LiVolsi A, Ed., *Endocrine Pathology*. Churchill Livingston, Philadelphia, PA, 2002.

Baloch ZW, LiVolsi VA. Tumor-to-tumor metastasis to follicular variant of papillary carcinoma of thyroid. *Arch Pathol Lab Med* 1999;123:703–706.

Banner BF, Myrent KL, Memoli VA, Gould VE. Neuroendocrine carcinoma of pancreas diagnosed by aspiration cytology. *Acta Cytol* 1985;29:442–448.

Batasakis JG, Bautina E. Metastases to major salivary glands. *Ann Otol Rhinol Laryngol* 1990;99:501–503.

Benning TL, Silverman JF, Berns LA, Geisinger KR. Fine needle aspiration of metastatic and hematologic malignancies clinically mimicking pancreatic carcinoma. *Acta Cytol* 1992;36:471–476.

Bourtsos EP, Bedrossian CWM, De Frias DVS, Nayar R. Thyroid plasmacytoma mimicking medullary carcinoma: A potential pitfall in aspiration cytology. *Diagn Cytopathol* 2000;23:354–358.

Carson HJ, Green LK, Castelli MJ, Reyes CV, Prinz RA, Gattuso P. Utilization of fine-needle aspiration biopsy in the diagnosis of metastatic tumors to the pancreas. *Diagn Cytopathol* 1995;12:8–13.

Cristallini EG, Peciarolo A, Bolis GB, Valenti L. Fine needle aspiration biopsy diagnosis of a splenic metastasis from a papillary serous ovarian adenocarcinoma. *Acta Cytol* 1991;35:560–562.

Elit LM, Cunnane MF. Breast metastasis from ovarian carcinoma: report of two cases and literature review. *J Surg Pathol* 1995;1:69–74.

Elsheikh TM, Herzberg AJ, Silverman JF. Fine needle aspiration cytology of metastatic malignancies involving unusual sites. *Am J Clin Pathol* 1997;108 (suppl 1):S12–S21.

Elsheikh TM. Salivary gland aspiration cytopathology. In: Atkinson BF, Silverman JF, Eds. *Atlas of Difficult Diagnoses in Cytopathology*. WB Saunders, Philadelphia, PA, 1998, pp. 451–480.

Font RL, Ferry AP. Carcinoma metastatic to the eye and orbit: III. A clinicopathologic study of 28 cases metastatic to the orbit. *Cancer* 1976;38:1326–1335.

Frias-Hidvegi D. *Guides to Clinical Aspiration Biopsy: Liver and Pancreas*. Igaku-Shoin, New York, 1988, pp. 205–321.

Gattuso P, Ramzy I, Truong LD, Lankford KL, Green L, Kluskens L, Spitz DJ, Reddy VB. Utilization of fine needle aspiration in the diagnosis of metastatic tumors to the kidney. *Diagn Cytopathol* 1992;21:35–38.

Gnepp DR. Metastatic disease to the major salivary glands. In: Ellis GL, Auclair PL, Gnepp DR, eds. *Surgical Pathology of the Salivary Glands*. WB Saunders, Philadelphia, PA, 1991, pp. 560–569.

Green LK, Ro JY, Mackay B, Ayala AG, Luna MA. Renal cell carcinoma metastatic to the thyroid. *Cancer* 1989;63:1810–1815.

Hajdu SI, Urban JA. Cancers metastatic to the breast. *Cancer* 1972;29:1691–1696.

Halbauer M, Kardum-Skelin I, Vranesic D, Crepinko I. Aspiration cytology of renal-cell carcinoma metastatic to the thyroid. *Acta Cytol* 1991;35(4):443–446.

Healy JH, Turnbull ADM, Miedema B, Lane JM. Acrometastases: a study of twenty-nine patients with osseous involvement of the hands and feet. *J Bone Joint Surg* 1986;68-A:743–746.

Khuraana KK, Powers CN. Basaloid squamous carcinoma metastatic to renal cell carcinoma: fine needle aspiration cytology of tumor-to-tumor metastasis. *Diagn Cytopathol* 1997;17:379–382.

Kline TS. *Handbook of Fine Needle Aspiration Biopsy Cytology*. 2nd ed. Churchill Livingstone, New York, 1988, pp. 495–465.

Knapp, Abdul-Karim FW. Fine needle aspiration cytology of acrometastasis: a report of two cases. *Acta Cytol* 1994;38:589–591.

Lernard TWJ, Wadehra V, Farndon JR. Fine needle aspiration biopsy in diagnosis of metastasis to thyroid gland. *JR Soc Med* 1984;77:196–197.

Linsk JA, Franzen S. Diseases of the lymph node and spleen. In: Linsk JA, Franzen S, Eds., *Clinical Aspiration Cytology*, 2nd ed. JB Lippincott, Philadelphia, 1989, pp. 354–358.

Lisbon E, Bloom RA, Husband JE, Stoker DJ. Metastatic tumors of bones of the hand and foot: a comparative review and report of 43 additional cases. *Skeletal Radiol* 1987;16:387–392.

Michelow PM, Leiman G. Metastases to the thyroid gland: diagnosis by aspiration cytology. *Diagn Cytopathol* 1995;13(3):209–213.

Nassar DL, Raab SS, Silverman JF, Kennerdell JS, Sturgis CD. Fine needle aspiration for the diagnosis of orbital hematolymphoid lesions. *Diagn Cytopathol* 2000;23:314–317.

Page DL, Anderson TJ. *Diagnostic Histopathology of the Breast*. Churchill Livingstone, New York, 1987.

Palgon NM, Novetsky AD, Fogler RJ, Lichter SM. Lung carcinoma presenting as a breast tumor. *NY State J Med* 1983;11–12:1188–1189.

Palma O, Canali N, Scaroni P, Torri AM. Fine needle aspiration biopsy: its use in the management of orbital and intraocular tumors. *Tumori* 1989;75:589–593.

Richardson JF, Katayama I. Neoplasm to neoplasm metastasis: an acidophilic adenoma harboring metastatic carcinoma: a case report. *Arch Pathol Lab Med* 1971;91:135–139.

Seifert G, Hennings K, Caselitz J. Metastatic tumors to the parotid and submandibular glands: analysis and differential diagnosis of 108 cases. *Pathol Res Pract* 1986;181:684–692.

Shields JA, Shields CL, Ehya H, Eagle RC, Potter PD. Fine needle aspiration biopsy of suspected intraocular tumors. *Ophthalmology* 1993;100:1677–1684.

Silverman JF, Feldman PS, Covell JL, Frable WJ. Fine needle aspiration cytology of neoplasms metastatic to breast. *Acta Cytol* 1987;31:281–300.

Silverman JF, Geisinger KR, Raab SS, Stanley MW. Fine needle aspiration biopsy of the spleen in the evaluation of neoplastic disorders. *Acta Cytol* 1993;2:158–162.

Sneige N, Zachariah S, Fanning TV, Dekmezian RH, Ordonez NG. Fine needle aspiration cytology of metastatic neoplasms in the breast. *Am J Clin Pathol* 1989;92:27.

Soderstrom N. Anatomy and histology of the spleen. In: Basal S, Ed., *Aspiration Biopsy Cytology*. Monographs in Clinical Cytology, vol. 7, part 2. Cytology of Infradiaphragmatic Organs, Karger, Basel, 1979, pp. 224–247.

Taavitsainen M, Koivuniemi A, Helminen J. Bondestam S, Kivisarri L, Pamilo M, Tierala E, Tiitinen H. Aspiration biopsy of the spleen in patients with sarcoidosis. *Acta Radiol* 1987;28:723–725.

Zhang C, Cohen J, Cangiarella JF, Waisman J, McKenna BJ, Chhieng DC. Fine needle aspiration of secondary neoplasms involving the salivary glands. *Am J Clin Pathol* 2000;113:21–28.

9

FNA of Soft Tissue and Bone

Lester J. Layfield

SOFT TISSUE AND BONE

LIPOMA

Clinical History
- Rare before third decade of life
- Higher incidence in men
- Superficial solitary lipomas most common in back, neck, shoulder, or abdomen
- Present as an asymptomatic slowly growing soft mass

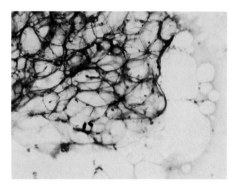

9-1. Lipoma. Lace-like fragment of tissue obtained from a lipoma. Note small, bland nuclei with dark homogeneous chromatin pattern. There is no evidence of nuclear atypia or lipoblasts. (modified Giemsa stain)

Cytopathologic Features
- Smears are grossly oily with free lipid in the background
- Lace-like tissue fragments composed of large fat cells admixed with branching blood vessels
- Individual fat cells have abundant clear cytoplasm, low nuclear: cytoplasmic ratio and small, bland, dark nuclei compressed to edge of cell
- Foamy histiocytes and multinucleated giant cells may be present (trauma)
- No true lipoblasts or mitotic figures

Special Stains and Immunohistochemistry
- Tumor cells are S-100 protein and vimentin positive

Modern Techniques for Diagnosis
- Lipomas lack amplification of MDM2 and CDK-4 genes

Differential Diagnosis
- Well-differentiated liposarcoma
  - Lace-like pattern of adipose tissue
  - True lipoblasts (may be rare)
  - Amplification of MDM2 and CDK-4 genes in many cases

PEARLS
- Lipomas may show areas of fat necrosis with necrotic debris and foamy histiocytes
- When reactive histiocytes contain lipid vacuoles they may be mistaken for lipoblasts
- Cannot separate lipomas from normal subcutaneous adipose tissue

INTRAMUSCULAR LIPOMA

Clinical Features
- Most common in patients between thirty and sixty years of age
- Large deep-seated mass
- Men more often affected than women
- Involves large muscles of thigh, shoulder, and upper arm

Cytopathologic Findings

- Smears have oily background with lipid droplets
- Fragments of "lace-like" tissue admixed with fragments of striated muscle
- Individual fat cells have abundant optically clear cytoplasm
- Nuclei are small with dark compressed chromatin and eccentrically placed
- Lipoblasts and mitotic figures are absent

Special Stains and Immunohistochemistry

- Fat cells are vimentin and S-100 protein positive

Modern Techniques for Diagnosis

- Intramuscular lipomas lack amplification for the MDM2 and CDK-4 genes

Differential Diagonsis

- Well-differentiated liposarcoma
  - ➤ Lace-like fragments of adipose tissue
  - ➤ True lipoblasts (may be rare)
  - ➤ Amplification of MDM2 and CDK-4 genes common

SPINDLE CELL LIPOMA

Clinical Features

- Characteristically occurs in men over forty-five years of age
- Most common locations are posterior neck, shoulder, and back
- Slowly growing, painless, solitary mass

Cytopatholgic Features

- Hypocellular smears, occasionally with myxoid background
- Small- to medium-sized fragments of spindle-shaped or polygonal stromal cells admixed with large adiocytes
- Individual fat cells have abundant clear cytoplasm
- Nonfatty stromal cells may run in bands or short bundles
- Minimal nuclear atypia in most cells but occasional cells may show significant nuclear atypia
- Absence of mitotic figures and true lipoblasts

Special Stains and Immunohistochemistry

- Spindle cells are strongly CD34 positive
- Spindle cells are S-100 protein negative but fat cells are strongly positive

Modern Techniques for Diagnosis

- Noncontributory

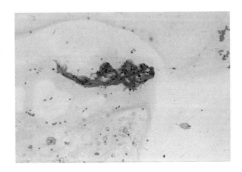

Differential Diagnosis

- Well-differentiated liposarcoma
  - ➤ Smears contain prominent numbers of lace-like tissue fragments
  - ➤ True lipoblasts present (rare)
  - ➤ Lack of CD34 positivity

9-2. Spindle cell lipoma. Tissue fragment obtained from a spindle cell lipoma. Scattered lipid droplets are seen in the background surrounding an aggregate of bland spindle cells. Nuclear atypia is absent and lipoblasts are not present (H&E)

★ CD34 positivity in stromal cells of a fatty tumor strongly favors spindle cell lipoma or pleomorphic lipoma

PLEOMORPHIC LIPOMA

Clinical Features
- Most common in men over forty-five years of age
- Most frequent sites of occurrence are neck, shoulder, and back
- Painless, slow-growing mass

Cytopathologic Features
- Smears are moderately cellular
- Large multivacuolated giant cells with round or ovoid nuclei often in a wreath-like arrangement (floret-type)
- Nuclei of giant cells and some mononuclear cells may be hyperchroamtic with a coarse chromatin pattern
- Nuclear molding may be prominent in giant cells
- Background may have myxoid appearance
- Mitotic figures are absent

Special Stains and Immunohistochemistry
- Neoplasms are strongly CD34 positive
- Fat cells are S-100 protein positive

Modern Techniques for Diagnosis
- Noncontributory

Differential Diagonsis
- Pleomorphic liposarcoma
  - ➤ Anaplastic giant cells with irregular arrangement of nuclei
  - ➤ S-100 protein positivity
  - ➤ Sarcomas are CD34 negative
  - ➤ Rare true lipoblasts are found in smears
  - ➤ Necrosis may be prominent in smears

★ Pleomorphic lipomas have floret-type giant cells
★ Lack true lipoblasts
★ Pleomorphic lipomas are CD34 positive

MYELOLIPOMA

Clinical Features
- Tumor-like growth of mature fat and bone marrow elements most commonly but not exclusively arising in the adrenal gland/retroperitoneum

- May occur as purely soft tissue mass
- Must distinguish from extramedullary hematopoiesis
- Patients with myelolipomas do not have hematopoietic abnormalities

Cytopathologic Features
- Smears contain an admixture of trilineage bone marrow elements and clusters of mature vacuolated adipose tissue
- Megakaryocytes often prominent

Special Stains and Immunohistochemistry
- Noncontributory

Modern Diagnostic Techniques
- Noncontributory

Differential Diagnosis
- Inadvertent aspirate of bone marrow
  - ➤ Must confirm location of aspiration within soft tissues
- Extramedullary hematopoietic tumors
  - ➤ Extramedullary hematopoietic tumors are associated with hepatosplenomegally as well as abnormalities of bone marrow

PEARLS

⭐ To adequately diagnosis soft tissue myelolipoma one must confirm absence of hematologic abnormalities and presence of lesion within soft tissue rather than bone marrow or adrenal

LIPOSARCOMA

Clinical Features
- Most common sarcoma of the adult life, peak incidence in sixth and seventh decades of life
- Men and women equally affected
- Majority occur in deep muscles of extremities followed by retroperitoneum
- Slowly growing, painless mass

Cytopathologic Features
- Well-differentiated liposarcoma
  - ➤ Smears of low to moderate cellularity
  - ➤ Abundant free lipid in background
  - ➤ Mixture of mature fat cells and fibroblasts forming lace-like tissues aggregates
  - ➤ Extremely rare or absent lipoblasts
  - ➤ True lipoblasts have one or multiple clear vacuoles displacing nucleus to edge of cell
- Myxoid liposarcoma
  - ➤ Myxoid background with magenta material lying free (air-dried, Giemsa-stained material)

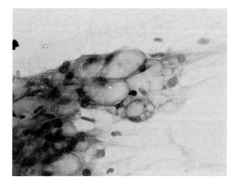

9-3. Liposarcoma. Tissue fragment obtained by needle aspiration from a liposarcoma. A multivacuolated lipoblast is present near the center of the field. The lipoblast has multiple lipid vacuoles displacing the nucleus to the edge of the cell (H&E)

➤ Tissue fragments composed of magenta-colored stroma with entrapped branching plexiform vascular network and round or ovoid cells
➤ True lipoblasts with two or more vacuoles displacing the nucleus to one side of the cell
➤ Myxoid matrix may have fibrillar appearance
➤ Single discohesive round, short spindle and vacuolated cells in background
▪ Round cell liposarcoma
➤ Granular background with dispersed single cells and tissue fragments
➤ Moderate to highly cellular smears
➤ Predominate cell is round with a foamy, vacuolated, or granular cytoplasm
➤ Cytoplasm present in moderate to scant amounts
➤ Nuclei are enlarged with prominent nucleoli
➤ Mitotic figures present but infrequent
▪ Pleomorphic liposarcoma
➤ Moderately cellular smears with a "dirty" granular background
➤ Neoplastic cells show marked nuclear pleomorphism
➤ Mononuclear or multinucleated anaplastic giant cells with granular or vacuolated cytoplasm
➤ True lipoblasts are uncommon
▪ Dedifferentiated liposarcoma
➤ Areas of well-differentiated liposarcoma intermixed with pleomorphic sarcoma or well-differentiated fibrosarcoma
➤ Multiple aspirates at multiple sites necessary to establish diagnosis (diagnosis usually not possible by FNA)

Special Stains and Immunocytochemistry
▪ Liposarcomas are S-100 protein and vimentin positive

Modern Techniques for Diagnosis
▪ Well-differentiated and dedifferentiated liposarcomas show amplification of the MDM2 and CDK-4 genes demonstrable by fluorescence in situ hybridization (FISH) techniques
▪ Myxoid and round cell liposarcomas demonstrate FUS-CHOP gene fusion products/translocations demonstrable by FISH techniques

Differential Diagnosis
Well-differentiated liposarcoma
▪ Lipoma
➤ Lace-like fragments of adipose tissue
➤ Absence of lipoblasts
➤ Absence of MDM2 and CDK-4 gene amplification
▪ Spindle cell lipoma
➤ Mixture of short spindle-shaped cells, oval cells, and mature fat cells
➤ CD34 positivity
➤ Lack of true lipoblasts
➤ Location within shoulder and back
▪ Fat necrosis
➤ Necrotic debris in background
➤ Presence of foamy histiocytes
➤ Fragments of lace-like mature adipose tissue
➤ Absence of true lipoblasts

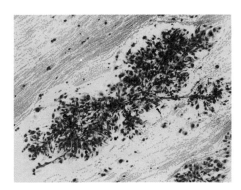 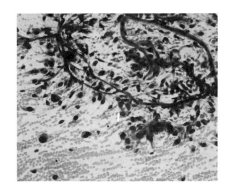

9-4. Myxoid liposarcoma *(left)*. A tissue fragment demonstrates the complex anastomosing capillary pattern characteristic of myxoid liposarcoma. The individual cells are predominately round or ovoid with hyperchromatic nuclei. The background red blood cells are arranged in an "Indian file" pattern due to free myxoid ground substance (modified Giemsa stain)

9-5. Myxoid liposarcoma *(right)*. High-power view of a tissue fragment from a myxoid liposarcoma demonstrating complex capillary network with entrapped short spindle and oval cells (modified Giemsa stain)

Myxoid Liposarcoma
- Myxoma
  - ➤ Hypocellular smears
  - ➤ Stellate and short spindle cells
  - ➤ Absence of tissue fragments with complex vascular pattern
  - ➤ Absence of vacuolated lipoblasts
- Myxoid malignant fibrous histiocytoma
  - ➤ Myxoid background
  - ➤ Scattered anaplastic mono- and multinuclear cells
  - ➤ Absence of true lipoblasts
- Myxoid chondrosarcoma
  - ➤ Myxoid background
  - ➤ Occasional chondroid matrix
  - ➤ Absence of true lipoblasts
  - ➤ Dominance within smears of small round cells
  - ➤ Absence of CHOP gene translocation

ROUND CELL LIPOSARCOMA

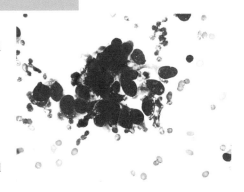

- Synovial sarcoma
  - ➤ Mixture of discohesive single cells and three-dimensional cell clusters
  - ➤ Numerous "naked" nuclei
  - ➤ Keratin and EMA immunohistochemical positivity
  - ➤ SYT-SSX translocation demonstrable by FISH

- Rhabdomyosarcoma
  - ➤ Cellular smears
  - ➤ Basic small cell morphology with expansion of cell types and sizes to include bi- and multinucleated giant cells
  - ➤ Filamentous or granular cytoplasm, rarely true cross-striations
  - ➤ Immunohistochemical positivity for desmin, muscle actins, myogenin and MyoD-1

9-6. Round cell liposarcoma. Aggregate of round to oval cells with modest amounts of cytoplasm and large hyperchromatic nuclei. Some cells contain finely vacuolated cytoplasm characteristic of round cell liposarcoma (modified Giemsa stain)

PLEOMORPHIC LIPOSARCOMA

- Malignant fibrous histiocytoma
  - ➤ Markedly pleomorphic cell population with spindle-shaped, polygonal, and giant cell forms
  - ➤ Lack of true lipoblasts

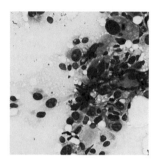

9-7. Pleomorphic liposarcoma. Material aspirated from a pleomorphic liposarcoma. Free lipid vacuoles are in the background and aggregate around the tissue fragment. The neoplastic cells show considerable variation in size and shape with mononuclear anaplastic giant cells being present. These cells have a foamy cytoplasm characteristic of pleomorphic liposarcoma (modified Giemsa stain)

PEARLS

★ Definitive diagnosis of liposarcoma depends on demonstration of lipoblasts
★ Myxoid stromal fragments with complex anastomosing vascular pattern highly specific for myxoid liposarcoma
★ FISH helpful in establishing diagnosis of myxoid and round cell liposarcoma by demonstrating CHOP gene rearrangements

SYNOVIAL SARCOMA

Clinical Features

■ Fourth most frequent type of soft tissue sarcoma
■ Most common in adolescents and young adults
■ Slightly more frequent in males than females
■ Occurs in a wide variety of body sites including head and neck, trunk, and upper and lower extremities. Most common site is the thigh/knee area
■ Presents clinically as palpable, deep-seated mass associated with pain or tenderness. Duration of symptoms before clinical diagnosis two to four years

Cytopathologic Features

■ Moderate to highly cellular smears
■ Mixture of tight three-dimensional cell clusters and dispersed single cells
■ Tissue fragments may display a fine vascular network and basement membrane material
■ At periphery of tissue fragments, cells may fray and fall off tissue fragments
■ Some smears are dominated by single cell pattern
■ Single discohesive cells have a round to ovoid appearance and are often represented by "naked" nuclei
■ Individual cells are of a small to medium size, approximating the size of a neutrophil
■ Nuclei appear bland with finely granular chromatin and small or inconspicuous nucleoli
■ Mitotic figures are easily identifiable, including atypical forms
■ In some cases, the cells comprising the tissue fragments have a spindle cell appearance

Cytopathologic Features for Biphasic Synovial Sarcoma

■ In addition to features characteristic of monophasic synovial sarcoma, biphasic synovial sarcomas may show cuboidal to columnar cells arranged in gland-like configurations or squamous cell clusters

9-8. Monophasic synovial sarcoma *(left).* Smear from a monophasic synovial sarcoma characterized by thick, three-dimensional cell clusters surrounded by numerous single cells. The disassociated cells often are represented by "naked" nuclei. The individual cells have round, ovoid or short spindle-shaped nuclei, which are associated with scanty amounts of cytoplasm (modified Giemsa stain)

9-9. Biphasic synovial sarcoma *(right).* Tissue fragment aspirated from a biphasic synovial sarcoma. A central gland-like structure is surrounded by short, spindle-shaped-and ovoid cells. The individual nuclei have a fine chromatin pattern and indistinct nucleoli (H&E)

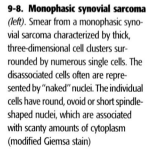

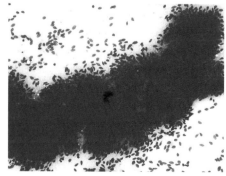

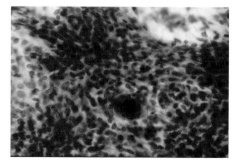

Immunohistochemistry

▦ Monophasic fibrous variants react uniformly with antibodies directed against vimentin

▦ Between 50% and 95% of monophasic fibrosynovial sarcomas will show weak focal staining with antibodies directed against cytokeratins and EMA

▦ 10–35% of synovial sarcomas are immunohistochemically reactive with S-100 protein

▦ 40–70% of monophasic fibrous synovial sarcomas are reactive with antibodies directed against CD99

▦ Approximately 100% of biphasic synovial sarcomas show focally strong immuno-histochemical staining with antibodies directed against vimentin, EMA and cytoker-atin. Staining for CD99 and S-100 protein is similar to that seen with the monophasic fibrous variant

Modern Techniques for Diagnosis

▦ FISH demonstrates the characteristic translocation t(X;18)(p11.2;11.2), which results in the fusion product SYT-SSX

▦ Two forms of the SYT-SSX fusion product exist, with biphasic tumors showing only the SYT-SSX 1 rearrangement, while monophasic fibrous types may show either the SYT-SSX 1 or the SYT-SSX 2

Differential Diagnosis

▦ Ewing's sarcoma and primitive neuroectodermal tumor
  ➤ Predominantly discohesive pattern of individual small cells
  ➤ Lack tissue fragments with vascular network
  ➤ Immunohistochemical positivity for O13 (CD99), FLI-1, and demonstration by FISH of the EWSR translocations
▦ Malignant peripheral nerve sheath tumors
  ➤ Prominent spindle cell component
  ➤ Unipolar or bipolar wavy cytoplasmic processes
  ➤ Moderate to marked degree of nuclear pleomorphism
  ➤ Wavy, bent, or folded nuclear membranes
  ➤ Immunohistochemical positivity for S-100 protein (<50%), PGP 9.5 and N-cam.
▦ Fibrosarcoma
  ➤ Majority of cells lie in tight clusters composed of spindle-shaped cells
  ➤ Lack of prominent discohesive cellular pattern
  ➤ Basillary to ovoid nuclei
  ➤ Higher degrees of nuclear atypia and pleomorphism present in fibrosarcomas Grades II and III

PEARLS

★ Prominent pattern of three-dimensional cell clusters amid a sea of round to ovoid, relatively small discohesive cells

★ Immunohistochemical positivity at least focally for EMA and cytokeratins

★ FISH demonstration of the SYT-SSX fusion product

GRANULAR CELL TUMOR

Clinical Features

▦ Most frequently occurs in the fourth, fifth, and sixth decades of life

▦ Twice as common in women as men

▦ Most common sites of presentation include dermis or subcutis. Less frequently found in the submucosa or striated muscle (tongue)

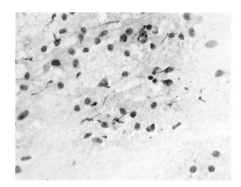

9-10. Granular cell tumor. Smear of a granular cell tumor. Within the granular background are dispersed round or oval nuclei lacking intact cytoplasm. Some cells form sheets with a granular syncytial cytoplasm. The nuclei are predominately round and may contain prominent nucleoli (Papanicolaou stain)

- Majority of cases are smaller than 3 cm at time of presentation
- Present as solitary painless nodule, usually of less than six months duration

Cytopathologic Features
- Cellular smears with cells lying singly and in syncytial clusters
- Intact cells show abundant granular cytoplasm
- Relatively bland nuclei containing prominent nucleoli
- Cells are fragile with many single cells being represented as "naked" nuclei
- Smear background has a dirty granular appearance due to abundant cytoplasmic debris
- Mitotic figures are not present

Special Stains, Immunohistochemistry
- Almost always positive for vimentin, S-100 protein, and MK1-C3
- Granular cell tumors are characteristically negative for HMB-45 and GFAP

Modern Techniques for Diagnosis
- Noncontributory

Differential diagnosis
- Rhabdomyoma
  - Individually dispersed and clusters of round to ovoid cells with fibrillary cytoplasm
  - Frequent cross-striations within cytoplasm
  - Cells contain multiple peripherally placed bland nuclei
  - Immunohistochemical positivity for desmin, myogenin and MyoD-1
- Rhabdomyosarcoma
  - Predominant small cell population with mono- and multinucleate giant cell forms
  - Significant degrees of nuclear pleomorphism present
  - Cytoplasm often appears fibrillar, rare cells with cross-striations may be present
  - Immunohistochemical positivity for desmin, myogenin, and MyoD-1
- Alveolar soft part sarcoma
  - Scanty to moderately cellular smears with bloody background
  - Large vesicular nuclei with prominent nucleoli
  - Occasional binucleated or even multinucleated forms present
  - Immunohistochemical positivity for desmin, negative for S-100 protein

PEARLS
- Numerous cells lie singly and in syncytial clusters
- Abundant granular debris in background with many "naked" nuclei
- Immunohistochemical positivity for S-100 protein

ALVEOLAR SOFT PART SARCOMA

Clinical Features
- Rare neoplasm representing at most 1% of all soft tissue sarcomas
- Occurs most commonly in adolescents and young adults (age range fifteen to thirty-five years)
- Female patients outnumber males

- Sarcoma occurs predominantly in lower extremity, especially buttocks and thigh
- Alveolar soft part sarcoma usually presents as slowly growing painless mass

Cytopathologic Features

- Variably cellular smears with hemorrhagic or "flocculant" debris-laden background
- Majority of cells lie singly, but some form three-dimensional clusters
- Marked cytoplasmic fragility with many "naked" nuclei
- Preserved cells show abundant granular cytoplasm and eccentrically located nuclei
- Cytoplasm often shows zonation pattern with central paranuclear granular component surrounded by a clear or vacuolated zone
- Nuclei are large with single prominent nucleolus
- Smooth nuclear membranes in most cases, but some cells with nuclear grooves
- Binucleated and multinucleated cells may be present
- Some tissue fragments preserve a pseudoalveolar or alveolar pattern
- Intranuclear cytoplasmic pseudoinclusions may be prominent

Special Stains and Immunohistochemistry

- Approximately 80% of cases are positive for desmin by immunocytochemistry
- Approximately 40% of cases show immunohistochemical positivity for vimentin
- Alveolar soft part sarcomas uniformly negative for EMA, myogenin, and MyoD-1

Modern Techniques for Diagnosis

- Noncontributory

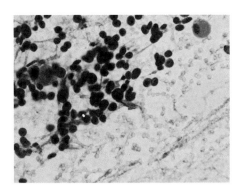

9-11. Alveolar soft part sarcoma.
Smears of material obtained from alveolar soft part sarcomas are characterized by single or poorly cohesive cells. These cells are frequently represented by "naked" nuclei or small, poorly cohesive cell clusters. Intact cells have a predominately granular cytoplasm. The nuclei are large with a vesicular to granular chromatin and characteristically huge nucleoli. Histiocytes may be scattered in the background (H&E)

Differential Diagnosis

- Alveolar rhabdomyosarcoma
  - ➤ Prominent round cell pattern with scattering of larger cells including multinucleated giant cells
  - ➤ Many cells show a fibrillary appearance to cytoplasm
  - ➤ Rare cells show cross striations
  - ➤ Immunohistochemical positivity for desmin, actins, myogenin, and MyoD-1
  - ➤ Cytogenetics and fluorescence in situ hybridization analysis will show specific translocations t(2;13)(q35;q14) or the t(1;13)(p36;q14)
- Rhabdomyoma
  - ➤ Individually dispersed cells with occasional small clusters
  - ➤ Granular cytoplasm frequently with evidence of cross-striations
  - ➤ Round to ovoid, bland, peripherally placed nuclei
  - ➤ Nuclei are frequently multiple
  - ➤ Very low nuclear:cytoplasmic ratio
- Granular cell tumor
  - ➤ Cellular smears with markedly granular dirty background
  - ➤ Many naked nuclei in background
  - ➤ Immunohistochemical positivity for S-100 protein, negative for desmin

PEARLS

- ★ Large round to polygonal cells with low nuclear:cytoplasmic ratio
- ★ Round to ovoid uniform nuclei with vesicular chromatin pattern and prominent nucleolus

★ Immunohistochemical positivity for desmin but nonreactivity for myogenin and S-100 protein

EPITHELIOID SARCOMA

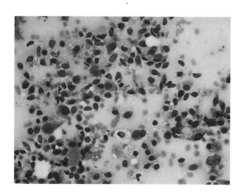

9-12. Epitheliod sarcoma. Epithelioid sarcomas of the distal extremities are characterized by moderately cellular smears containing predominately single cells and loose cell aggregates. The individual cells have a polygonal shape with moderate amounts of granular cytoplasm. The nuclei are large, ovoid, and often contain prominent nucleoli (modified Giemsa stain)

Clinical Features
- Most common soft tissue sarcoma of the hand and wrist
- Most commonly occurs in adolescents and young adults (ten to thirty-five years of age)
- Males outnumber females by approximately 2:1
- Most frequent sites are finger, hand and forearm, with knee and leg being less frequent sites. Proximal type exists
- Sarcoma may arise in subcutaneous or deeper tissues
- Sarcoma presents as painless solitary or multiple nodules

Cytopathologic Features
- Smears of variable cellularity but usually moderately to highly cellular
- Cellular component is usually single dispersed cells. Cell clusters are infrequent
- Neoplastic cells are large and round or polygonal with lesser numbers of interspersed spindle-shaped cells
- Mild to moderate pleomorphism present
- Large round to ovoid nuclei with variably prominent nucleoli
- Granular to vesicular chromatin pattern
- Eccentric location of nuclei giving an overall plasmacytoid appearance
- Binucleate cells may be present
- Intracytoplasmic vacuoles present in a minority of cells
- Pale zone within peripheral cytoplasm occasionally observed
- In a minority of cases, granuloma-like structures identified
- Proximal type has "rhabdoid" morphology

Special Stains and Immunohistochemistry
- Overwhelming majority of cells positive for vimentin
- Between 70% and 95% of cases will express cytokeratin and epithelial membrane antigen. S-100 protein and HMB-45 usually not expressed

Modern Techniques for Diagnosis
- Noncontributory

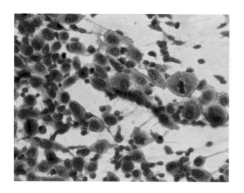

9-13. Epitheliod sarcoma. Epithelioid sarcomas of proximal type yield smears containing cells with a rhabdoid morphology. The cells are polygonal in shape with eccentrically placed nuclei and a dense or granular cytoplasm. The nuclei may have irregular nuclear membranes and contain small to moderately sized distinct nucleoli (H&E)

Differential Diagnosis
- Metastatic carcinoma
  - ➤ Prominence of cell clusters potentially showing tubular or glandular formations
  - ➤ Presence of true keratinization or metaplastic cytoplasm
  - ➤ Squamous cell carcinomas usually present as syncytial clusters, lacking intercellular spaces
- Melanoma
  - ➤ Presence of staining for melan A, HMB-45, and S-100 protein
  - ➤ Aspirates of many melanomas show marked nuclear pleomorphism
  - ➤ Melanin pigment present in some cases
- Granulomatous inflammation
  - ➤ Histiocytes of granulomatous inflammation show lesser degrees of nuclear atypia than do cells of epithelioid sarcomas
  - ➤ Granulomatous inflammation is nonreactive with antibodies directed against EMA and cytokeratin

■ Synovial sarcoma
   ➤ Prominent pattern of three-dimensional cell clusters surrounded by large numbers of noncohesive single cells
   ➤ Aspirates of synovial sarcomas usually highly cellular
   ➤ Synovial sarcomas are CD34 negative, while half of epithelioid sarcomas are CD34 positive
■ Extrarenal rhabdoid tumor
   ➤ May be cytologically impossible to distinguish from epithelioid sarcoma, proximal type
   ➤ Extrarenal rhabdoid tumors are almost always positive immunohistochemically for vimentin, S-100 protein, and neuron-specific enolayse

PEARLS

✸ Most epithelioid sarcomas are located in the distal extremities, particularly the hands and feet
✸ Immunohistochemical positivity for vimentin, keratins, and EMA
✸ A majority of cells lie singly and have a polygonal or plasmacytoid appearance.
✸ Binucleate forms may be present
✸ Dichotomous staining of cytoplasm with pale and darker zones
✸ Proximal form has "rhabdoid" morphology

CLEAR CELL SARCOMA OF SOFT TISSUES

Clinical Features
■ Rare sarcoma type, primarily affects young adults (age range twenty to forty years)
■ Majority occur within lower extremity, particularly the foot and ankle
■ Sarcoma is more common in women than men
■ Sarcoma presents as slowly enlarging mass causing pain or tenderness in up to 50% of cases
■ Average duration of symptoms is two years

Clinicopathologic Features
■ Highly cellular smears
■ Numerous intact noncohesive single cells
■ Rare three-dimensional cell clusters, often showing a microacinar pattern
■ Background may be bloody or "tigroid"
■ Some tumors may contain abundant melanin
■ Tumor cells are large and round to oval, with ill-defined cell margins and abundant clear cytoplasm
■ Nuclei are generally eccentrically located with a fine chromatin pattern and prominent central nucleolus
■ Binucleate and multinucleated cells may be present
■ Intranuclear cytoplasmic pseudoinclusions present in many cases

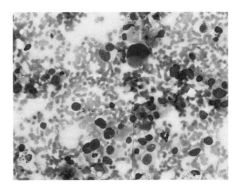

Special Stains and Immunohistochemistry
■ Most clear cell sarcomas of soft tissue are positive for vimentin and HMB-45
■ Between two-thirds and 80% of cases are S-100 protein positive
■ Clear cell sarcomas are nonreactive for CD31 and CD34

Modern Techniques for Diagnosis
■ More than 75% of clear cell sarcomas show a translocation involving the 12 and 22 chromosomes: t(12;22)(q13;q12), resulting in the ATF1-EwSS fusion product

9-14. Clear cell sarcoma. Smears prepared from aspirates of clear cell sarcoma of soft tissue show a predominately discohesive cell pattern. The component cells are oval or polygonal and show considerable nuclear pleomorphism. The nuclei may be displaced to one edge of the cell. The cytoplasm has a granular appearance. Scattered foamy and pigment-laden histiocytes may be present in the background (modified Giemsa stain)

Differential Diagnosis

■ Metastatic malignant melanoma

➤ Clear cell sarcoma of soft tissues cannot be distinguished from metastatic malignant melanoma on a purely cytologic basis

➤ Some malignant melanomas show significantly greater degrees of nuclear pleomorphism than is seen in clear cell sarcomas

➤ Malignant melanomas lack the translocation involving the 12 and 22 chromosomes characteristic of clear cell sarcoma of soft tissues

■ Synovial sarcoma

➤ Synovial sarcomas are characterized by highly cellular smears containing large numbers of noncohesive cells and a prominent number of three-dimensional cell clusters

➤ Synovial sarcomas are at least focally keratin and EMA positive

➤ Synovial sarcomas are nonreactive with antibodies directed against HMB-45 and melan A

➤ Synovial sarcomas lack melanin pigment seen in some clear cell sarcomas

➤ Synovial sarcomas reveal vascular networks within tissue fragments

■ Epithelioid sarcoma

➤ Highly cellular smears with granular necrotic debris in the background

➤ Cells lie both singly and in cohesive three-dimensional clusters

➤ Individual cells have abundant granular cytoplasm with eccentric nuclei

➤ Cells react with antibodies directed against EMA and the cytokeratins

■ Extrarenal rhabdoid tumor

➤ Moderate to highly cellular smears with cells lying in variably sized sheets and clusters as well as individually

➤ Cells are uniform, round to polygonal, with moderate to abundant cytoplasm

➤ Nuclei are round to slightly irregular and contain prominent nucleoli

➤ Chromatin is peripherally arranged, giving a distinctive chromatinic ring

➤ Mitotic figures are abundant

➤ Cytoplasm contains a homogenous inclusion-like area located in a perinuclear distribution

➤ Immunohistochemistry reveals positivity for vimentin and cytokeratin

PEARLS

⋆ Foamy background material in a band-like arrangement (tigroid)
⋆ Rare microacinar arrangements
⋆ Melanin pigment present in some neoplasms and may be abundant
⋆ Immunohistochemical positivity for S-100 protein and HMB-45
⋆ Characteristic translocation of chromosomes 12 and 22

EXTRARENAL RHABDOID TUMOR

Clinical Features

■ Broad age range but most occur in children
■ Variable clinical behavior
■ Wide distribution in soft tissue sites

Cytopathologic Features

■ Moderate to highly cellular smears
■ Cells lie in variably sized sheets and clusters surrounded by large numbers of noncohesive single cells

Single cells retain their cytoplasm, which is present in moderate to abundant amounts

Cytoplasm contains homogeneous inclusions, which may indent nucleus

Nuclei are round to slightly irregular and characteristically contain prominent nucleoli

Chromatin is peripherally arranged with a prominent chromatinic ring and vesicular pattern

Special Stains and Immunohistochemistry

Cells show reactivity for vimentin, cytokeratins, and EMA

Two-thirds of cases show actin positivity, one-third desmin positivity, and the majority demonstrate CD99

Modern Techniques for Diagnosis

The majority of cases reveal abnormalities of chromosome 22(q11–12)

Differential Diagnosis

Epithelioid sarcoma, proximal type

➤ Characteristic location within proximal portion of lower limbs, including inguinal area

➤ May be indistinguishable from malignant extrarenal rhabdoid tumors

Alveolar soft part sarcoma

➤ Cells lie singly and in variably sized clusters

➤ Cells are large and polygonal with finely granular cytoplasm

➤ Cytoplasm shows zonation pattern of pale and dark cytoplasm

➤ Binucleated and multinucleated cells may be present

➤ Some tissue fragments retain a pseudoalveolar or alveolar pattern

➤ Moderate number of cells show intranuclear cytoplasmic pseudoinclusions

➤ Alveolar soft part sarcomas are reactive with antibodies directed against desmin and muscle actins but are negative for cytokeratin and epithelial membrane antigen

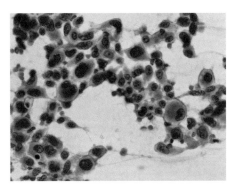

9-15. Rhabdoid tumor. Smears of rhabdoid tumors are cellular with large numbers of single or loosely cohesive cells. The cells are polygonal with only occasional spindle-shaped forms being present. The characteristic cell has a large eccentrically placed nucleus which may be indented by a paranuclear dense inclusion. Mitotic figures are present in the majority of smears (H&E)

PEARLS

★ The diagnosis of malignant extrarenal rhabdoid tumor is in most cases one of exclusion

★ Perinuclear inclusions are usually positive for vimentin, CD99, cytokeratin, EMA, and muscle actins

LANGERHANS CELL HISTIOCYTOSIS

Clinical Features

Langerhans cell histiocytosis is most frequent below five years of age

Males are more frequently affected than females

Bones are the most frequent site of involvement, including the femur, pelvis, ribs and spine

Extraosseous lesions can occur, including deposits in the central nervous system, skin, lung, liver, and lymph nodes

Bony lesions may be associated with pain

Cytopathologic Features

Smears are hypercellular and contain eosinophils and ovoid mononuclear and multinuclear histiocytes

9-16. Langerhan's cell histiocytosis *(left)*. Langerhans cell histiocytosis is characterized by highly cellular smears containing histiocytes, eosinophils, and multinucleated histiocyte-type giant cells. The histiocytes have moderate to abundant amounts of granular cytoplasm (H&E)

9-17. Langerhan's cell histiocytosis *(right)*. High-power view of Langerhans cell histiocytosis demonstrates mononuclear histiocytes with oval nuclei often displaying a prominent nuclear fold or cleft. Bilobed eosinophils are easily seen (H&E)

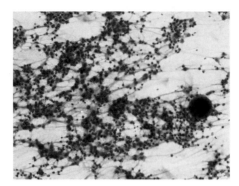
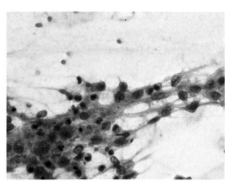

- Histiocytes have a bland chromatin with multiple small nucleoli
- Nucleus characteristically kidney shape with distinct membrane fold
- Langerhans cells frequently have abundant pale cytoplasm with well-defined borders
- Histiocytic cytoplasm may be vacuolated or foamy and may contain phagocytized debris
- Eosinophils present in variable numbers and in some smears may be sparse

Special Stains and Immunohistochemistry
- Histiocytes are immunohistochemically positive for S-100 protein and CD1A
- Electron microscopy demonstrates the characteristic Birbeck's granules

Modern Techniques for Diagnosis
- Noncontributory

Differential Diagnosis
- Osteomyelitis
  - Osteomyelitis is characterized by an admixture of inflammatory cells in which eosinophils do not dominate the picture
  - Histiocytes within chronic and granulomatous osteomyelitis do not show the characteristic nuclear folds of Langerhans histiocytes
- Melanoma
  - Large polygonal cells showing marked nuclear atypia
  - Mitotic figures common
  - Melan A and HMB-45 positivity. Lack CD1A staining

PEARLS

★ Langerhans cell histiocytosis may contain significant number of lymphocytes, plasma cells, and neutrophils within the inflammatory infiltrate, causing confusion with osteomyelitis
★ Immunohistochemical positivity for CD1A and S-100 protein strongly supports diagnosis

PSEUDOSARCOMATOUS SPINDLE CELL LESIONS (NODULAR FASCIITIS, PROLIFERATIVE FASCIITIS, AND PROLIFERATIVE MYOSITIS)

Clinical Features
- Majority of reported lesions arise in patients between the ages of fifteen and fifty years
- Males and females equally affected
- One of the most common soft tissue lesions
- History of rapid growth with preoperative duration of one month or less

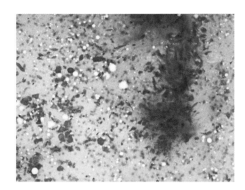 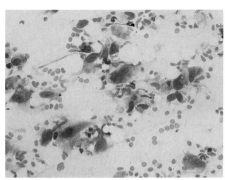

9-18. Nodular fasciitis *(left).* Smeared material characteristic of nodular fasciitis shows cell aggregates with a "tissue culture" appearance admixed with acute and chronic inflammatory cells and spindle cells. These spindle cells often show bipolar wispy processes, which are often fragile and disrupted by the smearing process (modified Giemsa stain)

9-19. Nodular fasciitis *(right).* The individual cells of nodular fasciitis have moderate to abundant cytoplasm. This cytoplasm has a delicate, wispy appearance with one or two cytoplasmic processes. The cells may lie singly or in clusters. The nuclei are large, but have smooth nuclear membranes and a generally fine chromatin pattern. Nucleoli can be prominent. Mitotic figures may be present (modified Giemsa stain)

■ Most common sites include upper extremities, trunk, chest wall, and back
■ Proliferative myositis and proliferative fasciitis occur in older age group (median age fifty years)

Cytopathologic Features
■ Low to moderate smear cellularity with cohesive groups of short spindled or stellate cells. Prominent number of single cells lying in background
■ Cells in tissue aggregates distributed around small delicate branching capillaries
■ Cellular aggregates show loose arrangement of cells with peripheral cells fraying off tissue aggregates (reparative appearance)
■ Tissue aggregates may have storiform appearance
■ Individual cells have "spindle" or stellate shape
■ Cytoplasm of cells present in moderate amounts, often with foamy appearance
■ Nuclei are large but retain open chromatin pattern, small nucleoli present
■ "Ganglion-like" cells minor component in nodular fasciitis but prominent in proliferative fasciitis
■ "Ganglion-like" cells and fragments of regenerating striated muscle prominent in proliferative myositis
■ Appearance of background variable; may be myxoid or granular
■ Scattered inflammatory cells, particularly lymphocytes and macrophages present.
■ Mitotic figures may be present but are all mirror image in form

Special Stains and Immunohistochemistry
■ Tumor cells show positivity for actins and desmin

Modern Techniques for Diagnosis
■ Noncontributory

Differential Diagnosis
■ Myxoma
➤ Characterized by abundant myxoid matrix
➤ Low cellularity with few vascularized tissue fragments
■ Fibromatosis
➤ Majority of cells are bland spindle-shaped cells with tapering cytoplasmic processes
➤ No evidence of mitotic activity
➤ Spindle cells admixed with mature-appearing adipose tissue and dengerating striated muscle
➤ Cellular forms may show mild to moderate nuclear hyperchromasia but no evidence of mitotic figures
➤ Fragments of hyalinized material and collagen bundles present in smears
■ Low-grade spindle cell sarcomas
➤ Generally lack tissue fragments with "tissue culture" appearance

➤ Mild to moderate nuclear atypia with rare to occasional mitotic figures
➤ Clinical history of larger size at presentation and slower rate of growth

★ Pseudosarcomatous spindle cell lesions of soft tissue show rapid growth over a few weeks to two months
★ Most cases present at a size of 1–2 cm
★ "Tissue culture" appearance with well-vascularized tissue fragments characteristic of pseudo-sarcomatous spindle cell lesions

MYOSITIS OSSIFICANS

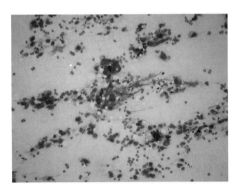

9-20. Myositis ossificans. Aspirate smears of myositis ossifficans contain a moderate number of oval to short spindle-shaped cells lying both singly and in small, loose clusters. A characteristic but not invariable component is background osteoid. This osteoid will surround some of the oval cells and has a magenta appearance in air dried preparations (modified Giemsa stain)

Clinical Features
■ Benign solitary well-circumscribed nodule arising most commonly in the musculature
■ Lesion often arises following injury
■ Initial history of pain and tenderness followed by rapid growth of doughy soft tissue swelling
■ Develop over several weeks to form a firm to stony hard mass averaging 3 to 6 cm in greatest dimension
■ Tumor most commonly found in active adolescents and young adults, predominantly males
■ 80% of cases involve the limbs, particularly quadriceps and gluteus muscles

Cytopathologic Features
■ Smears of variable cellularity with granular background
■ Dispersed spindle-shaped cells with fragments of striated muscle, round to ovoid osteoblasts, and multinucleated giant cells
■ Osteoid may be present in smears but is often not a prominent finding
■ Dominant cell type is either ovoid to polygonal or a short spindle-shaped cell
■ Cytoplasm is moderately abundant, often with feathery or wispy edges
■ Nuceli are usually round to ovoid and eccentrically located resembling osteoblasts

Special Stains and Immunohistochemistry
■ Noncontributory

Modern Techniques for Diagonsis
■ Noncontributory

Differential Diagnosis
■ Nodular fasciitis, proliferative fasciitis, and proliferative myositis
  ➤ Absence of osteoid/chondroid aids in separation of these lesions from myositis ossificans
■ Fibromatosis
  ➤ Predominant cell type is bland spindle-shaped cell with wispy cytoplasmic processes
  ➤ Fragments of dense collagen or hyaline material present
  ➤ Smears lack osteoid and chondroid matrix
■ Low-grade spindle cell sarcomas
  ➤ Lack osteoid and cartilaginous matrix
  ➤ Lack "tissue culture" appearance with round or ovoid osteoblast cells

★ Correlation with radiographic findings showing characteristic ossification zonation pattern greatly aids in the specific cytologic diagnosis of myositis ossificans

ELASTOFIBROMA

Clinical Features

▨ Majority of patients are elderly with peak incidence during the sixth and seventh decades of life
▨ Women affected more frequently than men
▨ Presents as slow-growing, deep-seated mass rarely associated with pain or tenderness
▨ Most common site is lower portion of scapula and chest wall deep to rhomboid major and latissimus dorsi muscles

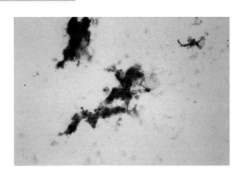

Cytopathologic Features

▨ Markedly hypocellular smears
▨ Fragments of adipose tissue intermingled with collagen fibers, elastic fiber fragments and bland spindle-shaped cells
▨ Characteristic gray spherical globules with serrated borders (petaloid globules) representing degenerated elastic fibers
▨ Degenerated elastic fibers often have a "braid-like" globular or stellate appearance

9-21. Elastofibroma. Smears obtained from elastofibromas are characteristically extremely hypocellular. Small fragments of disrupted elastic tissue and collagen are found occasionally associated with a cellular component. The cellular component is bland, with small dark nuclei (H&E)

Special Stains and Immunohistochemistry

Verhoeff elastin stain demonstrates elastic fibers

Modern Techniques for Diagnosis

▨ Electron microscopy demonstrates characteristic degenerating elastic fibers

Differential Diagonsis

▨ Hypocellular/acellular smears from other lesions
➤ Presence of characteristic altered elastic fibers (petaloid globules) separates nondiagnostic smears from material obtained from elastofibromas

★ Characteristic clinical history of slowly-growing mass in region of scapula of elderly individual key to diagnosis
★ Recognition of petaloid globules using wet-fixed H&E-stained material or Verhoeff elastin stain confirmatory for diagnosis

FIBROMATOSES (ABDOMINAL AND EXTRAABDOMINAL DESMOID TUMORS)

Clinical Features

▨ Common lesion occurring at a variety of body sites including palm, plantar surface of foot, penis, anterior abdominal wall, and connective tissue of muscles of the shoulder, thigh, and pelvic girdle
▨ Extraabdominal form most common in patients between puberty and 40 years of age. Women most commonly affected
▨ Abdominal fibromatosis most common in young women, frequently following child birth

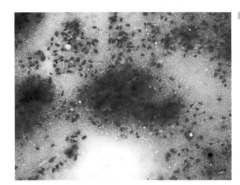
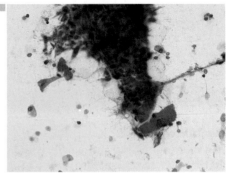

9-22. Fibromatosis *(left)*. Smears obtained from examples of fibromatosis may have a slightly myxoid or mucoid background. Smears may be cellular with the dominant cells being short, spindle shaped, or ovoid. The cells have enlarged but bland nuclei with small often distinct nucleoli. Mitotic figures are not seen. Frequently admixed with the "spindle" cell component are small fragments of striated muscle (central), which are a characteristic finding (modified Giemsa stain)

9-23. Fibromatosis *(right)*. Tissue fragment obtained from a case of cervical fibromatosis arising in an infant. The spindle cell component is characteristically bland and lacks mitotic figures. The nuclei of the cellular component are ovoid to spindle shaped and have absent or small, indistinct nucleoli. Characteristically fragments of striated muscle are entrapped within the tissue aggregates (H&E)

■ Abdominal and extraabdominal subtypes showing significant risk for local recurrence

■ Most abdominal and extraabdominal tumors measure 3–10 cm at clinical recognition

Cytopathologic Features
■ Two forms recognized cytologically
■ Low cellularity smears
  ➢ Smears of low to moderate cellularity
  ➢ Component cells have bland spindle-shaped appearance with oval or elongated nuclei
  ➢ Cells predominantly lie individually or in small loose clusters
  ➢ Majority of cells display tapering cytoplasmic processes
  ➢ Small polygonal cells interspersed with spindle forms
  ➢ Scattered inflammatory cells in background
  ➢ No evidence of nuclear atypia or mitotic activity
  ➢ Spindle cells admixed with fragments of mature appearing adipose tissue and degenerating striated muscle represented by multinucleated giant cells with cross-striations or fibrillar cytoplasm
■ Hypercellular fibromatoses
  ➢ Smears of moderately to high cellularity
  ➢ Predominant cell type is spindle shaped, frequently with a plump appearance
  ➢ Cells show mild cytologic atypia characterized by increased nuclear:cytoplasmic ratio and moderate nuclear hyperchromasia
  ➢ Nuclear membrane irregularity present
  ➢ Mitotic figures not present
  ➢ Spindle-shaped cells admixed with fragments of hyalinized material and collagen bundles along with small numbers of lymphocytes
  ➢ Cellular component may be mixed with fragments of mature adipose tissue and striated muscle

Special Stains and Immunohistochemistry
■ Noncontributory

Modern Techniques for Diagnosis
■ Noncontributory

Differential Diagnosis:
■ Nodular fasciitis and other pseudosarcomatous lesions
  ➢ "Tissue culture" appearance with vascularized tissue fragments
  ➢ Tissue fragments have cells "exfoliating" from edges
  ➢ Immunohistochemistry frequently positive for muscle actins

- Low-grade spindle cell sarcomas
  - ➤ Smear cellularity slightly higher than that seen in fibromatosis
  - ➤ Greater degrees of nuclear atypia
  - ➤ Rare to occasional mitotic figures seen in smears
  - ➤ Immunohistochemistry may display strong reactivity for actin, smooth muscle actin, desmin, PGP 9.5 or N-cam depending on type of sarcoma present
- Schwannoma
  - ➤ Strongly positive for S-100 protein
  - ➤ Wavy, bent, or grooved nuclei frequent
  - ➤ Filamentous cytoplasm
  - ➤ Verocay bodies may be present

PEARLS

★ Spindle cell population showing little or at most moderate nuclear atypia associated with dense fragments of hyalinized or collagenous material highly suggestive of fibromatosis

SOLITARY FIBROUS TUMOR

Clinical Features
- Most commonly arises in middle-aged adults
- No sex predilection
- May be found at any location with 40% occurring in subcutaneous tissues
- Most tumors present as well-demarcated, slowly growing, painless masses

Cytopathologic Features
- Smears of variable cellularity ranging from scant to moderate
- Background contains small number of red blood cells and inflammatory cells but no necrosis
- Ropy fragments of collagen may be entangled with cell clusters and short segments of blood vessels
- Cells may lie within tissue aggregates or be dispersed singly
- Edges of cell aggregates have feathery appearance with cells "dropping off"
- Majority of cells are of a short "spindle" or polygonal shape
- "Naked" nuclei commonly present in background
- Nuclei are round to oval in shape and may show some degree of angulation
- Moderate pleomorphism may be present but marked anaplasia is absent
- Chromatin pattern is finely granular and uniformly distributed throughout the nucleus
- Mitotic figures generally absent

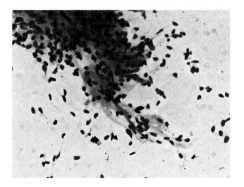 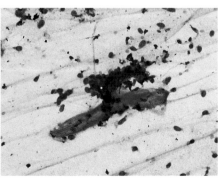

9-24. Solitary fibrous tumor (left). Smears obtained from solitary fibrous tumors contain a prominent number of three-dimensional tissue aggregates. These aggregates are often associated with ropey fragments of matrix/collagen tissue. The individual nuclei are oval or short "spindle" in shape. Various degrees of nuclear hyperchromasia and irregularity may be seen, but in most smears the nuclei have rather bland features with smooth nuclear membranes (modified Giemsa stain)

9-25. Solitary fibrous tumor (right). Characteristic of solitary fibrous tumors, the tissue fragments are often associated with ropey or string-like aggregates of collagenous tissue. In addition to the tissue aggregates, disassociated spindle cells are seen in the background. These cells may be largely stripped of their cytoplasm (modified Giemsa stain)

Special Stains and Immunohistochemistry

■ Cellular component demonstrates strong immunohistochemical positivity for CD34 and often for CD99

■ Immunohistochemical stains for desmin, cytokeratin, and S-100 protein usually negative

Modern Techniques for Diagnosis

■ Noncontributory

Differential Diagnosis

■ Fibromatosis, abdominal and extraabdominal
  ➤ Variable cellularity dominated by spindle-shaped cells
  ➤ Fragments of collagen bundles may be present
  ➤ Neoplastic cells may be admixed with fragments of benign adipose tissue and degenerating striated muscle
  ➤ Absence of staining for CD34

PEARLS

✶ Benign and malignant forms cannot be distinguished cytologically

✶ CD34 positivity in a nonendothelial vascular proliferation is strongly supportive of a diagnosis of solitary fibrous tumor

✶ Some cellular fragments may show a prominent vascular network

DERMATOFIBROSARCOMA PROTUBERANS AND GIANT CELL FIBROBLASTOMA

Clinical Features

■ Typically presents during early or middle adult life
■ Presents as nodular cutaneous mass
■ Indolent growth with long preclinical duration
■ Males affected more often than females
■ Occur most frequently on trunk and proximal extremities
■ Giant cell fibroblastoma may represent juvenile form of dermatofibrosarcoma protuberans

Cytopathologic Features

■ Smears of moderate to high cellularity
■ Cells lie both individually as well as in three-dimensional cell clusters
■ Background contains metachromatic stromal fragments of collagenous matrix material frequently associated with tightly cohesive cell clusters
■ Occasional cell clusters have a "storiform" pattern

9-26. Dermatofibroma *(left)*. Smears obtained from dermatofibromas are of moderate cellularity. Characteristically they contain cell clusters, which may have a storiform appearance. The individual nuclei are spindle shaped with blunt to slightly pointed ends. The nuclear chromatin is finely granular and the nuclei may have a vesicular appearance. Nucleoli vary in size. Mitotic figures are usually absent. Nuclear membranes as seen in this photograph may be irregular (H&E)

9-27. Giant cell fibroblastoma *(right)*. Characteristic multinucleated giant cells obtained by aspiration from a case of giant cell fibroblastoma. The nuclei overlap and frequently show considerable nuclear molding. The nuclei are bland, with smooth nuclear membranes and may have a kidney bean shape. Nuclear chromatin is usually finely granular and nucleoli may be prominent (modified Giemsa stain)

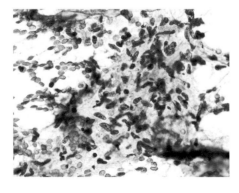
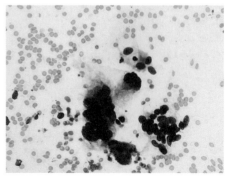

■ Individual cells are oval to spindle shaped

■ Nuclei are bland with fine chromatin pattern

■ Cells containing moderate amounts of cytoplasm, which appears pale and finely granular and may be distributed into bipolar cell processes

■ Mitotic figures are infrequent and always typical in form

■ Nuclei of cells from giant cell fibroblastoma may contain clefts, grooves, and folds in the nuclear membrane

■ Giant cell fibroblastomas contain a population of multinucleated giant cells with bland oval nuclei arranged in a floret or wreath-like pattern

Special Stains and Immunohistochemistry

■ Neoplastic cells are diffusely and strongly positive for CD34 and vimentin

■ Immunohistochemistry for S-100 protein and muscle specific actin is variably positive but desmin and cytokeratin staining is absent

Modern Techniques for Diagnosis

■ Noncontributory

Differential Diagnosis

■ Solitary fibrous tumor
  ➤ Spindle cell neoplasm with strong and diffuse CD34 positive staining
  ➤ Ropy matrix material and collagen fibers present in background and embedded in cell clusters
  ➤ Multinucleated giant cells not a component of sample
■ Fibromatosis, abdominal and extraabdominal
  ➤ Smears are of lower cellularity than seen in dermatofibrosarcoma protuberans
  ➤ Lack multinucleated giant cells
  ➤ Lack immunohistochemical positivity for CD34
■ Malignant fibrous histiocytoma
  ➤ Pleomorphic neoplasm with spindle, polygonal, and anaplastic giant cell forms
  ➤ Mitotic figures numerous and may be atypical in form
  ➤ CD34 negative

PEARLS

★ Superficial presentation as a nodular cutaneous mass helpful in specific diagnosis

★ CD34 positivity in a lesion with spindle cells and giant cells strongly suggest diagnosis of dermatofibrosarcoma protuberans/giant cell fibroblastoma

★ Translocations of chromosomes 17 and 22 may, in the future be diagnostically important

FIBROSARCOMA

Clinical Features

■ Most frequently occur between the ages of thirty and fifty-five years

■ Slightly more frequent in women than men

■ Preoperative duration of symptoms varies greatly from weeks to years

■ Probably infrequent sarcoma

■ Most commonly arises in deep soft tissues of lower extremities followed by upper extremities and trunk

Clinicopathologic Features

■ Cytologic features depend greatly on grade

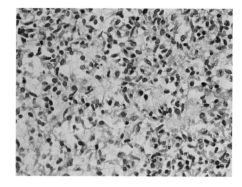

9-28. Fibrosarcoma. Aspirates from fibrosarcomas are frequently cellular and are characterized by a population of spindle-shaped cells. Because of the trauma of aspiration, these cells occasionally appear ovoid. Nuclear appearance depends on the grade of the fibrosarcoma. Moderate and poorly differentiated fibrosarcomas have enlarged hyperchromatic nuclei, often with irregular nuclear membranes and prominent nucleoli. Low-grade fibrosarcomas show only modest nuclear atypia with a finely granular chromatin pattern and indistinct nucleoli (H&E)

- Low-grade fibrosarcomas yield smears of relatively low cellularity while high-grade fibrosarcomas are associated with highly cellular smears
- Smears characterized by discohesive single cells admixed with three-dimensional highly cellular clusters showing significant nuclear overlap
- Cell clusters demonstrate interweaving of cells to form fascicles
- Low-grade lesions are cytologically bland, similar to fibromatoses
- High-grade fibrosarcomas show significant nuclear pleomorphism closely resembling that seen in malignant fibrous histiocytoma
- Relatively little collagenous tissue present in background or in cell clusters
- Majority of cells are oval or spindle shaped with ovoid or basillary nuclei containing tapered ends
- Nuclear membrane irregularities are frequent in high-grade lesions
- Chromatin is usually finely granular and nucleoli are not prominent except in high-grade lesions
- Mitotic figures usually identifiable in moderate and poorly differentiated fibrosarcomas, atypical forms may be found
- Aspirate smears from Grade III fibrosarcomas frequently contain necrotic material in the background admixed with blood

Special Stains and Immunohistochemistry

- Noncontributory, important only for nonreactivity for antibodies directed against specific markers such as CD34, desmin, S-100 protein, and actins

Modern Techniques for Diagnosis

- Noncontributory

Differential Diagnosis

- Fibromatoses, abdominal and extraabdominal
  - Nuclear features are more bland than seen in moderate and high-grade fibrosarcomas
  - Mitotic figures are not seen
  - Fragments of adipose tissue, collagenous matrix and striated muscle commonly admixed with spindle cell component
- Solitary fibrous tumor
  - Prominent number of cell clusters with intimate admixture of collagenous matrix material
  - Some cell clusters contain prominent vascular network
  - CD34 positivity by immunohistochemistry
  - Lesser degrees of nuclear atypia than seen in grade II and III fibrosarcomas
- Dermatofibrosarcoma protuberans/giant cell fibroblastoma
  - Nuclear atypia overlaps that of Grade I and Grade II fibrosarcomas
  - CD34 positivity
  - Tissue fragments may show storiform pattern
  - Multinucleated giant cells often present and may have wreath-like arrangement of nuclei

PEARLS

★ Fibrosarcoma may be inseparable on a cytologic basis from other spindle cell neoplasms. Absence of immunohistochemical positivity for tissue-specific markers is suggestive of the diagnosis of fibrosarcoma

★ Nuclei of spindle cells often have more sharply tapered ends than seen in leiomyosarcoma and most examples of malignant fibrous histiocytoma

SCHWANNOMA (NEURILEMMOMA)

Clinical Features
▧ Most common age of presentation between twenty and fifty years of age
▧ Males and females equally affected
▧ Schwannomas have predilection for head, neck, and flexor surfaces of upper and lower extremities
▧ Usually solitary sporadic lesions
▧ Slow-growing tumor usually present for years before diagnosis
▧ Pain and neurologic symptoms are uncommon

Cytopathologic Features
▧ Smears of variable cellularity with 52% highly cellular, 21% moderately cellular, and 27% poorly cellular
▧ Smear background clean or contains small numbers of red blood cells
▧ Majority of cells lie in tissue aggregates
▧ Tissue fragments vary in cellularity from highly cellular to predominantly myxoid
▧ Tumor cells both those in clusters and lying singly show indistinct cytoplasmic borders and a vaguely fibrillar cytoplasmic appearance
▧ Cell nuclei may be wavy, bent, or grooved
▧ Nuclear chromatin usually dark and condensed
▧ Intranuclear cytoplasmic pseudoinclusions may be present
▧ Verocay bodies found in approximately 10% of smears
▧ Occasional schwannomas show degenerative changes with characteristic nuclear enlargement, irregularity, and hyperchromasia
▧ The degenerative pleomorphic cells occasionally show large intranuclear inclusions (Kern–Loche)
▧ Mitotic figures not present

Special Stains and Immunohistochemistry
▧ Strong, diffuse immunohistochemical positivity for S-100 protein Leu-7 usually positive
▧ Variable expression of glial fibrillary acidic protein

Modern Techniques for Diagnosis
▧ Noncontributory

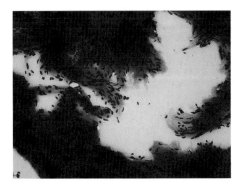 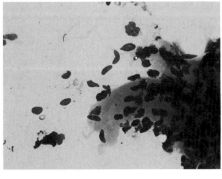

9-29. Schwannoma *(left)*. Schwannomas characteristically are associated with smears of low to moderate cellularity. The majority of cells form three-dimensional tissue fragments. These tissue fragments display a bundled or fascicular pattern. The component cells have filamentous cytoplasm often forming a syncytium. The nuclei are bland and hyperchromatic and are characterized by nuclear folds, bends, and undulations (modified Giemsa stain)

9-30. Schwannoma *(right)*. High-power view of a tissue fragment aspirated from a schwannoma. The tissue fragment has a syncytial appearance to the cytoplasm and spindle-shaped nuclei often with a bent conformation or nuclear folds and clefts. Mitotic figures are not seen (modified Giemsa stain)

Differential Diagnosis

■ Fibromatosis
- ➤ Lack wispy filamentous cytoplasm
- ➤ Lack prominent nuclear folds, bends, and sharply tapered ends
- ➤ Lack S-100 protein and Leu-7 immunohistochemical expression

■ Solitary fibrous tumor
- ➤ Lack wispy filamentous cytoplasmic processes
- ➤ Lack sharp tapered nuclear ends and prominent nuclear folds, bends, and clefts
- ➤ Lack strong diffuse S-100 positivity
- ➤ Express CD34

■ Pseudosarcomatous proliferations
- ➤ Show tissue culture arrangement of tissue fragments
- ➤ Frequently show actin immunohistochemical positivity
- ➤ Cell clusters may contain prominent vessels
- ➤ Background may contain inflammatory cells

PEARLS

★ Strong diffuse S-100 positivity
★ Wispy and filamentous bipolar cytoplasmic processes
★ Nuclei show prominent membranous bends, folds, and clefts

MALIGNANT PERIPHERAL NERVE SHEATH TUMOR

Clinical Features

■ Represent 5–10% of all soft tissue sarcomas
■ Occur in a background of neurofibromatosis type I
■ Most occur in patients between twenty and fifty years of age
■ Equal male/female incidence
■ Frequently arise as large fusiform mass associated with major nerve

Cytopathologic Findings

■ Cellular smears composed of tightly highly cellular aggregates of spindle-shaped cells
■ Background contains smaller number of individual spindle-shaped cells
■ Background may contain necrotic granular debris
■ Tissue fragments may show a storiform or fascicular pattern
■ Rarely tissue fragments have a palisading appearance

9-31. Malignant peripheral nerve sheath tumor *(left)*. Aspirates of malignant peripheral nerve sheath tumors are generally highly cellular. The cells lie in both tight, three-dimensional cell clusters as well as singly in the background. The cytoplasm of these cells is frequently filamentous. The cells run in bundles and fascicles and on occasion will show nuclear palisading. The nuclei have sharply pointed tips and are frequently bent, folded or comma-shaped (modified Giemsa stain)

9-32. Malignant peripheral nerve sheath tumor *(right)*. High-power view of a malignant peripheral nerve sheath tumor showing hyperchromatic nuclei with sharply pointed ends and nuclear folds or bends (modified Giemsa stain)

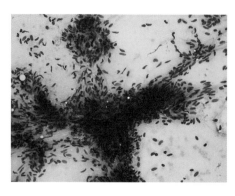
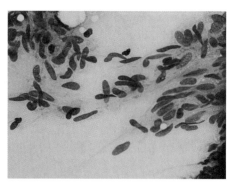

- Discohesive single cells are most numerous around tissue fragments
- Individual cells show prominent tapered cytoplasmic processes, frequently with a wavy filamentous appearance
- Cytoplasmic borders indistinct in cell clusters
- Nuclei are spindle shaped with sharply pointed ends and a prominence of nuclear folds, bends, or wavy appearance
- Nuclear pleomorphism variable but may be marked in high-grade cases
- Intranuclear cytoplasmic pseudo-inclusions found in many cases
- Epithelioid variant of malignant peripheral nerve sheath tumor is characterized by highly cellular smears and a bloody, frequently necrotic background
- Majority of cells in epithelioid variant lie singly and are oval or polygonal in shape
- Epithelioid variant cells have abundant cytoplasm with finely granular appearance
- Epithelioid variant cells occasionally show fine cytoplasmic vacuoles and indistinct cell borders
- Nuclei are hyperchromatic with a coarse chromatin, but nucleoli are usually absent or indistinct
- Prominent number of mitotic figures present in most patterns

Special Stains and Immunohitsochemistry
- Only half of malignant peripheral nerve sheath tumors express S-100 protein
- Many malignant peripheral nerve sheath tumors express PGP 9.5 and/or N-cam

Modern Diagnostic Techniques
- Noncontributory

Differential Diagonosis
- Schwannoma, particularly cellular and ancient forms
  - Strongly and diffusely express S-100 protein
  - Mitotic figures absent
  - Lower overall cellularity
  - Except in ancient forms, significant nuclear pleomorphism is absent
- Fibromatoses
  - Only low to moderate cellularity
  - Absence of mitotic figures
  - Prominence of hyaline and collagenous matrix, both free in the background and in cell clusters
  - Frequent presence of fragments of benign adipose tissue and degenerating striated muscle
- Solitary fibrous tumor
  - Overall lower cellularity than malignant peripheral nerve sheath tumor.
  - Absence of mitotic figures
  - Strong CD34 positivity
  - Tissue fragments frequently have prominent vascular network
  - Absence of prominent nuclear membrane folds, bends, and clefts
- Fibrosarcoma
  - Cytoplasm lacks filamentous wispy character
  - Nuclei lack membrane bends, folds, and clefts
  - Lack of positive staining for S-100 protein, N-cam, or PGP 9.5

PEARLS

- Nuclei with membrane folds, bends, and clefts highly suggestive of neural differentiation
- Frequent high mitotic figure counts helps define malignant potential

★ Immunohistochemical positivity for PGP 9.5, N-cam, or S-100 protein helps establish neural differentiation

LEIOMYOSARCOMA

Clinical Features
▧ Leiomyosarcomas occur in both cutaneous (dermal) and soft tissue forms
▧ Majority of soft tissue leiomyosarcomas arise within the retroperitoneal space and abdominal cavity
▧ Two-thirds of retroperitoneal leiomyosarcomas occur in women, with a median age at time of presentation of sixty years
▧ At the time of clinical detection, most retroperitoneal leimyosarcomas are of large size

Cytopathologic Features
▧ Smears obtained from leiomyosarcomas are of variable cellularity dependent on grade
▧ Well-differentiated leiomyosarcomas are usually of low to moderate cellularity with the majority of cells lying in tightly cohesive, three-dimensional cell clusters
▧ Cells are closely spaced and run in parallel, resulting in a side-by-side arrangement of the nuclei
▧ Moderate and poorly differentiated leiomyosarcomas are associated with smears of higher cellularity
▧ Moderate and high-grade leiomyosarcomas form three-dimensional cell clusters of more irregular appearance, with cells lying both in bundles and haphazardly arranged without demonstrable fascicular pattern
▧ Cells within bundles often have a syncytial appearance
▧ Small numbers of individual cells are seen in the background, often most numerous around cells clusters
▧ Individual cells may present as "naked" basillary shaped nuclei
▧ Nuclear appearance depends on grade with well-differentiated tumors showing an even homogeneous chromatin pattern, with small indistinct nucleoli
▧ Moderate and poorly differentiated leiomyosarcomas show hyperchromasia and nuclear membrane irregularity
▧ Basic nuclear shape is basillary with blunt nuclear tips
▧ Mitotic figures are usually infrequent to absent in low grade neoplasms

Special Stains and Immunohistochemistry
▧ Leiomyosarcomas show immunohistochemical staining for vimentin, actin, smooth muscle actin, desmin, and h-caldesmon
▧ Occasionally, focal staining for S-100 protein and CD117 is seen. Staining for cytokeratin and EMA is rare but has been reported

9-33. Leiomyosarcoma *(left)*. Aspirates of leiomyosarcomas are characterized by three-dimensional tissue fragments having a bundled or fascicular appearance. Small numbers of individual spindle shaped or ovoid cells are seen in the background (modified Giemsa stain)

9-34. Leiomyosarcoma *(right)*. The nuclei of moderately differentiated leiomyosarcomas are spindle shaped with rounded or blunt tips. The nuclei are hyperchromatic with smooth to slightly irregular nuclear membranes (modified Giemsa stain)

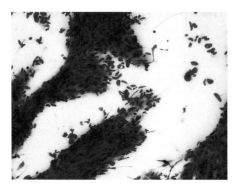
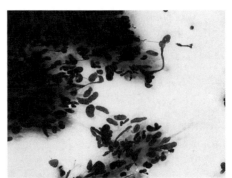

Modern Techniques for Diagonsis
- Noncontributory

Differential Diagonsis
- Fibrosarcoma
  - ➤ Frequently impossible to separate leiomyosarcoma from fibrosarcoma purely on cytomorphology
  - ➤ Fibrosarcomas are vimentin positive but are negative for muscle markers including muscle-specific actin and smooth muscle actin
- Neurofibrosarcoma
  - ➤ Majority of neurofibrosarcomas show nuclei with more pointed ends as well as folds, bends and irregularities of nuclear membrane
  - ➤ Malignant periopheral nerve sheath tumors show positive staining for S-100 protein (50%), PGP 9.5, and N-cam
- Solitary fibrous tumor
  - ➤ Smears are usually of lower cellularity than seen in leiomyosarcoma
  - ➤ Solitary fibrous tumors often associated with ropy collagenous stroma
  - ➤ Solitary fibrous tumors generally stain for CD34
- Fibromatosis (abdominal and extrabdominal desmoids tumors)
  - ➤ Smears from fibromatoses are usually of lower cellularity
  - ➤ Nuclear atypia is generally less in examples of fibromatosis than in leiomyosarcoma
  - ➤ Fibromatoses often associated with fragments of reactive striated muscle

PEARLS

★ Epithelioid variants of leiomyosarcoma exist in which the smears are dominated by polygonal or oval cells rather than the spindle-shaped cells characteristic of classical leiomyosarcoma

★ Staining patterns of epithelioid leiomyosarcoma are identical to those of spindle-shaped leiomyosarcomas

PLEOMORPHIC RHABDOMYOSARCOMA

Clinical Features
- Rare pleomorphic sarcoma of adult life
- Pleomorphic type arises most frequently in trunk and extremities, less commonly in retroperitoneum
- Men more frequently affected than women
- Most arise in patients over the age of fifty years

Cytopathologic Findings
- Smears are usually highly cellular and composed of markedly pleomorphic spindle cells, polygonal cells, and giant cells
- Nuclei are enlarged, hyperchromatic, and contain irregular nuclear contours and coarse chromatin
- Rare cells contain cytoplasmic cross-striations; filamentous cytoplasm more common

Special Stains and Immunohistochemistry
- Sarcomas are usually positive for muscle markers including desmin, actins, myogenin, and MyoD-1

Modern Techniques for Diagnosis
- Noncontributory

Differential Diagnosis

■ Malignant fibrous histiocytoma
➤ Pleomorphic sarcoma with anaplastic mono- and multinucleated giant cells showing no definitive direction of differentiation
➤ Lack of cytoplasmic cross-striations or filamentous character
➤ Lack of staining for muscle markers including desmin, actins, myogenin, and MyoD-1
■ Pleomorphic leiomyosarcoma
➤ Greater prominence of spindle cell component
➤ No evidence of cross-striation
➤ Less frequently express desmin and myogenin than do pleomorphic rhabdomyosarcomas

PEARLS

★ The presence of cytoplasmic cross-striations or a prominent whirling filamentous appearance within the cytoplasm suggests rhabdomyosarcomatous differentiation
★ While not specific, the strong expression of desmin, myogenin and/or MyoD-1 suggests rhabdomyosarcomatous differentiation, as these markers are more weakly and less frequently expressed in myofibroblastic and leiomyosarcomatous lesions

MALIGNANT FIBROUS HISTIOCYTOMA

Clinical Features

■ Majority of patients are older than fifty years
■ Males are affected more commonly than females
■ Majority of cases occur in deep soft tissues with the lower extremity and retroperitoneum being the most frequent sites
■ Patients present with a large growing soft tissue mass, occasionally associated with pain

Cytopathologic Features

■ Majority of cases yield smears of moderate to high cellularity
■ Majority of cells lie in loose aggregates with single discohesive cells scattered through smears but concentrated around tissue fragments
■ Background frequently bloody or may contain some necrotic debris
■ While not diagnostic of malignant fibrous histiocytoma, some tissue fragments may show a prominent storiform pattern
■ Majority of smears contain three cell types: plump spindle-shaped fibroblasts with long cytoplasmic processes; mono- or binucleated bizarre histiocyte-like cells with

9-35. Malignant fibrous histiocytoma *(left)*. Aspirates from malignant fibrous histiocytomas are usually highly cellular. The cells lie both singly and in cohesive cell clusters. Characteristically significant nuclear pleomorphism is present and the background may have a dirty, lacy, or granular appearance (modified Giemsa stain)

9-36. Malignant fibrous histiocytoma *(right)*. Material aspirated from malignant fibrous histiocytomas is characterized by a pleomorphic cell population of round, polygonal, oval, and spindle-shaped cells. Nuclei vary markedly in size and shape. Multinucleated giant cell forms are not infrequent (modified Giemsa stain)

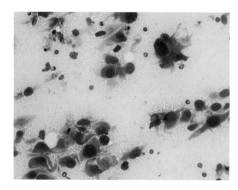 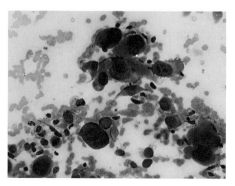

indistinct cytoplasmic borders and cytoplasmic vacuoles or phagocytized debris; and multinucleated anaplastic giant cells
▨ Mitotic figures present in a minority of cases, but when seen may be of typical or atypical form
▨ Necrotic debris present in background of <10% of the case

Special Stains and Immunohistochemistry
▨ Strong immunohistochemical expression of vimentin
▨ Weak or absent expression of histiocytic markers
▨ Absence of staining for other lineage markers including muscle actins, desmin, or S-100 protein

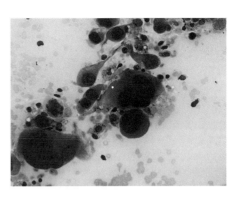

9-37. Malignant fibrous histiocytoma. Aspirates of malignant fibrous histiocytomas frequently contain anaplastic binucleated and multinucleated giant cells. Cell shape varies greatly from "spindle" to round (modified Giemsa stain)

Differential Diagnosis
▨ The diagnosis of malignant fibrous histiocytoma as a specific entity is currently questionable. Other pleomorphic sarcomas including pleomorphic liposarcoma, leiomyosarcoma, chrondrosarcoma, and rhabdomyosarcoma should be ruled out using appropriate lineage markers

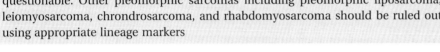
PEARLS

★ The diagnosis of storiform pleomorphic malignant fibrous histiocytoma is questionable as specific differentiation markers are absent and the storiform pattern is nonspecific. Perhaps these high-grade tumors without demonstrable direction of differentiation should be simply characterized as pleomorphic sarcomas

TENOSYNOVIAL GIANT CELL TUMOR, NODULAR AND DIFFUSE TYPES

Clinical Features
▨ Diffuse type
➢ Most commonly affects patients between twenty and forty years of age
➢ May affect any joint, but knee is most frequently involved, followed by ankle, hip, and shoulder
➢ May involve intra- and extraarticular space
➢ May be associated with localized pain and tenderness, joint effusion or limitation of motion
➢ Usually only one joint is involved, but polyarticular forms are known

▨ Localized form, tenosynovial giant cell tumor:
➢ Most commonly affects patients between thirty and fifty years of age
➢ Slight predilection for females
➢ Most commonly occurs in hands, especially fingers, but also can involve toes, ankles, knee, and wrists

9-38. Tenosynovial giant tumor *(left).* Aspirates from tenosynovial giant cell tumors of both localized and diffuse type are characterized by cellular smears. The smears are composed of round or ovoid mononuclear cells and a lesser number of multinucleated histiocytic type giant cells. Scattered foamy and pigment-laden histiocytes are seen in the background (modified Giemsa stain)

9-39. Tenosynovial giant cell tumor *(right).* Smears of tenosynovial giant cell tumor often contain hemosiderin in the background as well as in foamy histiocytes. The mononuclear cell component has round or ovoid nuclei often with distinct nucleoli. The multinucleated giant cells have overlapping nuclei usually numbering from two to ten (modified Giemsa stain)

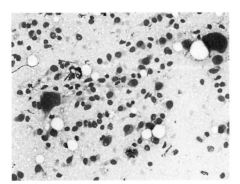
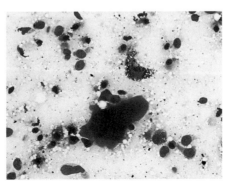

➤ Slow-growing lesion that may be associated with pain, limitation of motion, or soft tissue swelling

Cytopathologic Findings
- Cellular smears characterized by a dominant population of individually dispersed round or plump spindle-shaped cells
- Mononuclear cells have smooth, round nuclei with fine chromatin and single small nucleoli
- Nuclei are often eccentrically located within cells
- Variable number of multinucleated giant cells present
- Giant cells may contain fifty or more nuclei
- Mitotic figures infrequent but when present are of typical form
- Necrosis absent
- Foamy and pigment-laden histiocytes present in many cases
- Intranuclear inclusions and nuclear folds frequently present

Special Stains and Immunohistochemistry
- Noncontributory

Modern Techniques for Diagnosis
- Noncontributory

Differential Diagnosis
- Conventional giant cell tumor of bone
  ➤ Radiographic imaging studies serve to define site of origin and aid in distinction of conventional giant cell tumor of bone from localized and diffuse forms of tenosynovial giant cell tumor
- Dermatofibrosarcoma protuberans and giant cell fibroblastoma
  ➤ Location within subcutis or superficial soft tissue helps distinguish dermatofibrosarcoma from tenosynovial giant cell tumor
  ➤ Spindle cells and cohesive tissue fragments more prominent in dermatofibrosarcoma protuberans than in tenosynovial giant cell tumor
  ➤ CD34 positivity in both dermatofibrosarcoma protuberans and giant cell fibroblastoma
- Pleomorphic malignant fibrous histiocytoma
  ➤ Marked nuclear pleomorphism involving both spindle cells, polygonal cells, and giant cell component
  ➤ Nonmirror image (atypical) mitotic figures may be found in MFH but are invariably absent from tenosynovial giant cell tumor, both localized and diffuse subtypes

PEARLS

★ Location and pattern of growth predict biological potential

MALIGNANT FIBROUS HISTIOCYTOMA, GIANT CELL TYPE

- Giant cell malignant fibrous histiocytoma clinically and cytologically resembles pleomorphic malignant fibrous histiocytoma except for the prominence of osteoclast-like and pleomorphic giant cells. Currently, this category is regarded as a diagnosis of exclusion, after ruling out other pleomorphic sarcomas (please see discussion of pleomorphic MFH above)

CONVENTIONAL GIANT CELL TUMOR OF BONE

Clinical Features

▦ Represent approximately 5% of all primary bone neoplasms

▦ Distinct predilection for women

▦ Majority of patients are skeletally mature and over the age of eighteen years, with most cases being recognized in patients between twenty and forty years of age

▦ Majority of cases occur within long bones, particular distal femur, proximal tibia, distal radius, and proximal humerus

▦ May present with pathologic fracture

▦ Radiographic findings reveal eccentric osteolytic lesion centered on epiphysis of bone

9-40. Conventional giant cell tumor. Conventional giant cell tumors of bone are characterized by aggregates of mononuclear spindle-shaped cells and individual spindle-shaped mononuclear cells lying free in the background. Associated with the cell clusters are a number of multinucleated giant cells. The arrangement of cell clusters and multinucleated giant cells has a "checkerboard" appearance. The multinucleated giant cells may have up to fifty nuclei. The nuclei of the giant cells resemble those of the mononuclear cells (H&E)

Cytopathologic Findings

▦ Moderate to highly cellular smears with numerous tissue fragments lying in a bloody background

▦ Bimorphic cell population composed of mononuclear and multinucleated osteoclast-like giant cells

▦ Mononuclear cells frequently form cohesive tissue fragments to which variable numbers of giant cells are attached (checkerboard pattern)

▦ Mononuclear cell component has ovoid to spindle-shaped morphology

▦ Mononuclear cells have small to moderate amounts of cytoplasm, and when cells are in clusters, give a sycytial appearance

▦ Mononuclear cells have round, ovoid, or elongated nuclei, often eccentrically located

▦ Nuclei of mononuclear cells and multinucleated giant cells appear similar

▦ Multinucleated giant cells contain large numbers of nuclei, frequently fifty or more

▦ Foamy histiocytes may be found in some cases

▦ Mitotic figures may be found in the mononuclear component, but are always typical in form

Special Stains and Immunohistochemistry

▦ Noncontributory

Modern Techniques for Diagnosis

▦ Noncontributory

Differential Diagonsis

▦ Giant cell-rich osteosarcoma

➤ Osteosarcomas display distinct nuclear anaplasia in spindle or osteoblastic component

➤ Osteoclast-like giant cell nuclei are bland in comparison to stromal cell nuclei

➤ Osteoid present within smears

➤ Radiographic features help distinguish osteosarcoma from conventional giant cell tumor of bone

▦ Aneurysmal bone cyst

➤ Hypocellular bloody smears containing only rare spindle cells, osteoblast-like cells and osteoclast-like giant cells

➤ Characteristic radiographic appearance

▦ Chondroblastoma

➤ Occurs at younger age with most patients being skeletally immature and under age of eighteen years

➤ Mononuclear cells tend to be more round or ovoid in shape
➤ Mononuclear cell component frequently S-100 positive
➤ Giant cells contain fewer nuclei than those characteristic of conventional giant cell tumor

PEARLS

★ Radiographic–cytologic correlation imperative for accurate diagnosis
★ Osteoclast-like multinucleated giant cells may be seen in a variety of lesions including conventional giant cell tumor of bone, chondroblastoma, aneurysmal bone cyst and giant cell–rich osteosarcoma
★ Radiographs and nature of mononuclear cell component aids in distinction of the other lesions from conventional giant cell tumor of bone

CHONDROBLASTOMA

Clinical Features
▨ Osteolytic lesion centered in epiphysis of long bones
▨ 75% involve long bones of extremity, with most common anatomic sites being in the distal or proximal femur, proximal tibia, or proximal humerus
▨ Most patients are between ten and twenty-five years of age
▨ Lesion shows a predilection for males

Cytopathologic Findings
▨ Smears are usually hypercellular and contain a uniform population of round cells
▨ Cells have a moderate amount of cytoplasm surrounding a centrally or eccentrically located nucleus
▨ Nucleus shows prominent grooving and inconspicuous nucleoli
▨ Chondroid material frequently present but does not dominate smears
▨ Variable numbers of osteoclast-like giant cells present
▨ Occasional cells will show intranuclear cytoplasmic pseudoinclusions
▨ Inflammatory cells and necrotic debris absent

Special Stains and Immunohistochemistry
▨ Neoplastic mononuclear cells express S-100 protein and vimentin

Modern Diagnostic Techniques
▨ Noncontributory

9-41. Chondroblastoma *(left)*. Material obtained from chondroblastomas is usually of moderate cellularity. The cell population is composed predominately of small ovoid or round mononuclear cells and lesser numbers of multinucleated giant cells. The multinucleated giant cells contain fewer nuclei than seen in conventional giant cell tumor of bone (Papanicolaou)

9-42. Chondroblastoma *(right)*. The mononuclear cells of chondroblastomas have round nuclei, which may contain a distinct nuclear fold (Papanicolaou)

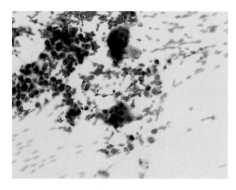
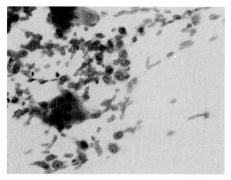

Differential Diagnosis
- Conventional giant cell tumor of bone
  - Cells are more spindle shaped than the round to ovoid cells of chondroblastoma
  - Multinucleated giant cells contain larger number of nuclei than seen in chondroblastoma
  - Skeletally mature individual
- Osteoclast-rich osteosarcoma
  - Stromal cells are spindle shaped, ovoid, or polygonal and possess greater degrees of nuclear atypia than seen in chondroblastoma
  - Stromal cells are not S-100 positive
  - Osteoid present in most smears
- Aneurysmal bone cyst
  - Smears are hypocellular, containing mostly blood with few spindle-shaped cells and multinucleated osteoclast-like giant cells

⋆ Radiographs are of great aid in disinguishing chondroblastoma from other giant-cell containing lesions of bone
⋆ Ovoid to round morphology of chondroblasts aids in their distinction from the spindle-shaped stromal cells of giant cell tumor of bone
⋆ Chondroblastomas occur in skeletally immature individuals

INTRAMUSCULAR MYXOMA

Clinical Features
- Predominantly affect adults, most commonly women
- Lesion appears as a slowly growing, painless mass
- Lesion occurs predominantly in lower extremities
- Majority are solitary, but rare multiple forms have been reported

Cytopathologic Features
- Abundant myxoid matrix comprising the majority of aspirated material
- Small population of spindle-shaped, stellate, or ovoid cells with bland nuclear features
- Nuclei are small, with a condensed chromatin and lack nucleoli
- Mitotic figures absent
- Small numbers of foamy histiocytes and lymphocytes may be present
- Scattered tissue aggregates may contain small segments of capillaries, occasionally showing branching

9-43. Intramuscular myxoma *(left)*. Smears prepared from aspirates of intramuscular myxoma are hypocellular with abundant myxoid material in the background. Dispersed in the smear are rare tissue fragments dominated by a myxoid matrix. Entrapped within these tissue fragments are occasional small segments of capillaries. These capillaries do not show a prominent anastomosing pattern. Also within the tissue fragments are bland, spindle-shaped, or stellate mononuclear cells (modified Giemsa stain)

9-44. Intramuscular myxoma *(right)*. The stromal cells of intramuscular myxomas are bland with smooth nuclear membranes and a dark chromatin pattern. Nuclear atypia is absent as are mitotic figures (modified Giemsa stain)

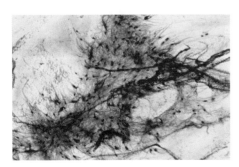 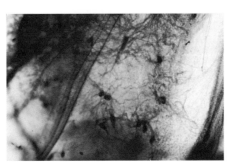

Special Stains and Immunohistochemistry
▦ Noncontributory

Modern Diagnostic Techniques
▦ Noncontributory

Differential Diagnosis
▦ Ganglion cyst
  ➤ Abundant myxoid/mucinous material in background
  ➤ Cellular component comprised histiocytes and occasional lymphocytes
  ➤ Absence of tissues fragments with capillary component
▦ Myxoid liposarcoma
  ➤ Abundant myxoid matrix, both in background and in tissue aggregates
  ➤ Tissue aggregates contain complex plexiform capillary network surrounding and entrapping ovoid cells, a component of which are true lipoblasts
  ➤ Lipoblasts and ovoid cells frequently S-100 positive
▦ Myxoid malignant fibrous histiocytoma
  ➤ Abundant myxoid background in which are admixed polygonal and spindle-shaped cells
  ➤ Component of anaplastic mononuclear and multinucleated giant cells present

PEARLS

★ Presence of abundant myxoid matrix with small number of tissue fragments and individual spindle-shaped and stellate cells characterizes myxoma
★ Myxomas may contain tissue fragments with branching capillaries, but lack the complex anastomosing capillary networks seen in myxoid liposarcomas

EWING SARCOMA (PRIMITIVE NEUROECTODERMAL TUMOR)

Clinical Features
▦ Most commonly affects children and adolescents between five and twenty-five years of age
▦ Males are more commonly affected than females
▦ In addition to mass lesion, patients may present with systemic symptoms including fever and an elevated erythrocyte sedimentation rate
▦ When arising in bone, radiographs show bone lysis with patchy bone sclerosis and "onion-skining" new periosteal bone formation
▦ Sarcoma usually involves diaphysis of long bones with most frequent sites of involvement being femur, humerus, and tibia
▦ Extraskeletal involvement occurs most commonly in the chest wall and paravertebral region as well as lower extremities and retroperitoneum

9-45. Ewing sarcoma *(left)*. Highly cellular smears characterize aspirates from Ewing's sarcomas. The overall pattern is that of a classic small cell malignancy. The cells lie both individually and in clusters. The individual cells have scant to absent cytoplasm and round hyperchromatic nuclei. Nucleoli are not prominent. Some nuclei will show nuclear molding, particularly within the tight cell clusters (modified Giemsa stain)

9-46. Ewing sarcoma *(right)*. Some Ewing's sarcomas show a bimodal cell population with a small, dark-cell component and a larger pale-cell component. Within the pale-cell component, the chromatin pattern is looser and nucleoli are more prominent. Both cell types have scanty cytoplasm (modified Giemsa stain)

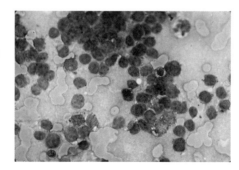

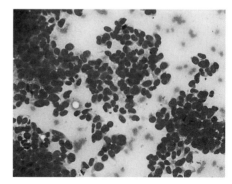

Cytopathologic Features

- Cellular smears composed of small round cells
- Bimodal population of light and dark cells in many smears
- Light cells possess fine open chromatin, while dark cells have condensed chromatin pattern
- Background may be extremely bloody or have a proteinaceous lace-like or fibrillary appearance
- Intracytoplasmic glycogen and rosette-like structures variably present
- Cell nuclei are round with one to two small nucleoli
- Cytoplasm is scanty and appears as a thin rim surrounding the nucleus

Special Stains and Immunohistochemistry

- Cells show immunohistochemical positivity for vimentin, CD99, FLI-1, and variable positivity for neuron specific enolase
- Some cases demonstrate cytokeratin positivity and soft tissue forms may show reactivity with antibodies directed against desmin, muscle specific actin, S-100 protein and synaptophysin

Modern Techniques for Diagnosis

- Ewing's sarcoma and PNET are associated with several translocations involving chromosome 22. The most frequent ones are t(11;22)(q24;q12), t(21;22)(q12;q12), and t(7;22)(p22;q12). These result in the EWS/FLI-1 fusion transcript

Differential Diagnosis

- Malignant lymphoma
  - ➤ Cellular smears with numerous lymphoglandular bodies in the background
  - ➤ Monomorphous population of lymphoid cells of varying sizes depending on histologic type
  - ➤ Demonstration of monoclonality and the presence of specific T- and B-cell markers important for diagnosis
- Rhabdomyosarcoma
  - ➤ Round cell population showing greater variability in cell size and shape
  - ➤ Some cells have tadpole shape or are represented by mono- or multinucleated giant cells
  - ➤ Cytoplasm more abundant than in Ewing's sarcoma and frequently shows a filamentous appearance and very rarely cytoplasmic cross-striations
  - ➤ Immunohistochemical positivity for desmin, muscle actins, and myogenin
- Mesenchymal chondrosarcoma
  - ➤ Population of small round cells showing slightly greater variability in size than is characteristic of Ewing's sarcoma
  - ➤ Some smears contain fragments of chondroid matrix
  - ➤ Cells associated with chondroid matrix are frequently S-100 protein positive
- Metastatic neuroblastoma
  - ➤ Examples of neuroblastoma may show background neuropil and ganglion cells
  - ➤ Occasional Homer-Wright rosettes may be seen
  - ➤ Neuroblastomas have cellular aspirates composed of individual small cells with some forming cohesive groups
  - ➤ Nuclear molding often seen
  - ➤ A second cell component of slightly larger cells with greater amounts of cytoplasm may be seen
  - ➤ Neuroblastomas are usually nonspecific enolase and S-100 protein positive and show no evidence of translocations on cytogenetic analysis

PEARLS

★ Relatively uniform small round cell population sometimes showing a slightly bimodal size distribution

★ Cytogenetic or fluorescence in-situ hybridization analysis to demonstrate EWSR-related translocations

RHABDOMYOSARCOMA (EMBRYONAL AND ALVEOLAR SUBTYPES)

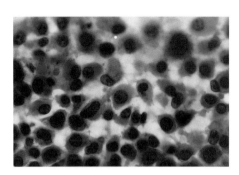

9-47. Embryonal/alveolar pattern of rhabdomyosarcoma. Aspiration smears of embryonal and alveolar pattern rhabdomyosarcomas are of moderate to high cellularity. The cells show considerable variability ranging from small, round cells with scanty cytoplasm to large cells with moderate or abundant cytoplasm. These larger cells have a granular or even filamentous appearance. Cell shape varies from round to ovoid or "tadpole" (H&E)

Clinical Features

■ Most common soft tissue sarcoma of childhood

■ Most patients younger than ten years of age at diagnosis

■ Most common manifestation is that of a soft tissue mass or swelling

■ Botryoid form of embryonal rhabdomyosarcoma arises in submucosa and tends to involve bladder, vagina, rectum, nasal cavity, and nasopharynx

■ Embryonal rhabdomyosarcoma most commonly occurs in children under ten years of age and involves genitourinary tract, head and neck, and retroperitoneum

■ Alveolar subtype most commonly affects adolescents and arises in extremities, paranasal sinuses, and retroperitoneum

Cytopathologic Findings

■ Embryonal subtype

➤ Smears usually cellular but botryoid subtype may be characterized by scanty cellularity in a myxoid background

➤ Smears usually contain three cell types, varying from early rhabdomyoblasts to larger, late rhabdomyoblasts. In most cases the predominant cell type is a small round cell with scanty cytoplasm

➤ Variability in cell size and shape is hallmark of rhabdomyosarcoma

➤ Cross-striations seen only in occasional cells. Filaments within cytoplasm are much more common

➤ Mitoses present in variable numbers but are usually identifiable in most smears

➤ Nuclei are round to oval and often eccentrically located. Chromatin pattern is finely granular and some degree of nuclear folding and irregularity is seen in most cases

➤ Nucleoli are often present and my be multiple

➤ Background may contain myxoid material or necrosis, yielding a "tigroid" appearance

■ Alveolar subtype

➤ Smears are of high cellularity

➤ Predominant cell type is small, early rhabdomyoblast, but multinucleated giant cell forms are characteristically found in smears

9-48. Rhabdomyosarcoma (left). Characteristic of rhabdomyosarcomas is a basically small cell pattern showing more marked variability in cell size and shape than is characteristic of other small cell malignancies. These cells may have a "tadpole," spindle shaped, or ovoid appearance. Binucleated and multinucleated giant cells are not infrequent (modified Giemsa stain)

9-49. Rhabdomyosarcoma (right). The presence of multinucleated tumor giant cells in a smear otherwise characteristic of a small cell malignancy strongly suggests the diagnosis of rhabdomyosarcoma (modified Giemsa stain)

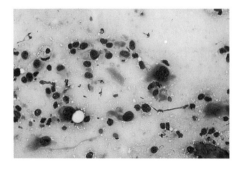
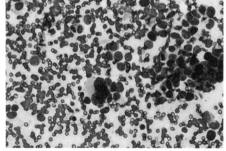

➤ Nuclei have moderately coarse chromatin with one or more nucleoli

➤ Nuclei are often variable in size with irregularity of nuclear contour

➤ A second population of cells showing strap-like appearance along with tadpole-shaped cells and multinucleated giant cells, often with peripherally located nuclei giving a "floret" appearance

➤ Cytoplasmic cross-striations very rare or absent

➤ Necrotic debris present in background

Special Stains and Immunohistochemistry

▢ Tumor cells are positive for vimentin, desmin, and muscle-specific actin in over 90% of cases

▢ Immunohistochemical positivity for MyoD-1 and myogenin are sensitive and relatively specific for rhabdomyosarcomatous differentiation

Modern Techniques for Diagnosis

▢ Alveolar subtype shows specific translocation, either t(2;13)(q35;q14) or t(1;13)(p36;q14)

Differential Diagnosis

▢ Malignant lymphoma

➤ Monomorphic infiltrate of lymphoid cells

➤ Numerous lymphoglandular bodies present in the background

➤ Positive staining with markers for either B-cell or T-cell differentiation

▢ Ewing's sarcoma/PNET

➤ Immunohistochemical staining for FLI-1 or O13

➤ More uniform population with some smears showing bimodal distribution of cell size, but prominent variability of cell size and shape as seen in rhabdomyosarcoma is absent

➤ Characteristic EWSR translocation seen

PEARLS

★ Alveolar rhabdomyosarcoma shows specific translocations, resulting in the PAX3/FKH fusion or the PAX7/FKHR fusion

★ Of all small cell malignancies, rhabdomyosarcomas show the greatest variability in cell size and shape, including the prominence of binucleate and multinucleated giant cell forms

CHONDROMA

Clinical Features

▢ Common benign neoplasm of bone with peak age of occurrence in the second decade of life

▢ Most common sites of occurrence small tubular bones of hands and feet, femur, and humerus

Cytopathologic Features

▢ Smears of low cellularity contain globules of hyaline cartilage

▢ Tissue fragments are of low cellularity with chondrocytes lying singly within lacunae

▢ Chondrocytes contain single small rounded nuclei with a condensed chromatin

▢ Binucleated chondrocytes extremely rare or absent

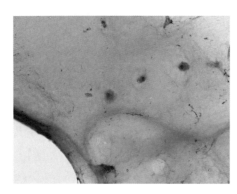

9-50. Chondroma. Smears obtained from chondromas are of low cellularity and characterized by fragments of hyaline cartilage. These tissue fragments have abundant stromal tissue with scattered bland mononuclear chondrocytes. The chondrocyte nuclei are small and round to ovoid. Nuclear crowding and binucleation are not characteristics of chondroma (H&E)

Special Stains and Immunohistochemistry
■ Noncontributory

Modern Techniques for Diagnosis
■ Noncontributory

Differential Diagnosis
■ Chondrosarcoma
  ➤ Enchondromas are essentially inseparable from well-differentiated chondrosarcomas by cytologic analysis
  ➤ Higher grade chondrosarcomas show greater cellularity with more nuclear atypia and a prominent population of single cells lying free in the background
  ➤ Chondrosarcomas more frequently show myxoid matrix, in addition to hyaline cartilage
■ Chordoma
  ➤ Abundant myxoid/chrondroid substance
  ➤ Presence of physaliferous cells

PEARLS

★ Radiographic correlation essential for accurate cytologic diagnosis
★ Presence of a spindle cell component is more suggestive of chondrosarcoma than chondroma

CHONDROSARCOMA

Clinical Features
■ Majority of patients over forty years of age and present with pain or local swelling
■ Most commonly arise in pelvis, ribs, femur, and humerus

Cytopathologic Features
■ Smear cellularity and appearance depends on chondrosarcoma grade
■ Low-grade chondrosarcomas are dominated by fragments of hyaline cartilage with low to at most moderate cellularity
■ Nuclei in grade I sarcomas appear bland and overlap pattern seen in chondroma
■ Small uniform chondrocytes may be found loose in background, but tissue fragments dominate smears
■ Grade I chondrosarcomas have binucleated cells that may be slightly larger or more spindle shaped than seen in chondromas
■ Grade II and III chondrosarcomas contain large fragments of hyaline cartilage or chondromyxoid matrix in which are dispersed large numbers of atypical chondrocytes, including spindle forms

9-51. Grade II Chondrosarcoma *(left).* This aspirate obtained from a grade II chondrosarcoma shows a tissue fragment composed of hyaline cartilage in which are dispersed an increased number of chondrocytes forming small aggregates. Some chondrocytes are binucleated. Overall cellularity is higher than seen in chondromas and nuclear hyperchromasia and size are greater than is characteristic of chondromas (H&E)

9-52. Grade II Chondrosarcoma *(right).* Grade II chondrosarcoma show abundant myxoid/chondroid ground substance, which entraps and partially obscures the neoplastic chondrocytes. Neoplastic chondrocytes have hyperchromatic nuclei with slightly irregular nuclear membranes. Overall cellularity is greater than that seen in chondromas (modified Giemsa stain)

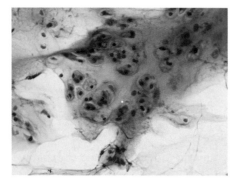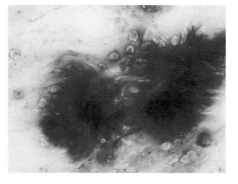

■ Myxoid/chondroid matrix may be so prominent as to obscure nuclear features

■ Grade III chondrosarcomas show marked nuclear atypia with prominent numbers of spindle shaped and pleomorphic malignant chondrocytes

Special Stains and Immunohistochemistry
■ Positive staining for S-100 protein is helpful in high-grade lesions

Modern Diagnostic Techniques
■ Noncontributory

Differential Diagnosis
■ Enchondroma
➤ Enchondromas may be inseparable from grade I chondrosarcomas
➤ Enchondromas are dominated by fragments of hyaline cartilage containing only uninucleated chondrocytes
➤ Bland nuclear features with absence of binucleated cells
■ Chordoma
➤ More abundant myxoid/chondroid background substance with entrapped round, ovoid and polygonal stromal cells
➤ Physaliferous cells prominent in chordomas
■ Chondroblastic oteosarcoma
➤ Radiographic and clinical features help separate these lesions, with osteosarcomas occurring in a younger age group

9-53. High-grade chondrosarcoma. High-grade chondrosarcomas are characterized by cellular smears containing round to polygonal cells. These cells have moderate to abundant cytoplasm. The nuclei are hyperchromatic and in high-grade lesions may contain distinct nucleoli. In high-grade chondrosarcomas, the chondroid matrix may be scant. When present it has a myxoid/chondroid appearance rather than classic hyaline cartilage (modified Giemsa stain)

PEARLS
★ Clinical and radiographic correlation essential for accurate diagnosis
★ Importance of aspirate is to document a cartilaginous lesion with radiologist usually able to separate enchondroma from chondrosarcoma

CHORDOMA

Clinical Features
■ Low-grade neoplasm with wide age distribution between twenty and eighty years and equal sex incidence
■ Most frequent sites of occurrence are base of skull, spheno-occipital area, and sacrococcygeal area

Cytopathologic Features
■ Abundant myxoid/chondroid matrix lying free in background and as tissue clumps
■ Large cells with abundant, multiply vacuolated cytoplasm (physaliphorous cells)
■ Second population of small, round, ovoid cells with modest amounts of granular cytoplasm
■ Nuclei within both vacuolated and granular cells are bland with fine chromatin and small nucleoli
■ Some cells may have a signet ring appearance

Special Stains and Immunohistochemistry
■ Neoplastic cells are immunoreactive for both S-100 protein and cytokeratin

9-54. Chordoma. Aspirates from chordomas are characterized by abundant background myxoid material. This myxoid material often obscures the cellular component in air-dried material. Characteristic of chordomas is the presence of physaliferous cells. These cells characteristically have magenta intracytoplasmic inclusions, which displace the nucleus to one edge of the cell (modified Giemsa stain)

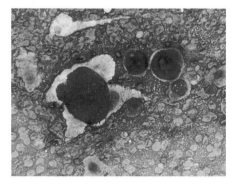

Modern Diagnostic Techniques
■ Noncontributory

Differential Diagnosis
■ Chondrosarcoma
➤ Lack physaliphorous cells characteristic of chordoma
➤ Lack keratin positivity while they express S-100 protein
■ Mucin-rich adenocarcinoma
➤ May contain prominent number of signet ring cells but lack true multivacuolated physaliphorous cells
➤ Express cytokeratins but lack S-100 protein expression

PEARLS

★ Recognition of physaliphorous cells caught in an abundant myxoid/chondroid matrix is characteristic of these lesions
★ Immunohistochemical expression of both S-100 protein and cytokeratins in a myxoid lesion is virtually diagnostic of chordoma

OSTEOSARCOMA

Clinical Features
■ After myeloma, osteosarcoma is the most common malignant tumor of bone
■ Majority of patients are male, most frequently between the ages of ten and twenty years
■ Presents with pain or palpable mass
■ Most common bones involved are femur, tibia, humerus, and pelvis

Cytopathologic Features
■ Moderate to highly cellular smears containing fragments of osteoid and cartilaginous matrix in background
■ Conventional intramedullary type shows a prominent population of pleomorphic spindle-shaped and ovoid cells
■ Subpopulation of plasmacytoid cells containing cytoplasmic vacuoles and intracytoplasmic small red granules (air-dried smears)
■ Anaplastic multinucleated giant cells present
■ Many smears contain a prominent number of mitotic figures, some of which are atypical in form
■ Matrix material appears as clumps and streamers of pink matrix representing osteoid (air-dried smears)
■ Chondroblastic osteosarcomas are dominated by myxoid/chondroid material with little true osteoid being present in smears

9-55. Osteosarcoma *(left)*. Aspirates of osteosarcomas are of moderate to high cellularity. Characteristically, they are composed of atypical round to ovoid cells. Of diagnostic importance is the presence of osteoid matrix, often having a filamentous appearance or forming aggregates, which entrap the neoplastic osteoblasts. Osteoid has a characteristic magenta appearance (modified Giemsa stain)

9-56. Osteosarcoma *(right)*. Fragments of osteoid frequently entrap neoplastic osteoblasts, but may lie free of a cellular component. The neoplastic osteoblasts have hyperchromatic nuclei which may be displaced to one edge of the cell (modified Giemsa stain)

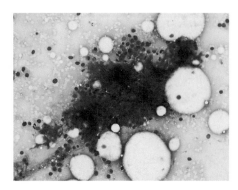
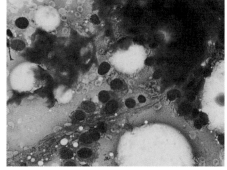

▪ Telangiectatic osteosarcomas are dominated by a bloody background with scattered ovoid, polygonal, or spindle-shaped cells showing moderate to marked nuclear atypia
▪ Rare fragments of pink, dense matrix (osteoid) best seen in air-dried smears
▪ Paraosteal and low-grade central osteosarcomas reveal osteoblasts with mild to moderate nuclear atypia
▪ Streamers of dense, pink osteoid matrix (air-dried smears)

Special Stains and Immunohistochemistry
▪ Neoplastic cells stain strongly for alkaline phosphotase

Modern Diagnostic Techniques
▪ Noncontributory

Differential Diagnosis
▪ Chondrosarcoma
  ➤ May be cytologically indistinguishable from chondroblastic osteosarcoma; age and radiographic findings may help separate these two lesions
▪ Pleomorphic sarcoma, not otherwise specified
  ➤ The finding of clumps of osteoid or osteoid streamers directly associated with malignant cells establishes the diagnosis of osteosarcoma; anaplastic mesenchymal malignancies without demonstrable osteoid formation cannot be definitively diagnosed as oteosarcoma, but diagnosis may be suggested by radiographic features

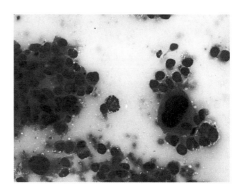

9-57. Intramedullary osteosarcoma. Conventional high-grade intramedullary osteosarcomas show considerable pleomorphism with multinucleated and binucleated tumor giant cells being present. Mitotic figures including atypical forms are found. Many osteoblasts have a slightly vacuolated cytoplasm which may be associated with small dark purple matrix granules (modified Giemsa stain)

PEARLS

★ Clinical, radiographic, and cytologic correlation essential for accurate diagnosis
★ The finding of direct osteoid production by neoplastic cells establishes the diagnosis of osteosarcoma in the appropriate radiographic background

HEMANGIOMA

Clinical Features
▪ Capillary hemangioma most common form and typically occurs in infants and young children
▪ Females more often affected than males
▪ Most commonly occurs in skin and subcutaneous tissue of head and neck region
▪ Initial rapid growth phase followed by stabilization then involution in a majority of cases

Cytopathologic Features
▪ Smears are dominated by red blood cells in which are scattered rare clusters of spindle-shaped cells and spindle cells lying singly
▪ Spindle cells may for short branching tube-like structures in which a central lumen containing red blood cells can be seen
▪ Nuclei are ovoid to spindle shaped, bland with a fine uniform chromatin

Special Stains and Immunohistochemistry
▪ Cells are immunohistochemically positive for CD31, CD34, and Factor VIII

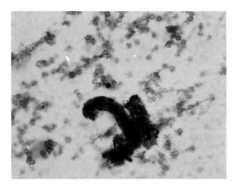

9-58. Hemangioma. Hemangiomas are characteristically dominated by red blood cells. Scattered among the red blood cells are rare capillary segments. The segments have an internal lumen, which may contain red blood cells. The tubular segments are composed short spindle-shaped cells with bland hyperchromatic nuclei (H&E)

Modern Diagnostic Techniques
- Noncontributory

Differential Diagnosis
- Low-grade angiosarcoma
  - ➤ May be cytologically inseparable but clinical features are usually helpful in distinguishing these two lesions
  - ➤ Angiosarcomas are associated with smears of slightly greater cellularity and larger numbers of single cells
- Kaposi's sarcoma
  - ➤ Clinical setting with immunosuppressed individual supports diagnosis of Kaposi's sarcoma
  - ➤ Low to moderate cellularity smears containing both single spindle-shaped cells and three-dimensional clusters showing mild nuclear atypia
  - ➤ Tissue fragments may show slit-like vascular spaces
  - ➤ Scattered hemosiderin granules within cellular component and background

PEARLS

★ Tissue fragments composed of cytologically bland spindle-shaped cells and epithelioid cells forming tubular clusters with internal red blood cells is essentially diagnostic of hemangioma in the appropriate clinical setting

ANGIOSARCOMA

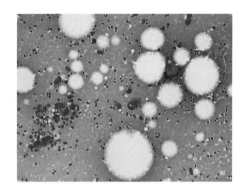

9-59. Angiosarcoma. Aspirates of angiosarcomas contain abundant blood. Amid the sea of red blood cells are scattered atypical spindle-shaped, polygonal, or ovoid neoplastic cells. In high grade angiosarcomas, the component cells frequently have an ovoid or epithelioid appearance with moderate amounts of cytoplasm. The cytoplasm may contain a single vacuole that displaces the nucleus to one side. In high-grade angiosarcomas, the nuclei are hyperchromatic and frequently contain huge nucleoli (modified Giemsa stain)

Clinical Features
- More common in women than men
- Wide age range, with the majority of cases occurring between 40 and 90 years of age
- Occur in a wide variety of body sites including skin of face and scalp and upper arm and axilla (post mastectomy)

Cytopathologic Features
- Cellularity variable, ranging from low to high
- All cases characterized by hemorrhagic background
- Tumor cells are polymorphous and composed of spindle-shaped, round, oval, or polygonal epithelial-like cells
- Occasional giant cells present
- Nuclear atypia varies widely, with cutaneous lesions in the elderly showing mild to at most moderate nuclear atypia; angiosarcoma of deep soft tissues show higher degrees of atypia, including nuclear anaplasia
- Polygonal epithelioid cells may show single large cytoplasmic vacuole
- Erythrophagocytosis and hemosiderin deposition may be seen
- Mitotic figures rare and necrosis generally absent

Special Stains and Immunohistochemistry
- Majority of cases are CD31, CD34, and Factor VIII positive

Modern Diagnostic Techniques
- Noncontributory

Differential Diagnosis

- Hemangioma
  - ➤ Hemangiomas are generally less cellular and lack any significant nuclear atypia
- Melanoma
  - ➤ Some melanomas may have a markedly hemorrhagic background containing discohesive cells
  - ➤ Melanin pigment may be present and must be separated from hemosiderin (iron stain)
  - ➤ Melanomas are S-100 protein, HMB-45, and melan A positive and lack staining for vascular markers

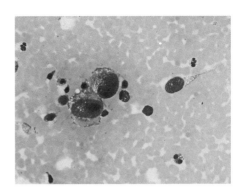

9-60. High-grade angiosarcoma.
In high-grade angiosarcomas, the individual cells often have an oval appearance with moderate amounts of cytoplasm surrounding hyperchromatic nuclei with huge nucleoli. The cytoplasm may have a slightly foamy appearance. The background contains a mixture of lymphocytes and plasma cells along with numerous red blood cells (modified Giemsa stain)

PEARLS

✭ Some angiosarcomas are characterized by single anaplastic cells with an oval, epithelioid, or polygonal appearance and do not show formation of vascular channels

✭ Some high-grade angiosarcomas will show formation of intracytoplasmic lumen, requiring separation from signet ring cell adenocarcinomas and hemangioendotheliomas

✭ Immunohistochemistry for CD31, CD34, and Factor VIII helpful in diagnosis

REFERENCES

PLEOMORPHIC LIPOMA

Akerman M, Rydholm A. Aspiration cytology of lipomatous tumors: a 10-year experience at an orthopedic oncology center. *Diagn Cytopathol* 1987; 3:295–301.

Guo Z, Voytovich M, Kurtycz DFI, Hoerl HD. Fine-needle aspiration diagnosis of spindle-cell lipoma: a case report and review of the literature. *Diagn Cytopathol* 2000; 23:362–365.

Lew WYC. Spindle cell lipoma of breast: a case report and literature review. *Diagn Cytopathol* 1993; 9:434–437.

Lopez-rios F, Albert N, Perez-Barrios A, de Agustin PP. Fine-needle aspiration of pleomorphic lipoma. *Diagn Cytopathol* 2001; 24:296–297.

Rigby HS, Wilson YG, Cawthorn SJ, Ibrahim NB. Fine needle aspiration of pleomrophic lipoma: a potential pitfall of cyto-diagnosis. *Cytopathology* 1993; 4:55–58.

Walaas L, Kindblom L-G. Lipomatous tumors: a correlative cytologic and histologic study of 27 tumors examined by fine needle aspiration cytology. *Human Pathol* 1985; 16:6–18.

MYELOLIPOMA

Saboorian MH, Timmerman TG, Ashfaqu R, Maiese RL. Fine-needle aspiration of a presacral myelolipoma: a case presentation with flow cytometry and immunohistochemical studies. *Diagn Cytopathol* 1999; 20:47–51.

PLEOMORPHIC LIPOSARCOMA

Akerman M, Rydholm A. Aspiration cytology of lipomatous tumors: a 10 year experience at an orthopedic oncology center. *Diagn Cytopathol* 1987; 3:295–301.

Attal H, Jensen J, Reyes CV. Myxoid liposarcoma of the anterior mediastinum. Diagnosis by fine-needle aspiration biopsy. *Acta Cytol* 1995; 39:511–513.

Dalla Palma P, Barbazza R. Well-differentiated liposarcoma of the paratesticular areas: report of a case with fine-needle aspiration preoperative diagnosis and review of the literature. *Diagn Cytopathol* 199; 6:421–426.

Shattuck MC, Victor TA. Cytologic features of well-differentiated sclerosing liposarcoma in aspirated samples. *Acta Cytol* 1988; 32:896–901.

Vicandi B, Jimenez-Hefferman J, Lopez-Ferrer P, Gonzalez-Permato P, Viguer JM. Cytologic features of round cell liposarcoma. A report on five patients. *Cancer (Cancer Cytopathol)* 2003; 99:28–32.

SYNOVIAL SARCOMA

Akerman M, Ryd W, Skytting B. Fine-needle aspiration of synovial sarcoma: criteria for diagnosis. Retrospective reexamination of 37 cases, including ancillary diagnostics. A Scandinavian Sarcoma Group study. *Diagn Cytopathol* 2003; 28:232–238.

Bergman S, Brownlee NA, Geisinger KR, Ward WG, Pettinati MJ, Katy P, Ellis E, Beaty MW, Kilpatrick SE. Diagnostic pitfalls associated with fine-needle aspiration biopsy in a patient with the myxoid variant of monophasic fibrous synovial sarcoma. *Diagn Cytopathol* 2006; 34:761–767.

Kilpatrick SE, Teat LA, Stanley MW, Ward WG, Savage PD, Geisinger KR. Fine-needle aspiration biopsy of synovial sarcoma: a cytomorphologic analysis of primary, recurrent and metastatic tumors. *Am J Clin Pathol* 1996; 106:769–775.

Klijanienko J, Caillaud J-M, Lagace R, Viehl P. Cytohistologic correlations in 56 synovial sarcomas in 36 patients. The Institut Curie experience. *Diagn Cytopathol* 2002; 27:96–102.

GRANULAR CELL TUMOR

Glant MD, Wall RW, Ransburg R. Endobronchial granular cell tumor: cytology of a new case and review of the literature. *Acta Cytol* 1979; 23:477–482.

Liu K, Madden JF, Olatidoye BA, Dodd LG. Features of benign granular cell tumor on fine-needle aspiration. *Acta Cytol* 1999; 43:552–557.

Mazur MT, Shultz JJ, Myers JL. Granular cell tumor. Immunohistochemical analysis of 21 benign tumors and one malignant tumor. *Acta Pathol Lab Med* 1990; 114:692–696.

ALVEOLAR SOFT PART SARCOMA

Fukuda T, Saito M, Nakaima T. Giemsa staining for alveolar soft part sarcoma. *Acta Cytol* 1999; 43:519–521.

Husein M, Nguyen G-K. Alveolar soft part sarcoma. Report of a case diagnosed by needle aspiration cytology and electron microscopy. *Acta Cytol* 1995; 39:951–954.

Lograno R, Wojtowycz MM, Wunderlich DW, Warner TF, Kurtycz DFI. Fine needle aspiration cytology and core biopsy in the diagnosis of alveolar soft part sarcoma presenting with lung metastatases. *Acta Cytol* 199; 464–470.

Lopez-Ferrer P, Jimenez-Hefferman JA, Vicardi B, Gonzalez-Peramato P, Viguer JM. Cytologic features of alveolar soft part sarcoma: report of three cases. *Diagn Cytopathol* 2002; 27: 115–119.

EPITHELIOID SARCOMA

Hasegawa T, Matsuno Y, Shimoda T, Umeda T, Yokoyama R, Hirohashi S. Proximal type epithelioid sarcoma: a clinicopathologic study of 20 cases. *Mod Pathol* 2001; 14:655–663.

Hernandez-Ortiz MJ, Valensuela-Ruiz P, Gonzalez-Estecha A, Santana-Acosta A, Ruiz-Villaepesa A. Fine needle aspiration of cytology of primary epithelioid sarcoma of the vulva. A case report. *Acta Cytol* 1995; 39:100–103.

Jogai S, Gupta SK, Goel A, Ahluwali J, Joshi K. Epithelioid sarcoma. Report of a case with fine needle aspiration diagnosis. *Acta Cytol* 2001; 45:271–273.

Pohar-Marinsek Z, Zidar A. Epithelioid sarcoma in FNAB smears. *Diagn Cytopathol* 1994; 11:367.

Zeppa P, Errico ME, Palombini L. Epithelioid sarcoma: report of two cases diagnosed by fine-needle aspiration biopsy with immunocytochemical correlation. *Diagn Cytopathol* 1999; 21:405–408.

CLEAR CELL SARCOMA OF SOFT TISSUES

Almeida MM, Nunes AM, Frable WJ. Malignatn melanoma of soft tissue. A report of three cases with diagnosis of fine needle aspiration cytology. *Acta Cytol* 1994; 38:241–246.

Caraway NP, Fanning CV, Wojcik EM, Staerkel GA, Benjamin RS, Ordonez NG. Cytology of malignant melanoma of soft parts: fine-needle aspirates and exfoliative specimens. *Diagn Cytopathol* 1993; 9:632–638.

Rau AR, Kini H, Verghese R. "Tigroid" background in fine-needle aspiration cytology of clear cell sarcoma. *Diagn Cytopathol* 2006; 34:355–357.

Schwartz JC, Zollars PR. Fine needle aspiration cytology of malignant melanoma of soft parts. Report of two cases. *Acta Cytol* 1990; 34:347–400.

Shabb NS, Boulos F, Tawil A, Hassein M, Hourani M. Clear cell sarcoma (malignant melanoma of soft parts): fine-needle aspiration cytology of highly pigmented tumor. *Diagn Cytopathol* 2003; 28:313–315.

Tong TR, Chow T-C, Chan OW-H, Lee K-C, Yeung S-H, Lam A, Yu C-K. Clear cell sarcoma diagnosis by fine-needle aspirative cytologic, histology and ultrastructural features; potential pitfalls; and literature review. *Diagn Cytopathol* 2002; 26:174–180.

EXTRARENAL RHABDOID TUMOR

Akhtar M, Kfoury H, Haider A, Sackey K, Ali MA. Fine-needle aspiration biopsy diagnosis of extrarenal malignant rhabdoid tumor. *Diagn Cytopathol* 1994; 11:271–276.

Perez JS, Perez-Guillermo M, Bernal AB, Lopez TM, Lopez FC. Malignant rhabdoid tumor of soft tissues: a clinicopathological and immunohistochemical study. *Diagn Cytopathol* 1992; 8:369–373.

White FV, Dehner LP, Belchis DA, et al. Congenital disseminated malignant rhabdoid tumor: a distinct clinicopathologic entity demonstrating abnormalities of chromosome 22q11. *Am J Surg Pathol* 1999; 23:249.

LANGERHANS CELL HISTIOCYTOSIS

Elsheikh T, Silverman JF, Wakely PE Jr, Holbrook CT, Jushi VV. Fine needle aspiration cytology of Langerhans cell histiocytosis (eosinophilic granuloma) of bone in children. *Diagn Cytopathol* 1991; 7:261–266.

Kilpatrick SE, Wenger DE, Gilchrist GS, et al. Langerhans cell histiocytosis (histiocytosis X) of bone: a clinicopathologic analysis of 263 pediatric and adult cases. *Cancer.* 1995;76:2471.

Shabb N, Fanning CV, Carrasco CH, Guo SQ, Katz RL, Ayala AG, Raymond AK, Cangir A. Diagnosis of eosiniophilic granuloma of bone by fine needle aspiration with concurrent institution of therapy. *Diagn Cytopathol* 1993; 9:3–12.

Van Heerde P, Maarten Egler R. The cytology of Langerhans cell histiocytosis (histiocytosis X). *Cytopathology* 1991; 2:149–158.

PSEUDOSARCOMATOUS SPINDLE CELL LESIONS

Anglo-Henry MR, Seaquist MB, Marsh WL. Fine needle aspiration of proliferative fasciitis. A case report. *Acta Cytol* 1985; 29:882–886.

Dahl I, Akerman M. Nodular fasciitis: a correlative cytologic and histologic study of 13 cases. *Acta Cytol* 1981; 25:215–223.

Dodd LG, Martinez S. Fine-needle aspiration cytology of pseudosarcomatous lesions of soft tissue. *Diagn Cytopathol* 2001; 24:28–35.

Kaw YT, Cuesta RA. Nodular fasciitis of the orbit diagnosed by fine needle aspiration cytology. A case report. *Acta Cytol* 1993; 37:957–960.

Layfield LJ, Crim J, Gupta D. Fine-needle aspiration findindgs in nodular myositis: a case report. *Diagn Cytopathol* 2000; 13:343–346.

Stanley MW, Skoog L, Tani EM, Horwitz CA. Nodular fasciitis: spontaneous resolution following diagnosis by fine-needle aspiration. *Diagn Cytopathol* 1993; 9:322–324.

MYOSITIS OSSIFICANS

de Almeida MM, Abecassis N, Almeida MO, Mendonca ME. Fine-needle aspiration cytology of myositis ossificans: a case report. *Diagn Cytopathol* 1994; 10:41–43.

Popok SM, Naib ZM. Fine-needle aspiration cytology of myositis ossificans. *Diagn Cytopathol* 1985; 1:236–240.

Röösen B, Herrlin K, Rydholm A, Akerman M. Pseudomalignant myositis ossificans. Clinical, radiologic and cytologic diagnosis. *Acta Orthop Scand* 1989; 60:457–460.

Wakely PE, Almedia M, Frable WJ. Fine-needle aspiration biopsy cytology of myositis ossificans. *Mod Pathol* 1994; 7:23–25.

ELASTOFIBROMA

Domanski HA, Carlen B, Sloth M, Rydholm A. Elastofibroma dorsi has distinct cytomorphologic features, making diagnostic surgical biopsy unnecessary: cytomorphologic study with clinical, radiologic and electron microscopic correlations. *Diagn Cytopathol* 2003: 29:327–333.

Harigupal M, Seshan SV, DeLellis RA, Yankelevitz D, Vazquez M. Aspiration cytology of elastofibroma dorsi: case report with ultrastructural and immunohistochemical findings. *Diagn Cytopathol* 2002; 26:310–313.

Nakamara Y, Ohta Y, Ztoh S, Nano, Y, Umeda A, Shima H, Tomada N. Elastofibroma dorsi: cytologic, histologic, immunohistochemical and ultrastructural studies. *Acta Cytol* 1992; 36:559–562.

FIBROMATOSES

Apple SK, Nieberg RK, Hirschowitz SL. Fine needle aspiration diagnosis of fibromatosis colli: a report of three cases. *Acta Cytol* 1997; 41:1373–1376.

Kurtycz DF, Logrono R, Hoerl HD, Heatley DG. Diagnosis of fibromatosis colli by fine-needle aspiration. *Diagn Cytopathol* 2000; 23:338–342.

McLeod DL, Geisinger KR, Hopkins MB III, Silverman JF. Fine needle aspiration cytology of the fibromatoses: a clinical and cytopathologic assessment. *Acta Cytol* 1987; 31:683.

Raab SS, Silverman JF, McLeod DL, Benning TL, Geisinger KR. Fine needle aspiration biopsy of fibromatoses. *Acta Cytol* 1993; 37:323–328.

Wakely PE Jr, Prince WG, Frable WJ. Sternomastoid tumor of infancy (fibromatosis colli): diagnosis by aspiration cytology. *Mod Pathol* 1989; 2:378–381.

Zaharopoulos P, Wang JY. Fine-needle aspiration cytology in fibromatoses. *Diagn Cytopathol* 1992; 8:73–78.

SOLITARY FIBROUS TUMOR

Ali SZ, Hoon V, Hoda S, Heelan R, Zakowski MF. Solitary fibrous tumor. A cytologic-histologic study with clinical, radiologic, and immunohistochemical correlations. *Cancer* 1997; 81:116–121.

Clayton AC, Salomao DR, Keeney GL, Mascimento AG. Solitary fibrous tumor: a study of cytologic features of six cases diagnosed by fine-needle aspiration. *Diagn Cytopathol* 2001; 25:172–176.

Drachenberg CB, Bourquin PM, Cochran LM, Burke KC, Kumar D, White CS, Papadimitriou JC. Fine needle aspiration biopsy of solitary fibrous tumors. Report of two cases with histologic, immunohistochemical and ultrastructural correlation. *Acta Cytol* 1998; 42:1003–1010.

Dusenbery D, Grimes MM, Frable WJ. Fine-needle aspiration cytology of localized fibrous tumor of pleura. *Diagn Cytopathol* 1992; 8:444–450.

DERMATOFIBROSARCOMA PROTUBERANS AND GIANT CELL FIBROBLASTOMA

Domanski HA, Gustafson P. Cytologic features of primary, recurrent, and metastatic dermatofibrosarcoma protuberans. *Cancer* 2002; 96:351–361.

Enjoji M, Hashimoto HL. Diagnosis of soft tissue sarcomas. *Pathol Res Pract* 1984; 178: 215–226.

Kim K, Goldblatt PJ. Fine needle aspiration cytology of sarcomas metastatic to the lung. *Acta Cytol* 1986; 30:688–694.

Layfield LJ, Gopez EV. Fine-needle aspiration cytology of giant cell fibroblastoma: case report and review of the literature. *Diagn Cytopathol* 2002; 26:398–403.

Perry MD, Furlong JW, Johnston WW. Fine-needle aspiration cytology of metastatic dermatofibroma protuberans. A case report. *Acta Cytol* 1986; 30:507–512.

Powers CN, Hurt MA, Frable WJ. Fine-needle aspiration biopsy: dermatofibrosarcoma protuberans. *Diagn Cytopathol* 1993; 9:145–250.

FIBROSARCOMA

Enjoji M, Hashimoto HL. Diagnosis of soft tissue sarcomas. *Pathol Res Pract* 1984; 178: 215–226.

Kim K, Goldblatt PJ. Fine needle aspiration cytology of sarcomas metastatic to the lung. *Acta Cytol* 1986; 30:688–694.

SCHWANNOMA (NEURILEMMOMA)

Dahl I, Hagmar B, Idvall I. Benign solitary neurilemoma (schwannoma). A correlative cytological and histological study of 28 cases. *Acta Pathol Microbiol Immunol Scand [A]* 1984;
92:91–101.

Domanski HA, Akerman M, Engellau J, Gustafson P, Mertens F, Rydholm A. Fine-needle aspiration of neruilemmoma (schwannoma). A clinicocytopathologic study of 116 patients. *Diagn
Cytopathol* 2006; 34:403–412.

Kapila K, Mathur S, Verma K. Schwannomas: a pitfall in the diagnosis of pleomorphic adenomas
on fine-needle aspiration cytology. *Diagn Cytopathol* 2002; 27:53–59.

Klijanienko J, Caillaud JM, Lagace R. Cytohistologic correlations in schwannomas (neurilemmomas) including "ancient", cellular, and epithelioid variants. *Diagn Cytopathol* 2006;
34:517–522.

Laforga JB. Cellular schwannoma: report of a case diagnosed intraoperatively with the aid of
cytologic imprints. *Diagn Cytopathol* 2003; 29:95–100.

Mooney EE, Layfield LJ, Dodd LG. Fine-needle aspiration of neural lesions. *Diagn Cytopathol*
1999; 20:1–5.

Ramzy I. Benign schwannoma: demonstration of Verocay bodies using fine needle aspiration.
Acta Cytol 1977; 21:316–319.

Zbieranowski I, Bedard YC. Fine needle aspiration of schwannomas. Value of electron
microscopy and immunocytochemistry in the preoperative diagnosis *Acta Cytol* 1989;
33:381–384.

MALIGNANT PERIPHERAL NERVE SHEATH TUMOR

Dodd LG, Scully S, Layfield LJ. Fine-needle aspiration of epithelioid malignant peripheral nerve
sheath tumor (epithelioid malignant schwannoma). *Diagn Cytopathol* 1997; 17:200–204.

Ducatman BS, Scheithauer BW, Piepgras DG, Reiman HM, Ilstrup DM. Malignant peripheral
nerve sheath tumors. A clinicopathologic study of 120 cases. *Cancer* 1986; 57:2006–2021.

McGee RS, Ward WG, Kilpatrick SE. Malignant peripheral nerve sheath tumor: a fine-needle
aspiration biopsy study. *Diagn Cytopathol* 1997; 17:298–305.

Vendraminelli R, Cavazzana AO, Poletti A, Galligioni A, Pennelli N. Fine needle aspiration cytology of malignant nerve sheath tumors. *Diagn Cytopathol* 1992; 559–562.

Wang AR, Weiss SW, Reed JA, Scott G. PGP 9.5 and N-CAM are sensitive markers for malignant
peripheral nerve sheath tumors (MPNSTs). *Mod Pathol* 2000; 13:16A.

LEIOMYOSARCOMA

Dahl I, Hagmar B, Angervall L. Leiomyosarcoma of the soft tissue. A correlative cytological and
histologic study of 11 cases. *Acta Pathol Microbiol Scand (Sect A)* 1981: 89:285–291.

Tao LC, Davidson DD. Aspiration biopsy cytology of smooth muscle tumors: a cytologic approach
to the differentiation between leiomyosarcoma and leiomyoma. *Acta Cytol* 1993; 37:300.

PLEOMORPHIC RHABDOMYOSARCOMA

Ali F, Smilari TF, Teichberg P, Hajdu SI. Pleomorphic rhabdomyosarcoma of the heart metastatic to bone. Report of a case with fine-needle aspiration biopsy findings. *Acta Cytol* 1995;
39:555–558.

MALIGNANT FIBROUS HISTIOCYTOMA

Berardo MD, Powers CN, Wakely PE Jr, Almeida MO, Frable WJ. Fine-needle aspiration cytopathology of malignant fibrous histiocytoma. *Cancer (Cancer Cytopathol)* 1997; 81:228–237.

Kim K, Goldblatt PJ. Malignant fibrous histiocytoma: cytologic, light microscopic and ultrastructural studies. *Acta Cytol* 1982; 26:507–511.

Klijanienko J, Caillaud J-M, Lagace R, Vielh P. Comparative fine-needle aspiration and pathologic
study of malignant fibrous histiocytoma: cytodiagnostic features of 95 tumors in 71 patients.
Diagn Cytopathol 2003; 29:320–326.

Liu K, Dodge RK, Dodd LG, Layfield LJ. Logistic regression analysis of high-grade spindle cell
neoplasms: a cytologic study. *Acta Cytol* 1999; 43:593–600.

Walaas L, Angervall L, Hagmar B, Säve-Söderbergh J. A correlative cytologic and histologic study
of malignant fibrous histiocytoma: an analysis of 40 cases examined by fine-needle aspiration
cytology. *Diagn Cytopathol* 1986; 2:46–54.

TENOSYNOVIAL GIANT CELL TUMOR, NODULAR AND DIFFUSE TYPES

Agarwal PK, Gupta M, Srivestava A, Agarwal S. Cytomorphology of giant cell tumor of tendon sheath. A report of two cases. *Acta Cytol* 1997; 41:587–589.

Dodd LG, Major NM. Fine-needle aspiration cytology of articular and periarticular lesions. *Cancer (Cytopathology)* 2002; 96:157–165.

Gangane N, Anshu, Skivkumar VB, Sharma SM. Intranuclear inclusions in a case of pigmented villonodular synovitis of the ankle. *Diagn Cytopathol* 2003; 29:349–351.

Lyer VK, Kapila K, Verma K. Fine-needle aspiration cytology of giant cell tumor of tendon sheath. *Diagn Cytopathol* 2003; 29:105–110.

Wakely PE, Frable WJ. Fine-needle aspiration biopsy cytology of giant cell tumor of tendon sheath. *Am J Clin Pathol* 1994; 102:87–90.

Yu GH, Staerkel GA, Kershisnik MM, Varma DGK. Fine-needle aspiration of pigmented villonodular synovitis of the temporomandibular joint masquerading as a primary parotid gland lesion. *Diagn Cytopathol* 1997; 16:47–50.

CONVENTIONAL GIANT CELL TUMOR OF BONE

Sanerkin Ng, Jeffree GM. *Cytology of Bone Tumours. A Colour Atlas with Text.* Philadelphia: J.B. Lippincott Co., 1980, pp. 91–100.

Sneige N, Ayala AG, Carrasco CH, Murray J, Raymond AK. Giant cell tumor of bone: a cytologic study of 24 cases. *Diagn Cytopathol* 1985; 2:111–117.

Vertani A, Fulciniti F, Boshci R, Marino G, Zeppa P, Troncone G, Palombini L. Fine needle aspiration biopsy diagnosis of giant-cell tumor of bone. An experience with nine cases. *Acta Cytol* 1990; 34:863–867.

CHONDROBLASTOMA

Ascoli V, Facciolo F, Muda AO, Martelli M, Nardi F. Chondroblastoma of the rib presenting as an intrathoracic mass. Report of a case with fine needle aspiration biopsy, immunocytochemistry and electron microscopy. *Acta Cytol* 1992; 36:423–429.

Kilpatrick SE, Pike EJ, Geisinger KR, Ward WG. Chondroblastoma of bone: use of fine-needle aspiration biopsy and potential diagnostic pitfalls. *Diagn Cytopathol* 1997; 16:65–71.

Pohar-Marinsek Z, Us-Krasovec M, Lamovec J. Chondroblastoma in fine needle aspirates. *Acta Cytol* 1992; 36:367–370.

INTRAMUSCULAR MYXOMA

Akerman M, Rydholm A. Aspiration cytology of intramuscular myxoma. A comparative clinical, cytologic and histologic study of ten cases. *Acta Cytol* 1983; 27:505–510.

Caraway NP, Staerkel GA, Fanning CV, et al. Diagnosing intramuscular myxoma by fine-needle aspiration: a multidisciplinary approach. *Diagn Cytopathol* 1994; 11:255.

Schwartz HS, Walker R. Recognizable magnetic resonance imaging characteristics of intramuscular myxoma. *Orthopedics* 1997; 20:431.

EWING'S SARCOMA (PRIMITIVE NEUROECTODERMAL TUMOR)

Akhtar M, Ali MA, Sabbah R. Aspiration cytology of Ewing's sarcoma: light and electron microscopic correlation. *Cancer* 1985: 556:2051–2060.

Dahl I, Akerman M, Angerval L. Ewing's sarcoma of bone: a correlative cytological and histological study of 14 cases. *Acta Pathol Microbiol Immunol Scand (Sect A)* 1986; 94:363–369.

Fanning TV, Katz RL, Ayala AG. Fine needle aspiration of Ewing's sarcoma of bone: an analysis of 57 specimens. *Acta Cytol* 1985; 29:932.

Renshaw AA, Perez-Atayde AR, Fletcher JA, et al. Cytology of typical and atypical Ewing's sarcoma/PNET. *Am J Clin Pathol* 1996; 106:620.

RHABDOMYOSARCOMA (EMBRYONAL AND ALVEOLAR SUBTYPES)

Akhtar M, Ali MA, Bakry M, Hug M, Sackey K. Fine-needle aspiration biopsy diagnosis of rhabdomyosarcoma: cytologic, histologic and ultrastructural correlations. *Diagn Cytopathol* 1992; 8:465–474.

Das K, Mirani N, Hameed M, Pliner L, Aisner SC. Fine-needle aspiration cytology of alveolar rhabdomyosarcoma utilizing ThinPrep® liquid-based sample and cytospin preparations: a case confirmed by FKHR break-apart rearrangement by FISH probe. *Diagn Cytopathol* 2006; 34:704–706.

de Jong ASH, van Kessel-van Vark M, van Heerde P. Fine-needle aspiration biopsy diagnosis of rhabdomyosarcoma; an immunocytochemical study. *Acta Cytol* 1987; 31:573–577.

Seidal T, Walaas L, Kindblom LG, Angervall L. Cytology of embryonal rhabdomyosarcoma: a cytologic light microscopic, electron microscopic and immunohistochemical study of serum cases. *Diagn Cytopathol* 1988; 4:242–299.

CHONDROMA

Xiaojing P, Xiangcheng Y. Cytodiagnosis of bone tumors by fine-needle aspiration. *Acta Cytol* 1985; 29:570–575.

Walaas L, Kindblom LG, Gunterberg B, Bergh P. Light and electron microscopic examination of fine-needle aspirates in the preoperative diagnosis of cartilaginous tumors. *Diagn Cytopathol* 1990; 5:396–468.

CHONDROSARCOMA

Dodd LG. Fine-needle aspiration of chondrosarcoma. *Diagn Cytopathol* 2006; 34:413–418.

Lerma E, Tani E, Brosjo O, Bauer H, Söderlund V, Skoog L. Diagnosis and grading of chondrosarcoma on FNA biopsy material. *Diagn Cytopathol* 2003; 28:13–17.

Xiaojing P, Xiangcheng Y. Cytodiagnosis of bone tumors by fine-needle aspiration. *Acta Cytol* 1985; 29:570–575.

Walaas L, Kindblom LG, Gunterberg B, Bergh P. Light and electron microscopic examination of fine-needle aspirates in the preoperative diagnosis of cartilaginous tumors. *Diagn Cytopathol* 1990; 5:396–468.

CHORDOMA

Layfield LJ. Cytologic differential diagnosis of myxoid and mucinous neoplasms of the sacrum and parasacral soft tissues. *Diagn Cytopathol* 2003; 28:264–271.

Walaas L, Kindblom LG. Fine-needle aspiration biopsy in the preoperative diagnosis of chordoma: a study of 17 cases with application of electron microscopic, histochemical and immunocytochemical examination. *Hum Pathol* 1991; 22:22–28.

OSTEOSARCOMA

Dodd LG, Scully SP, Cothran RL, Harrelson JM. Utility of fine-needle aspiration in the diagnosis of primary osteosarcoma. *Diagn Cytopathol* 2002; 27:350–353.

Layfield LJ, Glasgow BJ, Anders KH, Mirra JM. Fine needle aspiration of primary bone lesions. *Acta Cytol* 1987; 31:177–184.

Nicol KK, Ward WG, Savage PD, Kilpatrick SE. Fine-needle biopsy of skeletal versus extraskeletal osteosarcoma. *Cancer* 1998; 84:176–185.

Ward WG, Kilpatrick S. Fine needle aspiration biopsy of primary bone tumors. *Clin Orthop Rel Res* 2000; 373:80–87.

HEMANGIOMA

Layfield LJ, Mooney EE, Dodd LG. Not by blood alone: diagnosis of hemangiomas by fine-needle aspiration. *Diagn Cytopathol* 1998; 19:250–254.

Sharm SG, Aron M, Kapila K, Ray R. Epithelioid hemangioma: morphological presentation on aspiration smears. *Diagn Cytopathol* 2006; 34:830–833.

ANGIOSARCOMA

Gagner J-P, Yim JH, Yang G-CH. Fine-needle aspiration cytology of epithelioid angiosarcoma: a diagnostic dilemma. *Diagn Cytopathol* 2005; 33:429–433.

Klijanienko J, Caillaud J-M, Lagace R, Vielh P. Cytohistologic correlations in angiosarcoma including classic and epithelioid variants: Institut Curie's Experience. *Diagn Cytopathol* 2003; 29:140–145.

Minimo C, Zakowski M, Lin O. Cytologic findings of malignant vascular neoplasms: a study of twenty-four cases. 2002; 26:349–355.

10

Thyroid Gland

Paolo Gattuso, Kristin Galan, and Odile David

ACUTE THYROIDITIS

Clinical Features
- Rare clinical entity
- Majority of patients (60%) have a preexisting thyroid disease, usually goiter
- In children, predisposing factors include pyriform sinus fistula or thyroglossal duct remnant
- Fever, pain, neck swelling, and tender thyroid on palpation
- Majority of the cases are bacterial

Cytologic Features
- Neutrophil exudate
- Histiocytes
- Granulation tissue, reparative changes
- Necrotic debris
- Microorganisms may be present: most common – bacteria; rarely viral inclusions, fungal forms, and *Pneumocystis carinii* have been reported

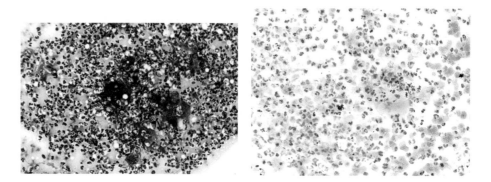

10-1A. Acute thyroiditis *(left)*. Neutrophilic exudade (modified Giemsa stain)

10-1B. Acute thyroiditis *(right)*. Gram stain showing Gram-positive cocci

Special Stains and Immunohistochemistry

- Gram stain: positive for bacterial forms
- PAS and GMS: positive for fungal forms and *P. carinii*

Modern Techniques for Diagnosis

- Noncontributory

Differential Diagnosis

- Necrotic tumor
  - ➤ Necrotic material
  - ➤ Acute inflammatory cells
  - ➤ Presence of viable tumor cells
- Giant cell carcinoma
  - ➤ Numerous neutrophils may be present in the aspirate of anaplastic carcinoma
- Granulomatous thyroiditis
  - ➤ Early phase may show numerous neutrophils
- Neck cyst
  - ➤ Contents show necrotic debris and neutrophils
- Necrotizing lymphadenitis
  - ➤ Necrotic material, neutrophils
  - ➤ Reparative changes
  - ➤ Microorganisms may be present

PEARLS

- ★ Most common microorganism: Gram-positive *Staphylococcus aureus*
- ★ Tender thyroid gland on palpation
- ★ Yellow–green purulent material seen on aspiration
- ★ Neutrophilic exudate on the smear

GRANULOMATOUS THYROIDITIS (DE QUERVAIN'S THYROIDITIS)

Clinical Features

- Fever, malaise, severe tenderness in thyroid area, and sore throat
- Affects women considerably more often than men (3:1 to 5:1)
- Transient hyperthyroidism with high levels of T_3 and T_4 and low serum TSH level
- Association with HLA-B35
- Believed to be associated with a viral infection (mumps, adenovirus, influenza, coxsackie, Epstein–Barr)
- Majority of cases show complete resolution
- Rarely aspirated because the diagnosis is usually clinical apparent

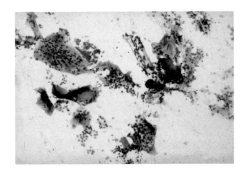 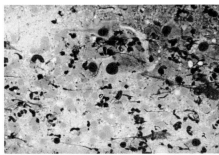

10-2A. De Quervain's thyroiditis *(left)*. Numerous multinucleated giant cells are seen in the background of the smear (Papanicolaou stain)

10-2B. De Quervain's thyroiditis *(right)*. Numerous acute inflammatory cells and reactive follicular cells (modified Giemsa stain)

Cytologic Features
- Prominence of multinucleated giant cells
- Plasma cells, lymphocytes
- Granulomas composed of epithelioid histiocytes
- Degenerating follicular cells
- Cellular debris and colloid material
- Acute phase-presence of atypical follicular cells

Special Stains and Immunohistochemistry
- Acute phase: Carcinoembryonic antigen (CEA) positive in center of granuloma
- Chronic phase: CA19-9 positive

Modern Techniques for Diagnosis
- Noncontributory

Differential Diagnosis
- Hashimoto's thyroiditis
  - ➤ Oxyphilic metaplasia (Hürthle cells)
  - ➤ Tingible body macrophages
  - ➤ Lymphoplasmacytic infiltrate
  - ➤ Lymphoid tangles
  - ➤ Multinucleated giant cells
- Acute suppurative thyroiditis
  - ➤ Neutrophils
  - ➤ Necrotic debris
  - ➤ Bacterial colonies may be seen
  - ➤ Atypical follicular cells
  - ➤ Aspirate consists of yellow–green pus
- Sarcoidosis
  - ➤ Well-organized granulomas
  - ➤ No inflammatory response
- Tuberculosis
  - ➤ Caseation necrosis

PEARLS

★ Multinucleated giant cells with more than 200 nuclei containing ingested colloid material
★ Cellular debris and colloid material
★ Most likely a viral infection

HASHIMOTO'S THYROIDITIS

Clinical Features
- Most common cause of hypothyroidism in areas of the world where iodine levels are sufficient
- More common in middle-aged white females
- 5–10% of patients present with a dominant nodule
- Association with HLA-D3 and HLA-DR5
- Patients are at higher risk of developing other autoimmune diseases
- Increased risk of developing non-Hodgkin's lymphoma, large cell type, B-cell phenotype
- Increased risk of thyroid cancer still controversial (papillary, follicular)
- Production of autoantibodies: antithyroglobulin, anti-TSH, and antimicrosomial

Cytopathologic Features
- Oxyphilic metaplasia (Hürthle cells)
- Multinucleated giant cells
- Lymphoplasmacytic infiltrate
- Tingible body macrophages
- Lymphoid tangles
- Lymphoglandular bodies in the background
- Rarely squamous metaplasia
- Frequent aggregates of histiocytes
- Rare granulomas
- Nononcocytic follicular epithelium

Special Stains and Immunohistochemistry
- Noncontributory

Modern Techniques for Diagnosis
- Noncontributory

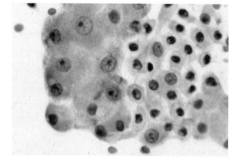
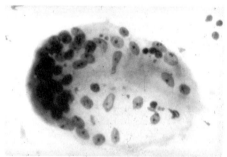
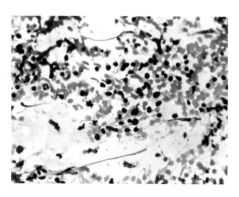
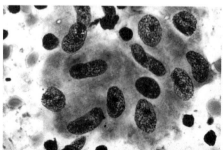

10-3A. Hashimoto's thyroiditis *(top, left)*. Hürthle cells metaplasia with abundant eosinophilic granular cytoplasm. Prominent nucleoli are visiable (Papanicolaou stain)

10-3B. Hashimoto's thyroiditis *(top, right)*. Multinucleate giant cell (modified Giemsa stain)

10-3C. Hashimoto's thyroiditis *(bottom, left)*. Mature lymphoid cells and lymphoid tangle (modified Giemsa stain)

10-3D. Hashimoto's thyroiditis *(bottom, right)*. Cluster of epitheliod histocytes and rare lymphoid cells in the background (modified Giemsa stain)

Differential Diagnosis
- Malignant lymphoma
  - Monomorphic infiltrate of lymphoid cells
  - Difficult to make the diagnosis of malignant lymphoma when thyroid is partially involved by Hashimoto's thyroiditis
- Follicular neoplasm, Hürthle cell type
  - Lack of lymphohistiocytic cells
  - Absence of giant cells
  - Extremely difficult to recognize follicular neoplasm in the background of thyroiditis
- Diffuse goiter
  - Paucity of lymphoid cells and oncocytes
  - Abundant colloid material
  - Sheets of ordinary follicular cells

PEARLS

- ☆ Autoimmune disease
- ☆ HLA-DR3 and HLA-DR5
- ☆ Increased risk of malignant lymphoma
- ☆ Multinucleated giant cells, histiocytic aggregates, lymphoplasmacytic infiltrate, Hürthle cells, and lymphoid tangles

RIEDEL'S THYROIDITIS

Clinical Features
- Synonyms: fibrous thyroiditis, Riedel's struma, or invasive thyroiditis
- Uncommon disease, slight predilection for middle-aged women
- Extremely firm enlargement of the thyroid gland
- Slowly progressive clinical course
- May be related to other progressive fibrosing diseases, for example, diseases of the mediastinum, retroorbital, and retroperitoneum
- Negative or low levels of autoantibody titers
- Most current studies refute the possibility of progression from a highly fibrosing form of Hashimoto's thyroiditis to Reidel's thyroiditis

Cytopathologic Features
- Scant cellularity
- Fibroconnective tissue
- Rare oncocytic cells
- Sparse follicular center lymphocytes
- Neutrophils and eosinophils
- Absence of squamous metaplasia
- Rare multinucleated giant cells
- Bland spindle-shaped cells and myofibroblasts

Special Stains and Immunohistochemistry
- Noncontributory

Modern Techniques for Diagnosis
- Noncontributory

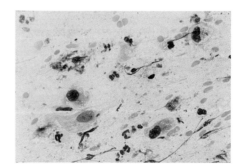

10-4. Riedel's thyroiditis. myofibroblasts and rare acute inflammatory cells (modified Giemsa stain)

Differential Diagnosis

■ Fibrosing variant of Hashimoto's thyroiditis
➤ Abundant follicular center cells
➤ Hürthle cell metaplasia
➤ Squamous metaplasia may be present
➤ Sparse eosinophils and neutrophils
➤ Aggregates of histiocytes
■ Granulomatous thyroiditis (de Quervain's subacute thyroiditis)
➤ Numerous multinucleated giant cells
➤ Granulomas composed of epithelioid histiocytes
➤ Cellular debris and colloid material
➤ Degenerating follicular cells
➤ Atypical follicular cells in the acute phase

PEARLS

★ Scant cellularity, and often unsatisfactory aspirate
★ Presence of neutrophils and eosinophils
★ Related to other fibrosing diseases, for example, there of the mediastinum, retro-orbital, and retroperitoneal

DIFFUSE NONTOXIC (SIMPLE GOITER) AND MULTINODULAR GOITER

Clinical Features

■ Enlargement of the thyroid gland or goiter is the most common manifestation of thyroid disease
■ Diffuse and multinodular goiter reflect impaired synthesis of thyroid hormone
■ Most commonly secondary to dietary iodine deficiency
■ Endemic goiter (Alps, Andes, and Himalayas)
■ High levels of TSH
■ Airway obstruction, dysphagia

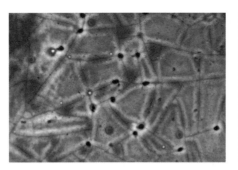
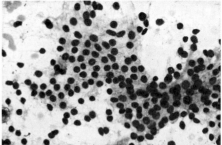
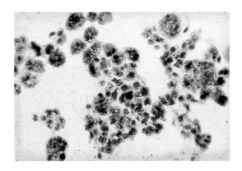
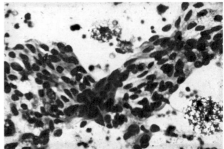

10-5A. Goiter *(top, left).* Colloid material with stain glass appearance (modified Giemsa stain)

10-5B. Goiter *(top, right).* Uniform sheet of monolayered follicular cells (modified Giemsa stain)

10-5C. Goiter *(bottom, left).* Numerous pigmented-laden macrophages (Papanicolaou stain)

10-5D. Goiter *(bottom, right).* Classic reparative changes of the follicular epithelium. Hemosiderin-laden macrophages seen in the background (modified Giemsa stain)

Cytopathologic Features

- Scant to moderate cellularity
- Large amount of watery colloid material
- Follicular cells adhering at the periphery of tissue fragments
- Large sheets of monolayer follicular cells
- Minimal or absent microfollicle formation
- Hürthle cell metaplasia may be seen
- Multinucleated giant cells may be present
- Pigment-laden and foamy macrophages may be seen if cystic changes occur
- Repair can be also present
- The follicular cells usually have round uniform nuclei and inconspicuous nucleoli
- Papillae may be present; however, the cytologic features of papillary carcinoma are not present
- Dystrophic stromal calcifications

Special Stains and Immunohistochemistry

- Most goiters stain negative for Leu-7 (CD57)

Modern Techniques for Diagnosis

- Polyclonality of hyperplastic nodules in contrast to monoclonality of follicular adenomas (cytogenetic analysis)

Differential Diagnosis

- Thyroid cyst
  - Sparse follicular epithelial cells
  - Watery brown fluid
  - Foamy and pigmented macrophages
  - Giant cells with foamy cytoplasm
  - Cholesterol crystals
  - Reparative changes
  - Degenerating red blood cells
  - Psammoma bodies, presence of numerous follicular epithelial cells, papillae, etc., may be an indication for a cystic papillary carcinoma
  - A simple thyroid cyst should collapse after FNA. Any residual mass should be re-biopsied
- Follicular adenoma, non-Hürthle cell type
  - Scanty colloid material
  - Very cellular cytologic smears
  - Microfollicular pattern
  - Usually one single cell type
  - Rarely Hürthle cell metaplasia, macrophages
  - Loss of honeycomb pattern
  - Usually a solitary nodule
- Adenomatous or cellular nodule
  - Highly cellular smears, acinar formation, and marginal vacuoles
  - The cytologic features may overlap with that of a follicular neoplasm
  - Cytopathologist's experience may play a role in minimizing the number of surgical interventions

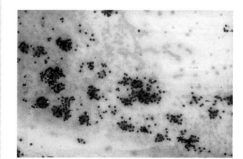

10-5E. Adenomatous nodule. Cellular smear with microfollicular pattern. Abundant colloid material seen in the background (modified Giemsa stain)

- Large amount of watery colloid material
- Lack of microfollicular pattern

★ Follicular cells usually have round uniform nuclei and inconspicuous nucleoli
★ Different type of cells, follicular, histiocytes, Hürthle cells, repair

FOLLICULAR ADENOMA

Clinical Features

▦ Discrete solitary masses
▦ Large nodules may produce local symptoms such as difficulty in swallowing
▦ Usually appear as cold nodules on radionucleotide scanning
▦ Up to 10% of cold nodules are malignant lesions
▦ By contrast hot nodules are rarely malignant
▦ 20% of follicular adenomas have mutations in the RAS family oncogenes
▦ Associated with Cowden syndrome (multiple hamartomas)
▦ Predilection for middle-aged women

Cytopathologic Features

▦ Highly cellular smears
▦ Microfollicular pattern
▦ Uniform size of follicles
▦ Scanty colloid material
▦ Nuclear enlargement may be seen
▦ Nucleoli variable
▦ Syncytial clusters
▦ Scanty Hürthle cell metaplasia may be present

Special Stains and Immunochemistry

▦ Follicular adenomas: Positive for thyroglobulin, low-molecular-weight cytokeratin and TTF-1 but not for high-molecular-weight cytokeratins, calcitonin, or neuroendocrine markers
▦ Vimentin: Often positive
▦ Most adenomas are negative for Leu-7 (CD-57)

Modern Technique for Diagnosis

▦ Trisomy 7 is the most frequent clonal cytogenetic aberration detected
▦ Most common structural aberration reported involves translocation of chromosome 19 (19q13) and of the short arm of chromosome 2 (2p21)
▦ Mutations of RAS genes have been detected

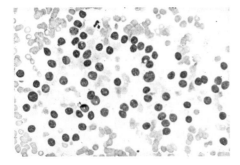

10-6. Follicular adenoma. Microfollicular pattern. No nuclear overlapping present. Absence of colloid material in the background (modified Giemsa stain)

Differential Diagnosis

▪ Adenomatous or cellular nodule
➤ Most difficult diagnosis to make on FNA material because of the overlapping of cytologic features with a follicular adenoma
➤ Some have a lot of epithelial cells and scanty colloid material
➤ Very subjective diagnosis
➤ Cytopathologist's experience may play a role in reducing false positive cases
▪ Goiter
➤ Large amount of watery colloid
➤ Minimal or absent microfollicular pattern
➤ Pigment laden and foamy macrophages
➤ Hürthle cell metaplasia may be seen
➤ Tissue fragments
➤ Large sheets of monolayered follicular cells

➤ Reparative changes
➤ Dystrophic stromal calcifications

✳ Cellular smears
✳ Microfollicular pattern is highly suggestive of a follicular neoplasm
✳ Scanty colloid material
✳ Syncytial clusters
✳ Usually single cold nodule
✳ Difficult to differentiate from an adenomatous or cellular goiter on FNA material
✳ Accurate diagnosis of a follicular neoplasm requires several cytologic features enumerated above

HÜRTHLE CELL ADENOMA

Clinical Features
▧ Solitary nodules
▧ Multiple adenomas may occur particularly in young women
▧ More common in women in the fifth decade
▧ Cold nodules on a thyroid scintigram
▧ Hürthle cells are also named Askanazy cells, oxyphilic cells, and oncocytic cells

Cytopathology Features
▨ Once single cell type, Hürthle cells
▨ Single cells are usually conspicuous
▨ Three-dimensional clusters
▨ Nuclear pleomorphism may be present
▨ Cells with abundant granular eosinophilic cytoplasm
▨ Presence of prominent nucleoli
▨ Scant or absent colloid material

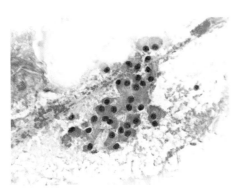

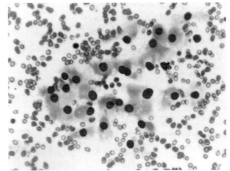

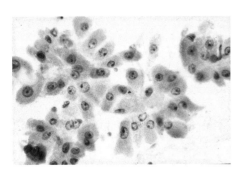

10-7A. Hürthle cell adenoma
(top, left). Sheet of follicular cells with a large amount of eosinophilic granular cytoplasm (Papanicolaou stain)

10-7B. Hürthle cell adenoma *(top, right).* Loosely cohesive follicular cells with abundant dense cytoplasm (modified Giemsa stain)

10-7C. Hürthle cell adenoma *(opposite).* Clusters of Hürthle cells with dense granular cytoplasm. The nuclei contain prominent nucleoli (modified Giemsa stain)

- Minimal or absent microfollicular pattern
- Binucleation is common
- Plasmacytoid cells
- Multinucleation may suggest malignancy
- Intranuclear cytoplasmic inclusions have been reported
- Absence of lymphoid cells

Special Stains and Immunohistochemistry

- Thyroglobulin: Positive
- Cytokeratins: Positive
- TTF-1: Positive
- Cytokeratin 19: Negative
- Cytochrome C oxidase: Positive (highlights mitochondria)

Modern Technique for Diagnosis

- Electron microscopy: Cells contain packed mitochondria having abnormal size, shape, and content
- P_{21} RAS oncogen product
- Aneuplody and chromosal losses (10_q) may be associated with a worse diagnosis
- Some lesions show PPARγ rearrangements

Differential Diagnosis

- Hashimoto's thyroiditis with predominant Hürthle cell nodule
  - Numerous Hürthle cells
  - Background of the smear contains lymphocytes plasma cells, follicular cells, and histocytes
- Goiter
  - Colloid material
  - Scattered Hürthle cells
  - Flat sheets with honeycomb pattern
  - Tissue fragments
  - Foamy cells and hemosiderin-laden macrophages if cystic changes occurred
  - Reparative changes

PEARLS

- ⋆ Solitary nodules
- ⋆ One single cell type (Hürthle cells)
- ⋆ Prominent nucleoli
- ⋆ Abundant granular eosinophilic cytoplasm
- ⋆ Scant colloid material
- ⋆ Binucleation
- ⋆ A follicular Hürthle cell neoplasm is unlikely if you have changes of Hashimoto's thyroiditis in the background

MEDULLARY CARCINOMA

Clinical Features

- Neuroendocrine tumor derived from the parafollicular cells, or C cells of the thyroid gland
- C-cells produce calcitonin

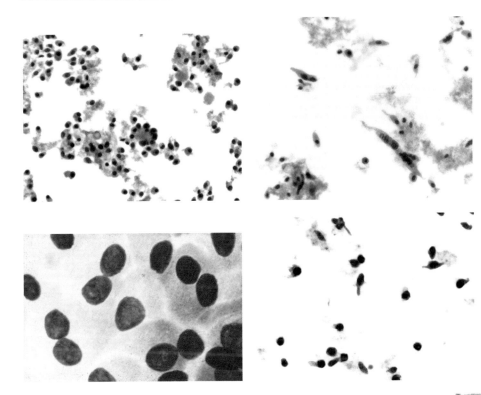

10-8A. Medullary carcinoma *(top, left)*. Cellular smear containing small plasmacytoid cells (Papanicolaou stain)

10-8B. Medullary carcinoma *(top, right)*. Medullary carcinoma with prominent spindle cell component (Papanicolaou stain)

10-8C. Medullary carcinoma *(bottom, left)*. Eosinophilic granular cytoplasm. Binucleation is appreciated (modified Giemsa stain)

10-8D. Medullary carcinoma *(bottom, right)*. Calcitonin positive cells in medullary carcinoma cells

- 80% sporadic
- Associated with MEN syndrome IIA or IIB
- Familial form of medullary thyroid carcinoma (FMTC)
- MEN-II form occurs in younger patients
- Sporadic and FMTC forms occur in adults
- Multicentricity is seen in familial cases

10-8E. Medullary carcinoma. Synaptophysin-positive cells in medullary carcinoma cells

Cytopathologic Features

- Typically hypercellular cytologic smears with single or loosely cohesive cells
- Cells vary in shape: spindle, plasmacytoid, and granular
- Binucleation and multinucleation may be seen
- Salt and pepper chromatin pattern
- Cytoplasm contains red granules (modified Giemsa stain)
- Amyloid material (magenta in color on modified Giemsa stain)
- Occasionally papillae and follicles can be appreciated
- Cytoplasm is basophilic and granular (on Papanicolaou stain)
- Intranuclear cytoplasmic inclusions in up to 20% of the cases
- Oncocytic variant
  - The majority of the cells contain a large amount of granular cytoplasm
  - May be difficult to differentiate this variant from Hürthle cell neoplasms without special stains (calcitonin)
- Spindle cell variant
  - Composed predominantly of spindle cells
  - May be difficult to differentiate this variant from metastatic sarcoma, spindle cell carcinoma (squamous), or primary anaplastic carcinoma

- Papillary variant
  - True papillae with fibrovascular cores are rarely seen
  - Intranuclear cytoplasmic inclusions may be present and can be confused with papillary carcinoma
  - Medullary and papillary carcinomas can coexist in the same gland
- Clear cell variant
  - Rare variant
  - Clear cytoplasm
  - Can be confused with other clear cell tumors
- Small cell variant
  - Poorly differentiated medullary carcinoma
  - Identical cytologic features as small cell carcinoma of the lung
  - Metastases from the lung should be excluded
- Giant cell variant
  - Presence of giant and spindle cells in medullary carcinoma may be misinterpreted as an anaplastic carcinoma

Special Stains and Immunochemistry
- Calcitonin: Positive
- Chromogranin: Positive
- Carcinoembryonic antigen (CEA): Positive in tumor cells and serum
- Congo red: Positive in amyloid material
- Thyroglobulin: Negative
- Synaptophysin: Positive
- TTF-1: Positive
- Low-molecular-weight keratins: Positive

Modern Technique for Diagnosis
- Cytogenetics: Gene for the MEN-IIA present near the centromere of chromosome 10
- Elevated levels of H-RAS and N-MYC oncogenes
- RET mutations (Mq18T) occur in 20–80% of sporadic medullary carcinoma
- Electron microscopy: Cytoplasmic dense-core secretory granules

Differential Diagnosis
- Hürthle cell neoplasms
  - Large amount of eosinophilic granular cytoplasm
  - Prominent nucleoli
  - Nuclei lack the characteristic salt and pepper chromatin
  - Binucleation and multinucleation may be seen
- Anaplastic carcinoma
  - More pleomorphic cells than in the classic medullary carcinoma
- Metastatic tumors
  - Sarcomas
  - Spindle cell carcinomas
  - Small cell carcinoma of the lung

PEARLS

- ✦ MEN syndrome IIA and IIB
- ✦ Multicentric cases seen in familial cases
- ✦ Cytoplasm contains red granules on modified Giemsa stain (calcitonin)
- ✦ Amyloid material

★ Intranuclear cytoplasmic inclusions can be seen up to 20% of the cases
★ Salt-and-pepper nuclear chromatin pattern
★ Usually single cold nodule
★ Medullary carcinoma can mimic several metastatic neoplasms; special studies and clinical history may be helpful in separating medullary carcinoma from metastatic tumors

PAPILLARY CARCINOMA

Clinical Features

▨ Asymptomatic thyroid nodule
▨ Cold nodule on thyroid scintiscans
▨ Excellent prognosis, ten-year survival rate in excess of 95%
▨ More common in women (in Japan 9:1)
▨ Well-documented association with radiation exposure
▨ Poor prognostic features include
  ➤ Male sex
  ➤ Older age
  ➤ Extrathyroid growth
  ➤ Large size

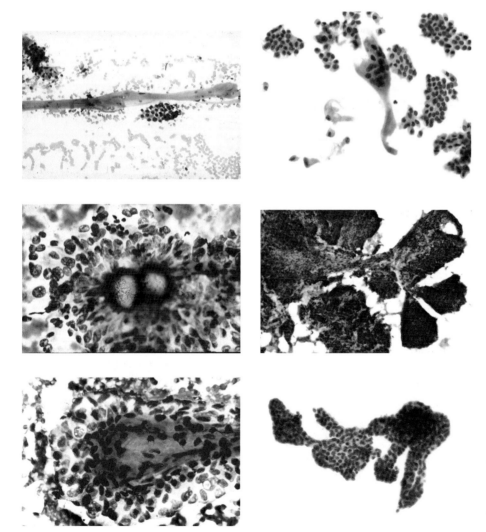

10-9A. Papillary carcinoma *(top, left)*. Bubble gum colloid material pattern is appreciated (modified Giemsa stain)

10-9B. Papillary carcinoma *(top, right)*. Multinucleated giant cells are present in the background (Papanicolaou stain)

10-9C. Papillary carcinoma *(middle, left)*. Cluster of papillary carcinoma cells containing a psammoma body (modified Giemsa stain)

10-9D. Papillary carcinoma *(middle, right)*. Papillary tissue fragments (Papanicolaou stain)

10-9E. Papillary carcinoma *(bottom, left)*. Papillary cluster with central vascular core (modified Giemsa stain)

10-9F. Papillary carcinoma *(bottom, right)*. Complex avascular papillae (Papanicolaou stain)

■ Coexistence with Hashimoto's thyroiditis
■ Association with familial adenomatous polyposis coli (FAP), Cowden syndrome, and perhaps Carney complex

Cytopathologic Features
■ Bubble gum colloid pattern
■ Multinucleated foreign body–type giant cells
■ Psammoma bodies
■ Papillary tissue fragments
■ Monolayered sheets of cells
■ Intranuclear cytoplasmic inclusions
■ Linear chromatin ridge (groove)
■ Dense, metaplastic, and septate cytoplasm
■ Fusiform/oval nuclei with fine powdery chromatin
■ Inconspicuous multiple nucleoli
■ Follicular variant of papillary carcinoma
  ➤ Neoplastic follicles instead of papillae showing intranuclear cytoplasmic inclusions and linear chromatin ridge (groove)
■ Sclerosing papillary carcinoma
  ➤ Abundant psammoma bodies
  ➤ Squamous metaplasia
  ➤ Marked lymphoid response
  ➤ Fragments of fibrous tissue
■ Tall cell papillary carcinoma
  ➤ Occurs in older patients
  ➤ Tall cells with large amount of eosinophilic cytoplasm
  ➤ Nuclear changes similar to that of classic papillary carcinoma
  ➤ Psammoma bodies rarely seen
■ Columnar cell papillary carcinoma
  ➤ Tall columnar cells with stratified nuclei having fine chromatin pattern and longitudinal nuclear grooves
  ➤ The cytoplasm tends to be clear
■ Hürthle cell papillary carcinoma
  ➤ This diagnosis can be made when the vast majority of the cells are Hürthle cells

Special Studies and Immunohistochemistry
■ Thyroglobulin: Positive
■ Cytokeratin 19: Positive
■ Vimentin: Positive
■ S-100 protein: Often positive

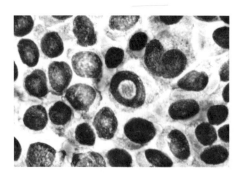

10-9G. Papillary carcinoma. Well formed intranuclear–cytoplasmic inclusion (modified Giemsa stain)

Modern Techniques Diagnosis
■ Oncogene alteration : PTC, TRK, and R-RAS mutations
■ BRAF mutations
■ PTC oncogene is thought to represent a re-arranged form of RET-proto-oncogene on chromosome 10q11-q12

Differential Diagnosis
■ Follicular neoplasms/carcinomas
  ➤ Lack of papillae
  ➤ Absence of psammoma bodies
  ➤ Sparse nuclear grooves
  ➤ Absence of intranuclear cytoplasmic inclusions
  ➤ Absence of squamoid cytoplasm

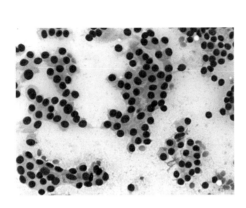 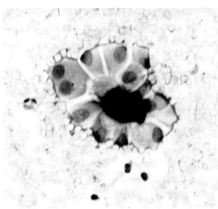

10-9H. Follicular variant of papillary carcinoma *(left)*. Sheets of follicular cells with focal microfollicular differentiation. Nuclear grooving and small not-well-formed intranuclear cytoplasmic inclusions (modified Giemsa stain)

10-9I. Tall cell variant of papillary carcinoma *(right)*. Papillary cluster of tall cells surrounding a psammoma body (Papanicolaou stain)

➤ Characteristic microfollicular pattern
➤ Lack of lymphoid cells in the background

PEARLS

★ Psammoma bodies
★ Intranuclear cytoplasmic inclusions
★ Nuclear grooves
★ Papillary tissue fragments
★ Bubble gum colloid material
★ Papillary carcinoma should never be diagnosed solely on the basis of one or two cytologic features as described above
★ Several cytologic criteria must be present before a definitive diagnosis of papillary carcinoma can be rendered

ANAPLASTIC CARCINOMA

Clinical Features
▦ Mean age at diagnosis in the sixth and seventh decades
▦ More common in women (3:1)
▦ Presents as a rapidly enlarging neck mass
▦ High likelihood of cervical lymph nodes or distant metastases at presentation
▦ Cold nodule on radioactive iodine scan
▦ Death usually within a year of diagnosis
▦ Most arise from a preexisting thyroid neoplasm, usually a papillary carcinoma

Cytopathology Features
▦ Highly cellular cytologic smear
▦ Cells usually are distributed singly or in clusters
▦ Marked nuclear pleomorphism
▦ Squamoid, giant, and spindle cells
▦ Coarse chromatin pattern, prominent nucleoli
▦ Necrotic debris in the background
▦ Numerous mitotic figures, including abnormal forms
▦ Osteoclastic giant cells may be present

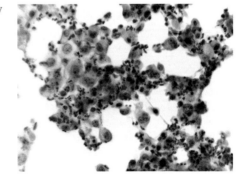

10-10. Anaplastic carcinoma. Large pleomorphic cells numerous acute inflammatory cells are present in the background (Papanicolaou stain)

Special Stains and Immunohistochemistry
▦ AE1/AE3 cytokeratin: Expressed in 80% of the cases
▦ Thyroglobulin: Negative

▥ TTF-1: Rarely positive
▥ CEA: Uncommonly expressed <10%

Modern Techniques for Diagnosis
▥ Oncogene expression (p21 RAS)
▥ Strong association with TP 53 mutations
▥ β-Catenin (CTNNB$_1$) mutations have also been described
▥ Electron microscopy can demonstrate the presence of epithelial cell junctions and tonofilaments

Differential Diagnosis
▥ Metastatic sarcoma, such as fibrosarcoma or malignant fibrous histio-cytoma
▥ Primary sarcomas and/or metastatic sarcomas to the thyroid gland are extremely rare
▥ Medullary carcinoma
  ➤ Can mimic anaplastic carcinoma because of the presence of spindle cells, binucleation and multinucleation. However, neuroendocrine chromatin pattern, presence of amyloid material and clinical features should help in reaching the correct diagnosis
▥ Metastatic neoplasms that may have a spindle cell pattern (squamous cell carcinoma, melanoma, and renal cell carcinoma)
▥ Benign reactive processes seen in thyroiditis, goiters, epithelial repair, and radiation changes. However, in these conditions, despite the marked nuclear pleo-morphism, the nuclear chromatin pattern is pale and bland

PEARLS

✶ Large pleomorphic cells
✶ Spindle cells
✶ Binucleation, multinucleation
✶ High mitotic rate, some abnormal forms
✶ Necrotic debris
✶ Rapidly growing lesion
✶ Usually elderly female patients
✶ Can be confused on cytologic smears with spindle cell carcinoma, sarcoma, melanoma, medullary carcinoma, and benign reactive processes

FOLLICULAR CARCINOMA

Clinical Features
▥ 5% of thyroid cancers
▥ Between 25% and 40% of thyroid cancers in iodine-deficient areas
▥ Cold nodule on isotopic scan
▥ More common in women
▥ Distant metastases in up to 20% of patients at presentation with the most common sites of involvement being bone and lungs

Cytologic Features
▥ Hypercellular smears
▥ Dispersed microfollicular pattern
▥ Prominent nucleoli
▥ The cells lining the follicles usually are stratified, with loss of nuclear polarity, increased nuclear chromatin density, and some atypia

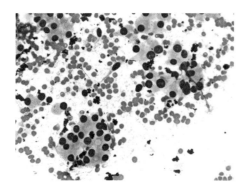

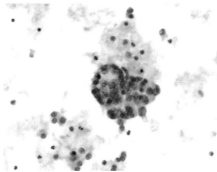

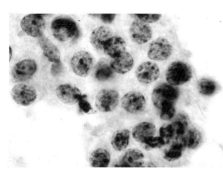

10-11A. Follicular carcinoma *(top, left)*. Microfollicular pattern with minimal stratification and loss of polarity (modified Giemsa stain)

10-11B. Follicular carcinoma *(top, right)*. Follicular differentiation with nuclear stratification – single neoplastic cells are seen in the background (Papanicolaou stain)

10-11C. Follicular carcinoma *(opposite)*. Loosely cohesive cells with coarse chromatin pattern. Single mitosis is appreciated (Papanicolaou stain)

- Crowding of cells, three-dimensional groups, and irregular follicles speak in favor of carcinoma
- Scant colloid material
- Increased number of single cells
- Hürthle cell carcinoma
  - Frequent multinucleation
  - Macronucleoli
  - Marked pleomorphism
  - Crowed sheets of cells with ill-defined cell borders

Special Stains and Immunohistochemistry
- TTF-1: Positive
- Low-molecular-weight cytokeratin: Positive
- Galectin-3, HBME-1, CD15, and CD44v6: May be positive
- BCL-2: usually positive

Modern Techniques for Diagnosis
- PPry gene rearrangement found in 20–50% of cases
- RAS gene mutation in 20–50% of cases

Differential Diagnosis
- Follicular variant of papillary carcinoma
  - Intranuclear cytoplasmic invaginations
  - Nuclear grooves
  - Powdery chromatin pattern
  - Irregular nuclear membranes
- Follicular adenoma
  - Distinguishing between follicular adenoma and a well-differentiated follicular carcinoma is not an easy task on FNA material

★ The distinction between a follicular adenoma and a follicular carcinoma on FNA material is not always possible because follicular carcinoma may have a bland cytologic appearance. In addition, follicular adenoma may show nuclear atypia, enlargement, and pleomorphism

POORLY DIFFERENTIATED CARCINOMA (INSULAR CARCINOMA)

- More common in women
- Very rare in United States; originally reported in Italy
- Morphologic variant of follicular carcinoma
- Mean age at diagnosis in the fifth and sixth decades
- Frequent metastases to bone, lungs, and regional lymph nodes
- Poor prognosis

Cytologic Features
- Highly cellular smears
- High number of single cells
- Small to intermediate-sized cells
- Sparse microfollicular pattern
- Bland appearance of the cells
- High nuclear/cytoplasmic ratios
- Nuclei with fine chromatin pattern
- Necrosis and mitosis are common

Special Stains and Immunohistochemistry
- Thyroglobulin: Positive
- TTF-1: Positive
- Ki-67 index: Increased
- BCL-2: Positive in 80% of the cases
- Calcitonin: Negative

Modern Techniques for Diagnosis
- TP53 exons five to nine mutations in 20–30% of cases
- H-K or N-RAS mutations occur in about 50% of cases

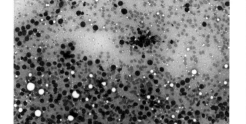

10-12. Insular carcinoma. Mostly single follicular cells. Vague follicular pattern in appreciated (modified Giemsa stain)

Differential Diagnosis
- Medullary carcinoma
  - Predominantly dispersed cell pattern
  - Spindle, small, clear, oncocytic, papillary, giant cell morphology
  - Salt-and-pepper chromatin pattern
  - Presence of red cytoplasmic granules (calcitonin) on modified Giemsa stain
  - Binucleation
  - Amyloid material
- Malignant lymphoma
  - Cells dispersed as single cells
  - Lack of cohesive groups of cells
  - Lymphoglandular bodies in the background
  - Absent follicular pattern
- Papillary carcinoma
  - Psammoma bodies
  - Papillae

➤ Squamoid metaplasia
➤ Nuclear grooves
➤ Powdery chromatin, irregular nuclear membranes, and intranuclear cytoplasmic inclusions are cytologic features that can be seen in both insular and papillary carcinoma

PEARLS

★ Predominantly small to intermediate-sized single cells with high nuclear cytoplasmic ratios
★ Necrosis and high cellularity
★ Numerous mitotic figures
★ Low grade cytologic atypia
★ Trabeculae and/or clusters of cells with poorly defined cytoplasm

MALIGNANT LYMPHOMA

Clinical Features
▪ 1–2% of all primary thyroid cancers
▪ Secondary involvement of the thyroid gland by malignant lymphoma is more common (15%)
▪ Rare before the age of forty years
▪ Strong association with Hashimoto's thyroiditis
▪ Thyroid is considered to be a (MALT) site and low-grade and high-grade lymphomas can occur
▪ Majority are large B-cell type
▪ Prognosis is better when confined to the thyroid gland

Cytopathologic Features
▪ Monophormic population of lymphoid cells
▪ Single cells with scant to moderate amount of cytoplasm
▪ Nuclear membranes can be either cleaved or noncleaved
▪ Karyorrhexis can be prominent
▪ Presence of lymphoglandular bodies in the background
▪ Small cell lymphoma (small lymphocytic and small cleaved) difficult to distinguish from chronic thyroiditis

Special Stains and Immunochemistry
▪ LCA: Positive
▪ CD20: Positive
▪ CD79a: Positive
▪ BCL-2: Positive

Modern Technique for Diagnosis
▪ For subtyping refer to lymph node chapter

Differential Diagnosis
▪ Hashimoto's thyroiditis
  ➤ Lymphoid cells at different stages of maturation
  ➤ Hürthle cell metaplasia
  ➤ Plasma cells

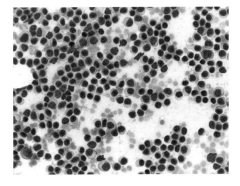

10-13. Malignant lymphoma. Monomorphic population of lymphoid cells (modified Giemsa stain)

■ Undifferentiated small cell carcinoma
  ➤ Primary undifferentiated small cell carcinoma of the thyroid gland is rare; mostly are metastases from lungs
  ➤ Cohesive groups of cells that show nuclear molding
  ➤ Scant cytoplasm, fine chromatin pattern
  ➤ Lack of lymphoglandular bodies
■ Small cell variant of medullary carcinoma
  ➤ Difficult to differentiate from malignant lymphoma
  ➤ Amyloid material and demonstration of calcitonin helps to confirm the diagnosis of medullary carcinoma

PEARLS

⋆ Strong association with Hashimoto's thyroiditis
⋆ Mostly large B-cell type
⋆ Prominent karyorrhectic index
⋆ Difficult at times to differentiate on cytologic material from Hashimoto's thyroiditis, small cell variant of medullary carcinoma and small cell carcinoma

GRAVES DISEASE

Clinical Features
▨ Autoimmune thyroid disease
▨ Most common in young women, rare in children
▨ Increased T_3 and T_4
▨ Decreased TSH
▨ IgG antibodies to TSH receptor
▨ Ophthalmopathy (exophthalmos), dermopathy (pretibial edema)

Cytopathologic Features
▨ High cellularity
▨ Flame cells
▨ Lymphocytes may be present
▨ Hürthle cells, giant cells also can be present
▨ Usually scant colloid material
▨ Three-dimensional cell groups and papillary clusters are often seen

Special Stains and Immunochemistry
▨ Noncontributory

Modern Technique for Diagnosis
▨ Noncontributory

Differential Diagnosis
▨ Hashimoto's thyroiditis
  ➤ Prominent germinal center cells
  ➤ Hürthle cells usually are more conspicuous than in Graves disease aspirates
  ➤ Flame cells usually are absent
▨ Papillary carcinoma
  ➤ Papillae with classic nuclear changes
  ➤ Few Hürthle cells
  ➤ Lymphocytes and giant cells can be seen in both papillary carcinoma and Graves disease

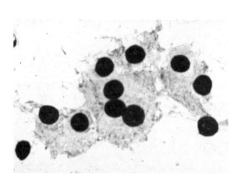

10-14. Graves disease. Cluster of follicular cells with abundant red granular cytoplasma (modified Giemsa stain)

> ➤ Flame cells usually are seen in benign thyroid conditions; however, they have sporadically been reported with thyroid malignancies
> ◼ Toxic nodular goiter
> ➤ The cytologic features are similar to those of thyroid hyperplasia (flame cells, Hürthle cells, cellular smears)
> ➤ Giant cells and lymphocytes are rarely seen

✳ Flame cells
✳ Rarely aspirated unless there is a predominant nodule
✳ Can be confused on cytology with papillary carcinoma

METASTATIC TUMORS

Clinical Features
◼ Metastases to the thyroid gland may occur as direct extension of malignancies from contiguous organs or as a result of hematogenous/lymphatic spread from distant sites
◼ Autopsy studies show up to 25% of cases with metastases to the thyroid gland (most often multifocal)
◼ Usually solitary nodule (clinical practice)
◼ The most common tumors to metastasize to the thyroid gland are: kidney, lungs, breast, hematologic malignancies, and melanoma

Cytopathologic Features
◼ Clinical history is one of the most important factors in the differential diagnosis of these lesions
◼ Difficult to differentiate these lesions from a poorly differentiated or undifferentiated thyroid cancer

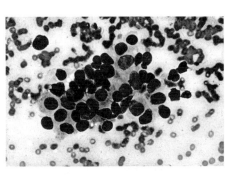

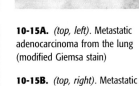

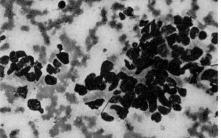

10-15A. *(top, left)*. Metastatic adenocarcinoma from the lung (modified Giemsa stain)

10-15B. *(top, right)*. Metastatic signet ring carcinoma from the stomach (Papanicolaou stain)

10-15C. *(opposite)*. Metastatic undifferentiated small cell carcinoma from the lung (modified Giemsa stain)

Special Stains and Immunochemistry
- HMB-45 and S-100 protein: Positive in malignant melanoma
- CD10 and vimentin: Positive in renal cell carcinoma
- Thyroglobulin: Negative in all metastatic tumors

Modern Technique for Diagnosis
- Noncontributory

Differential Diagnosis

- Majority of primary thyroid cancers are papillary, follicular, medullary, and anaplastic spindle or giant cell variant. Any neoplasm with cytologic features that look different from those of four neoplasms, strongly favor the possibility of a metastatic tumor

PEARLS

⋆ Clinical history probably is one of the most important factors in the differential diagnosis of primary versus metastatic tumors

REFERENCES

ACUTE THYROIDITIS

Battan R, Mariuz P, Raviglione Mc, et al. *Pneumocystis carinii* infection of the thyroid in a hypothyroid patient with AIDS: Diagnosis by fine needle aspiration biopsy. *J Clinical Endocrinol Metab* 1991 72:724–726.

Chi H, Lee YJ, Chiu NC, Huang FY, Huang CY, Lee KS, Shih SL, Shih BF. Acute suppurative thyroiditis in children. *Pediatr Infect Dis J* 2002 May;21(5):384–7.

Fukata S, Miyauchi A, Kuma K, Sugawara M. Acute suppurative thyroiditis caused by an infected piriform sinus fistula with thyrotoxicosis. *Thyroid* 2002 Feb;12(2):175–8.

Hopwood NJ, Kelch RP. Thyroid Masses. Approach to diagnosis and management in childhood and adolescence. *Pediatr Rev* 1993; 14:481–7.

Lin JD, Huang BY, Huang HS, Juang JH, Jeng LB. Ultrasonography and fine needle aspiration cytology of acute suppurative thyroiditis. *Changgeng Yi Xue Za Zhi* 1993 Jun;16(2):93–8.

Nishihara E, Miyauchi A, Matsuzuka F, Sasaki I, Ohye H, Kubota S, Fukata S, Amino N, Kuma K. Acute suppurative thyroiditis after fine-needle aspiration causing thyrotoxicosis. *Thyroid* 2005 Oct;15(10):1183–7.

Shukla HS. Fine needle aspiration cytology in the management of acute suppurative thyroiditis. *Ear Nose Throat J* 1994 Jun;73(6):415–7.

Singh SK, Agrawal JK, Kumar M, Hopwood NJ, Kelch RP. Thyroid Masses. Approach to diagnosis and management in childhood and adolescence. *Pediatr Rev* 1993; 14:481–7.

GRANULOMATOUS THYROIDITIS (DE QUERVAIN'S THYROIDITIS)

Berger SA, Zonszein J, Villamena P, et al. Infectious diseases of the thyroid gland. *Rev Infect Dis* 1983 5:108–22.

Chang TC, Lai SM, Wen CY, Hsiao YL. Three-dimensional cytomorphology in fine needle aspiration biopsy of subacute thyroiditis. *Acta Cytol* 2004 Mar–Apr;48(2):155–60.

Garcia Solano J, Gimenez Bascunana A, Sola Perez J, Campos Fernandez J, Martinez Parra D, Sanchez Sanchez C, Montalban Romero S, Perez-Guillermo M. Fine-needle aspiration of subacute granulomatous thyroiditis (De Quervain's thyroiditis): a clinico-cytologic review of 36 cases. *Diagn Cytopathol.* 1997 Mar;16(3):214–20.

Lu CP, Chang TC, Wang CY, Hsiao YL. Serial changes in ultrasound-guided needle aspiration cytology in subacute thyroiditis. *Acta Cytol.* 1997 Mar–Apr;41(2):238–43.

Ofner C, Hittmair A, Kroll I, Bangerl I, Zechmann W, Totsch M, Ladurner D, Bocker W, Schmid KW. Fine needle aspiration cytodiagnosis of subacute (de Quervain's) thyroiditis in an endemic goitre area. *Cytopathology.* 1994 Feb;5(1):33–40.

Shabb NS, Salti I. Subacute thyroiditis: fine-needle aspiration cytology of 14 cases presenting with thyroid nodules. *Diagn Cytopathol.* 2006 Jan;34(1):18–23.

Shabb NS, Tawil A, Gergeos F, Saleh M, Azar S. Multinucleated giant cells in fine-needle aspiration of thyroid nodules: their diagnostic significance. *Diagn Cytopathol.* 1999 Nov; 21(5):307–12.

HASHIMOTO'S THYROIDITIS

Arguelles R, Rigla M, Otal C, Cubero JM, Bague S, Carreras AM, Eulalia E, Gonzalez-Campora R, Galera H, Prat J. Comparative findings of lymphocytic thyroiditis and thyroid lymphoma. *Acta Cytol.* 2003 Jul–Aug;47(4):575–80.

Carson HJ, Castelli MJ, Gattuso P. Incidence of neoplasia in Hashimoto's thyroiditis: a fine-needle aspiration study. *Diagn Cytopathol.* 1996 Feb;14(1):38–42.

Lui LH, Bakhos R, Wojcik EM. Concomitant papillary carcinoma and Hashimoto's thyroiditis. *Semin Diagn Pathol.* 2001 May;18(2):99–103.

MacDonald K, Yazdi HM. Fine needle aspiration biopsy of Hashimoto's thyroiditis. Sources of diagnostic error. *Acta Cytol.* 1999 May–Jun;43(3):400–6.

Nguygen GK, Ginsberg J, Crockford PM, Villanueva RR. Hashimoto's thyroiditis; cytodiagnostic accuracy and pitfalls. *Diagn Cytopathol.* 1997 Jun;16(6)531–6.

Poropatich C, Marcus D, Oertel YC. Hashimoto's thyroiditis: a fine-needle aspiration of 50 asymptomatic cases. *Diagn Cytopathol.* 1994;11(2):141–5.

Tseleni-Balafouta S, Kyroudi-Voulgari A, Paizi-Biza P, Papacharlampous NX. Lymphocytic thyroiditis in fine-needle aspirates: differential diagnostic aspects. *Diagn Cytopathol.* 1989;5(4):362–5.

RIEDEL'S THYROIDITIS

Beham A, Langsteger W, Schmid C, Lind P, Kronberger D. [Chronic invasive fibrous thyroiditis (Riedel struma). Case report with special reference to preoperative diagnosis]. *Wien Klin Wochenschr* 1988 Apr 1;100(7):210–5.

Harigopal M, Sahoo S, Recant WM, DeMay RM. Fine-needle aspiration of Riedel's disease: report of a case and review of the literature. *Diagn Cytopathol.* 2004 Mar;30(3):193–7.

Papi G, Corrado S, Carapezzi C, De Gaetani C, Carani C. Riedel's thyroiditis and fibrous variant of Hashimoto's thyroiditis a clinicopathological and immunohistochemical study. *J Endocrinol Invest.* 2003 May;26(5):444–9.

Papi G, Corrado S, Cesinaro AM, Novelli L, Smerieri A, Carapezzi C. Riedel's thyroiditis: clinical, pathological and imaging features. *Int J Clin Pract.* 2002 Jan–Feb;56(1):65:7.

Riedel's thyroiditis associated with high titers of antimicrosomal and antithyroglobulin antibodies and hypothyroidism. *J Endocrinol Invest.* 1994 Oct;17(9):733–7.

Schwaegerle SM, Bauer TW, Esselstyn CB Jr. Riedel's thyroiditis. *Am J Clin Pathol.* 1988 Dec;90(6):715–22.

Yasmeen T, Khan S, Patel SG, Reeves WA, Gonsch FA, de Bustros A, Kaplan EL. Clinical case seminar: Riedel's thyroiditis: report of a case complicated by spontaneous hypoparathyroidism, recurrent laryngeal nerve injury, and Horner's syndrome. *J Clin Endocrinol Metab.* 2002 Aug;87(8):3543–7.

Zelmanovitz F, Zelmanovitz T, Beck M, Cerski CT, Schmid H, Czepielewski MA.

DIFFUSE NONTOXIC (SIMPLE GOITER) AND MULTINODULAR GOITER

Das DK, Khanna CM, Tripathi RP, Pant CS, Mandal AK, Chandra S, Chachra K, Sharma S, Sodhani P, Singh H, Thusoo TK. Solitary nodular goiter. Review of cytomorphologic features in 441 cases. *Acta Cytol.* 1999 Jul–Aug;43(4):563–74.

Dumitriu L, Mogos I, Calin E. Fine-needle aspiration biopsy of the thyroid correlated with clinical scintigraphic, echographic and pathologic data in nodular and diffuse goiter. *Endocrinologie* 1984 Oct–Dec;22(4):261–8.

Fiorella RM, Isley W, Miller LK, Kragel PJ. Multinodular goiter of the thyroid mimicking malignancy: diagnostic pitfalls in fine-needle aspiration biopsy. *Diagn Cytopathol.* 1993;9(3):351–5; discussion 355–7.

Harach HR, Zusman SB, Saravia Day E. Nodular goiter: a histo-cytological study with some emphasis on pitfalls of fine-needle aspiration cytology. *Diagn Cytopathol.* 1992;8(4):409–19.

Kung IT, Yuen RW. Fine needle aspiration of the thyroid. Distinction between colloid nodules and follicular neoplasms using cell blocks and 21-gauge needles. *Acta Cytol.* 1989 Jan–Feb;33(1): 53–60.

Layfield LJ, Wax T, Jones C. Cytologic distinction of goiterous nodules from morphologically normal thyroid: analyses of cytomorphologic features. *Cancer* 2003 Aug 25;99(4):217–22.

Lucas A, Sanmarti A, Salinas I, Llatjos M, Foz M. Amyloid goiter. Diagnosis by fine-needle aspiration biopsy of the thyroid. *J Endocrinol Invest* 1989 Jan;12(1):43–6.

FOLLICULAR ADENOMA

Baloch ZW, Fleisher S, LiVolsi VA, Gupta PK. Diagnosis of "follicular neoplasm": a gray zone in thyroid fine-needle aspiration cytology. *Diagn Cytopathol.* 2002 Jan;26(1):41–4.

Barbaro D, Simi U, Lopane P, Pallini S, Orsini P, Piazza F, Pasquini C, Soriani G. Thyroid nodules with microfollicular findings reported on fine-needle aspiration: invariably surgical treatment? *Endocr Pract.* 2001 Sep–Oct;7(5):352–7.

Chen H, Dudley NE, Westra WH, Sadler GP, Udelsman R. Utilization of fine-needle aspiration in patients undergoing thyroidectomy at two academic centers across the Atlantic. *World J Surg.* 2003 Feb;27(2):208–11.

Ersoz C, Firat P, Uguz A, Kuzey GM. Fine-needle aspiration cytology of solitary thyroid nodules: how far can we go in rendering differential cytologic diagnoses? *Cancer* 2004 Oct 25;102(5): 302–7.

Goldstein RE, Netterville JL, Burkey B, Johnson JE. Implications of follicular neoplasms, atypia, and lesions suspicious for malignancy diagnosed by fine-needle aspiration of thyroid nodules. *Ann Surg* 2002 May;235(5):656–62; discussion 662–4.

Greaves TS, Olvera M, Florentine BD, Raza AS, Cobb CJ, Tsao-Wei DD, Groshen S, Singer P, Lopresti J, Martin SE. Follicular lesions of thyroid: a 5-year fine-needle aspiration experience. *Cancer* 2000 Dec 25;90(6):335–41.

Kelman AS, Rathan A, Leibowitz J, Burstein DE, Haber RS. Thyroid cytology and the risk of malignancy in thyroid nodules: importance of nuclear atypia in indeterminate specimens. *Thyroid* 2001 Mar;11(3):271–7.

Kollur SM, El Sayed S, El Hag IA. Follicular thyroid lesions coexisting with Hashimoto's thyroiditis: incidence and possible sources of diagnostic errors. *Diagn Cytopathol* 2003 Jan;28(1): 35–8.

Sidawy MK, Del Vecchio DM, Knoll SM. Fine-needle aspiration of thyroid nodules: correlation between cytology and histology and evaluation of discrepant cases. *Cancer* 1997 Aug 25;81(4):253–9.

Tulecke MA, Wang HH. ThinPrep for cytologic evaluation of follicular thyroid lesions: correlation with histologic findings. *Diagn Cytopathol* 2004 Jan;30(1):7–13.

Zeppa P, Benincasa G, Lucariello A, Palombini L. Association of different pathologic processes of the thyroid gland in fine needle aspiration samples. *Acta Cytol* 2001 May–Jun;45(3):347–52.

HÜRTHLE CELL ADENOMA

Alaedeen DI, Khiyami A, McHenry CR. Fine-needle aspiration biopsy specimen with a predominance of Hurthle cells: a dilemma in the management of nodular thyroid disease. *Surgery* 2005 Oct;138(4):650–6; discussion 656–7.

Blumenfeld W, Nair R, Mir R. Diagnostic significance of papillary structures and intranuclear inclusions in Hurthle-cell neoplasms of the thyroid. *Diagn Cytopathol* 1999 Apr;20(4):185–9.

Elliott DD, Pitman MB, Bloom L, Faquin WC. Fine-needle aspiration biopsy of Hürthle cell lesions of the thyroid gland: a cytomorphologic study of 139 cases with statistical analysis. *Cancer.* 2006 Feb 1; [Epub ahead of print]

Giorgadze T, Rossi ED, Fadda G, Gupta PK, Livolsi VA, Baloch Z. Does the fine-needle aspiration diagnosis of "Hurthle-cell neoplasm/follicular neoplasm with oncocytic features" denote increased risk of malignancy? *Diagn Cytopathol.* 2004 Nov;31(5):307–12.

Gonzalez JL, Wang HH, Ducatman BS. Fine-needle aspiration of Hurthle cell lesions. A cytomorphologic approach to diagnosis. *Am J Clin Pathol.* 1993 Sep;100(3):231–5.

Kini SR, Miller JM, Hamburger JI. Cytopathology of Hurthle cell lesions of the thyroid gland by fine needle aspiration. *Acta Cytol* 1981 Nov–Dec;25(6):647–52.

McIvor NP, Freeman JL, Rosen I, Bedard YC. Value of fine-needle aspiration in the diagnosis of Hurthle cell neoplasms. *Head Neck* 1993 Jul–Aug;15(4):335–41.

Nguyen GK, Husain M, Akin MR. Cytodiagnosis of benign and malignant Hurthle cell lesions of the thyroid by fine-needle aspiration biopsy. *Diagn Cytopathol* 1999 May;20(5):261–5.

Renshaw AA. Hurthle cell carcinoma is a better gold standard than Hurthle cell neoplasm for fine-needle aspiration of the thyroid: defining more consistent and specific cytologic criteria. *Cancer* 2002 Oct 25;96(5):261–6.

Yang YJ, Khurana KK. Diagnostic utility of intracytoplasmic lumen and transgressing vessels in evaluation of Hurthle cell lesions by fine-needle aspiration. *Arch Pathol Lab Med* 2001 Aug;125(8):1031–5.

MEDULLARY CARCINOMA

Aulicino MR, Szporn AH, Dembitzer R, Mechanick J, Batheja N, Bleiweiss IJ, Burstein DE. Cytologic findings in the differential diagnosis of C-cell hyperplasia and medullary carcinoma by fine needle aspiration. A case report. *Acta Cytol* 1998 Jul–Aug;42(4):963–7.

Cakir M, Altunbas H, Balci MK, Karayalcin U, Karpuzoglu G. Medullary thyroid carcinoma, follicular variant. *Endocr Pathol.* 2002 Spring;13(1):75–9.

Dedivitis RA, Di Giovanni JH, Silva GF, Marinho LC, Guimaraes AV. [Oncocytic variant of medullary thyroid carcinoma: case report]. *Arq Bras Endocrinol Metabol* 2004 Apr;48(2):315–7. Epub 2004 Jul 7.

Duskova J, Janotova D, Svobodova E, Novak Z, Tretinik P. Fine needle aspiration biopsy of mixed medullary-follicular thyroid carcinoma. A report of two cases. *Acta Cytol.* 2003 Jan–Feb; 47(1):71–7.

Forrest CH, Frost FA, de Boer WB, Spagnolo DV, Whitaker D, Sterrett BF. Medullary carcinoma of the thyroid: accuracy of diagnosis of fine-needle aspiration cytology. *Cancer* 1998 Oct 25;84(5):295–302.

Ibarrola de Andres C, Castellano Megias VM, Ballestin Carcavilla C, Alberti Masgrau N, Perez Barrios A, De Agustin PA. Hepatic metastases from the spindle cell variant of medullary thyroid carcinoma: report of a case with diagnosis by fine needle aspiration biopsy. *Acta Cytol* 2001 Nov–Dec;45(6):1022–6.

Kakudo K, Miyauchi A, Ogihara T, Takai SI, Kitamura H, Kosaki G, Kumahara Y. Medullary carcinoma of the thyroid. Giant cell type. *Arch Pathol Lab Med* 1978 Sep;102(9):445–7.

Kini SR, Miller JM, Hamburger JI, et al. Cytopathologic features of medullary carcinoma of the thyroid. *Arch Pathol Med* 1984 108:156–9.

PAPILLARY CARCINOMA

Brandwein-Gensler M, Urken M, Wang B. Collision tumor of the thyroid: a case report of metastatic liposarcoma plus papillary thyroid carcinoma. *Head Neck* 2004 Jul;26(7):637–41.

Chuah KL, Hwang JS, Ng SB, Tan PH, Poh WT, Au VS. Cytologic features of cribriform-morular variant of papillary carcinoma of the thyroid: a case report. *Acta Cytol* 2005 Jan–Feb;49(1): 75–80.

Das DK, Mallik MK, Sharma P, Sheikh ZA, Mathew PA, Sheikh M, Mirza K, Madda JP, Francis IM, Junaid TA. Papillary thyroid carcinoma and its variants in fine needle aspiration smears. A cytomorphologic study with special reference to tall cell variant. *Acta Cytol* 2004 May–Jun;48(3):325–36.

Khurana KK, Truong LD, LiVolsi VA, Baloch ZW. Cytokeratin 19 immunolocalization in cell block preparation of thyroid aspirates. An adjunct to fine-needle aspiration diagnosis of papillary thyroid carcinoma. *Arch Pathol Lab Med* 2003 May;127(5):579–83.

Lam AK, Lo CY. Diffuse sclerosing variant of papillary carcinoma of the thyroid: a 35-year comparative study at a single institution. *Ann Surg Oncol* 2006 Feb;13(2):176–81. Epub 2006 Jan 17.

Mesonero CE, Jugle JE, Wilbur DC, Nayar R. Fine-needle aspiration of the macrofollicular and microfollicular subtypes of the follicular variant of papillary carcinoma of the thyroid. *Cancer.* 1998 Aug 25;84(4):235–44.

Moreira AL, Waisman J, Cangiarella JF. Aspiration cytology of the oncocytic variant of papillary adenocarcinoma of the thyroid gland. *Acta Cytol.* 2004 Mar–Apr;48(2):137–41.

Ohori NP, Schoedel KE. Cytopathology of high-grade papillary thyroid carcinomas: tall-cell variant, diffuse sclerosing variant, and poorly differentiated papillary carcinoma. *Diagn Cytopathol.* 1999 Jan;20(1):19–23.

Punthakee X, Palme CE, Franklin JH, Zhang I, Freeman JL, Bedard YC. Fine-needle aspiration biopsy findings suspicious for papillary thyroid carcinoma: a review of cytopathological criteria. *Laryngoscope* 2005 Mar;115(3):433–6.

Wu HH, Jones JN, Grzybicki DM, Elsheikh TM. Sensitive cytologic criteria for the identification of follicular variant of papillary thyroid carcinoma in fine-needle aspiration biopsy. *Diagn Cytopathol.* 2003 Nov;29(5):262–6.

Ylagan LR, Dehner LP, Huettner PC, Lu D. Columnar cell variant of papillary thyroid carcinoma. Report of a case with cytologic findings. *Acta Cytol.* 2004 Jan–Feb;48(1):73–7.

ANAPLASTIC CARCINOMA

Bauman ME, Tao LC. Cytopathology of papillary carcinoma of the thyroid with anaplastic transformation. A case report. *Acta Cytol.* 1995 May–Jun;39(3):525–9.

Cameselle-Teijeiro J, Febles-Perez C, Sobrinho-Simoes M. Cytologic features of fine needle aspirates of papillary and mucoepidermoid carcinoma of the thyroid with anaplastic transformation. A case report. *Acta Cytol* 1997 Jul–Aug;41(4 Suppl):1356–60.

Fortson JK, Durden FL Jr, Patel V, Darkeh A. The coexistence of anaplastic and papillary carcinomas of the thyroid: a case presentation and literature review. *Am Surg* 2004 Dec;70(12):1116–9.

Guarda LA, Peterson CE, Hall W, Baskin HJ. Anaplastic thyroid carcinoma: cytomorphology and clinical implications of fine-needle aspiration. *Diagn Cytopathol.* 1991;7(1).63–7.

Kumar PV, Torabinejad S, Omrani GH. Osteoclastoma-like anaplastic carcinoma of the thyroid gland diagnosed by fine needle aspiration cytology. Report of two cases. *Acta Cytol* 1997 Jul–Aug;41(4 Suppl):1345–8.

Luze T, Totsch M, Bangerl I, Hittmair A, Sandbichler P, Ladurner D, Schmid KW. Fine needle aspiration cytodiagnosis of anaplastic carcinoma and malignant haemangioendothelioma of the thyroid in an endemic goitre area. *Cytopathology* 1990;1(5):305–10.

Mai DD, Mai KT, Shamji FM. Fine needle aspiration biopsy of anaplastic thyroid carcinoma developing from a Hurthle cell tumor: a case report. *Acta Cytol* 2001 Sep–Oct;45(5):761–4.

Saunders CA, Nayar R. Anaplastic spindle-cell squamous carcinoma arising in association with tall-cell papillary cancer of the thyroid: A potential pitfall. *Diagn Cytopathol* 1999 Dec;21(6):413–8.

FOLLICULAR CARCINOMA

Carling T, Udelsman R. Follicular neoplasms of the thyroid: what to recommend. *Thyroid.* 2005 Jun;15(6):583–7 [Review].

Clary KM, Condel JL, Liu Y, Johnson DR, Grzybicki DM, Raab SS. Interobserver variability in the fine needle aspiration biopsy diagnosis of follicular lesions of the thyroid gland. *Acta Cytol* 2005 Jul–Aug;49(4):378–82.

Giorgadze T, Rossi ED, Fadda G, Gupta PK, Livolsi VA, Baloch Z. Does the fine-needle aspiration diagnosis of "Hurthle-cell neoplasm/follicular neoplasm with oncocytic features" denote increased risk of malignancy? *Diagn Cytopathol* 2004 Nov;31(5):307–12.

Harach HR, Zusman SB, Day ES. Nodular Goiter: A histo-cytological study with some emphasis on pitfalls of fine-needle aspiration cytology. *Diagn Cytopathol* 1992 8:409–19.

Harach HR, Zusman SB. Necrotic debris in thyroid aspirates: a feature of follicular carcinoma of the thyroid. *Cytopathology* 1992 3:359–64.

Kini SR, Miller JM, Hamburger JI, et al. Cytopathology of Follicular Lesions of the Thyroid Gland. *Diagn Cytopathol.* 1985 1:123–132.

Kini SR, Miller JM, Hamburger JI. Cytopathology of hurthle cell lesions of the thyroid gland by fine needle aspiration. *Acta Cytol* 1981 25:647–52.

Smith J, Cheifetz RE, Schneidereit N, Berean K, Thomson T. Can cytology accurately predict benign follicular nodules? *Am J Surg* 2005 May;189(5):592–5; discussion 595.

POORLY DIFFERENTIATED CARCINOMA (INSULAR CARCINOMA)

Gong Y, Krishnamurthy S. Fine-needle aspiration of an unusual case of poorly differentiated insular carcinoma of the thyroid. *Diagn Cytopathol* 2005 Feb;32(2):103–7.

Guiter GE, Auger M, Ali SZ, Allen EA, Zakowski MF. Cytopathology of insular carcinoma of the thyroid. *Cancer* 1999 Aug 25;87(4):196–202.

Kuhel WI, Kutler DI, Santos-Buch CA. Poorly differentiated insular thyroid carcinoma. A case report with identification of intact insulae with fine needle aspiration biopsy. *Acta Cytol* 1998 Jul–Aug;42(4):991–7.

Layfield LJ, Gopez EV. Insular carcinoma of the thyroid: report of a case with intact insulae and microfollicular structures. *Diagn Cytopathol* 2000 Dec;23(6):409–13.

Pereira EM, Maeda SA, Alves F, Schmitt FC. Poorly differentiated carcinoma (insular carcinoma) of the thyroid diagnosed by fine needle aspiration (FNA). *Cytopathology.* 1996 Feb;7(1):61–5.

Pietribiasi F, Sapino A, Papotti M, Bussolati G. Cytologic features of poorly differentiated 'insular' carcinoma of the thyroid, as revealed by fine-needle aspiration biopsy. *Am J Clin Pathol* 1990 Dec;94(6):687–92.

Sironi M, Collini P, Cantaboni A. Fine needle aspiration cytology of insular thyroid carcinoma. A report of four cases. *Acta Cytol* 1992 May–Jun;36(3):435–9.

MALIGNANT LYMPHOMA

Al-Marzooq YM, Chopra R, Younis M, Al-Mulhim AS, Al-Mommatten MI, Al-Omran SH. Thyroid low-grade B-cell lymphoma (MALT type) with extreme plasmacytic differentiation: report of a case diagnosed by fine-needle aspiration and flow cytometric study. *Diagn Cytopathol* 2004 Jul;31(1):52–6.

Cha C, Chen H, Westra WH, Udelsman R. Primary thyroid lymphoma: can the diagnosis be made solely by fine-needle aspiration? *Ann Surg Oncol* 2002 Apr;9(3):298–302.

Das DK, Gupta SK, Francis IM, Ahmed MS. Fine-needle aspiration cytology diagnosis of non-Hodgkin lymphoma of thyroid: a report of four cases. *Diagn Cytopathol* 1993 Dec;9(6):639–45.

Gupta N, Nijhawan R, Srinivasan R, Rajwanshi A, Dutta P, Bhansaliy A, Sharma S. Fine needle aspiration cytology of primary thyroid lymphoma: a report of ten cases. *Cytojournal.* 2005 Dec 9;2:21.

Lu JY, Lin CW, Chang TC, Chen YC. Diagnostic pitfalls of fine-needle aspiration cytology and prognostic impact of chemotherapy in thyroid lymphoma. *J Formos Med Assoc* 2001 Aug;100(8):519–25.

Matsuzuka F, Miyauchi A, Katayama S, Narabayashi I, Ikeda H, Kuma K, Sugawara M. Clinical aspects of primary thyroid lymphoma: diagnosis and treatment based on our experience of 119 cases. *Thyroid* 1993 Summer;3(2):93–9.

Sangalli G, Serio G, Zampatti C, Lomuscio G, Colombo L. Fine needle aspiration cytology of primary lymphoma of the thyroid: a report of 17 cases. *Cytopathology* 2001 Aug;12(4): 257–63.

GRAVES DISEASE

Anderson SR, Mandel S, LiVolsi VA, Gupta PK, Baloch ZW. Can cytomorphology differentiate between benign nodules and tumors arising in Graves' disease? *Diagn Cytopathol* 2004 Jul;31(1):64–7.

Cantalamessa L, Baldini M, Orsatti A, Meroni L, Amodei V, Castagnone D. Thyroid nodules in Graves disease and the risk of thyroid carcinoma. *Arch Intern Med* 1999 Aug 9–23;159(15): 1705–8.

Carnell NE, Valente WA. Thyroid nodules in Graves' disease: classification, characterization, and response to treatment. *Thyroid* 1998 Jul;8(7):571–6.

Das DK. Marginal vacuoles (fire-flare appearance) in fine needle aspiration smears of thyroid lesions: does it represent diffusing out of thyroid hormones at the base of follicular cells? *Diagn Cytopathol* 2006 Apr;34(4):277–83.

Jayaram G, Singh B, Marwaha RK. Grave's disease. Appearance in cytologic smears from fine needle aspirates of the thyroid gland. *Acta Cytol* 1989 Jan–Feb;33(1):36–40.

Liel Y, Zirkin HJ, Sobel RJ. Fine needle aspiration of the hot thyroid nodule. *Acta Cytol* 1988 Nov–Dec;32(6):866–7.

Mishra A, Mishra SK. Thyroid nodules in Graves' disease: implications in an endemically iodine deficient area. *J Postgrad Med* 2001 Oct–Dec;47(4):244–7.

Sahin M, Guvener ND, Ozer F, Sengul A, Ertugrul D, Tutuncu NB. Thyroid cancer in hyperthyroidism: incidence rates and value of ultrasound-guided fine-needle aspiration biopsy in this patient group. *J Endocrinol Invest* 2005 Oct;28(9):815–8.

Slowinska-Klencka D, Klencki M, Sporny S, Popowicz B, Lewinski A. Cytologic appearance of toxic nodular goiter after thyrostatic treatment. A karyometric study. *Anal Quant Cytol Histol* 2003 Feb;25(1):39–46.

Wang CY, Chang TJ, Chang TC, Hsiao YL, Chen MH, Huang SH. Thyroidectomy or radioiodine? The value of ultrasonography and cytology in the assessment of nodular lesions in Graves' hyperthyroidism. *Am Surg* 2001 Aug;67(8):721–6.

METASTATIC TUMORS

Bozbora A, Barbaros U, Kaya H, Erbil Y, Kapran Y, Ozbey N, Ozarmagan S. Thyroid metastasis of malignant melanoma. *Am J Clin Oncol* 2005 Dec;28(6):642–3.

Hanna WC, Ponsky TA, Trachiotis GD, Knoll SM. Colon cancer metastatic to the lung and the thyroid gland. *Arch Surg* 2006 Jan;141(1):93–6.

Kihara M, Yokomise H, Yamauchi A. Metastasis of renal cell carcinoma to the thyroid gland 19 years after nephrectomy: a case report. *Auris Nasus Larynx* 2004 Mar;31(1):95–100.

Loo CK, Burchett IJ. Fine needle aspiration biopsy of neuroendocrine breast carcinoma metastatic to the thyroid. A case report. *Acta Cytol* 2003 Jan–Feb;47(1):83–7.

Maly A, Meir K, Maly B. Isolated carcinoid tumor metastatic to the thyroid gland: report of a case initially diagnosed by fine needle aspiration cytology. *Acta Cytol* 2006 Jan–Feb;50(1): 84–7.

Michelow PM, Leiman G. Metastases to the thyroid gland: diagnosis by aspiration cytology. *Diagn Cytopathol* 1995 Oct;13(3):209–13.

Nenkov R, Radev R, Hristosov K, Krasnaliev I, Vicheva S, Sechanov T. Locally advanced papillary thyroid carcinoma with coexistent metastasis from hepatocellular carcinoma in the thyroid gland and parathyroid adenoma. *Thyroid* 2005 Dec;15(12):1415–6.

Owens CL, Basaria S, Nicol TL. Metastatic breast carcinoma involving the thyroid gland diagnosed by fine-needle aspiration: a case report. *Diagn Cytopathol* 2005 Aug;33(2):110–5.

11

FNA of Kidney and Adrenal Gland

Luan D. Truong and Rose Anton

KIDNEY

NORMAL/NONNEOPLASTIC KIDNEY

Clinical Features
■ Noncontributory

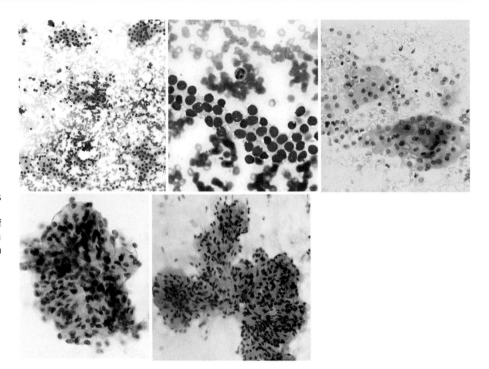

11-1. Non-neoplastic elements.
Upper left, middle, and right: Abundant clusters of proximal tubular cells in flat sheets with abundant cytoplasm, central nuclei, and absence of binucleation. The cell uniformity is a key feature differentiating them from oncocytoma cells. Lower left: A glomerulus with characteristic features including outer smooth contour imparted by the glomerular capillaries. Lower right: Isolated glomeruli may artifactually aggregate (Papanicolaou, modified Giemsa stains and H&E stains)

Cytologic Features

- Low (often) or high (unusual) cellularity
- Most cells from proximal tubules, since they normally account for about 90 of tubular cross-sections in the cortex
  - Small mostly flat sheets, rare single cells, three-dimensional (3-D) clusters often associated with intact tubular basement membrane
  - Well-defined cell border; homogeneous, ample cytoplasm; characteristic cell junction when seen
  - Round uniform central nuclei with small nucleoli; bare nuclei rare but sometimes numerous
- Few cells from other tubular segments
  - Intact slender tubules, flat sheets, or single cells (rare) with smaller nuclei and scanty cytoplasm
- Glomeruli
  - Often seen: Pathognomonic features

Special Stains and Immunohistochemistry

- Proximal tubular cells positive for the renal cell carcinoma marker (RCCM) antigen, PAX2, and CD10; negative for kidney-specific cadherin
- Distal tubular cells negative for RCCM and CD10; positive for kidney-specific cadherin and PAX2

Modern Techniques for Diagnosis

- Noncontributory

Differential Diagnosis

- RCC
  - Feature NOT favoring tubular cells: Large 3-D clusters, abundant isolated cells, loose aggregates, few rare cells with binucleation, larger nuclei, spindle shape, cytoplasmic clearing or vacuolization, clusters with vascular cores
  - Imunostain not helpful: Positive for both RCCM and CD10

- Renal oncocytoma
  - ➤ Same type of cytoplasm as proximal tubular cells; more variable cell, nuclear, and nucleolar sizes; better preserved cell border
  - ➤ RCCM and CD10: negative for oncocytoma, but positive for proximal tubular cells

- ✶ Rather frequent in renal FNAs
- ✶ One of the most frequent causes of false-positive diagnosis of RCC (59% interpreted as RCC in a CAP educational program)
- ✶ Normal epithelial cells may simulate epithelioid component of renal neoplasms characterized (and diagnosed) by the presence of both stromal and epithelioid components, for example, Wilms' tumor or clear cell sarcoma.
- ✶ Can be abundant in FNA of simple cyst, leading to the diagnosis of cystic RCC

SIMPLE CYST

Clinical Features
- Up to 50% renal masses are cystic
- Most frequent lesion: Simple cyst, cystic RCC, cystic nephroma, cystic partially differentiated nephroblastoma, mixed stromal epithelial tumor, acquired cystic kidney disease-associated RCC
- If imaging typical for simple cyst (unilocular, smooth/thin wall, no mural nodule, no intracystic density): No need for FNA or treatment
- Atypical imaging: Cystic lesions other than simple cyst considered, and a specific diagnosis, best provided by FNA, often needed before treatment

Cytopathologic Features
- Macrophages almost always present
- Cyst wall cells: About 50% of cases, isolated cells, small flat sheets usually <10 cells, no nuclear atypia, variable cytoplasm including clear
- Renal tubular cells (see below) less often
- Lymphocytes, neutrophils (suggesting cyst infection), crystals, reactive fibroblasts from cyst capsule, and Liesegang rings (smooth round or faceted acellular laminated bodies due to precipitation of intracystic proteinaceous debris)
- May be acellular
- The inflammatory cells may show necrosis, sometimes marked
- Any deviations from the above features should prompt alternative diagnoses

Special Stains and Immunohistochemistry
- See below

Modern Techniques for Diagnosis
- Noncontributory

Differential Diagnosis
- RCC
  - ➤ Macrophages may form small aggregates with atypical nuclei, simulating RCC
  - ➤ Immunostain: RCC cells keratin positive/CD68 negative; reverse profile for macrophages
- Infected simple cyst
  - ➤ Cystic features and variable neutrophils, single cystic lesion on imaging

■ Abscess
  ➤ Abundant neutrophils, organisms sometimes seen (bacteria, fungi); no cystic features, usually multiple lesions
■ Other cystic lesions
  ➤ See below

PEARLS

★ Gross appearance (clear, bloody, or cloudy) not indicating benign versus malignant
★ Macrophages may appear atypical and form clusters, simulating RCC (these cells have cytoplasmic inclusions and keratin negative/CD68 positive immunoprofile)
★ FNA of simple cyst may contain nonneoplastic tubular cells in about a quarter of cases; due to FNA of not only cyst content but also pericystic solid areas; tubular cells can be abundant causing confusion with cystic RCC
★ The diagnosis of simple cyst requires typical FNA and imaging findings. Any deviations should prompt alternative diagnosis
★ More than rare benign cyst wall lining epithelial cells even with ''benign'' imaging should be considered ''suspicious''
★ ''Typical'' FNA findings of benign cyst with ''atypical'' imaging should be considered ''Suspicious'': This may reflect sampling of ''benign'' locules in cystic nephroma, or in acquired cystic kidney disease

CYSTIC RENAL CELL CARCINOMA

Clinical Features
■ 15% of RCCs predominantly cystic
■ Single uni- or multilocular mass
■ Several distinct histologic types: mutilocular cystic RCC (almost all clear cell), unilocular (mostly papillary), extensively necrotic RCC (often clear cell, less frequently papillary); acquired cystic kidney disease–associated RCC

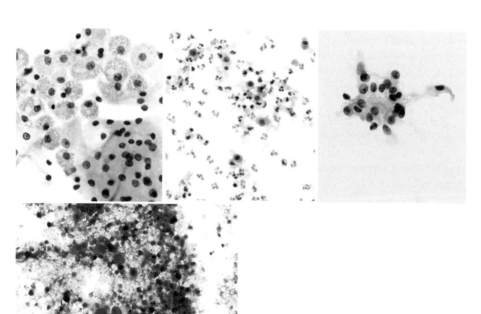

11-2. Cystic renal lesion.
Upper: Simple cyst showing macrophage aggregates, admixed with tubular cell cluster (*left*). Neutrophils may be abundant suggesting infection (*middle*). A rare benign cluster of epithelial cells with mild atypia, which may represent cyst epithelial cells (*right*). Lower: Cystic renal cell carcinoma with cystic background, abundant necrotic debris, and a few mildly atypical epithelial cells (Papanicolaou and modified Giemsa stains)

Cytopathologic Features
■ Cystic background: Cystic fluid (cloudy /bloody), macrophages, necrotic cells, inflammatory cells, and
■ Clear cell or papillary RCC features (see below)

Special Stains and Immunohistochemistry
■ See RCC types

Modern Techniques for Diagnosis
■ Noncontributory

Differential Diagnosis
■ Simple cyst
➤ Imaging very helpful: Unilocular, smooth thin wall is usually a simple cyst: multilocular, thickened/shaggy/calcified wall, mural nodules, dense intracystic content, and necrosis
■ Other cystic lesions, including cystic RCC
➤ Strict FNA and imaging criteria for simple cyst: Any deviation should raise the possibility of cystic RCC: look for features of RCC against a cystic background
■ Cystic nephroma
➤ See below
■ Acquired cystic kidney disease (ACK)–associated RCC
➤ ACK is defined as diffuse renal cystic changes of associated with long-term dialysis for end-stage renal disease
➤ Mass lesions may develop against the ACK background including abscess, hematoma, fibrosis, adenoma, and carcinoma; FNA may potentially help in their differentiation
➤ Limited experience with one FNA showing clear cell RCC admixed with numerous macrophages and lymphocytes and another with features of benign simple cyst

PEARLS

★ High false-negative FNAs (up to 75%) due to scant tumor bulk, sampling of cysts devoid of tumor cell lining, or low nuclear grade of tumor cells
★ Mutilocular cystic clear cell RCC almost always low nuclear grade (Furhman 1 or 2), virtually never metastasize
★ Clinical communication that *"a negative result is not reliable"* imperative

CYSTIC NEPHROMA

Clinical Features
■ Rare benign tumor
■ Bimodal age distribution (<4 and >30 years)
■ Striking female dominance (F/M = 8:1)
■ Circumscribed multilocular cystic mass, not distinguishable from other renal cystic masses by imaging, thus FNA
■ Cystic nephroma and mixed epithelial and stromal tumor may belong to a same tumor type composed of various combinations of epithelial and stromal components

Cytopathologic Features
■ *Hypocellular,* few isolated polygonal cells or small clusters of epithelial cells
■ Variable cytoplasm: Ample, granular, partially vacuolated, clear

- Nuclei: Benign or enlarged, hyperchromatic, irregular contour
- Cystic background: Abundant macrophages
- No necrosis or inflammation

Special Stains and Immunohistochemistry
- Noncontributory

Modern Techniques for Diagnosis
- Noncontributory

Differential Diagnosis
- Simple cyst
  - FNA of cystic nephroma reminiscent of simple cyst, but with more epithelial cells and more nuclear atypia
- Cystic RCC
  - Low cellularity, absence of necrosis, paucity of single cells favor cystic nephroma
- Cystic partially differentiated nephroma
  - Clinical and imaging features practically identical to that of cystic nephroma
  - Blastema element (see nephroblastoma) is a feature of cystic partially differentiated nephroma but not cystic nephroma; this, however, is not always present in FNA

PEARLS

★ Although the FNA is often obviously benign, a specific diagnosis may not be possible without tissue core

CYSTIC PARTIALLY DIFFERENTIATED NEPHROBLASTOMA

Clinical Features
- Almost always in children (<2 years)
- Asymptomatic abdominal mass (tumor usually very large, considering the young age of the patients), usually incidental finding
- Single mutilocular cystic mass, without solid area
- Histologically similar to cystic nephroma, except for the additional presence microscopic foci of nephroblastoma tissue in the septa
- Considered benign variant of nephroblastoma, cured by excision, including partial nephrectomy, thus a need for preoperative diagnosis by FNA

Cytopathologic Features
- Low or moderate cellularity
- Two cell populations
  - Epithelial cells (from cyst lining): Similar to those from cystic nephroma (see above)
  - Blastemal cells: Isolated cell or small loose clusters, with scant cytoplasm and hyperchromomatic nuclei (see also "nephroblastoma")
- Cystic background with macrophages

Special Stains and Immunohistochemistry
- The nephroblastoma component has the same immunoprofile as nephroblastoma

Modern Techniques for Diagnosis
▨ Noncontributory

Differential Diagnosis
▨ Cystic nephroma
➤ Clinical and imaging features identical for these tumor types; blastemal element not seen in cystic nephroma
▨ Nephroblastoma
➤ Low cellularity and cystic background are not features of nephroblastoma (see also nephroblastoma below)

PEARLS

★ Diagnosis often missed since blastemal component is usually minor and not sampled

MIXED EPITHELIAL STROMAL TUMOR (MEST)

Clinical Features
▨ Rare adult neoplasm composed of variable combination of epithelial and stromal components
▨ Incidental findings or mass effects
▨ Striking female prominence (F/M = 6/1)
▨ Solid or cystic by imaging
▨ Benign, cured by excision

Cytopathologic Features
▨ Two cell types: spindle and epithelial
▨ Cohesive or loose clusters, or single spindle cells, associated with extracellular matrix; benign nuclei; moderate cytoplasm, indistinct cell border; few bare nuclei
▨ Small clusters of epithelial cells; benign nuclei; scanty cytoplasm

Special Stains and Immunohistochemistry
▨ Stromal component: positive for actin, desmin, vimentin, estrogen receptor, progesterone receptor
▨ Epithelial components positive for keratin, vimentin

Modern Techniques for Diagnosis
▨ Noncontributory

Differential Diagnosis
▨ Sarcomatoid RCC
➤ Both spindle and epithelial cells present; usually marked nuclear atypia for both, in contrast with benign features of MEST
➤ The epithelial component may show features of RCC of a specific type
▨ Cystic partially differentiated nephroblastoma
➤ Benign epithelial cells in both
➤ Blastemal cells, but not spindle cells as in cystic partially differentiated nephroblastoma
▨ Primary renal sarcoma
➤ Spindle cells may be the predominant component in mixed epithelial stromal tumor; but without marked nuclear atypia as in renal sarcoma

■ Leiomyoma

➤ Smooth muscle cells, for example, benign cigar-shaped nuclei and ample dense cytoplasm

➤ Absence of epithelial component; but an epithelial component may not be sampled in MEST

■ Congenital mesoblastic nephroma

➤ Single or loose cluster of benign spindle cells with minimal nuclear atypia

➤ Probably not distinguishable from mixed epithelial stromal tumor, unless epithelial component also present

➤ Congenital mesoblastic nephroma is limited to infants (<3 months); MEST previously called "adult mesoblastic nephroma", a misnomer

PEARLS

⭑ Significant atypical cytologic features rule out MEST

⭑ Nonneoplastic tubular cells may be included in FAN of purely spindle cell tumors, for example, leiomyoma, sarcoma, congenital mesoblastic nephroma, primitive neuroectodermal tumor, clear cell sarcoma, not to be confused with neoplastic epithelial component

CLEAR CELL RCC

Clinical Features

■ Most frequent type of RCCs (75%)

■ Adult tumor; RCC regardless of subtypes very rare (< 1%) in children.

■ Genetic changes: 3p deletion, von Hippel Lindau gene mutations, in both familial and sporadic tumors

■ Small incidental renal tumors removed by laparoscopic partial nephrectomy: One-third are benign and two-thirds are RCCs (equal clear cell and papillary). These diagnoses are reflected in FNA, increasingly indicated for these tumors.

■ Granular cell variant, typical features for clear RCC, but with most tumor cells showing granular eosinophilic cytoplasm

■ The multilocular cystic variant, almost always low nuclear grade, virtually never metastasize

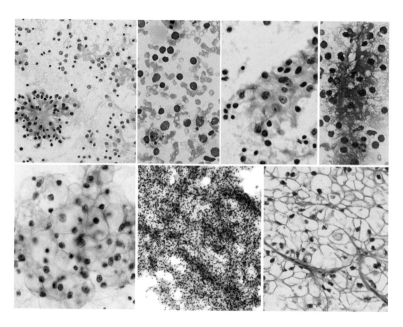

11-3. Clear cell renal cell carcinoma. Upper left: A cell cluster and abundant bare nuclei, a characteristic feature. Upper middle: FNA may be composed predominantly of bare nuclei, and this is usually more pronounced in air-dried modified Giemsa stained smears. Upper middle: Characteristic cytoplasm, that is, abundant, with both clear and solid portion. Upper right: Cytoplasm may be uniformly vacuolated, simulating adrenocortical cells. Lower left: Cytoplasm may be uniformly clear, with well-defined cell membrane, and mildly atypical nuclei, characteristic features of a low-grade renal cell carcinoma. Lower middle: A large cluster of tumor cells traversed by a capillary network. Lower right: The corresponding cell block shows the same features. (Papanicolaou, modified Giemsa stains and H&E)

Cytopathologic Features

▪ Often bloody but highly cellular, isolated cells, large 3-D groups, focally anchoring to capillaries, irregular contours with tumor cells "dangling" out; some clusters reminiscent of papillary formation; abundant isolated bare nuclei in some cases

▪ Polygonal cells with *indistinct* border; variable cytoplasm: abundant, clear, wispy/feathery, vacuolated, granular (best appreciated in modified Giemsa stain), combined features in a single FNA typical

▪ Clear cytoplasm, usually dissolved in alcohol fixation, giving rise to abundant isolated bare nuclei

▪ Cytoplasmic globules rare but characteristic for RCC

▪ Low N/C ratio; small round uniformly hyperchromatic nuclei without nucleoli (Furhman grade 1); large slightly irregular nuclei with abnormal chromatin, and small nucleoli (Furhman grade 2); large frequent pronounced irregular contour and large eosinophilic nucleoli (Furhman grade 3); or huge, bizarre mutilobated nuclei (Furhman grade 4); more than one grade in the same FNA often

▪ Rarely numerous tumor cells with characteristic cytoplasmic and nuclear features of clear cell RCC, but with spindle cell morphology, not to be confused with sarcomatoid RCC or sarcoma

▪ Necrosis or cystic changes (fluid specimen, abundant macrophages, inflammatory cells) infrequent in solid tumors, but prominent in cystic tumors (see "Cystic RCC")

Special Stains and Immunohistochemistry

▪ Negative mucin stains

▪ Distinctive immunoprofile
  ➤ Positive for low molecular-weight keratins, EMA, vimentin, CD10, RCCM, PAX-2 (nuclear)
  ➤ Negative for high-molecular-weight keratins, CEA, kidney-specific cadherin, p63

▪ Immunostain usually not needed for diagnosis, but indispensable for diagnosing clear cell RCCs metastatic to other organs, or tumors metastatic to kidney

Modern Techniques for Diagnosis

▪ Noncontributory

Differential Diagnosis

▪ Normal tubular cells
  ➤ Present by themselves or admixed with tumor cells; large, 3-D clusters NOT seen (refer also to normal tubular cells above).

▪ Oncocytoma
  ➤ Typical "oncocytoma" cells (see Oncocytoma) may be seen, especially in the granular cell variant; but note other cells diagnostic for clear cell RCC, often present even in the granular cell variant
  ➤ Oncocytoma positive for kidney-specific cadherin, paralbumin. (These are negative in RCC), but negative for RCCM, CD10, vimentin. (These are positive in RCC)

▪ Normal/hyperplastic adrenal cortex or adrerocortical adenoma
  ➤ Uniform cell population
  ➤ "Isometric" (small vacuoles of equal size) cytoplasmic vacuolization rather than clear (best appreciated in modified Giemsa stain), or granular; uniform, benign nuclei
  ➤ Absence of large 3-D clusters
  ➤ Adrenocartical cells positive for melan A, calretinin, inhibin, synaptophysin (these are negative for RCC); but negative for RCCM, CD10, keratin, EMA (these are positive in RCC); both positive for vimentin

■ Adrenal cortical carcinoma
  ➤ Infrequent, yet problematic
  ➤ Cytoplasmic spectrum, but granular more frequent than clear
  ➤ Often severe nuclear atypia (more nuclear atypia than in RCC). Immunostain essential (see above)
■ Urothelial carcinoma
  ➤ Denser cytoplasm, better defined cell border, frequent spindle cells, absence of capillaries associated with tumor cell clusters
  ➤ Urothelial carcinoma cells positive for high-molecular-weight keratin, CK7, CK20, p63 (nuclear), thrombomodulin, uroplakin, CEA (These are negative for RCC); but negative for RCCM, vimentin (These are positive for RCC); both positive for CD10)
■ Renal infarct
  ➤ May simulate RCC on imaging
  ➤ Smear composed entirely of necrotic tubular cells, necrotic glomeruli, if present, very characteristic feature
  ➤ Regenerative renal tubular cells may be atypical, simulating RCC cells
■ Xanthogranulomatous pyelonephritis
  ➤ Foamy macrophages (see also below)
■ Malakoplakia
  ➤ von Hannseman cells (macrophages with abundant granular cytoplasm
  ➤ Michelis–Gutmann bodies (see also "Malakoplakia")
■ Angiomyolipoma
  ➤ See "Angiomyolipoma"

PEARLS

★ Tissue cores and or cell block very helpful (may be the only diagnostic materials), amenable to immnunostain (see also "Metastatic Tumor")

★ The diagnosis of RCC should be followed by cell typing and nuclear grading. This is often possible by FNA (75% of cases). Tumor grade reflects the highest grade (multiple grades in about 15% of FNAs of RCC)

★ Not infrequently, the diagnosis of RCC is unequivocal, but *typing is not possible*, especially for high-grade tumors

PAPILLARY RCC

Clinical Features

▦ About 15% of RCCs. More frequent in FNA of small incidental renal tumors
▦ More likely to be bilateral (4%), or multifocal (22%) than other types of RCC
▦ May appear as a cystic (often unicystic) mass, confused with simple cyst by imaging
▦ Two histologic subtypes (1 and 2). Type 2 characterized by more abundant eosinophilic cytoplasm, higher nuclear grade, and worse prognosis. However, subtyping has not been characterized in FNA
▦ Genetic changes: Trisomy or tetrasomy 7, trisomy 17, loss of Y chromosome

Cytopathologic Features

▦ Low-grade tumors: Typical features
  ➤ Highly cellular, many complex, 3-D, papillary clusters with or without fibrovascular cores, and smooth contours; relatively few isolated tumor cells; bare nuclei much less frequent than clear cell RCC
  ➤ Rather scant cytoplasm, without the features of clear cell RCC (see above), may contain hemosiderin
  ➤ Usually low nuclear grades (Furhman grade 1 or 2); nuclear grooves often

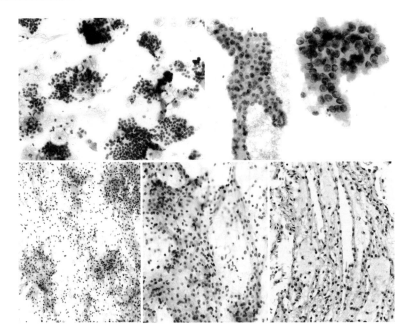

11-4. Papillary renal cell carcinoma (upper) and tubular mucinous renal cell carcinoma (lower). Upper left: Abundant papillary clusters with smooth contour focally associated with foamy macrophages. Upper middle: A papillary cluster with smooth border and uniform cells with mild nuclear atypia. Upper right: Low–grade nuclei with cytoplasmic hemosiderin, a characteristic feature. Lower left: Abundant papillary clusters with irregular contour, together with dispersed cells. Lower middle: Cells with minimal nuclear atypia forming ill-defined papillary solid clusters or thin parallel cords (left), a characteristic feature. A background mucin should be present but not observable in Pap stain. Lower right: The cell block shows thin cell cords or glands separated by mucin. (Courtesy of Nancy Caraway, MD, MD Anderson Hospital, Houston, Tx). (Papanicolaou and H&E stains)

➤ Abundant macrophages (with or without hemosiderin) frequent and often *prominent* in both solid and cystic variant; psammoma bodies

▪ High-grade tumor (probably including the subtype 2) may be indistinguishable from high-grade clear cell RCC

Special Stains and Immunohistochemistry

▪ Distinctive immunoprofile

➤ Positive for RCCM, CD10, vimentin, EMA, low-molecular-weight keratins, PAX-2 (nuclear)

➤ CK7 and alpha-methylacyl-CoA racemase (AMACR) positive in papillary RCC, but not other RCC subtypes

Modern Techniques for Diagnosis

▪ Noncontributory

Differential Diagnosis

▪ Papillary adenoma

➤ Should have FNA features identical to low-grade papillary RCC. By definition, less than 0.5 cm, thus not subjected to FNA

▪ Urothelial carcinoma

➤ Papillary clusters often in low-grade tumor; but denser cytoplasm, better defined cell border, frequent spindle cells, absence of abundant macrophages.

➤ Different immunoprofiles (see Urothelial Carcinoma)

▪ Collecting duct RCC

➤ Papillary clusters usually a component of multiple patterns (single cells, variably sized clusters, necrotic tumor cells, fibroblasts)

➤ Often marked nuclear atypia

➤ Immunostain important for differential diagnosis

➤ Collecting duct RCC positive for high-molecular-weight keratin (this is negative in papillary RCC) and low-molecular-weight keratins, CK7, EMA, CEA, PAX-2 (nuclear), ulex lectin, peanut lectin

➤ Collecting duct RCC negative for RCCM, CD10, vimentin (these are positive in papillary RCC)

■ Metanephric adenoma

➤ Papillary structures can be seen in FNA of metanephric adenoma. But there is also the background of "small round cell tumor" (see below)

➤ Component cells small, scant cytoplasm, with minimal atypia

➤ Characteristic immunoprofile (WT-1 and CD57 are positive, AMACR is negative; opposite profile for papillary RCC

■ Mucinous tubular and spindle cell carcinoma

➤ Cellular smears, low nuclear atypia and focal papillary structures seen: this tumor is even considered a variant of papillary RCC

➤ Several typical features not seen in papillary RCC, including:

Irregular border of the papillary clusters (vs. smooth border in papillary RCC)

Amorphous, metachromatic, myxoid, focally bubbly stroma, reminiscent of those in pleomorphic adenoma; admixed with interconnected epithelial aggregates

Loose sheet of parallel, low-grade ovoid cells as the mirror images of the compressed parallel tubules in tissue

PEARLS

★ Both macrophages and tumor cells can contain hemosiderin, but tumor cell hemosiderin is very characteristic for papillary RCC and not seen in other renal tumors

CHROMOPHOBE RCC

Clinical Features

■ 5% of RCCs

■ Genetic changes: Extensive chromosomal loss (1, 2, 6, 10, 13, 17, 21), TP53 gene mutation

■ Single well-circumscribed mass without necrosis or calcification by imaging

■ Better prognosis than clear cell or papillary RCC

■ Probably deriving from the intercalated cells of collecting duct

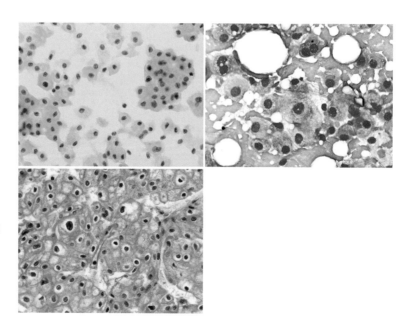

11-5. Chromophobe renal cell carcinoma. Upper left: Loose clusters of cells with abundant cytoplasm, perinuclear halo, well-defined cell membrane, mild nuclear atypia, and ocassional binucleation. (Papanicolaou stain). Upper right: Same features in modified Giemsa stain. Lower: Same features in the corresponding cell block. (H&E stains)

Cytopathologic Features

▨ Cellular smears, often markedly so, with abundant isolated or *small* clusters of polygonal cells

▨ Diagnostic cells but not always present: Abundant vacuolated, flocculent cytoplasm, perinuclear clearing/halo, well-defined/accentuated cell border

▨ Other cells with abundant granular cytoplasm but no other diagnostic features

▨ Low N/C ratio; usually Furhman nuclear grade 2, *irregular/raisinoid nuclear contour including grooves*, binucleation, intranuclear inclusion, small nucleoli: Characteristic for chromophobe RCC, rarely seen in other RCC types

▨ Rare isolated tumor cells with marked nuclear atypia against the background of more typical tumor cells

▨ Necrosis, inflammation, or cystic background not seen

Special Stains and Immunohistochemistry

▨ Diffuse strong cytoplasmic positivity by Hale's colloidal iron stain

▨ Distinctive immunoprofile

▨ Positive for low-molecular-weight keratins, CK7, EMA, CD117, kidney-specific cadherin, paralbumin

▨ Negative for high-molecular-weight keratins, RCCM, CK20, CD10, vimentin, S-100A1

Modern Techniques for Diagnosis

▨ Noncontributory

Differential Diagnosis

▨ Oncocytoma
  ➤ Much less cytoplasmic or nuclear pleomorphism than chromophobe RCC
  ➤ Uniform, round nuclei; no perinuclear clearing; no prominent cell membrane
  ➤ Focal or no cytoplasmic colloidal iron stain
  ➤ Immunostain perhaps not helpful: Immunoprofile practically identical to chromophobe RCC, except for S-100A1 (positive in oncocytoma, negative in chromophobe RCC)
▨ Renal hybrid oncocytic tumor
  ➤ Multifocal/bilateral tumors with "hybrid" features of oncocytoma and chromophobe RCC, characteristic for the Bird–Hogg–Dubre syndrome

PEARLS

★ Significant histologic, immunohistochemical and cytologic overlapping of oncocytoma and oncocytic variant of chromophobe RCC. Their differentiation may not be possible by FNA

COLLECTING DUCT RCC

Clinical Features

▨ < 1% of RCCs

▨ Derived from principal cells of collecting ducts

▨ Wide age ranges, often younger than other types of RCC

▨ Very aggressive, metastasis at presentation often (up to a half), often large potentially unresectable tumor, thus more prone to FNA

▨ A variant seen exclusive in those with sickle cell disease (renal medullary carcinoma)

▨ Imaging often suggesting TCC

▨ No constant genetic markers

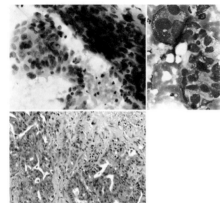

11-6. Collecting duct renal cell carcinoma. Upper: Highly atypical cells with focal necrosis, reminiscent of a high-grade carcinoma, rather than renal cell carcinoma. Lower: Cell block shows gland formation, solid clusters, desmoplastic stroma, (Papanicolaou and modified Giemsa and H&E stains)

Cytopathologic Features

■ Cellular; large 3-D aggregates, papillary clusters, or single cells, of rather uniform features; tumor cells with fibrous tissue fragments

■ Variable cytoplasmic volume, but often scanty granular cytoplasm (higher N/C ratio than other RCC), infrequently vacuolated, rare cells with cytoplasmic mucin

■ Highly atypical central or eccentric (hobnail) nuclei; large, hyperchromatic, prominent single or multiple nucleoli; irregular nuclear contour; frequent mitosis

■ The overall features more reminiscent of poorly differentiated adenocarcinoma than RCC

■ Necrosis, inflammation, macrophages usually not prominent

■ Tumor cells may be in urine, a very unusual feature for other RCC types (large tumor mass in renal medulla often invading renal pelvis wall)

■ FNA may be performed not for renal tumor but for metastases, with the same features

Special Stains and Immunohistochemistry

■ Cytoplasmic mucin occasionally

■ Distinctive immunoprofile

➤ Positive for high-molecular-weight keratins, low-molecular-weight keratins, CK7, EMA, CEA, PAX-2 (nuclear), Ulex lectin, peanut lectin

➤ Negative for RCCM, CD10, vimentin

Modern Techniques for Diagnosis

■ Noncontributory

Differential Diagnosis

■ Although a diagnosis of a high-grade carcinoma often obvious, further classification often not possible

■ Metastatic carcinoma

➤ Cytology closely simulating collecting duct RCC

➤ Cytoplasmic mucin rarely seen in both metastatic carcinoma and collecting duct RCC (mucin virtually not seen in other types of RCC)

➤ Clinical history, renal imaging (bilateral multifocal tumor for metastasis), and immunostain may help

■ Transitional cell carcinoma (TCC)

➤ Both can be predominantly in medulla area

■ Low-grade TCC

➤ No problem: This is characterized by large clusters of cells with dense ample cytoplasm, well defined cell borders, low nuclear grade, frequent spindle cells: Quite different from collecting duct RCC

■ High-grade TCC

➤ May not distinguishable from collecting duct RCC by cytology

➤ Some cells with retained "urothelial" features (dense ample cytoplasm, well-defined cell borders, frequent spindle cells) suggest the diagnosis

➤ Cell block/tissue core essential for definitive diagnosis

■ High-grade papillary RCC

➤ High-grade papillary clusters seen in both

➤ May not distinguishable from collecting duct RCC by cytology

➤ Cell block/tissue core essential for a definitive diagnosis

■ Renal medullary RCC

➤ Considered a variant of collecting duct RCC

➤ Seen almost exclusively in young African American males with sickle cell disease or trait
➤ Cytologic and immunoprofile essentially identical to those of collecting duct RCC; diagnosis added by characteristic demographic features

PEARLS

✦ Difficult diagnostic problem, but perhaps quite rare (collecting duct RCC accounting for <2% of all RCCs)

SARCOMATOID RCC

Clinical Features
▦ 3–5% of RCC
▦ Not considered a separate entity, but arising from (and seen together with) other types of RCC (de-differentiation)
▦ Sarcomatoid changes impart poor prognosis
▦ Often unresectable tumor, prompting FNA for diagnosis before nonsurgical treatment

Cytopathologic Features
▦ Cellular smears
▦ Spindle cells, most often single disperse, or less often in small clusters
▦ Clusters usually not "tight" but displaying stroma separating cells
▦ Epithelioid cells possible but usually not forming clusters
▦ Often highly atypical nuclei: Large nuclei with irregular contour and prominent nucleoli; spindle cells may be the only component
▦ Often (80% of FNAs) a component of non-sarcomatoid RCC present, usually high-grade clear cell RCC

Special Stains and Immunohistochemistry
▦ The background RCC component: Usual immunoprofile expected for the subtype
▦ Sarcomatoid component: Almost always vimentin positive; but also *keratin positive in most cases (85%)*

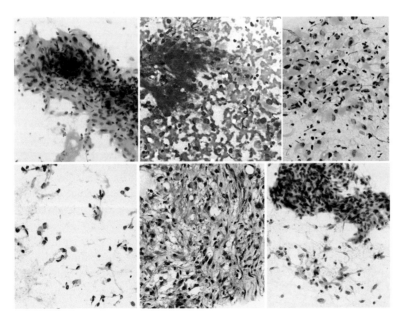

11-7. Sarcomatoid renal cell carcinoma. Upper left: Predominantly spindle cells forming a tight cluster. Upper middle: The modified Giemsa stain shows metachromatic stroma separating tumor cells, this feature is not obvious in the Pap stain, but is a characteristic "sarcomatoid" feature. Disperse cuboidal cells also seen. Upper right: Dispersed mostly cuboidal cells and few spindle cells. Lower left: Highly atypical spindle cells. Lower middle: Similar features in cell block. Lower right: A low-grade leiomyosarcoma with both dispersed and clustered spindle cells, indistinguishable from sarcomatoid renal cell carcinoma. (Papanicolaou and modified Giemsa and H&E stains)

Modern Techniques for Diagnosis
- Noncontributory

Differential Diagnosis
- Primary renal sarcomas
  - Very rare (<1% of renal tumors); leiomyosarcoma most often; other including rhadomyosarcoma, hemangiopericytoma, liposarcoma, malignant fibrous histiocytoma, osteosarcoma, angiosarcoma
  - FNA of these tumors not yet described or only as rare isolated cases; but probably similar to their counterparts elsewhere
  - Absence of an RCC component
  - Immunostain essential: Spindle cell component of sarcomatoid RCC often are keratin positive, but renal sarcomas are keratin negative
  - Many renal sarcomas are from renal capsule and may be predominantly perirenal
- Angiomyolipoma (see below)
- Adrenocortical carcinoma
  - Atypical spindle cells may be present
  - Tumor cells more typical for adrenocorcical carcinoma also seen
  - Typical immunoprofile for adrenocortical cells (see "Adrenal Tumors")
- High-grade transitional cell carcinoma (TCC)
  - TCC may have a spindle cell component
  - Cells more typical for TCC also often seen (polygonal, dense cytoplasm, well-defined cytoplasmic border, tight clusters)
  - Tumor cells also in urine specimens
  - Typical immunoprofile for TCC
- Leiomyoma, mixed epithelial and stromal tumor, classic variant of congenital mesoblastic nephroma
  - Only or predominantly spindle cells in FNA, minimal nuclear atypia

PEARLS

★ The vast majority (>90%) of renal malignant spindle cell tumors are sarcomatoid RCC

RENAL PELVIS TRANSITIONAL CELL CARCINOMA (TCC)

Clinical Features
- About 7% of renal neoplasms
- Elderly patients, about half with history of TCC elsewhere
- Low-grade TCC (two-third) usually not invading kidney: Diagnosed by urine cytology
- High-grade TCC (one-third) often shows extensive renal invasion, simulating renal neoplasms; urine cytology may be falsely negative or nondiagnostic, thus FNA

Cytopathologic Features
- Low-grade tumor (often urine cytology): Cellular, variable 3-D papillary clusters with characteristic "urothelial" features, that is, polygonal, dense cytoplasm, well-defined cytoplasmic border, frequent spindle cells; mild nuclear atypia
- High-grade tumor (FNA or urine cytology)
  - Cellular, 3-D clusters or single cells (often); necrosis sometime prominent
  - Obvious nuclear atypia; variable cytoplasm, but some cells with "urothelial" features still present; cells with cytoplasmic flattened tail ("cercariform" cells) reported to be characteristic for TCC; sometimes cells with squamous or glandular differentiation

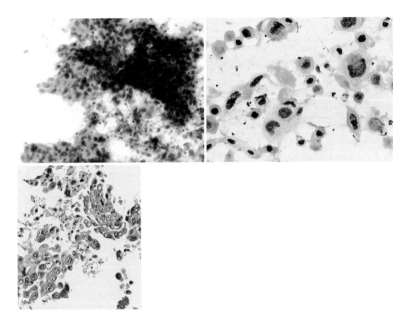

11-8. Poorly differentiated transitional cell carcinoma. Upper left: Large cluster composed of both cuboidal and spindle cells with "hard" cytoplasm and marked nuclear atypia. Upper right: Characteristic cells with atypical spindle nuclei and ample cyanophilic cytoplasm. Lower: Similar features noted in cell block. (Papanicolaou H&E and stains)

Special Stains and Immunohistochemistry

▦ Distinctive immunoprofile
  ➤ Positive for high-molecular-weight keratin, low-molecular-weight keratins, CK7, CK20, p63 (nuclear), thrombomodulin, uroplakin, CEA, CD10
  ➤ Negative for RCCM, vimentin

Modern Techniques for Diagnosis

▦ Noncontributory

Differential Diagnosis

▦ Low-grade TCC must be differentiated from reactive urothelial cells, just as for urinary bladder cytology (see the Urine chapter)
▦ High-grade TCC must be differentiated from:
▦ High-grade RCC
  ➤ RCC and TCC cells of high grade perhaps indistinguishable
  ➤ RCC, even of high grade, often has better differentiated areas with more typical features
  ➤ Different immunoprofiles (See RCC and TCC)
▦ Collecting duct RCC
  ➤ Both collecting duct RCC and TCC are in renal pelvic/medullary area
  ➤ Both have a quite similar cytologic spectrum
  ➤ High-grade TCC may still have better differentiated areas with more typical "urothelial" features (see above)
  ➤ Immunostain essential for differential diagnosis
▦ Sarcomatoid RCC
  ➤ Both tumor types may have focal malignant spindle cells; an "urothelial" versus "RCC" background may differentiate them
▦ Metastasis to kidney, and other types of primary renal pelvis carcinoma (squamous, adeno, and undifferentiated)
  ➤ All rare compared with renal pelvic TCC

PEARLS

★ Although the differential diagnosis include several tumor types, high-grade TCC remains the most frequent tumor among them
★ High-grade TCC: Obvious malignant, but tumor typing often problematic

LYMPHOMA

Clinical Features

▨ Four clinical forms: secondary, primary, posttransplant lymphoproliferative disorder (PTLD), and intravascular lymphoma

▨ Secondary: renal involvement in those with known lymphoma; renal masses other than lymphoma not infrequent in this context, including RCC (tenfold increases incidence of RCC in lymphoma patients)

▨ Primary: NOT rare, 3–6% primary renal tumors; characteristic imaging (diffuse bilateral enlargement, acute renal failure, multifocal/bilateral, marked perinal involvement; prominent hilar lymphadenopathy)

▨ PTLD: kidney probably the most frequently affected organ

▨ Intravascular lymphoma: kidney one of the most frequently affected organs

▨ Optimal treatment is chemo/radiation therapy, surgery contraindicated

▨ Clinical or imaging findings often suggestive of lymphoma, prompting FNA for confirmation

Cytopathologic Features

▨ Abundant lymphoid cells (scanty cytoplasm, round nuclei), dyshesive, evenly distributed; small clusters often, but cells in them showing typical lymphoid features as those in the background

▨ Lymphoglandular bodies (clustered cytoplasm without nuclei, repeatedly reported to be characteristic, but found not helpful in a large personal study)

▨ No necrosis; no cystic features

▨ Most often uniform lymphoid cells with large nuclei, fine chromatin, constant nuclei (reflecting large B-cell lymphoma); less often uniform small lymphoid cells or mixed large and small lymphoid cells

▨ Rare cases with spindle cells having more cytoplasm forming clusters, simulating carcinoma, but still with a more typical lymphoid background

Special Stains and Immunohistochemistry

▨ Positive lymphoid cell markers, B-cell lymphoma in almost all cases

▨ Negative epithelial markers

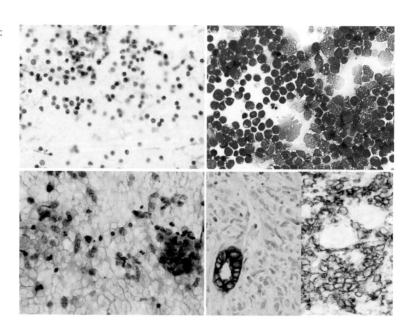

11-9. Renal lymphoma. Upper left: Abundant dispersed mostly small lymphocytes. Upper right: Cytospin is composed of typical small lymphocytes, but a few of them show artifactual changes reminiscent of small cell carcinoma cells. This type of change may be diffuse and creates confusion with small cell carcinoma. Lower left: Large cell lymphoma displaying dispersed cells without obvious lymphoid features. but with ample cytoplasm and spindle nuclei; there is also cell clustering; these features can simulate carcinoma. Lower right: The tumor cells in the corresponding cell block also display these atypical nuclear features, but they are negative for keratin and positive for common leukocyte antigen. (Papanicolaou, modified Giemsa stains and immunohistochemical stain)

Modern Techniques for Diagnosis
▪ Flow cytometry most helpful; if lymphoma suspected in adequacy check, material for "flow" imperative
▪ Gene arrangement as the last resort, rarely needed

Differential Diagnosis
▪ Small cell carcinoma
➤ Rare, described in either renal pelvis or kidney
➤ Primary or metastasis, with roughly the same frequency
➤ Differentiating features similar to those in more familiar sites, for example, lung: Bare nuclei, nuclear molding, hyperchromatic clump chromatin, isolated cell and small true epithelial clusters, necrotic background, apoptotic cells, absence, or inconspicuous nucleoli. Most of these features are not seen in lymphoma
▪ Other "small round cell tumors" of the kidney
➤ These include nephroblastoma, primitive neuroectodermal tumor, rhabdomyosarcoma, synovial sarcoma, neuroblastoma, desmoplastic small round cell tumor, neuroendocrine tumor including carcinoid tumor
➤ Rare in kidney; mostly in children
➤ See "Small Round Cell Tumors"
▪ Inflammatory renal masses
➤ Including abscess, pyelonephritis, inflammatory pseudotumor
➤ Polymorphic inflammatory cells: Small lymphocytes, large lymphocytes, plasma cells, macrophages, neutrophils; mostly T cells versus mostly B cells for lymphoma
▪ Acute rejection
➤ The same clinical and imaging of acute renal transplant rejection and PTLP in renal transplant in some cases
➤ If lymphoid cells in PTLP atypical and monomorphic with focal necrosis: No diagnostic problem
➤ If lymphoid tumor cells in PTLD polymorphic (in some cases): can be confused with rejection:
➤ Most of these cells are B cells versus T cells in rejection
➤ Most of these cells are positive for Epstein–Barr virus antigen or RNA

PEARLS

★ More frequent than suggested by literature
★ Incorrect diagnosis leading to unnecessary surgery
★ Lymphoma and RCC rarely coexist in the same kidney
★ Many differential diagnoses, but lymphoma accounting for the vast majority of them
★ Diagnosis of lymphoma usually obvious, if it is thought of and its characteristic clinical and imaging features known

METASTATIC CARCINOMA

Clinical Features
▪ Occult metatasis to kidney frequent (20% in autopsy of patients with disseminated tumor); symptomatic cases rare, usually bilateral and multifocal masses with the primary site known at time of renal presentation
▪ FNA done in atypical cases to rule out concomitant primary renal tumor or nonneoplastic mass
▪ Lung as the primary site in more than two-thirds, without preference for histologic types

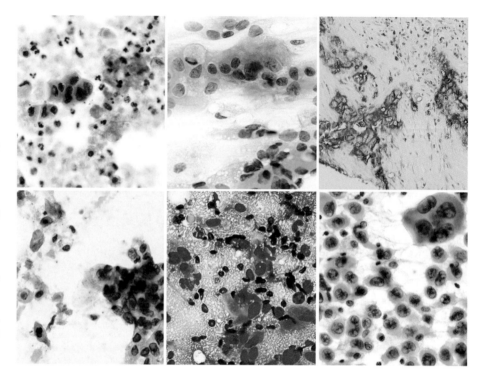

11-10. Metastatic tumors.
Upper left: Adenocarcinoma with highly atypical cells in small clusters against a prominent necrotic background. Upper middle: A rare tumor cell with cytoplasmic mucin. Upper right: Strong staining for CEA in cell block. Lower left: Squamous cell carcinoma displaying highly atypical cell clusters, together with squamous differentiation including a "hard" cyanophilic or orangiophilic cytoplasm in a few isolated cells. Lower middle: These features can also be seen in modified Giemsa stain. Lower right: Malignant melanoma characterized by dispersed cells with large nuclei and nucleioli, and a rare multinucleated tumor cells. (Papanicolaou modified Giemsa stains and immunoperoxidase stain)

Cytopathologic Features
- Cellular, clusters or isolated dispersed cells, bloody, mitoses
- Necrosis, often prominent
- Features reminiscent of high-grade adenocacinoma: Clusters reminiscent of gland formation; scanty cytoplasm, columnar cells, well-defined cell membrane; highly atypical nuclei
- Features reminiscent of small cell carcinoma or poorly differentiated squamous cell carcinoma
- No usual features of RCC

Special Stains and Immunohistochemistry
- Immunoprofiles reflecting primary sites
- Knowledge on potential primary site facilitates a focused immunohistochemical workup

Modern Techniques for Diagnosis
- Noncontributory

Differential Diagnosis
- Clinical history, renal imaging helpful; immunostain needed (and indispensable in some cases)
- Clear cell RCC
  - Typical RCC features (abundant clear, vacuolated, feathery cytoplasm; ill-defined cell border; bare nuclei) not seen in metastasis
  - Low-grade nuclear atypia in some RCCs, but constantly high grade in metastasis
- Collecting duct RCC
  - Cytology closely simulating metastasis adenocarcinoma; cytoplasmic mucin occassionaly seen in both metastatic carcinoma and collecting duct RCC (mucin virtually not seen in other types of RCC)
  - Immunostain essential

■ Renal pelvis primary squamous cell carcinoma
  ➤ Similar to metastatic squamous cell carcinoma, but very rare
■ High-grade TCC
  ➤ Few cells with typical "urothelial" features (dense ample cytoplasm, well-defined but not accentuated cell borders, frequent spindle cells), against the background of nondescript highly atypical cells

PEARLS

✶ High-grade nuclei without typical cytoplasmic features of RCC: Think about metastatic tumor
✶ Prominent necrosis: Think about metastatic tumor
✶ Symptomatic renal metastasis infrequent but accounting for a disproportionately high percentage of malignant renal FNAs (up to 20%)

ONCOCYTOMA

Clinical Features
■ Most frequent benign renal epithelial neoplasm
■ Often incidental in elderly man (mean age 70; M/F 2/1)
■ 5–10% of resected renal epithelial tumors
■ Increasing incidence in renal FNAs, reflecting a trend to diagnose before treatment for incidental renal mass
■ No specific genetic marker

Cytopathologic Features
■ Cellular smears, with abundant *small* clusters (some with associated vascular stroma) or isolated polygonal cells
■ Cytoplasm: abundant homogeneous granular; no cell border or perinuclear halo; bare nuclei possible
■ Nuclei: low N/C ratio; central or eccentric; mild or no pleomorphism, round smooth contour, without grooves; small or no nucleoli; binucleation possible, but less often than chromophobe RCC
■ No necrosis, inflammation, or cystic changes
■ Focal prominent nuclear atypia rarely seen (reported in 12% of oncocytoma in tissue studies)
■ Focal cells with typical nuclei but scanty cytoplasm "oncoblastic features" (reported in 10% of oncocytomas in tissue studies)

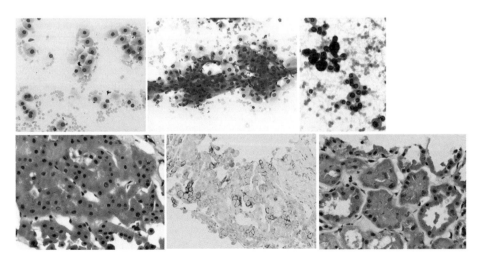

11-11. Oncocytoma. Upper left: Cells with abundant cytoplasm, mildly atypical central nuclei, in small clusters of dispersed cells, almost identical to proximal tubular cells, except for a subtle variation in cell shape and size. Upper middle: A tumor cell cluster traversed by capillaries, a feature not seen in tubular cell clusters. Upper right: Isolated highly atypical cells against the background of typical oncocytoma cells, a characteristic feature. Lower left: Similar features in the cell block. Lower middle: Tumor cells positive for kidney-specific cadherin. Lower right: Proximal tubular cells cytologically similar to oncocytoma cells in the same cell block (Papanicolaou and modified Giemsa stains, immunoperoxidase stain and H&E)

Special Stains and Immunohistochemistry
■ Negative or weak focal positive for colloidal iron stain
■ Distinctive immunoprofile
  ➤ Positive for low-molecular-weight keratins, CK7, EMA, CD117, kidney-specific cadherin, paralbumin, S-100A1
    ➤ Negative for high-molecular-weight keratins, RCCM, CK20, CD10, vimentin

Modern Techniques for Diagnosis
■ Noncontributory

Differential Diagnosis
■ Normal proximal tubular cells
  ➤ Same type of cytoplasm as oncocytoma; but with much less variation in the size of cell, nuclei, or nucleoli
  ➤ 3-D clusters with vascular stroma are not features of proximal tubular cells
  ➤ Differential immunoprofiles (see above)
■ Chromophobe RCC
  ➤ More cellular plemorphism; nuclear irregularities
  ➤ Well defined cell border, perinuclear clearing
  ➤ Immunoprofiles practically identical for oncocytoma and chromophobe RCC, except for S-100A1 (positive in oncocytoma, negative in chromophobe RCC)
■ Clear cell RCC
  ➤ Cells typical for oncocytoma may be seen; but other diagnostic cells also present even in the granular cell variant
  ➤ Differential immunoprofiles (see above)

PEARLS

★ One of the most frequent tumors incidentally in elderly patients who may have serious disease and not be surgical candidate
★ The FNA diagnosis of oncocytoma may justify watchful waiting: Correct FNA diagnosis imperative

ANGIOMYOLIPOMA (AML)

Clinical Features
■ Benign tumor composed of variable combinations of adipose tissue, blood vessels, and smooth muscle
■ Sporadic (80%) or associated with tuberous sclerosis (20%)
■ Sporadic form: Single, elderly, F/M=4/1
■ Tuberous sclerosis–associated form: Multifocal, bilateral, childhood–adulthood, F/M = 1/1, sometimes associated with renal cysts or RCC, epithelioid variant (see below) overrepresented
■ Epithelioid variant composed almost entirely of epithelioid smooth muscle cells; malignant (50% with distant metastasis)
■ Most diagnosed by imaging due to high fat content; others with low fat content confused with RCC
■ Often asymptomatic; increased incidence due to more frequent abdominal imaging; amenable to partial nephrectomy or watchful waiting; thus a need for pretreatment diagnosis by FNA
■ Extensively cystic in rare cases, simulating cystic RCC on imaging

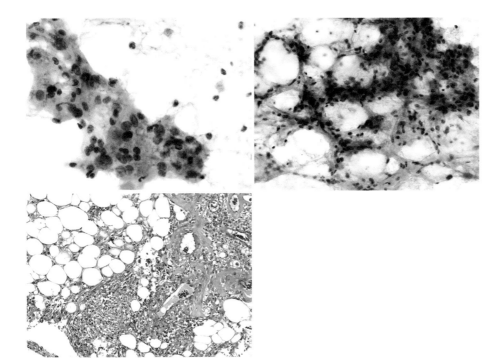

11-12. Angiomyolipoma. Upper left: A cluster of epithelioid cells closely simulating renal cell carcinoma. Upper right: A diagnostic cluster composed of both epithelioid/spindle cells and adipocytes also noted in the same smear. Lower: Similar features in the cell block. (Papanicolaou stain and H&E)

Cytopathologic Features
▪ Typical and diagnostic in a minority of cases. The diagnostic features including:
  ➢ Cellular smears; no necrosis, inflammation, or mitosis
  ➢ Isolated (more frequent) and small 3-D clusters of spindle cells; polygonal cells much less frequent
  ➢ Benign nuclei: Elongated, no or inconspicuous nucleoli, occasional intranuclear inclusion
  ➢ Adipose tissue less frequent: Adipocytes as small clusters, or *admixed with spindle cells*
  ➢ Large vessels quite unusual
▪ Nonspecific and problematic in most cases; especially epithelioid variant; almost identical to RCC (see Pearls)
  ➢ Cellular; single or small 3-D clusters of large epithelial cells; few spindle cells; few highly atypical epithelioid cells occasionally; dispersed, individual bare nuclei possible
  ➢ Round or irregular nuclei with large nucleoli, mitosis
  ➢ Abundant/adequate vacuolated or granular cytoplasm; well defined cell membrane but not accentuated
  ➢ Necrosis possible; often no fat; no blood vessels
  ➢ *However, diagnostic clusters (mixed adipocytes/ spindle/eptheloid cells) can also be seen*

Special Stains and Immunohistochemistry
▪ Distinctive immunoprofile; the spindle and epithelioid cells
  ➢ Positive for melanocytic markers (HMB-45, melan A, CD63, tyrosinase)
  ➢ Positive for smooth muscle markers (smooth muscle actin, muscle-specific actin, calponin)
  ➢ May be positive for estrogen receptor, progesterone receptor, S-100, and desmin
  ➢ Negative for epithelial markers
  ➢ Essential for differentiating from RCC

Modern Techniques for Diagnosis
▪ Noncontributory

Differential Diagnosis
- Clear cell RCC
  - More cells with clear cytoplasm, less spindle cells
  - More necrosis, cystic changes, inflammatory background
  - Diagnostic clusters (Spindle/round cells admixed with adipocytes may be seen even in epitheloid AML, but not in clear cell RCC
  - Clinical features helpful: The type of AML confused with RCC often of epithelioid type, and this often seen in younger patients with features of tuberous sclerosis
  - Immunostain essential for differential diagnosis
- Sarcomatoid RCC
  - More atypia than AML
  - Sarcomatoid cells against the background RCC cells
  - Clinical features helpful; immunostain essential
- Liposarcoma
  - More abundant adipose tissue; atypical adipocytes; spindle cells seen in the de-differentiated liposarcoma with a range of nuclear atypia (benign to monstrous)
  - Retroperitoneal tumor (rather than renal) by imaging
  - Immunostain essential

PEARLS

★ Very frequently misdiagnosed as RCC (always think of "AML" before diagnosing RCC). If AML thought of, careful review often reveals diagnostic clusters (mixed adipocytes/spindle/eptheloid cells)

★ AML with typical imaging findings (much fat), not subjected to FNA; AML with low or no fat content (epithelioid) not suspected by imaging subjected to FAN: Confused with RCC

★ AML of other organs (lymph node, liver, adrenal, spleen) rarely coexists with renal AML; multifocality, not metastasis; same FNA findings as renal AML

RENAL ABSCESS

Clinical Features
- One or multiple "masses" variably involving kidney, renal pelvis, perinephric soft tissue, simulating neoplasm
- Predisposing factors: Pyelonephritis, urinary tract obstruction, severe immunosuppression, AIDS
- Caused by bacteria (*Escherichia coli*, Proteus, Klebsiella, mycobacteria); fungi (actinomyces, candida, aspergillus)
- Flank pain, fever

Cytopathologic Features
- Cloudy fluid specimen
- Abundant neutrophils
- Other types of inflammatory cells less pronounced
- No cyst features (see "Simple Cyst")
- Usually no epithelial cells
- Organisms may be present, but may not be obvious in Pap or modified Giemsa stains even when abundant

Special Stains and Immunohistochemistry
- Specimen should be submitted for special stains and culture for organisms

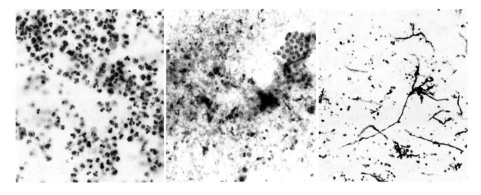

11-13. Renal abscess. Left: Abundant neutrophils and few macrophages. Middle: The FNA can be composed mostly of necrotic debris admixed with atypical tubular cells simulating necrotic tumor. Right: The GMS stain of the same FAN shows abundant fungal hyphae and yeasts not obvious in routine smears (Papanicolaou and modified Giemsa stain)

Modern Techniques for Diagnosis
■ Noncontributory

Differential Diagnosis
■ Infected simple cyst
  ➤ See "Simple Cyst"
■ Xanthogranulomatous pyelonephritis and malakoplakia
  ➤ Absence of abundant foamy macrophages or von Hansemann cells
■ Renal neoplasms
  ➤ Usually no epithelial cells in FNA of abscess, but a rare case with abundant necrotic or intact tubular cells

PEARLS

✶ Usually obvious diagnosis; but rare cases with numerous necrotic/atypical tubular cells and fewer neutrophils than typical: Confusion with tumor. Even in these cases, malignant nuclear features usually not seen

XANTHOGRANULOMATOUS PYELONEPHRITIS (XGP)

Clinical Features
■ A form of chronic pyelonephritis, characterized by extensive accumulation foamy macrophages, with fewer other inflammatory cells
■ Predisposing factors: Urinary obstruction, bacterial infection
■ Flank pain, fever, pyuria, renal lithiasis
■ Involvement of a portion or the whole kidney; can appear as renal masses with perirenal extension, closely simulating malignant neoplasm on imaging, thus a need for FNA

Cytopathologic Features
▨ Macrophages, isolated or in small flat clusters, with abundant foamy vacuolated (*not clear*) cytoplasm, no nuclear atypia, but may be multinucleated
▨ Background of inflammation
▨ Rare reactive fibroblasts
▨ Often necrotic background, rarely prominent
▨ Rarely, mature squamous cells (from associated renal pelvis squamous metaplasia)

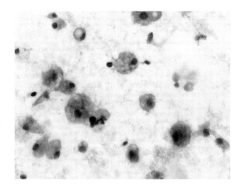

11-14. Xanthogranulomatous pyelonephritis. Disperse xanthoma cells with abundant vacuolated cytoplasm (Papanicolaou stain)

Special Stains and Immunohistochemistry
▓ Macrophages: CD68 positive/keratin negative on cell block sections

Modern Techniques for Diagnosis
▓ Noncontributory

Differential Diagnosis
■ Clear cell RCC
    ➤ Features of clear cell RCC not seen in XGP: Clear cytoplasm, large cohesive, 3-D sheets. More than minimal nuclear atypia, marked necrosis, marked inflammatory background, bare nuclei seen in both but only pronounced in RCC
■ Spindle cell lesions
    ➤ FNA of XGP may contain atypical fibroblasts; but they are few, and seen against the typical background of XGP
■ Malakoplakia
    ➤ See "Renal Malakoplakia"

PEARLS

★ Imaging usually quite "worrisome," in contrast with an inflammatory/"low-grade" appearance in FNA: A diagnostic clue

RENAL MALAKOPLAKIA

Clinical Feature
▓ Distinctive form of localized chronic inflammation, creating single or multifocal renal masses, simulating renal neoplasm
▓ Usually associated with urinary tract infection or severe immunosuppression
▓ Due to impaired phagolysosomes to digest phagocytized bacteria or other cellular elements, leaving partially digested glycolipids as the nidus for gradual deposition of calcium and iron salts, forming the diagnostic Michaelis–Gutmann bodies

Cytopathologic Features
▓ Macrophages with abundant granular (not clear or foamy) cytoplasm, disperse cells without clusters
▓ Michaelis–Gutmann bodies: Pathognomonic for malakoplakia. 2–5 micron, round, concentric multilayered, basophilic calcospherites; within or outside cell cytoplasm
▓ Inflammatory background

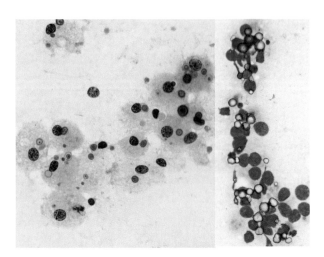

11-15. Renal malakoplakia.
Clusters of macrophages with abundant cytoplasm and moderate nuclear atypia, simulating renal cell carcinoma, but the diagnostic Michealis–Guttman bodies are obvious (Papanicolaou and modified Giemsa stains)

Special Stains and Immunohistochemistry
▨ The Michaelis–Gutmann bodies have a characteristic histochemical profile (positive for PAS, Perl's iron, von Kossa, alizarin red, GMS, mucicarmine, alcian blue, and toluidine)
▨ The macrophages are positive for CD68 and negative for keratin

Modern Techniques for Diagnosis
▨ Noncontributory

Differential Diagnosis
▨ See "Xanthogranulomatous Pyelonephritis"

PEARLS
★ Michaelis–Gutmann bodies usually abundant and easily identified, when present

NEPHROBLASTOMA

Clinical Features
▨ Mainly in children (<10 years); rarely in adults
▨ Accounting for 85% pediatric renal tumors
▨ Asymptomatic palpable mass, or mass effects; distant metastasis at presentation (25%), lung and liver most frequent, leading to FNA of metastatic lesions
▨ FNA rarely needed since the diagnosis obvious by clinical and imaging findings
▨ FNA indicated in uncertain clinical diagnosis (for preoperative radiation or chemotherapy), unresectable tumor (bilateral, marked local spreading, metastasis)

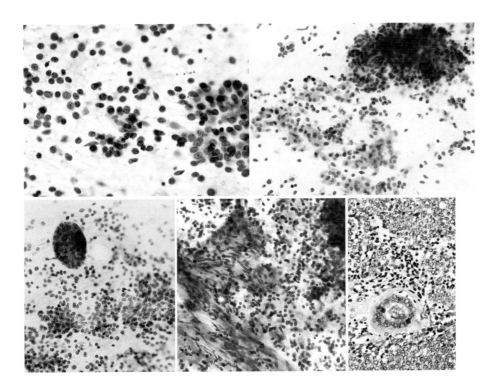

11-16. Nephroblastoma. All illustrations are from the same case. Upper left: Abundant blastema cells in disperse or in loose clusters, not readily distinguishable from other "small blue cell tumors". Upper right: Cells with similar nuclear features but more abundant cytoplasm are also seen, indicating characteristic tubular differentiation. Lower left: A tubule with intact basement membrane against the background of blastema cells. Lower middle: Stromal fragments adjacent to blastema cells. Lower right: The cell block shows blastema cells and a tubule. (Courtesy of Nancy Caraway, M.D., M. D. Anderson Hospital, Houston, TX)

Cytopathologic Features

- Similar for pediatric and adult variants; similar for primary and metastatic tumors
- Very cellular smears; necrosis and acute/chronic inflammation frequent
- Three cell types: Blastemal (virtually 100%), epithelial (60%), and stromal (33%). All three (40%); less than three (60%)
- Blastemal cells
    - Isolated or loose clusters; small cells (1.2 to 2× the size of small lymphocyte)
    - Round, oval, or less frequently spindle, hyperchromatic nuclei with fine chromatin; no or small nucleoli
    - Very scanty cytoplasm
- Epithelial cells
    - 3-D tight clusters, larger than blastemal cells
    - Forming tubules (occasionally surrounded by basement membrane, gland-like structures, cell nest) or glomeruli
    - Cuboidal or columnar cells with more cytoplasm
    - Large hyperchromatic nuclei
- Spindle stromal cells
    - Often isolated cells, small clusters
    - Spindle nuclei in loose (metachromatic in modified Giemsa stain) connective tissue matrix
    - Rarely specialized stromal cells (skeletal muscle, smooth muscle, cartilage, fat, bone, ganglion cells, neuroglial tissue/cells)
- Anaplastic cell changes (in anaplastic variant)
    - Large, pleomorphic mononuclear or multinucleated; at least 3× the size of adjacent cells in two perpendicular dimension (elongated cell not qualified)
    - Markedly hyperchromatic
    - Abnormal mitotic figures, often multipolar
    - Rather scant cytoplasm
    - Isolated cells against typical background of nephroblastoma (focal anaplasia), or the majority of cells (diffuse anaplasia)

Special Stains and Immunohistochemistry

- Immature cells (blastemal cells and primitive epithelial cells)
    - Positive for vimentin, NSE, WT-1, CD56; negative for cytokeratin
- Mature epithelial cells
    - Positive cytokeratin; negative for other markers above
- Stromal cells
    - Positive vimentin, negative for other markers above
- Anaplastic cells
    - Positive for p53
- All cells
    - Negative for common leukocyte antigen, CD99, S-100, desmin, myogenin (See also Table)

Modern Techniques for Diagnosis

- Noncontributory

Differential Diagnosis

- See "Small Round Cell Tumors" of the Kidney

PEARLS

- ★ Three components present: Definitive diagnosis
- ★ Less then three: potentially problematic since blastemal component (almost always present) can closely simulate small round cell tumors

★ The spindle cell component may be mistaken as fibrous stroma
★ The primitive tubular component often scanty and easily overlooked
★ Normal tubular epithelial cells may be sampled and confused with tumor epithelial component
★ Strict criteria for cellular anaplasia (elongated cells, enlarged but not hyperchromatic nuclei and megakaryocyte do not qualify as anaplasia)

"SMALL ROUND CELL TUMORS" OF THE KIDNEY

Clinical Features
▨ This group includes several tumors: Most of them are seen in children; aside from nephroblastoma, the others are very rare (nephroblastoma 90%; mesoblastic nephroma 5%; neuroblastoma, primitive neroectodermal tumor, synovial sarcoma, small cell carcinoma, lymphoma, neuroendocrine tumor including carcinoid, metanephric tumors, plasmacytoma, together 4%)
▨ Each of them has distinct clinical, histologic, immunohistochemical, cytogenetic features. However, they share common FNA features (see below)
▨ Differential diagnosis involving FNA often needed, since their treatment may involve tumor type–specific preoperative adjuvant therapy

Cytopathologic Features
▨ See Differential Diagnosis

Special Stains and Immunohistochemistry
▨ See Table and Differential Diagnosis

Modern Techniques for Diagnosis
▨ See Table and Differential Diagnosis

Differential Diagnosis
▨ All these tumor types share the same FNA features: "Small round cell features" including cellular smears, cells with small round/oval/spindle hyperperchomatic nuclei, absent or inconspicuous nucleoli, scanty cytoplasm (usually twice the size of RBC in modified Giemsa stain, and <10 micron in fixed smears)

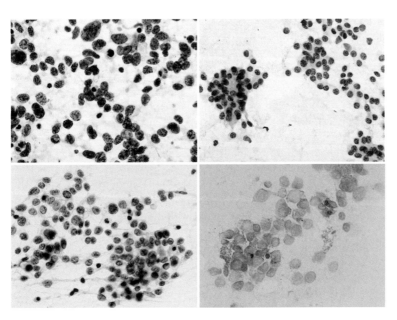

11-17. "Small round cell tumors". Upper left: Small cell carcinoma showing dispersed cells or small clusters with scanty cytoplasm, molded nuclei, and coarse chromatin. Upper right: Neuroblastoma: Note a rosette formation. Lower left: Primitive neuroectodermal tumor: Note diffuse mild chromatin clearing. Lower right: Primitive neuroectodermal tumor: Cytoplasmic glycogen granules (red) (Papanicolaou and modified Giemsa stains)

■ Some of these tumor types have additional diagnostic features (see below), but they are not always seen

■ A specific diagnosis usually not made by FNA smears alone, but requires correlation with histologic and immunohistochemical features on cell block or corresponding tissue cores (See Table)

■ Specialized studies for prognosis or diagnosis, suitable for FNA material, may be helpful

■ Nephroblastoma
  ➤ If all three components seen: Definitive diagnosis
  ➤ Differentiated mesenchymal cells, for example, cells with rhabdomyoblastic differentiation favor the diagnosis
  ➤ If only blastemal component seen, need ancillary studies
  ➤ Note that nephroblatoma accounts for the vast majority (90%) of "small round cell tumors" of the kidney

■ Neuroblastoma
  ➤ Rosette formation, metachromatic fibrillary matrix (neuropil) background, cytoplasmic processes, "salt-and-pepper" chromatin, ganglion cells (in case of ganglioneuroblastoma)
  ➤ N-myc amplification, deletion/amplification of chromosome 1p; detectable on FNA material
  ➤ The vast majority due extension from adrenal gland rather than true primary renal tumor

■ Lymphoma
  ➤ See "Lymphoma"

■ Primitive neuroectodermal tumor
  ➤ Rosette formation
  ➤ Large, irregular punched out large cytoplasmic vacuoles due to glycogen accumulation
  ➤ Chromosomal translocation (11;22) (q24; q12), detectable on FNA materials
  ➤ Benign tubular cells can be sampled by FNA, leading to misdiagnosis of nephroblastoma

■ Rhadomyosarcoma
  ➤ Strap or tadpole cells

■ Synovial Sarcoma
  ➤ Clusters of epithelial cells without atypia, reflecting sampling of microcysts lined by benign renal tubular type of cells frequently seen in this tumor
  ➤ Chromosomal translocation (X;18)(p11.2;q11)

■ Desmoplastic Small Round Cell Tumor
  ➤ Fragments of desmoplastic stroma
  ➤ Chromosomal translocation (11;12)(p13;q11.2)

■ Congenital mesoblastic nephroma
  ➤ Three histologic variants, that is, classic, cellular, and mixed
  ➤ FNA of the cellular variant shows "small round cell tumor" features
  ➤ The classic variant shows abundant clustered or disperse spindle/ovoid cell with cigar-shaped nuclei with minimal nuclear atypia
  ➤ The mixed variant shows both

■ Small cell carcinoma
  ➤ Can be either primary or metastatic, with roughly equal frequency, with similar FNA features as small cell carcinoma elsewhere
  ➤ Prominent nuclear molding

■ Metanephric adenoma or adenofibroma
  ➤ Cells may show more epithelial features, for example, compact follicular or acinar formation

■ Rhabdoid tumor
➤ Areas of "undifferentiated" tumor may be aspirated, accounting for the "small round cell tumor" features. However, more typical features also seen (see below)

✶ If the clinical differential diagnosis is "small round cell tumors", make sure to obtain enough material for cell block preparation, and fresh material in preservation fluid for cytogenetic/molecular studies
✶ The vast majority of these tumor are in children

RHABDOID TUMOR

Clinical Features
■ 2% of pediatric renal tumor
■ Almost always <5 years
■ Often presented with disseminated disease, leading to FNA for diagnosis
■ Aggressive (80% died within two years)
■ Rhabdoid tumor composed entirely of rhadoid component as a distinct clinicopathologic entity versus focal rhabdoid areas seen in 5% of RCCs, usually the high-grade ones

Cytopathologic Features
■ Cellular smears; mostly disperse cells, rare small clusters
■ Diagnostic "rhabdoid" cells: Large cells, abundant dense cytoplasm, large nuclei, vesicular chromatin, prominent (eosinophilic) nucleoli, large cytoplasmic inclusion
■ Cells with some but not all these features in the background
■ Similar cells with spindle shape possible

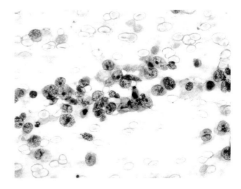

Special Stains and Immunohistochemistry
■ Strong vimentin staining, especially the paranuclear inclusion
■ Focal strong EMA and CK
■ Negative for muscle markers
■ Absence of nuclear staining for SMARCB1/INI1 protein (see below)

11-18. Rhabdoid tumor. Mostly disperses cells with prominent nucleoli and coarse chromatin. Cytoplasmic inclusion is noted in a rare cell (lower left). (Papanicolaou stain)

Modern Techniques for Diagnosis
■ Biallelic inactivation or deletion of the SMARCB1/INI1 tumor suppressor gene in chromosome 22 is the molecular hallmark
■ Cytogenetic detection of this deletion is of no practical diagnostic utility, but the deletion leads to uniform loss of the SMARCB1/INI1 protein, which is uniformly expressed in nuclei of normal tissue or neoplastic tissue other than rhabdoid tumor

Differential Diagnosis
■ Definitive diagnosis requiring the rather uniform presence characteristic cells, since many other pediatric and adults renal neolasms may have focal rhabdoid features, against the typical background of the parental tumors
■ Rhabdomyosarcoma or rhabdomyoblastic form of nephroblastoma
➤ These often feature rhamomyoblasts characterized by fibrillary cytoplasmic with possible cross-striation
➤ Other typical features of nephroblastoma may be seen

★ Differential diagnosis important since rhabdoid tumor almost uniformly fatal, in contrast to possible good outcome of its mimickers such as rhabdomyoblastic nephroblastoma

CLEAR CELL SARCOMA

Clinical Features
- Virtually limited to children (mean age three years)
- 3% of pediatric tumors
- 5% with metastasis at presentation
- Often late recurrence or metastasis (frequently to bone thus the name "bone metastasizing renal tumor of childhood"

Cytopathologic Features
- Cellular smears; three cell types
- "Cord" cells (corresponding with the main cell type forming cords in tissue): delicate, wispy cytoplasm, being sheared off in many cells leaving bare nuclei; round/oval nuclei with frequent grooves, delicate, dusty chromatin, not hyperchromatic, small nucleoli in some cells
- "Septal" cells corresponding with the spindle stromal cells in tissue: Spindle cells with mild nuclear atypia, isolated cells or more commonly embedding in vascularized myxoid stroma
- Small and pyknotic cells probably reflecting degeneration of the other cell types
- Metachromatic myxoid material, often abundant, without or with septal cells or blood vessels embedded in it
- Rare cases with anaplastic single cells

Special Stains and Immunohistochemistry
- Only vimentin is positive, negative for all other markers often used for renal tumors

Modern Techniques for Diagnosis
- Noncontributory

Differential Diagnosis
- Regardless of several described histologic variants, FNA shows all features above, albeit of different proportion, for example, cord cells predominantly in classic variant, septal cells with myxoid stroma predominant in spindle cell variant.
- Nephroblastoma
  ➤ "Small round cell features" are not seen in clear cell sarcoma; in contrast, the spectrum of myxoid matrix changes characteristic for clear cell sarcoma not seen in Wilms' tumor
  ➤ Anaplastic cells seen in both nephroblastoma and clear cell sarcoma, both are positive for p53: Diagnostic problem

★ Normal tubular epithelial cells often sampled, a source of confusion with other tumor such as nephroblastoma

	CK	CD45	S-100	CD99	Des	Myo	CD56	WT-1	Vim	Chro	Syna	Neuro
	Immunoprofiles of "small round cell tumors" of the kidney											
Nephroblastoma	+*	-	-	-!	+	-	+	+	+	-	-	-
Neuroblastoma	-	-	≈	-	-	-	+	-	+	+	+	+
Primitive neuroectodermal tumor	≈	-	-	+	-	-	-!	-	+	-	-	-
Rhabdomyosarcoma	-	-	-	-!	+	+	+	-	+	-	-	-
Desmoplastic small round cell tumor	+	-	-	≈	+	-	≈	+	+	-	-	-
Synovial sarcoma	≈	-	-!	+	-	-	+	-	+	-	-	-
Metanephric tumors	+	-	-	-	-	-	-	+	+	-	-	-
Congenital mesoblastic nephroma, cellular variant &	-	-	-	-	≈	-	-	-	+	-	-	-
Lymphoma	-	+	-	-[¢]	-	-	-	-	+	-	-	-
Small cell carcinoma	+	-	-	-	-	-	+	-	-	≈	≈	-
Rhabdoid tumor	≈	-	-	-	-	-	-	-	+	-	-	-
Clear cell sarcoma	-	-	-	-	-	-	-	-	+	-	-	-

Abbreviations: +* = See text; -! = Often negative, but occasionally positive; ≈ = Variable; ¢: positive in most lymphoblastic lymphomas; & = Positive for actin; Des = Desmin; Myo = Myogenin; Vit = Vimentin; Chro = Chromogranin; Syna = Synaptophysin; Neuro = Neurofilament.

ADRENAL GLAND

CORTICAL ADENOMA AND HYPERPLASIA

Clinical Features
- Smaller average size (2.75 cm) than cortical carcinoma (9 cm)
- Bilaterality favors hyperplasia over adenoma

Cytologic Features
- Variable cellularity; some cellular cohesion, mostly dyshesive
- Nuclei small, round with sometimes marked anisonucleosis but little pleomorphism, nucleoli usually small
- Scant to abundant foamy cytoplasm that is fragile, resulting in numerous naked nuclei
- Foamy background (lipid)
- No necrosis or mitoses

Special Stains and Immunohistochemistry
- Melan-A, calretinin, inhibin, synaptophysin, CD56 positive
- EMA, S-100, keratin, p53 usually negative

Modern Techniques for Diagnosis
- Noncontributory

Differential Diagnosis
- Adrenal cortical carcinoma (ACC)
  - Necrosis, mitoses, malignant-appearing chromatin present
  - Clinical and radiographic correlation helpful
- Small round blue cell tumor
  - Cortical cells, if stripped of their fragile cytoplasm, can resemble a small cell tumor
  - Anisonucleosis without pleomorphism, molding or necrosis suggests cortical cells
  - Immunocytochemistry can be helpful

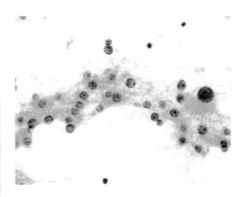

11-19. Cortical adenoma/ hyperplasia. Round, regular nuclei, with some anisonucleosis and abundant foamy cytoplasm (Papanicolaou stain)

■ Hepatocellular carcinoma
  ➤ Transgressing vessels and sinusoidal cells lining thickened trabecula present
  ➤ Immunocytochemistry can be helpful

PEARLS

★ Distinction between adenoma/hyperplasia and well differentiated ACC may be impossible
★ ACC does not characteristically show large sheets of cells and there is less of a foamy background

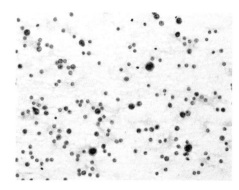

11-20. Cortical adenoma/ hyperplasia. These cells have been stripped of their cytoplasm, resulting in a foamy background. The marked anisonucleosis without pleomorphism is characteristic of an endocrine lesion and does not imply malignancy (Papanicolaou stain)

ADRENAL CORTICAL CARCINOMA

Clinical Features
■ Very rare, seen in middle-aged adults usually
■ More often functional than benign cortical lesions
■ Large (>6 cm) adrenal lesions are suspicious for malignancy

Cytologic Features
■ Cellular, poorly cohesive
■ Cells may be large and polygonal, spindled, or bizarre
■ Round-to-oval enlarged nucleus with prominent nucleolus, multinucleation may be present
■ Cells range from bland (well differentiated) to anaplastic
■ Abundant, sometimes foamy, to scant cytoplasm; few naked nuclei
■ Necrosis, mitoses present

Special Stains and Immunohistochemistry
■ Melan-A, calretinin, inhibin, synaptophysin, CD56 positive
■ EMA, S-100, keratin, p53 usually negative

11-21. Cortical adenoma/ hyperplasia *(left).* This lesion simulates a small blue cell tumor. Note the absence of nuclear molding and necrosis (Papanicolaou stain)

11-22. Adrenal cortical carcinoma *(right).* This can be very difficult to distinguish from cortical adenoma/ hyperplasia. There is a little more cytologic atypia and lesser amount of cytoplasm than benign cortical cells (Papanicolaou stain)

11-23. Adrenal cortical carcinoma *(left).* Identification of mitotic figures is very helpful in correctly establishing a malignant diagnosis (Papanicolaou stain)

11-24. Adrenal cortical carcinoma *(right).* This will show obvious cytologic features of malignancy (Papanicolaou stain)

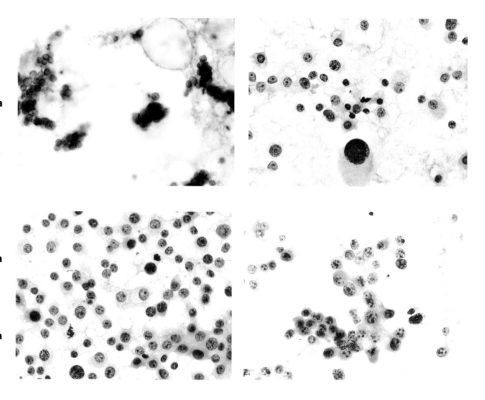

Modern Techniques for Diagnosis
■ Noncontributory

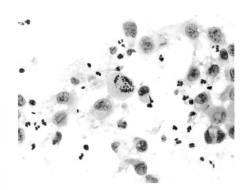

Differential Diagnosis
■ Adrenal cortical adenoma/hyperplasia
  ➤ No/rare mitoses or necrosis, no diffuse cytologic atypia
■ Pheochromocytoma
  ➤ More anisonucleosis, less pleomorphism
  ➤ Melan-A, calretinin, inhibin immunonegative (opposite for cortical lesions)
  ➤ p53, S-100 immunopositive (opposite for cortical lesions)
■ Renal cell carcinoma
  ➤ RCC, CD10, EMA immunopositive (opposite for cortical lesions)
  ➤ Melan-A, calretinin, inhibin immunonegative (opposite for cortical lesions)
■ Metastatic adenocarcinoma
  ➤ Mucin positive; immunocytochemical staining appropriate with primary source

11-25. Poorly differentiated adrenal cortical carcinoma (Papanicolaou stain)

PEARLS

★ If struggling between the diagnosis of a benign adrenal nodule versus well-differentiated carcinoma, presence of metastasis (liver, lung, lymph node usually) helpful in establishing malignant diagnosis

PHEOCHROMOCYTOMA

Clinical Features
■ If functional, sweating, flushing, palpitations, paroxysmal hypertension, headache, nervousness
■ Elevation of urinary vanillylmandelic acid and/or catecholamines
■ Wide age range
■ May be part of multiple endocrine neoplasia (MEN) syndrome

Cytologic Features
■ Polygonal or spindled cells, cohesive or dyshesive
■ Usually round nucleus with sometimes marked anisonucleosis but little pleomorphism
■ Variable chromatin, may have prominent nucleolus, mitoses rare, no necrosis
■ Large nuclear pseudoinclusions may be seen
■ Cytoplasm granular, can be scant to abundant

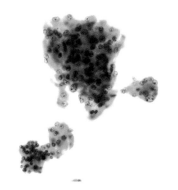
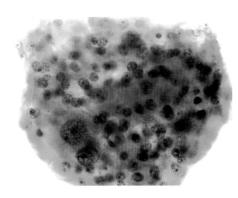

11-26. Pheochromocytoma *(left)*. Polygonal cells with anisonucleosis without pleomorphism. (Papanicolaou stain)

11-27. Pheochromocytoma *(right)*. Marked anisonucleosis without pleomorphism. Cytologic features typical of an endocrine lesion and does not imply malignancy. (Papanicolaou and modified Giemsa stain)

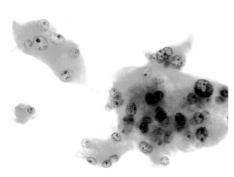

11-28. Pheochromocytoma.
Polygonal cells with anisonucleosis without pleomorphism. (Papanicolaou stain)

Special Stains and Immunohistochemistry
■ Synaptophysin, chromogranin, CD56, S-100 (sustentacular cells) positive
■ Melan-A, calretinin, inhibin, keratin usually negative

Modern Techniques for Diagnosis
■ Noncontributory

Differential Diagnosis
■ Adrenocortical carcinoma
➤ Melan-A, calretinin, inhibin immunopositive
➤ Necrosis and mitoses more often seen
■ Metastatic carcinoma
➤ Clinical findings are helpful
➤ Keratin and other epithelial markers usually immunopositive
■ Melanoma
➤ Clinical findings and immunohistochemistry are helpful

PEARLS

★ 10% rule: 10% bilateral; 10% malignant; 10% extraadrenal; 10% in children; 10% asymptomatic; 10% familial

METASTATIC TUMORS

Clinical Features
■ Lung, kidney, melanoma, breast, and GI tract are most common

Cytologic Features
■ Vary depending on the original tumor
■ Metastases more frequently show nuclear pleomorphism and mucin vacuoles than cortical lesions
■ Compare adrenal cytology with the previous known tumor

Special Stains and Immunohistochemistry
■ Mucin stains for adenocarcinoma
■ Immunophenotypic pattern consistent with primary tumor
■ Lymphoma work-up including flow cytometry for hematolymphoid processes

Modern Techniques for Diagnosis
■ Noncontributory

Differential Diagnosis
■ Primary adrenal lesions
➤ Melan-A, calretinin, inhibin usually positive in cortical lesions
➤ Synaptophysin, chromogranin, CD56, S-100 protein positive in pheochromocytoma

PEARLS

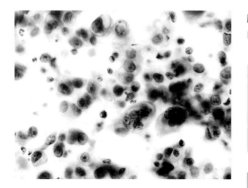

11-29. Metastatic adenocarcinoma.
This is a metastasis from lung to the adrenal gland. Mucin vacuoles are evident. (Papanicolaou stain)

★ Most adrenal masses represent metastasis, rather than an adrenal primary
★ Process all material for cell block for possible immunocytochemistry

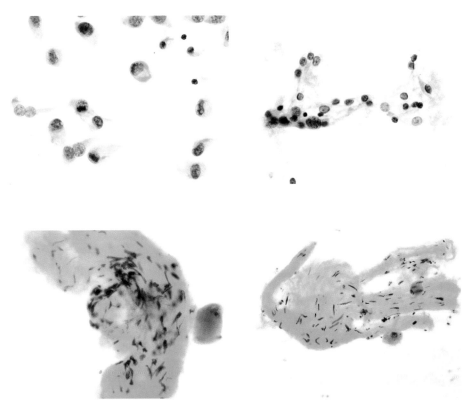

11-30. Metastatic tumor *(left)*. This is a metastasis to the adrenal gland. If melanin pigment/history is not evident/available, then immunocytochemistry and clinical correlation are essential. (Papanicolaou stain)

11-31. Metastatic tumor *(right)*. This carcinoma is a metastasis to the adrenal gland. Some cytoplasmic clearing is seen. Immunocytochemistry and clinical correlation may be required to establish the correct diagnosis. (Papanicolaou stain)

11-32. Ganglioneuroma *(left)*. Fragment of cohesive spindled cells and a single ganglion cell are seen. (Papanicolaou stain)

11-33. Ganglioneuroma *(right)*. Two mature ganglion cells are present adjacent to a fragment of bland spindled cells. (Papanicolaou stain)

NEUROBLASTIC TUMORS

Clinical Features
- Represents a spectrum from neuroblastoma (least differentiated) to ganglioneuroblastoma (intermediate) to ganglioneuroma (most differentiated)
- Neuroblastoma: second most common solid malignant tumor in children, usually less than five years old
- Ganglioneuroblastoma: Usually children; adrenal is an uncommon location
- Ganglioneuroma: Usually older people; like ganglioneuroblastoma, adrenal is a less common location than retroperitoneum or mediastinum

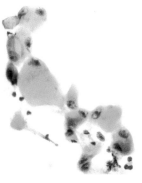

11-34. Ganglioneuroma. Mature ganglion cells show a vesicular nucleus, prominent nucleolus and abundant cytoplasm and are very helpful in establishing the correct diagnosis. (Papanicolaou stain)

Cytologic Features
- Neuroblastoma: hyperchromatic small cells with round to slightly oval nuclei, scant cytoplasm, pseudorosettes may be seen
- Ganglioneuroma: contains large ganglion cells, with fine chromatin, prominent nucleoli and abundant cytoplasm, fibrillary/myxoid background and cohesive and dyshesive spindled cells; absence of mitoses, necrosis, pleomorphism and neuroblasts (immature component)
- Ganglioneuroblastoma: mixture of mature (ganglioneuroma) and immature (neuroblastoma) components

Special Stains and Immunohistochemistry
- Synaptophysin, chromogranin, S-100 positive

Modern Techniques for Diagnosis
- Noncontributory

Differential Diagnosis

■ Neuroblastoma: any small blue cell tumor – synaptophysin/chromogranin will be immunonegative

➤ Lymphoma: Leukocyte common antigen (LCA) positive

➤ Rhabdomyosarcoma: Actin/desmin immunopositive

➤ Wilms' tumor: CD99 positive

➤ Ewing's sarcoma: CD99 positive

■ Ganglioneuroma

➤ Schwannoma: Presence of Verocay bodies, no ganglion cells

➤ Neurofibroma: no ganglion cells

PEARLS

★ Any immature forms exclude the diagnosis of ganglioneuroma

★ Ganglion cells when present are easy to recognize because of their large size, abundant cytoplasm and prominent nucleoli and are helpful in establishing the correct diagnosis. However, they may be absent on aspirates because of sampling artifact, making it difficult to render the correct diagnosis

MYELOLIPOMA

Clinical Features

■ Benign tumor of older individuals

■ Usually an incidental finding

■ Computerized tomography (CT) images show low density, consistent with fat

Cytologic Features

■ Mature adipose tissue

■ Hematopoietic cells with trilineage hematopoiesis

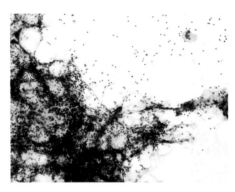 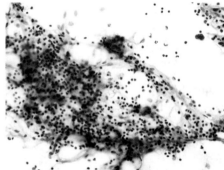

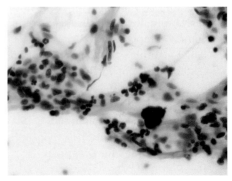

11-35. Myelolipoma *(top, left).* Adipose tissue and hematopoietic cells are present. (Papanicolaou stain)

11-36. Myelolipoma *(top, right).* Trilineage hematopoiesis. (Papanicolaou stain)

11-37. Myelolipoma *(opposite).* An adipocyte and hematopoietic cells are seen. (Papanicolaou stain)

Special Stains and Immunohistochemistry
■ Myeloid cells are myeloperoxidase, Sudan black, and chloroacetate esterase positive

Modern Techniques for Diagnosis
■ Noncontributory

Differential Diagnosis
■ Lymphoma
➤ Non-Hodgkin's lymphoma would not have the mixed background of eosinophils, neutrophils, megakaryoctes, and associated adipose tissue
➤ Hodgkin's lymphoma will not have associated adipose tissue
■ Lipomatous tumor
➤ Look for atypical lipocytes and vascular network
➤ Various hematopoietic elements not a component

PEARLS

★ The name describes what you should see

REFERENCES

NORMAL/NONNEOPLASTIC KIDNEY
Juul N, Torp-Pederson S, Gronvall S, Holm HH, Koch F, Larsen S. Ultrasonically guided fine needle aspiration biopsy of renal masses. *J Urol* 1985; 133:579–581.

Kim Y-J, Nast CC. Identification of tubular cell nephron segment origin in renal fine-needle aspirates. *Mod Pathol* 1993; 6: 150–154.

Renshaw AA, Granter SR, Cibas ES. Fine-needle aspiration of the adult kidney. *Cancer (Cancer Cytopathol)* 1997; 81: 71–88.

Truong LD, Todd TD, Dhurandhar B, Ramzy I. Fine-needle aspiration of renal masses in adults: Analysis of results and diagnostic problems in 108 cases. *Dignostic Cytopathol* 1999; 20: 339–349.

Young NAS, Mody DR, Davey DD. Fine-needle aspiration biopsy of lymphoproliferative disorders – interpretations based on morphologic criteria alone: results from the College of American Pathologists Interlaboratory Comparison Program in Nongynecologic Cytopathology. *Arch Pathol Lab Med* 2006; 130: 1766–1771.

SIMPLE CYST
Bosniak MA. Difficulties in classifying cystic lesions of the kidney. *Urol Radiol* 1991: 13: 91–93.

Renshaw AA, Granter SR, Cibas ES. Fine-needle aspiration of the adult kidney. *Cancer (Cancer Cytopathol)* 1997; 81: 71–88.

Todd TD, Dhurandhar B, Mody D, Ramzy I. Truong LD. Fine-needle aspiration of cystic lesions of the kidney. Morphologic spectrum and diagnostic problems in 41 cases. *Am J Clin Pathol* 1999; 111: 317–28.

Truong LD, Todd TD, Dhurandhar B, RamZy I. Fine-needle aspiration of renal masses in adults: analysis of results and diagnostic problems in 108 cases. *Diagn Cytopathol* 1999, 20: 339–49.

CYSTIC RENAL CELL CARCINOMA
Renshaw AA, Granter SR, Cibas ES. Fine-needle aspiration of adult kidney. *Cancer Cytopathol* 1997, 81: 71–88.

Todd TD, Dhurandhar B, Mody D, Ramzy I. Truong LD. Fine-needle aspiration of cystic lesions of the kidney. Morphologic spectrum and diagnostic problems in 41 cases. *Am J Clin Pathol* 1999; 111: 317–28.

Truong LD, Todd TD, Dhurandhar B, Ramzy I. Fine-needle aspiration of renal masses in adults: analysis of results and diagnostic problems in 108 cases. *Dignostic Cytopathol* 1999; 20: 339–349.

CYSTIC NEPHROMA
Clark SP, Kung IT, Tang SK. Fine-needle aspiration of cystic nephroma (multilocular cyst of the kidney). *Diagn Cytopathol* 1992; 8: 349–351.

Dey P, Das A, Radhika S. Fine needle aspiration cytology of cystic partially differentiated nephroblastoma. A case report. *Acta Cytol* 1996; 40: 770–772.

Drut R. Cystic nephroma: cytologic findings in fine-needle aspiration cytology. *Diagn Cytopathol* 1992; 8: 593–595.

Hughes JH, Niemann TH, Thomas PA. Multicystic nephroma: report of a case with fine-needle aspiration findings. *Diagn Cytopathol* 1996; 14: 60–63.

Nayak A, Iver VK, Agarwala S, Verma K. Fine needle aspiration cytology of cystic partially differentiated nephroblastoma of the kidney. *Cytopathology* 2006; 17:145–148.

Renshaw AA, Granter SR, Cibas ES. Fine-needle aspiration of the adult kidney. *Cancer (Cancer Cytopathol)* 1997; 81: 71–88.

Todd TD, Dhurandhar B, Mody D, Ramzy I, Truong LD. Fine-needle aspiration of cystic lesions of the kidney. Morphologic spectrum and diagnostic problems in 41 cases. *Am J Clin Pathol* 1999; 111: 317–328.

CYSTIC PARTIALLY DIFFERENTIATED NEPHROBLASTOMA

Dey P, Das A, Radhika S. Fine needle aspiration cytology of cystic partially differentiated nephroblastoma. A case report. *Acta Cytol* 1996; 40:770–772.

Katz RI. Kidney, adrenals, and retroperitoneum. In Bibbo M, Editor. *Comprehensive Cytopathology*, 2nd ed. Philadelphia: WB Saunders, 1997: pp. 781–797.

Nayak A, Iver VK, Agarwala S, Verma K. Fine needle aspiration cytology of cystic partially differentiated nephroblastoma of the kidney. *Cytopathology* 2006; 17:145–148.

MIXED EPITHELIAL STROMAL TUMOR (MEST)

Dey P, Srinivasan R, Nijhawan R, Rajwanshi A, Banerjee CK, Rao KL, Gupta SK. Fine needle aspiration cytology of mesoblastic nephroma. A case report. *Acta Cytol* 1992; 36: 404–406.

Iyer VK, Agarwala S, Verma K. Fine-needle aspiration cytology of clear cell sarcoma of the kidney: Studies of eight cases. *Diagn Cytopathol* 2005; 33: 83–89.

Kaw YT. Cytologic findings in congenital mesoblastic nephroma. A case report. *Acta Cytol* 1994; 38: 235–240.

Kumar N, Jain S. Aspiration cytology of mesoblastic nephroma in adult: Diagnostic dilemma. *Diag Cytopathol* 2000; 23: 124–126.

CLEAR CELL RCC

Fetsch PA, Powers CN, Zakowski MF, Abati A. Anti-alpha-inhibin: marker of choice for the consistent distinction between adrenocortical carcinoma and renal cell carcinoma in fine-needle aspiration. *Cancer* 1999; 87: 168–172.

Renshaw AA, Lee KR, Madge R, Granter SR. Accuracy of fine needle aspiration in distinguishing subtypes of renal cell carcinoma. *Acta Cytol* 1997; 41: 987–994.

Silverman JF, Gurley AM, Harris JP. Fine needles aspiration cytology of renal infarct. Cytomorphologic findings and potential diagnostic pitfalls in two cases. *Acta Cytol* 1991; 35: 736–741.

Simsir A, Chhieng D, Wei XJ, Yee H, Waisman J, Cangiarella J. Utility of CD10 and RCCma in the diagnosis of metastatic conventional renal-cell adenocarcinoma by fine-needle aspiration biopsy. *Diagn Cytopathol* 2005; 33: 3–7.

Unger P, Hague K, Klein G, Fine needle aspiration of a renal cell carcinoma with eosinophilic globules. A case report. *Acta Cytol* 1993; 37: 201–204.

Volpe A, Jewett MAS. The natural history of small renal masses. *Nat Clin Pract Urol* 2005; 2: 384–390.

Yang B, Ali SZ, Rosenthal DL. CD10 facilitates the diagnosis of metastatic renal cell carcinoma from primary adrenal cortical neoplasm in adrenal fine-needle aspiration. *Diagn Cytopathol* 2002; 27: 149–152.

Zaman MB. The kidneys, adrenals, and retroperitoneum. In Koss LG, Melemed MR, Editors. *Koss's Diagnostic Cytology and its Histopathologic Basis*, 5th ed., Philadelphia: Lippincott Wiliams & Wilkins (Chapter 40).

PAPILLARY RCC

Dekmezian R, Sneige N, Shabb N. Papillary renal cell carcinoma: fine-needle aspiration of 15 cases. *Diag Cytopathol* 1991; 7: 198–203.

Lim JC, Wojcik EM. Fine-needle aspiration cytology of papillary renal cell carcinoma: the association with concomitant secondary malignancies. *Diagn Cytopathol* 2006; 34:797–800.

Olgac S, Hutchinson B, Tickoo SK, Reuter VE. Alpha-methylacyl-CoA racemase as a marker in the differential diagnosis of metanephric adenoma. *Mod Pathol* 2006; 19: 218–224.

Ortega JA. Cytologic aspect of mucinous tubular and spindle-cell renal carcinoma in fine-needle aspirates. *Diagn Cytopathol* 2006; 34:660–662.

Wang S, Filipowicz EA, Schnadid VJ. Abundant intracytoplasmic hemosiderin in both histiocytes and neoplastic cells: a diagnostic pitfall in fine-needle aspiration of cystic papillary renal-cell carcinoma. *Diagn Cytopathol* 2001; 24: 82–85.

CHROMOPHOBE RCC

Adley BP, Schafernak KT, Yeldandi AV, Yang XJ, Nayar R. Cylogic and histologic findings in multiple hybrid oncocytic tumors in a patient with Birt-Hogg-Dube syndrome: a case report. *Acta Cytol* 2006: 584–588.

Akhtar M, Ali MA. Aspiration cytology of chrmophobe cell carcinoma of the kidney. *Diagn Cytopathol* 1995; 13: 287–294.

Granter SR, Renshaw AA. Fine-needle aspiration biopsy of chromophobe renal cell carcinoma. Analysis of six cases. *Cancer Cytopathol* 1997; 81: 122–128.

Liu J, Fanning CV. Can renal oncocytoma be distinguished from renal cell carcinoma on fine-needle aspiration specimens? A study of conventional smears in conjunction with anxillary studies. *Cancer Cytopathol* 2001; 93: 3909–3917.

Rocca PC, Brunelli M, Gobbo S, Eccher A, Bragantini E, Mina MM, Ficarra V, Zattoni F, Zamò A, Pea M, Scarpa A, Chilosi M, Menestrina F, Bonetti F, Eble JN, Martignoni Diagnostic utility of S100A1 expression in renal cell neoplasms: an immunohistochemical and quantitative RT-PCR study. *Mod Pathol* 2007; 20:722–728.

Salamaca J, Alberti N, Lopez-Rios F, Perez-Barrios A, Martinez-Gonzalez Ma, de Agustin P. Fine-needle aspiration of chromophobe renal cell carcinoma. *Acta Cytol* 2007; 51: 9–15.

Sun W, McGregor DK, Ordonez NG, Ayala AG, Caraway NP. Fine needle aspiration cytology of a low grade myxoid renal epithelial neoplasm: a case report. *Acta Cytol* 2005; 49: 525–529.

Wiatrowska BA, Zakowski MF. Fine-needle aspiration biopsy of chromophobe renal cell carcinoma and oncocytoma. Comparison of cytomorphologic features. *Cancer Cytopathol* 1999; 87: 161–167.

COLLECTING DUCT RCC

Assad L, Resetkova E, Oliveira VL, Sun W, Stewart JM, Katz RL, Caraway NP. Cytologic features of renal medullary carcinoma. *Cancer (Cancer Cytopathol)* 2005; 105: 28–34.

Bejar J, Szvalb S, Maly B, Munichor M, Cohen H. Collecting duct carcinoma of kidney: a cytological study and case report. *Diagn Cytopathol* 1996; 15: 136–138.

Caraway NP, Wojcik EM, Katz RL, Ro JY, Ordonez NG. Cytologic findings of collecting duct carcinoma of the kidney. *Diagn Cytopathol* 1995; 13: 304–309.

Layfield LJ. Fine-needle aspiration biopsy of renal collecting duct carcinoma. *Diagn Cytopathol* 1994; 11: 74–78.

Ono K, Nishino E, Nakamine H. Renal collecting duct carcinoma. Report of a case with cytologic findings on fine needle aspiration. *Acta Cytol* 2000;44: 380–384.

Sironi M, Salvina AG. New cytological findings on fine-needle aspiration of renal collecting duct carcinoma. *Diagn Cytopathol* 2003; 29: 239–240.

Zaman SS, Sack MJ, Ramchandani P, Tomaszewski JE, Gupta PK. Cytopathology of retrograde renal pelvis brush specimens: an analysis of 40 cases with emphasis on collecting duct carcinoma and low-intermediate grade transitional cell carcinoma. *Diagn Cytopathol* 1996; 15: 312–321.

SARCOMATOID RCC

Auger M, Katz RL, Sella A, Ordonez NG, Lawrence DD, Ro JY. Fine-needle aspiration cytology of sarcomatoid renal cell carcinoma: a morphologic and immunocytochemical study of 15 cases. *Diagn Cytopathol* 1993; 9: 46–51.

de Peralta-Venturina M, Moch H, Amin M, Tamboli P, Hailemariam S, Mihatsch M, Javidan J, Stricker H, Ro JY, Amin MB. Sarcomatoid differentiation in renal cell carcinoma: a study of 101 cases. *Am J Surg Pathol* 2001, 25: 275–284.

Wang J, Weiss LM, Hu B, Chu P, Zuppan C, Felix D, Rausei-Mills V, Chase DR. Usefulness of immunohistochemistry in delineating renal spindle cell tumours. A retrospective study of 31 cases. *Histopathology* 2004; 44:462–471.

RENAL PELVIS TRANSITIONAL CELL CARCINOMA (TCC)

DeMay R. The kidney. In *The Art and Science of Cytopathology*, pp. 1094–1095.

Juul N, Torp-Pederson S, Gronvall S, Holm HH, Koch F, Larsen S. Ultrasonically guided fine needle aspiration biopsy of renal masses. *J Urol* 1985; 133: 579–581.

Kannan V. Papillary transitional-cell carcinoma of the upper urinary tract: a cytological review. *Diagn Cytopathol* 1990; 6: 204–209.

Powers CN, Elbadawi A. Cercariform cells: a clue to the cytodiagnosis of transitional cell origin of metastatic neoplasms? *Diagn Cytopathol* 1995; 13:15–21.

Santamaría M, Jauregui I, Urtasun F, Bertol A. Fine needle aspiration biopsy in urothelial carcinoma of the renal pelvis. *Acta Cytol* 1995; 39:443–438.

Truong LD, Todd TD, Dhurandhar B, Ramzy I. Fine-needle aspiration of renal masses in adults: analysis of results and diagnostic problems in 108 cases. *Dignostic Cytopathol* 1999; 20: 339–349

LYMPHOMA

Desmoplastic small round cell tumor of the kidney in childhood. Wang LL, Perlman EJ, Vujanic GM, Zuppan C, Brundler MA, Cheung CR, Calicchio ML, Dubois S, Cendron M, Murata-Collins JL, Wenger GD, Strzelecki D, Barr FG, Collins T, Perez-Atayde AR, Kozakewich H. *Am J Surg Pathol* 2007; 31: 576–584.

Garcia M, Konoplev S, Morosan C, Abruzzo LV, Bueso-Ramos CE, Medeiros LJ. MALT lymphoma involving the kidney: a report of 10 cases and review of the literature. *Am J Clin Pathol* 2007; 128: 464–473.

Gattuso P, Castelli MJ, Peng Y, Reddy VB. Posttransplant lymphoproliferative disorders: a fine-needle aspiration biopsy study. *Diagn Cytopathol* 1997; 16: 392–395.

Hunter S, Samir A, Eisner B, Gervais D, Maher M, Hahn P, McGovern F, Mueller P. Diagnosis of renal lymphoma by percutaneous image guided biopsy: experience with 11 cases. *J Urol* 2006; 176: 1952–1956.

Truong LD, Caraway N, Ngo T, Laucirica R, Katz R, Ramzy I. Renal lymphoma. The diagnostic and therapeutic roles of fine-needle aspiration. *Am J Clin Pathol* 2001; 115:18–31.

METASTATIC CARCINOMA

Giashuddin S, Cangiarella J, Elgert P, Levine PH. Metastases to the kidney: eleven cases diagnosed by aspiration biopsy with histological correlation. *Diagn Cytopathol* 2005; 32: 325–329.

Marec-Bérard P, Crassard N, Schell M, Philip T, Thiesse P, Ranchin B, Frappaz D. Osteosarcoma metastatic to the kidney and iatrogenic hemorrhage. *Pediatr Blood Cancer.* 2008; 50: 690–692.

Gattuso P, Ramzy I, Truong LD, Lankford KL, Green L, Kluskens L, Spitz DJ, Reddy VB Utilization of fine-needle aspiration in the diagnosis of metastatic tumors to the kidney. *Diagn Cytopathol* 1999; 21: 35–38.

ONCOCYTOMA

Akhtar M, Ali MA. Aspiration cytology of chromophobe cell carcinoma of the kidney. *Diagn Cytopathol* 1995; 13: 287–294.

Granter SR, Renshaw AA. Fine-needle aspiration biopsy of chromophobe renal cell carcinoma. Analysis of six cases. *Cancer (Cancer Cytopathol)* 1997, 81: 122–128.

Liu J, Fanning CV. Can renal oncocytoma be distinguished from renal cell carcinoma on fine-needle aspiration specimens? A study of conventional smears in conjunction with anxillary studies. *Cancer (Cancer Cytopathol)* 2001; 93: 3909–3917.

Nguyen GK, Amy RW, Tsang S. Fine-needle aspiration biopsy cytology of renal oncocytoma. *Acta Cytol* 1985; 29: 33–36.

Rocca PC, Brunelli M, Gobbo S, Eccher A, Bragantini E, Mina MM, Ficarra V, Zattoni F, Zamò A, Pea M, Scarpa A, Chilosi M, Menestrina F, Bonetti F, Eble JN, Martignoni Diagnostic utility of S100A1 expression in renal cell neoplasms: an immunohistochemical and quantitative RT-PCR study. *Mod Pathol* 2007; 20:722–8.

Wiatrowska BA, Zakowski MF. Fine-needle aspiration biopsy of chromophobe renal cell carcinoma and oncocytoma. Comparison of cytomorphologic features. *Cancer Cytopathol* 1999; 87: 161–167.

ANGIOMYOLIPOMA

Cibas ES, Goss GA, Kulke MH, Demetri GD, Fletcher CD. Malignant epithelioid angiomyolipoma ('sarcoma ex angiomyolipoma') of the kidney: a case report and review of the literature. *Am J Surg Pathol* 2001; 25: 121–126.

Crapanzano JP. Fine-needle aspiration of renal angiomyolipoma: cytological findings and diagnostic pitfalls in a series of five cases. *Diagn Cytopathol* 2005; 32: 53–57.

Mai KT, Yazdi HM, Perkins DG, Thijssen A. Fine needle aspiration biopsy of epithelioid angiomyolipoma. A case report. *Acta Cytol* 2001; 45: 233–236.

Mojica WD, Jovanoska S, Bernacki EG. Epithelioid angiomyolipoma: appearance on fine-needle aspiration report of a case. *Diagn Cytopathol* 2000; 23: 192–195.

Pancholi V, Munjal K, Jain M, Munjal S, Agreawal R, Nandedkar S. Preoperative diagnosis of renal angiomyolipoma with fine needle aspiration cytology: a report of 3 cases. *Acta Cytol* 2006; 50: 466–468.

Sangawa A, Shintaku M, Nishimura M. Nuclear pseudoinclusions in angiomyolipoma of the kidney. A case report. *Acta Cytol* 1998; 42: 425–429.

Todd TD, Dhurandhar B, Mody D, Ramzy I, Truong LD. Fine needle aspiration of cystic lesions of the kidney: morphologic spectrum and diagnostic problems in 51 cases. *Am J Clin Pathol* 1999; 111: 317–328.

Truong LD, Todd TD, Dhurandhar B, Mody D, Ramzy I: Fine needle aspiration of renal masses: analysis of results and diagnostic problems in 113 cases. *Diagn Cytopathol* 1999; 20: 339–349.

Truong LD, Y-J Choi, Ayala G. Amato R, Shen S, Krishnan B. Renal cystic neoplasms and renal neoplasms associated with renal cystic diseases. Pathogenetic and molecular links. *Adv Diagn Pathol* 2003; 10:135–159.

Villari D, Grosso M, Vitarelli E, Tuccari G, Barresi G. Nuclear pseudoinclusions in fine-needle aspiration cytology of hepatic angiomyolipoma: case report. *Diagn Cytopathol* 2000; 22: 390–393.

RENAL ABSCESS

de Medeiros CR, Dantas da Cunha A. Jr., Pasquini R, Arns da Cunha C. Primary renal aspergillosis: extremely uncommon presentation in patients treated with bone marrow transplantation. *Bone Marrow Transplant* 1999; 24:113–114.

Hyldgaard-Jensen J, Sandstrøm HR, Pedersen JF. Hyldgaard-Jensen. Ultrasound diagnosis and guided biopsy in renal actinomycosis. *Br J Radiol* 1999; 72: 510–512.

Todd TD, Dhurandhar B, Mody D, Ramzy I. Truong LD. Fine-needle aspiration of cystic lesions of the kidney. Morphologic spectrum and diagnostic problems in 41 cases. *Am J Clin Pathol* 1999; 111: 317–328.

XANTHOGRANULOMATOUS PYELONEPHRITIS

Dhinga KK, Singal S, Jain S. Rare coexistence of keratinizing squamous metaplasia with xanthogranulomatous pyelonephritis. Report of a case with the role of immunohistochemistry in the diagnosis. *Acta Cytol* 2007; 51: 92–94.

Kumar N, Jain S. Aspiration cytology of focal xanthogranulomatous pyelonephritis: a diagnostic challenge. *Diagn Cytopathol* 2004; 30:111–114.

McKee G. The kidney and retroperitoneum. In *Diagnostic Cytopathology*, 2nd ed. Gray W and McKee G, Editors. Philadelphia, PA: Churchill Livinston, 2003.

Mollier S, Descotes JL, Pasquier D, Coquillat P, Michel A, Dalsoglio S, Rambeaud JJ. Pseudoneoplastic xanthogranulomatous pyelonephritis. A typical clinical presentation but unusual diagnosis and treatment. *Eur Urol* 1995; 27: 170–173.

RENAL MALAKOPLAKIA

Gupta M, Vantatesh SK, Kumoar A, Pandey R. Fine-needle aspiration cytology of bilateral renal malakoplakia. *Diagn Cytopathol* 2004; 31:116–117.

Kapasi II, Robertson S, Futter N. Diagnosis of renal malacoplakia by fine needle aspiration cytology. A case report. *Acta Cytol* 1998; 42: 1419–1423.

NEPHROBLASTOMA

Akhtar M, Ali MA, Sackey K, Sabbah R, Burgess A. Aspiration cytology of Wilms' tumor: correlation of cytologic and histologic features. *Diagn Cytopathol* 1989; 5: 269–74.

DeMay R. The kidney. In *The Art and Science of Cytopathology*. pp 1095–97 Geisinger KR, Wakely PE, Woford MM. Unresectable stage IV nephroblastoma: a potential indication for fine-needle aspiration biopsy in children. *Diagn Cytopathol* 1993; 9: 197–201.

Dey P, Radhika S, Rajwanhi A, Rao KL, Khajuria A, Nijhawan R, Banarjee CK. Aspiration cytology of Wilms' tumor. *Acta Cytol* 1993; 37: 477–82.

Iyer VK, Kapila K, Agsrwala S, Dinda AK, Verma K. Wilms' tumor. Role of fine needle aspiration and DNA ploidy by image analysis in prognostication. *Anal Quant Cytol Histol* 1999; 21: 505–11.

Peng L, Perle MA, Scholes JV, Yang GCH. Wilms' tumor in adults: Aspiration cytology and cytogenetics. *Diagnostic Cytopathol* 2002; 26: 99–103.

Quijano G, Drut R. Cytologic characteristics of Wilms' tumors in fine needle aspirates. A study of ten cases. *Acta Cytol* 1989; 33: 263–6.

"SMALL ROUND CELL TUMORS" OF THE KIDNEY

Barroca H, Carvalho JL, da Costa MJ, Cirnes L, Seruca R, Schmitt FC. Detection of N-myc amplification in neuroblastomas using Southern blotting on fine needle aspirates. *Acta Cytol* 2001; 45: 169–172.

Bosco M, Galliano D, La Saponara F, Pacchioni D, Bussolati G. Cytologic features of metanephric adenoma of the kidney during pregnancy: a case report. *Acta Cytol* 2007; 51: 468–472.

Das DK. Fine-needle aspiration cytology diagnosis of small round cell tumor: value and limitations. *Indian J Pathol Microbiol* 2004; 4: 309–318.

Fröstad B, Martinsson T, Tani E, Falkmer U, Darnfors C, Skoog L, Kogner P. The use of fine-needle aspiration cytology in the molecular characterization of neuroblastoma in children. *Cancer* 1999; 25; 87: 60–68.

Fröstad B, Tani E, Brosjö O, Skoog L, Kogner P. Fine needle aspiration cytology in the diagnosis and management of children and adolescents with Ewing sarcoma and peripheral primitive neuroectodermal tumor. *Med Pediatr Oncol* 2002; 38: 33–40.

Granja NM, Begnami MD, Bortolan J, Filho AL, Schmitt FC. Desmoplastic small round cell tumour: cytological and immunocytochemical features. *Cytojournal* 2005;18: 2–6.

Halliday BE, Slagel DD, Elsheikh TE, Silverman JF. Diagnostic utility of MIC-2 immunocytochemical staining in the differential diagnosis of small b Diagnostic utility of MIC-2 immunocytochemical staining in the differential diagnosis of small blue cell tumors. *Diagn Cytopathol* 1998; 19: 410–416.

Kang SH, Perle MA, Nonaka D, Zhu H, Chan W, Yang GC. Primary Ewing sarcoma/PNET of the kidney: fine-needle aspiration, histology, and dual color break apart FISH Assay. *Diagn Cytopathol* 2007; 35: 353–337.

Khayyata S, Grignon DJ, Aulicino MR, Al-Abbadi MA. Metanephric adenoma vs. Wilms' tumor: a report of 2 cases with diagnosis by fine needle aspiration and cytologic comparisons. *Acta Cytol* 2007; 51: 464–467.

Lane BR, Chery F, Jour G, Sercia L, Magi-Galluzzi C, Novick AC, Zhou M. Renal neuroendocrine tumours: a clinicopathological study. *BJU Int* 2007; 100: 1030–1035.

Maly B, Maly A, Reinhartz T, Sherman Y. Primitive neuroectodermal tumor of the kidney. Report of a case initially diagnosed by fine needle aspiration cytology. *Acta Cytol* 2004; 48: 264–268.

Miyake M, Fujimoto K, Tanaka M, Matsushita C, Tanaka N, Hirao Y. A case of small cell carcinoma of the kidney. *Hinyokika Kiyo* 2007; 53: 235–240.

Radhika S, Bakshi A, Rajwanshi A, Nijhawan R, Das A, Kakkar N, Joshi K, Marwaha RK, Rao KL. Cytopathology of uncommon malignant renal neoplasms in the pediatric age group. *Diagn Cytopathol* 2005; 32: 281–286.

Ravindra S, Kini U. Cytomorphology and morphometry of small round-cell tumors in the region of the kidney. *Diagn Cytopathol* 2005; 32: 211–216.

Serrano R, Rodríguez-Peralto JL, De Orbe GG, Melero C, de Agustín P. Intrarenal neuroblastoma diagnosed by fine-needle aspiration: a report of two cases. *Diagn Cytopathol* 2002; 27: 294–297.

Sharifah NA. Fine needle aspiration cytology characteristics of renal tumors in children. *Pathology* 1994; 26: 359–364.

Silverman JF, Joshi VV. FNA biopsy of small round cell tumors of childhood: cytomorphologic features and the role of ancillary studies. *Diagn Cytopathol* 1994; 10: 245–255.

Vesoulis Z, Rahmeh T, Nelson R, Clarke R, Lu Y, Dankoff J. Fine needle aspiration biopsy of primary renal synovial sarcoma. A case report. *Acta Cytol* 2003; 47: 668–672.

Wang LL, Perlman EJ, Vujanic GM, Zuppan C, Brundler MA, Cheung CR, Calicchio ML, Dubois S, Cendron M, Murata-Collins JL, Wenger GD, Strzelecki D, Barr FG, Collins T, Perez-Atayde AR, Kozakewich H. Desmoplastic small round cell tumor of the kidney in childhood. *Am J Surg Pathol* 2007; 31: 576–584.

RHABDOID TUMOR

Akhtar M, Ali MA, Sackey K, Bakry M, Johnson T. Fine-needle aspiration biopsy diagnosis of malignant rhabdoid tumor of the kidney. *Diagn Cytopathol* 1991; 7: 36–40.

Barroca HM, Costa MJ, Carvalho JL. Cytologic profile of rhabdoid tumor of the kidney. A report of 3 cases. *Acta Cytol* 2003; 47: 1055–1058.

Drut R. Cystic nephroma: cytologic findings in fine-needle aspiration cytology. *Diagn Cytopathol* 1992; 8: 593–595.

Radhika S, Bakshi A, Rajwanshi A, Nijhawan R, Das A, Kakkar N, Joshi K, Marwaha RK, Rao KL. Cytopathology of uncommon malignant renal neoplasms in the pediatric age group. *Diagn Cytopathol* 2005; 32: 281–286.

Sharifah NA. Fine needle aspiration cytology characteristics of renal tumors in children. *Pathology* 1994; 26: 359–364.

Sigauke E, Rakheja D, Maddox DL, Hladik CL, White CL, Timmons CF, Raisanen J. Absence of expression of SMARCB1/INI1 in malignant rhabdoid tumors of the central nervous system, kidneys and soft tissue: an immunohistochemical study with implications for diagnosis. *Mod Pathol* 2006; 19:717–725.

Sukov WR, Cheville JC, Lager DJ, Lewin JR, Sebo TJ, Lewin M. Malignant mixed epithelial and stromal tumor of the kidney with rhabdoid features: report of a case including immunohisto-chemical, molecular genetic studies and comparison to morphologically similar renal tumors. *Hum Pathol* 2007; 38: 1432–1437.

Yusuf Y, Belmonte AH, Tchertkoff V. Fine needle aspiration cytology of a recurrent malignant tumor of the kidney with rhabdoid features in an adult. A case report. *Acta Cytol* 1996; 40: 1313–1316.

CLEAR CELL SARCOMA

Akhtar M, Ali MA, Sackey K, Burgess A Fine-needle aspiration biopsy of clear-cell sarcoma of the kidney: light and electron microscopic features. *Diagn Cytopathol* 1989; 5; 181–187.

Drut R, Pomar M. Cytologic characteristics of clear-cell sarcoma of the kidney (CCSK) in fine-needle aspiration biopsy (FNAB): a report of 4 cases. *Diagn Cytopathol* 1991; 7: 611–614.

Iyer VK, Agarwala S, Verma K. Fine-needle aspiration cytology of clear-cell sarcoma of the kidney: study of eight cases. *Diagn Cytopathol* 2005; 33: 83–89.

Iyer VK, Kapila K, Verma K. Fine needle aspiration cytology of clear cell sarcoma of the kidney with spindle cell pattern. *Cytopathology* 2003; 14: 160–164.

Portugal R, Barroca H. Clear cell sarcoma, cellular mesoblastic nephroma and metanephric adenoma: cytological features and differential diagnosis with Wilms tumour. *Cytopathology* 2008; 19: 80–85.

ADRENAL GLAND CORTICAL ADENOMA AND HYPERPLASIA

Dusenbery D, Dekker A. Needle biopsy of the adrenal gland: retrospective review of 54 cases. *Diagn Cytopathol* 1996; 14: 126–134.

Fassina AS, Borsato S, Fedeli U. Fine needle aspiration cytology (FNAC) of adrenal masses. *Cytopathology* 2000; 11: 302–311.

Min KW, Song J, Bosenberg M, Aceby J. Adrenal cortical nodule mimicking small round cell malignancy on fine needle aspiration. *Acta Cytol* 1988; 32: 543–546.

Wadih GE, Nance KV, Silverman JF. Fine-needle aspiration cytology of the adrenal gland. Fifty biopsies in 48 patients. *Arch Pathol Lab Med* 1992; 116: 841–846.

Wu HHJ, Cramer HM, Kho J, Elsheikh TM. Fine needle aspiration cytology of benign adrenal cortical nodules. A comparison of cytologic findings with those of primary and metastatic adrenal malignancies. *Acta Cytol* 1998; 42: 1352–1358.

ADRENAL CORTICAL CARCINOMA

Dusenbery D, Dekker A. Needle biopsy of the adrenal gland: retrospective review of 54 cases. *Diagn Cytopathol* 1996;14:126–134.

Katz RL, Patel S, Mackay B, Zornoza J. Fine needle aspiration cytology of the adrenal gland. *Acta Cytol* 1984; 28: 269–282.

Saboorian MH, Katz RL, Charnsangavej C. Fine needle aspiration cytology of primary and metastatic lesions of the adrenal gland. A series of 188 biopsies with radiologic correlation. *Acta Cytol* 1995; 39: 843–851.

Wadih GE, Nance KV, Silverman JF. Fine-needle aspiration cytology of the adrenal gland. Fifty biopsies in 48 patients. *Arch Pathol Lab Med* 1992; 116: 841–846.

Wu HHJ, Cramer HM, Kho J, Elsheikh TM. Fine needle aspiration cytology of benign adrenal cortical nodules. A comparison of cytologic findings with those of primary and metastatic adrenal malignancies. *Acta Cytol* 1998; 42: 1352–1358.

PHEOCHROMOCYTOMA

de Agustin P, Lopez-Rios F, Alberti N, Perez-Barrios A. Fine-needle aspiration biopsy of the adrenal glands: a ten-year experience. *Diagn Cytopathol* 1999; 21: 92–97.

Deodhare S, Chalvardjian A, Lata A, Marcuzzi D. Adrenal pheochromocytoma mimicking small cell carcinoma on fine needle aspiration biopsy. A case report. *Acta Cytol* 1996;40:1003–1006.

Handa U, Khullar U, Mohan H. Pigmented pheochromocytoma: report of a case with diagnosis by fine needle aspiration. *Acta Cytol* 2005;49:421–423.

Nance KV, McLeod DL, Silverman JF. Fine-needle aspiration cytology of spindle cell neoplasms of the adrenal gland. *Diagn Cytopathol* 1992;8:235–241.

Shidham VB, Galindo LM. Pheochromocytoma. Cytologic findings on intraoperative scrape smears in five cases. *Acta Cytol* 1999; 43: 207–213.

METASTATIC TUMORS

Fassina AS, Borsato S, Fedeli U. Fine needle aspiration cytology (FNAC) of adrenal masses. *Cytopathology* 2000;11:302–311.

Sabooriah MH, Katz RL, Charnsangavej C. Fine needle aspiration cytology of primary and metastatic lesions of the adrenal gland. A series of 188 biopsies with radiologic correlation. *Acta Cytol* 1995;39:843–851.

Wadih GE, Nance KV, Silverman JF. Fine-needle aspiration cytology of the adrenal gland. Fifty biopsies in 48 patients. *Arch Pathol Lab Me.* 1992;116:841–846.

Wu HH, Cramer HM, Kho J, Elsheikh TM. Fine needle aspiration cytology of benign adrenal cortical nodules. A comparison of cytologic findings with those of primary and metastatic adrenal malignancies. *Acta Cytol* 1998;42:1352–1358.

Zhang PJ, Genega EM, Tomaszewski JE, Pasha TL, LiVolsi VA. The role of calretinin, inhibin, melan-A, BCL-2 and C-kit in differentiating adrenal cortical and medullary tumors: an immunohistochemical study. *Mod Pathol* 2003;16:591–597.

NEUROBLASTIC TUMORS

Domanski HA. Fine-needle aspiration of ganglioneuroma. *Diagn Cytopathol* 2005;32:363–336.

Frostad B, Tani E, Kogner P, Maeda S, Bjork O, Skoog L. The clinical use of fine needle aspiration cytology for diagnosis and management of children with neuroblastic tumors. *Eur J Cancer* 1998; 34: 529–536.

Joshi VV, Silverman JF. Pathology of neuroblastic tumors. *Semin Diagn Pathol* 1994;11:107–117.

Joshi VV, Silverman JF, Altshuler G, Cantor AB, Larkin EW, Neill JS, Norris HT, Shuster JJ, Holbrook CT, Hayes FA, et al. Systematization of primary histopathologic and fine-needle aspiration cytologic features and description of unusual histopathologic features of neuroblastic tumors: a report from the Pediatric Oncology Group. *Hum Pathol* 1993;24:493–504.

Kumar PV. Fine-needle aspiration cytologic diagnosis of ganglioneuroblastoma. *Acta Cytol* 1987;31:583–586.

MYELOLIPOMA

Deblois GG, De May RM. Adrenal myelolipoma diagnosis by computed-tomographic guided fine-needle aspiration. A case report. *Cancer* 1985;55:848–850.

Dunphy CH. Computed tomography-guided fine needle aspiration biopsy of adrenal myelolipoma. Case report and review of the literature. *Acta Cytol* 1991;35:353–356.

Katsuta K, Nakabayashi H, Kuroda Y, Liu PI. Adrenal myelolioma: preoperative diagnosis by fine-needle aspiration cytology. *Diagn Cytopathol* 1989;5:298–300.

Osborn M, Smith M, Senbanjo T, Crofton M, Robinson S, Rajan P. Adrenal myelolipoma – clinical, radiological and cytological findings: a case report. *Cytopathology* 2002;13:242–246.

Settakorn J, Sirivanchai C, Rangdaeng S, Chaiwum B. Fine-needle aspiration cytology of adrenal myelolipoma: case report and review of the literature. *Diagn Cytopathol* 1999;21:409–412.

12

Parathyroid Gland: Head and Neck

Aylin Simsir and Joan F. Cangiarella

PARATHYROID CYSTS

Clinical Features
- Fourth to sixth decade
- May present as a palpable neck mass, can be confused with a cystic nodule of the thyroid
- Usually solitary
- Usually arises from the inferior glands
- Majority are nonfunctioning; less than 10% associated with hyperparathyroidism
- Nonfunctioning cysts are more common in women, functioning more common in men
- Can produce compressive symptoms

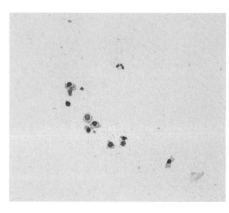

12-1. Parathyroid cyst.
Predominantly acellular smears with thin proteinaceous fluid and scattered mononuclear cells and macrophages (modified Giemsa stain)

Cytologic Features
■ Water clear to blood-tinged thin fluid
■ Acellular smears with mononuclear cells or macrophages

Special Stains and Immunohistochemistry
■ Parathyroid hormone (PTH) positive
■ Thyroglobulin negative

Modern Techniques for diagnosis
■ PTH C-terminal/mid-molecule assay shows markedly elevated levels of parathyroid hormone

Differential Diagnosis
■ Thyroid cyst
  ➤ Thick colloid, brownish to reddish cyst fluid
  ➤ Monolayered sheets of thyroid epithelium and colloid
■ Branchial cleft cyst
  ➤ Usually occurs in lateral neck
  ➤ Yellowish and viscous cyst fluid
  ➤ Squamous epithelial cells, neutrophils, and debris
■ Cystic parathyroid adenoma
  ➤ Bloody to brown cyst fluid
  ➤ Epithelial cells in three-dimensional groupings, papillary clusters, and microfollicles

PEARLS

★ Thin water clear fluid or thin slightly blood tinged fluid on aspiration should suggest a parathyroid cyst
★ Assaying parathyroid hormone levels of cyst fluid is essential

PARATHYROID ADENOMA

Clinical Features
■ Female to male ratio of 3:1
■ Most occur in the fourth decade
■ Can occur after radiation therapy of the head and neck
■ Cause of 80–85% of primary hyperparathyroidism
■ Hypoechoic nodule on ultrasound; usually not palpable
■ 75% involve an inferior gland

Cytologic Features
■ Variable cytologic features
■ Moderately cellular smears with numerous cohesive three-dimensional groups and dissociated cells
■ Disordered monolayered sheets, branched clusters with frayed edges, tissue fragments composed of epithelial cells arranged around capillary cores (papillary fragments), and microacinar arrangements may be seen
■ Naked nuclei in background
■ Small cells with small nuclei (1 to 2× size of a red blood cell) and mild to moderate anisokaryosis
■ Nuclear overlapping and nuclear molding common
■ Nuclei are round to oval with hyperchromasia, coarsely granular chromatin, and smooth nuclear membranes

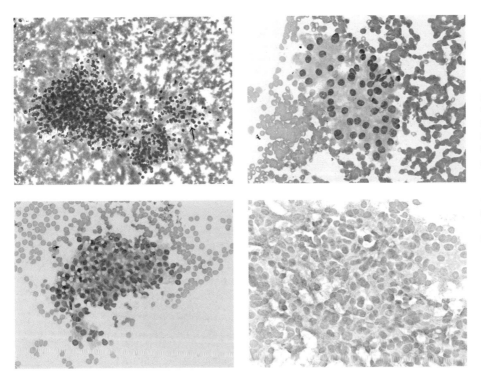

12-2A. Parathyroid adenoma *(top, left)*. Cohesive sheets of cells with microacinar arrangements (arrow). Colloid-like material (upper right) and naked nuclei are noted in the background (modified Giemsa stain)

12-2B. Parathyroid adenoma *(top, right)*. High magnification shows neoplastic cells with round nuclei, coarsely granular chromatin, smooth nuclear membranes and fine cytoplasmic granularity (modified Giemsa stain)

12-2C. Parathyroid adenoma *(bottom, left)*. Cytoplasmic vacuolation is noted (modified Giemsa stain)

12-2D. Parathormone stain *(bottom, right)*. Diffuse cytoplasmic positivity for parathormone is seen

- Predominantly ill-defined, scanty pink to pale blue cytoplasm with fine blue granularity on modified Giemsa stain corresponding to the chief cells
- Oxyphil cells resembling Hürthle cells rarely seen
- Cytoplasmic vacuoles and paravacuolar granulation in the minority
- Inconspicuous nucleoli and rare intranuclear inclusions can be seen
- Colloid-like material, macrophages, lymphocytes, and mast cells can be seen

Special Stains and Immunohistochemistry
- Silver stains identify the argyrophilic granules present in parathyroid cells
- Positivity for chromogranin, parathormone, neurospecific enolase and keratin; negativity for thyroglobulin

Modern Techniques for diagnosis
- PTH C-terminal/mid-molecule assay
- RT-PCR detection of PTH gene mRNA
- Ki-67 high in carcinoma in comparison to adenoma

Differential Diagnosis
- Thyroid-nodular goiter
  - Flat honeycomb sheets rather than three-dimensional fragments
  - Macrofollicle formations
  - Hürthle cells
  - Less anisokaryosis
  - Less naked nuclei
  - Larger cells with more cytoplasm, finely granular chromatin, and occasional small nucleoli
  - Abundant colloid
  - Hemosiderin-laden macrophages
- Papillary carcinoma of the thyroid
  - Nuclear grooves
  - Nuclear pseudoinclusions

> ➤ Papillary clusters
> ➤ Cell palisading
■ Lymphoid lesions
> ➤ Lymphoglandular bodies
■ Parathyroid hyperplasia
> ➤ Difficult to distinguish from adenoma, favored by cellular monomorphism
> ➤ Sheets and syncytial groups without microfollicles

✴ A history of hyperparathyroidism should suggest a diagnosis of a parathyroid adenoma

PARATHYROID CARCINOMA

Clinical Features
■ Palpable neck mass
■ Hyperparathyroidism with bone disease and renal stones
■ Only accounts for a small percentage of cases of hyperparathyroidism
■ Hypercalcemia
■ Markedly elevated parathyroid hormone
■ Can be nonfunctioning with normal calcium and PTH levels
■ Equal predilection for males and females
■ Fifth decade of life

Cytologic Features
■ Differentiation from adenoma may be difficult
■ Large number of dissociated cells
■ Pleomorphic large cells in loosely cohesive groupings
■ Indistinct cell borders
■ Anisokaryosis
■ Granular chromatin
■ Small nucleoli
■ Giant naked large cells
■ Some cases show little atypia

Special Stains and Immunohistochemistry
■ Cytokeratin and chromogranin positive
■ Ki-67 is high in carcinoma

Modern Techniques for Diagnosis
■ Loss of parafibromin, the protein product of the HRPT2 gene

Differential Diagnosis
■ Parathyroid adenoma
> ➤ Can be difficult to distinguish
> ➤ Less pleomorphism with absence of giant naked large cells
■ Thyroid carcinomas
> ➤ Lacks hypercalcemia
> ➤ Thyroglobulin positivity and chromogranin negativity in papillary and follicular carcinomas

⋆ High suspicion in a patient with hyperparathyroidism, a palpable neck mass, hypercalcemia, and bone or renal disease
⋆ Single case report of cutaneous seeding after FNA

SECONDARY TUMORS

Clinical Features
▪ At autopsy metastasis to the parathyroid gland found in 11.9% of patients with cancer
▪ Most common origin in decreasing frequency are breast, leukemia, melanoma, lung, and soft tissue
▪ Hypoparathyroidism as a result of tumorous involvement is uncommon

Cytologic features
▪ Depends on the primary site of origin

Special Stains
▪ Immunohistochemistry may be useful to determine primary site

Modern Techniques for diagnosis
▪ Depends on primary tumor

Differential Diagnosis
▪ Knowledge of clinical history is crucial

⋆ Metastatic involvement can occur through metastatic spread or by direct involvement of adjacent organs such as the thyroid gland
⋆ Knowledge of medical history is critical

BRANCHIAL CLEFT CYST

Clinical Features
▪ Presents as a swelling in the lateral aspect of the neck; anterior to the sternocleidomastoid muscle
▪ Most common location in the upper middle third of the neck
▪ May occur anywhere from the preauricular area to the clavicle
▪ Wide age variation: most common in the second to third decades of life
▪ Usually asymptomatic swelling; if inflamed/infected can be painful with rapid growth
▪ Origin: Congenital or acquired cyst; most likely cystic change in embryologic remnants of the branchial clefts/incomplete obliteration (congenital/developmental theory) or epithelial inclusions within cervical lymph nodes that become cystic (acquired theory)

Cytologic Features
▪ Turbid fluid
▪ Proteinaceous debris
▪ Crystals
▪ Squamous (nucleated or anucleated) and/or glandular (ciliated columnar) cells

12-3. Malignant melanoma metastatic to the parathyroid gland. Cellular smear with single cells with eccentric nuclei and abundant cytoplasm. Intranuclear inclusions and intracytoplasmic vacuoles are noted (modified Giemsa stain)

12-4A. Branchial cleft cyst *(top, left)*. Proteinaceous fluid, macrophages and numerous columnar glandular cells in clusters and singly (modified Giemsa stain)

12-4B. Branchial cleft cyst *(top, right)*. High magnification shows ciliated columnar cells (modified Giemsa stain)

12-4C. Branchial cleft cyst *(below)*. Branchial cleft cyst may be of scanty cellularity with numerous macrophages, proteinaceous debris and rare squamous cells (Ultrafast Papanicalaou stain)

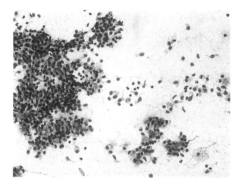
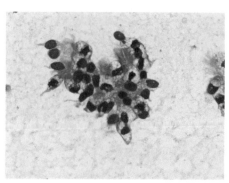

▦ Macrophages and lymphocytes, in variable amounts
▦ If inflamed, acute inflammatory cells or granulation tissue may be seen

Special Stains and Immunohistochemistry
▦ Neither special stains nor immunohistochemistry is used for the routine diagnosis of branchial cleft cyst
▦ P53 and GLUT-1 immunostaining may aid in differentiating metastatic squamous cell carcinoma from branchial cleft cyst

Modern Techniques for Diagnosis
▦ A higher percentage of metastatic squamous cell carcinomas tend to express p53 immunostaining as compared to benign squamous lesions
▦ Glucose transporter-1 (GLUT-1) immunostaining is observed in most metastatic squamous cell carcinomas whereas branchial cleft cysts show no staining
▦ Negative staining for GLUT-1 does not exclude malignancy; however, positive immunoreactivity for GLUT-1 aids in accurate diagnosis of malignancy

Differential Diagnosis
■ When encountered in unusual locations:
➤ Upper neck/preauricular or intrathyroid area – may be confused with salivary gland and thyroid gland lesions
■ Cystic metastatic squamous cell carcinoma
➤ Older age and the presence of large epithelial tissue fragments, nuclear pleomorphism/atypia, and necrosis favor a diagnosis of metastatic squamous cell carcinoma
■ Inflamed cysts
➤ Reactive squamous cell atypia may mimic metastatic well-differentiated squamous cell carcinoma
■ Epidermoid inclusion cyst
➤ Cheesy/paste like material containing numerous anucleated squamous cells

★ Turbid fluid showing proteinaceous debris, crystals, squamous (nucleated or anucleated) and/or glandular (columnar) cells, macrophages, and lymphocytes

★ If significant squamous atypia present, excision should be recommended as it may be impossible to distinguish from metastatic squamous cell carcinoma especially in the older age group

THYROGLOSSAL DUCT CYST

Clinical Features
▦ Painless swelling in the midline of the neck; anywhere from base of the tongue to the thyroid gland
▦ Most common location is at the level of the hyoid bone
▦ Most common in young children, but also seen in adults and elderly
▦ Usually asymptomatic swelling; moves with protrusion of the tongue
▦ If inflamed or infected can be painful
▦ Origin: Developmental cyst; failure of closure of the thyroglossal duct

Cytologic Features
▦ Clear to cloudy fluid
▦ Sparsely cellular smears with squamous, columnar/glandular, or ciliated respiratory type cells
▦ Thyroid follicular epithelial cells are rare
▦ Epithelial component may be sparse
▦ Cystic proteinaceous, thin watery, or thicker colloid-like background
▦ Macrophages and inflammatory cells (neutrophils and lymphocytes) usually present
▦ Cholesterol crystals may be seen

Special Stains and Immunohistochemistry
▦ Thyroid epithelium is positive for thyroid stimulating hormone (TSH)

Modern Techniques for Diagnosis
▦ Noncontributory

Differential Diagnosis
▦ Branchial cleft cyst
  ➤ Presents as lateral neck mass
  ➤ More cellular
  ➤ Proteinaceous debris
  ➤ Crystals
  ➤ Squamous (nucleated or anucleated) and/or glandular (columnar) cells
  ➤ Macrophages and lymphocytes
▦ Epidermoid inclusion cyst
  ➤ Cheesy/paste like material with abundant anucleated squamous cells
▦ Thyroid gland lesion (colloid nodule)
  ➤ Abundant colloid
  ➤ Variable amounts of macrophages and follicular cells
▦ Metastatic squamous cell carcinoma involving a lymph node
  ➤ Greater number of squamous cells with atypia

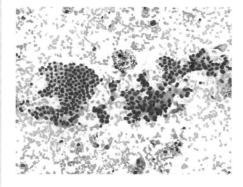

12-5. Thyroglossal duct cyst. Monolayered sheets of thyroid follicular epithelial cells, macrophages, and proteinaceous debris (modified Giemsa stain)

★ Clear to cloudy fluid with sparse cellularity
★ Cystic background containing a few if any epithelial cells
★ Some inflammatory cells and crystals
★ Cytologic features of thyroglossal duct cyst overlap with other cystic neck lesions; in the appropriate location and clinical setting, diagnosis is straightforward. However, due to overlapping cytologic features, FNA has been shown to have moderate sensitivity and positive predictive value for accurate preoperative diagnosis
★ Malignant transformation occurs but rare (1%)
★ Most common malignancy arising in thyroglossal duct cyst is papillary carcinoma followed by squamous cell carcinoma
★ FNA may be falsely negative due to sparse cellularity

EPIDERMOID INCLUSION CYSTS/DERMOID CYSTS

Clinical Features
■ Painless soft tissue/subcutaneous swelling anywhere in the head and neck area
■ Most common in the face and neck
■ Seen in children and in adults; more common in adults
■ Can become painful when inflamed/infected

Cytologic Features
■ Cheesy/pasty and foul smelling material
■ Cellular smears
■ Keratinaceous debris
■ Numerous anucleated and some nucleated squamous cells
■ Can contain skin appendages such as hair
■ If inflamed neutrophils, macrophages and lymphocytes may predominate

Special Stains and Immunohistochemistry
■ Noncontributory

Modern Techniques for Diagnosis
■ Noncontributory

Differential Diagnosis
■ Inflamed cysts
  ➤ May be confused with metastatic well differentiated squamous cell carcinoma based on the extent of squamous atypia
  ➤ Caution is advised when inflamed cyst contents are aspirated to avoid a false-positive diagnosis
  ➤ Excision may be unavoidable for a definitive diagnosis

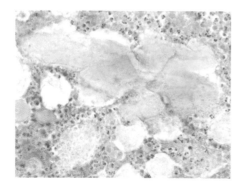

12-6. Epidermoid inclusion cyst. Anucleated squames surrounded by numerous neutrophils and histiocytes (Ultrafast Papanicalaou stain)

★ Cheesy/pasty material on aspiration
★ Numerous anucleated squamous cells and keratinous debris
★ Caution advised in inflamed cysts as not to overinterpret reactive squamous atypia

CYSTIC METASTASES

CYSTIC SQUAMOUS CELL CARCINOMA

Clinical Features
▩ Head and neck squamous cell carcinomas commonly metastasize to neck nodes
▩ A subset of SCC metastases becomes cystic – dilution of the specimen by aspirated cyst fluid may lead to false negative FNA diagnosis
▩ Most cystic nodal SCC metastases arise from small well-differentiated primaries in the oropharyngeal area (Waldeyer's ring-tonsil, base of tongue, nasopharynx)

Cytologic Features
▩ Cystic fluid
▩ Variable cellularity – may be sparsely cellular
▩ Keratinaceous debris
▩ Anucleated and nucleated squamous cells with variable atypia
▩ May have an inflammatory component mimicking an inflamed branchial cleft or epidermoid inclusion cyst

Special Stains and Immunohistochemistry
▩ P53 and GLUT-1 immunopositivity

Modern Techniques for Diagnosis
▩ P53 and GLUT-1 immunopositivity

Differential Diagnosis
▩ Inflamed branchial cleft or epidermoid inclusion cysts
➤ Reactive squamous cell atypia may mimic metastatic well differentiated squamous cell carcinoma
➤ Older age and the presence of large epithelial tissue fragments, nuclear pleomorphism, and necrosis favor a diagnosis of metastatic squamous cell carcinoma

PEARLS
★ Cystic material on aspiration
★ Variable celluarity
★ Anucleated and nucleated squamous cells with variable atypia and keratinaceous debris
★ FNA may be falsely negative
★ It is recommended that all adult patients over age 40 presenting with lateral cystic neck masses be evaluated by radiologic imaging and FNA followed by tissue biopsy if FNA is inconclusive

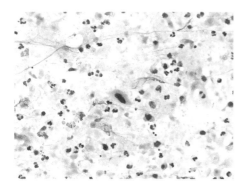 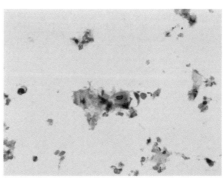

12-7A. Cystic squamous cell carcinoma *(left).* Proteinaceous debris, numerous neutrophils and histiocytes and a rare malignant squamous cell with hyperchromatic nuclei and dense abundant cytoplasm (modified Giemsa stain)

12-7B. Cystic squamous cell carcinoma *(right).* Papanicaloau stain shows a rare atypical squamous cell)

CYSTIC PAPILLARY THYROID CARCINOMA METASTASIS

Clinical Features

- Papillary thyroid carcinoma commonly metastasizes to cervical lymph nodes
- Neck node metastasis may be the initial presentation of occult primary thyroid carcinoma
- Papillary carcinoma metastasis can become cystic and lead to difficulties in diagnosis by FNA due to low cellularity secondary to dilution of the specimen by aspirated cyst fluid similar to cystic squamous cell carcinoma
- In rare cases, thyroidectomy fails to reveal a primary papillary carcinoma. Proposed scenarios to explain this situation are as follows:
  - ➤ Papillary carcinoma arising in aberrant thyroid tissue in a branchial cleft cyst
  - ➤ Papillary carcinoma arising in epithelial thyroid inclusions in cervical lymph nodes
  - ➤ Extremely small primary thyroid tumors that escape histologic sampling or complete regression of the primary tumor

Cytologic Features

- Cystic thin fluid
- Sparse cellularity
- Calcifications
- Lymphocytes
- Scant or no papillary carcinoma cells
- If neoplastic cells are present, the cytologic features include cells with oval enlarged nuclei with nuclear grooves and pseudoinclusions

Special Stains and Immunohistochemistry

- CK19 and thyroglobulin positivity

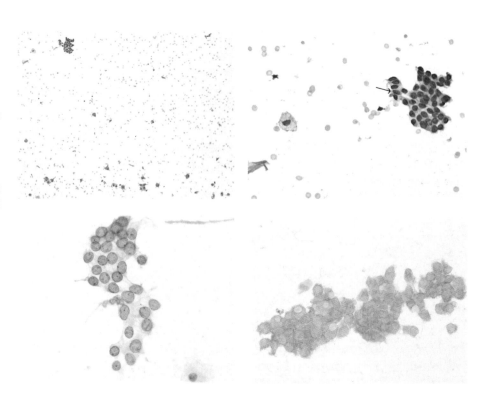

12-8A. Cystic papillary thyroid carcinoma *(top, left)*. Cystic thin fluid with numerous histiocytes and a single cluster of papillary epithelium (upper left) (modified Giemsa stain)

12-8B. Cystic papillary thyroid carcinoma *(top, right)*. Higher magnifications shows histiocytes and a cluster of neoplastic cells with oval nuclei and rare nuclear grooves (arrow) (modified Giemsa stain)

12-8C. Cystic papillary thyroid carcinoma *(bottom, left)*. Ultrafast papanicalaou stain shows characteristic grape-like clusters with nuclear clearing and nuclear grooves (Ultrafast Papanicalaou stain)

12-8D. Thyroglobulin stain *(bottom, right)*. Immunohistochemical staining for thyroglobulin shows diffuse cytoplasmic positivity)

Modern Techniques for Diagnosis
- RET/PTC oncogene rearrangement
- BRAF V599E mutation

Differential Diagnosis
- Branchial cleft cyst
  - ➤ Turbid fluid showing proteinaceous debris, crystals, squamous (nucleated or anucleated) and/or glandular (columnar) cells, macrophages, and lymphocytes
  - ➤ Absence of nuclear features of papillary carcinoma

PEARLS

★ Cystic material on aspiration

★ Variable cellularity with lymphocytes and calcification; if neoplastic cells are absent or sparse FNA may be falsely negative

★ It is recommended that all adult patients presenting with papillary carcinoma on FNA of a lateral neck mass undergo evaluation of the thyroid gland, which includes total thyroidectomy to identify a primary thyroid papillary carcinoma; some of these primary thyroid tumors are reported to be as small as 1.0 mm or they may have completely regressed leaving scar tissue only; thus no tumor may be found despite thorough histologic examination of the thyroid gland

NASOPHARYNGEAL CARCINOMA

Clinical Features
- Frequently presents as a lymph node metastasis in the neck
- Other symptoms can include nasal symptoms, ear symptoms and headache
- Affects men more often than women
- Bimodal age distribution with peak at fifteen to tewenty five years and second peak at sixty to seventy years
- Prevalent in Southeast Asia and Northern Africa
- Etiology is multifactorial but includes race, genetics, environmental factors, and Epstein–Barr virus infection

Cytologic Features
- Cellular smears
- Tumor cells in cohesive clusters and/or singly
- Large, ovoid, and overlapping nuclei
- Abundant naked large nuclei in background
- Multiple, large, prominent nucleoli
- Scarce cytoplasm
- Indistinct cell borders
- Lymphoid background
- Rarely eosinophils and granulomas

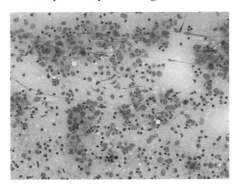 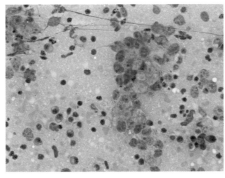

12-9A. Nasopharyngeal carcinoma *(left).* Neoplastic cells in clusters or dispersed as large naked nuclei. Small lymphocytes and plasma cells are noted in the background (modified Giemsa stain)

12-9B. Nasopharyngeal carcinoma *(right).* Neoplastic cells have large nuclei with multiple prominent nucleoli and scant cytoplasm. Numerous mitotic figures are seen (modified Giemsa stain)

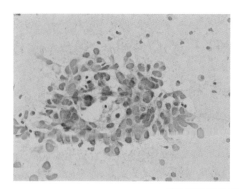

12-9C. EBV antigen stain. Immunohistochemical stain for Epstein–Barr virus early antigen shows strong cytoplasmic positivity in the neoplastic cells

Special Stains and Immunohistochemistry

- Cytokeratin positivity
- Epithelial membrane antigen is usually positive
- Carcinoembryonic antigen is variably positive
- Epstein–Barr virus early antigen and viral capsid antigen positivity

Modern Techniques for Diagnosis

- In situ hybridization for Epstein–Barr virus encoded early RNA
- IgG against early EBV antigen and IgA against viral capsid antigen; can have false positives

Differential Diagnosis

- Hodgkin's lymphoma
  - ➤ Eosinophils, histiocytes and granulomas are more prominent
  - ➤ Neoplastic cells are more irregular and have multinucleated and polylobulated forms
  - ➤ Reed–Sternberg cells have distinct vacuolated pale-gray cytoplasm
  - ➤ Positive for CD15 and CD30
- Non-Hodgkin's large cell lymphoma
  - ➤ Lack of cohesive groups
  - ➤ Monotonous lymphoid cell population
  - ➤ Positive for leukocyte common antigen
- Poorly differentiated large cell carcinoma
  - ➤ Immunohistochemistry is helpful

PEARLS

★ Most common presentation is metastasis to regional neck nodes and thus naso-pharyngeal carcinoma should be considered in all cases of cervical lymphadenopathy

MERKEL CELL CARCINOMA

Clinical Features

- Malignant primary neuroendocrine skin tumor
- Most common in older adults but can be seen in younger individuals
- Sun-exposed areas (head and neck and extremities) are the most common sites
- Presents as a rapidly enlarging firm skin nodule with discolored overlying skin
- Usually about 1.5 cm in size
- Clinically aggressive behavior with variable locoregional recurrence and lymph node and distant metastasis rates reported in the literature
- Most important prognostic factor is the stage of disease at presentation
- Treatment is surgical excision with clean margins followed by radiation therapy

12-10A. Merkel cell carcinoma *(left).* Cellular smears with abundant single cells and rare dyshesive small groups in a background of numerous stripped tumor nuclei (modified Giemsa stain)

12-10B. Merkel cell carcinoma *(right).* Tumor cells have round nuclei with finely granular chromatin and scant cytoplasm. Nuclear molding is evident. Mitotic figures are noted (modified Giemsa stain)

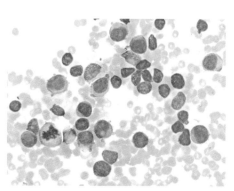

Cytologic Features
- Cellular aspirates
- Dyscohesive smears with abundant single cells and small loose groups
- Nuclear molding and overlapping of cells
- Monomorphic small to intermediate-sized cells
- Round nuclei, scant cytoplasm (thin rim)
- Finely granular cytoplasm with multiple small inconspicuous nucleoli
- Background contains necrosis and stripped nuclei

Special Stains and Immunohistochemistry
- Positive for low-molecular-weight cytokeratins (dotlike perinuclear staining) and neuroendocrine markers such as NSE
- Positive for CK20 and negative for TTF-1; aids in differentiating from pulmonary small cell carcinoma metastasis

Modern Techniques for Diagnosis
- Noncontributory

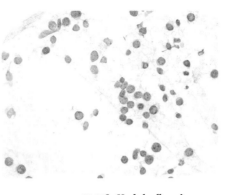

12-10C. Merkel cell carcinoma. The finely granular chromatin pattern of the Merkel cells is highlighted (Ultrafast Papanicalaou stain)

Differential Diagnosis
- Metastatic small cell carcinoma
  - ➤ Cytomorphology is similar; use immunohistochemistry (CK20 and TTF-1) and clinical history
- Malignant lymphoma
  - ➤ Merkel cell carcinoma lacks lymphoglandular bodies and displays loose clusters and nuclear molding; lymphoma cells are negative for cytokeratins whereas Merkel cell carcinoma cells are negative for LCA
- Pilomatrixoma
  - ➤ Uniformity of basaloid cells, lack of atypia and presence of ghost cells and keratin debris in pilomatrixoma
- Basal cell carcinoma
  - ➤ Basaloid cell clusters in basal cell carcinoma display tight clusters with central crowding and overlapping and peripheral palisading
- Melanoma
  - ➤ Melanoma can present as an undifferentiated small cell pattern; use immunohistochemistry (HMB-45, melan-A, MART-1; S-100 can be positive in Merkel cell carcinoma)

PEARLS
- ★ Cellular smears with dissociated cells and loose clusters and necrosis
- ★ Small cell carcinoma and other small blue round cell tumors enter the differential diagnosis
- ★ Routine use of immunohistochemistry is recommended for accurate diagnosis
- ★ Clinical history is important to differentiate this tumor from other small round cell tumors

PARAGANGLIOMA (CAROTID BODY TUMOR)

Clinical Features
- Rare among head and neck tumors
- Arises from the chemoreceptor organ located at the bifurcation of the carotid artery; usually firmly attached to the vessel
- Presents as an enlarging lateral neck mass

12-11A. Paraganglioma *(left).* Cellular aspirates with cohesive groups and small clusters of ovoid to spindled cells with marked pleomorphism (modified Giemsa stain)

12-11B. Paraganglioma *(right).* Tumor cells have oval to spindled-shaped nuclei with marked variation in size and shape, stippled chromatin and moderately abundant granular cytoplasm (modified Giemsa stain)

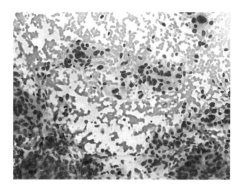 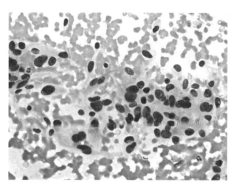

- May be pulsatile due to close relationship with the carotid artery
- Most are sporadic; familial tumors may be multifocal
- Imaging studies often helpful in diagnosis – Doppler ultrasonography, contrast computed tomography (CT), magnetic resonance imaging (MRI), magnetic resonance angiography (MRA)
- Usually nonfunctional
- Usually benign
- 10% behave aggressively with local invasion or metastasis to lymph nodes and lung
- Treatment is surgical excision

Cytologic Features
- Aspiration may be very bloody due to high vascularity
- Moderate to high cellularity in a bloody background; blood may dilute the specimen decreasing the cellularity of the smears
- Isolated and clusters of cells with acinar/rosette-like structures
- Round to oval, sometimes spindled or plasmacytoid cells with granular moderately abundant cytoplasm
- Round nuclei with stippled chromatin pattern
- Nucleoli may be prominent
- Nuclear grooves and inclusions may rarely be present
- Endocrine atypia may be present (anisocytosis, giant, and bizarre cells) – should not be interpreted as signs of malignancy
- No definitive histologic or cytologic features to predict malignancy

Special Stains and Immunohistochemistry
- Positive for S-100 (sustentacular cells), NSE, chromogranin, synaptophysin, serotonin, and various other peptide hormones
- Negative for keratin

Modern Techniques for Diagnosis
- Dense core cytoplasmic neurosecretory granules on electron microscopy

Differential Diagnosis
- Metastatic carcinoma
  - Immunohistochemistry is helpful
- Plasmacytoma
  - Immunohistochemistry and imaging findings helpful
- Medullary thyroid carcinoma
  - Immunohistochemistry and imaging findings helpful
- Papillary thyroid carcinoma
  - Papillary clusters
  - Nuclear grooves and inclusions
  - Psammoma bodies

★ Bloody material on aspiration
★ Variable cellularity with single and clusters of cells showing moderately abundant
cytoplasm with granularity
★ Acinar/rosette formation
★ Atypia should not be mistaken for malignancy

FIBROMATOSIS

Clinical Features
▥ Benign but locally aggressive proliferation of fibrous tissue
▥ Originating in musculoaponeurotic tissues
▥ Head and neck location accounts for 12% of cases
▥ Presents as an enlarging, painless swelling

Cytologic Features
▥ Low to moderately cellular smears
▥ Groups of loosely cohesive, bland, spindle-shaped cells
▥ Individual spindle-shaped or polygonal cells
▥ Oval to elongated plump nuclei
▥ Cytoplasmic tails
▥ Finely dispersed chromatin with no or few nucleoli
▥ Collagenized, finely fibrillar matrix in the background
▥ Rare inflammatory cells

Special Stains and Immunohistochemistry
▥ Smooth muscle actin (SMA) and desmin (most cases) positivity

Modern Techniques for Diagnosis
▥ Noncontributory

Differential Diagnosis
▥ Low-grade fibrosarcoma
➤ Increased cellularity
➤ Mitotic figures
➤ Cytologic atypia
▥ Schwannoma
➤ Wavy nuclei
➤ S-100 protein positivity
▥ Reparative process
➤ Less stromal cells

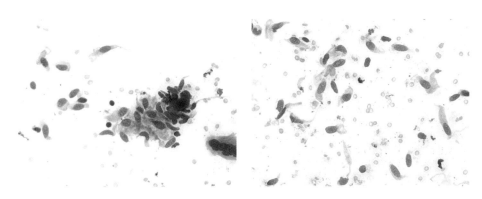

12-12A. Fibromatosis (left).
Loosely cohesive bland spindle-shape
cells and single spindle-shaped cells
intermixed with a finely fibrillar matrix
material (modified Giemsa stain)

12-12B. Fibromatosis (right).
The spindle-shaped cells have oval,
plump nuclei, finely dispersed
chromatin and cytoplasmic tails
(modified Giemsa stain)

➤ Cells have stellate configurations
➤ Inflammatory cells are prominent

PEARLS

★ Mild nuclear pleomorphism should not be misinterpreted as sarcoma
★ Treatment is wide local resection due to the local aggressiveness and high recurrence rate associated with fibromatosis

PILOMATRIXOMA (CALCIFYING EPITHELIOMA OF MALHERBE)

Clinical Features
- Benign hair matrix tumor
- Most common in children and young adults
- Head and neck and upper extremities are the most common sites
- Presents as a hard dermal nodule with normal or sometimes discolored overlying skin
- Clinical impression is usually a lesion other than pilomatrixoma such as infection, sebaceous cyst or other cutaneous and noncutaneous tumors
- Treatment is surgical excision

Cytologic Features
- Background of lymphocytes and amorphous debris
- Basaloid cells (uniform small cells with high nuclear to cytoplasmic ratios, round to oval nuclei, smooth nuclear borders, open chromatin pattern, prominent nucleoli) arranged singly and in cohesive to loosely cohesive sheets
- Ghost (shadow) epithelial cells
- Keratin debris
- Foreign body type giant cells
- Nucleated squamous cells
- Calcium deposits

Special Stains and Immunohistochemistry
- Noncontributory

Modern Techniques for Diagnosis
- Noncontributory

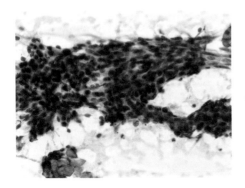

12-13. Pilomatrixoma. Basaloid uniform small cells arranged in cohesive sheets with ghost cells showing squamous features (lower left) (hematoxylin and eosin stain)

Differential Diagnosis
- Benign cysts containing squamous cells
- Epidermal inclusion and branchial cleft cysts specially if ruptured and inflamed
  ➤ Ghost cells, basaloid cells and calcific debris in pilomatrixoma
- Squamous cell carcinoma
  ➤ Uniformity of basaloid cells and lack of atypia in pilomatrixoma
- Basal cell carcinoma
  ➤ Basaloid cell clusters display central crowding and overlapping with peripheral palisading
  ➤ Mature squamous cells, shadow cells, and foreign body type giant cells are not seen in basal cell carcinomas

⋆ Look for basaloid cells and ghost cells
⋆ Ghost cells are sometimes more easily identified on cell blocks
⋆ Routine use of cell blocks is recommended for accurate diagnosis
⋆ Location of the lesion and the age of the patient are important to keep in mind in differentiating this lesion from other basaloid head and neck lesions

NODULAR FASCIITIS

Clinical Features
▪ Benign spindle cell proliferation of myofibroblasts
▪ Previously designated "subcutaneous pseudosarcomatous fibromatosis"
▪ Histologically and cytologically mimics sarcoma
▪ Presents as a rapidly growing subcutaneous/soft tissue mass
▪ Usually less than 5 cm in size
▪ Most common location is upper extremities
▪ Most common in young adults but can occur in any age
▪ Surgical excision is not necessary due to spontaneous resolution in most cases (resolution expected in eight to twelve weeks)

Cytologic Features
▪ Moderately to highly cellular smears
▪ Oval to spindled or stellate-shaped cells of myofibroblastic origin in clusters
▪ Similar single spindled and ganglion-like cells in the background
▪ Spindled cells with prominent nucleoli
▪ Nuclear chromatin is open and bland
▪ Small nucleoli
▪ Variable inflammation including neutrophils, lymphocytes, eosionophils, histiocytes
▪ Bi-and multinucleated giant cells
▪ Metachromatic myxoid stroma usually present
▪ Brisk mitotic activity may be present

Special Stains and Immunohistochemistry
▪ Vimentin, SMA, CD68 positive

Modern Techniques for Diagnosis
▪ Noncontributory

Differential Diagnosis
▪ Schwannoma
  ➤ Neoplastic cells have neural features

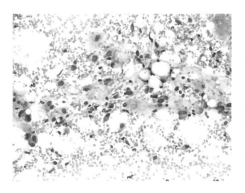
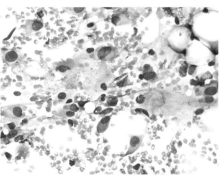

12-14A. Nodular fasciitis *(left).* Moderately cellular smears with stellate-shaped cells admixed within metachromatic myxoid material (modified Giemsa stain)

12-14B. Nodular fasciitis *(right).* Higher magnifications shows stellate cells with oval nuclei, finely granular chromatin and abundant cytoplasm admixed with metachromatic myxoid stroma (modified Giemsa stain)

> Spindled cells with pointed ends
> Hypercellular stromal fragments alternate with hypocellular areas
> Verrocay bodies may be seen
> Stroma is finely fibrillar
> No mitotic figures or inflammation
> S-100 positive
> CD68 and SMA negative
■ Sarcoma
> Cellular smears
> Atypical spindled cells with nuclear pleomorphism
> Mitotic figures (including atypical forms)
> Necrosis
> Coarse irregular nuclear chromatin
> Prominent nucleoli
> Small cellular tissue fragments and single cells

PEARLS

★ May mimic sarcoma due to high cellularity, prominence of nucleoi in ganglion-like cells, and brisk mitotic activity
★ Clinical history is very important – rapidly growing lesion in a young adult
★ Cytologic features of a cellular myofibroblastic proliferation in the background of metachromatic/myxoid stroma with variable numbers of inflammatory cells secure a diagnosis of nodular fasciitis

SCHWANNOMA

Clinical Features

■ Benign spindle cell tumor of schwann cell origin
■ Most common benign lesion arising from the peripheral nerves
■ Found in all sites but is more common in the head and neck area and the extremities
■ Affects all ages; most common in third through sixth decades
■ In the head and neck area presents most commonly as painless neck mass
■ Painful on aspiration – pain radiating along the nerve
■ Treatment is surgical excision
■ Malignant transformation is very rare

Cytologic Features

■ Cellularity varies: high cellularity in 40–79% of cases – poor cellularity in 12– 21% of cases; in one study, 23% of cases were insufficient for diagnosis
■ Tissue fragments of varying size and variable cellularity
■ Cellular areas correspond to Antoni A areas

12-15A. Schwannoma *(left).* Cellular smear containing tissue fragments with alternating hypercellular (Antoni A) and hypocellular (Antoni B) areas (modified Giemsa stain)

12-15B. Schwannoma *(right).* Nuclei appear wavy, comma shaped or have pointed ends (modified Giemsa stain)

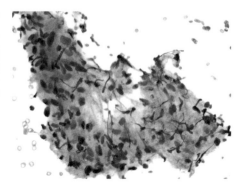

- Hypocellular areas and myxoid areas correspond to Antoni B areas
- Individual cells are spindled and wavy
- Comma-shaped cells are common
- Cells in tissue fragments have indistinct cell borders
- Embedded in fibrillar, collagenized, or myxoid matrix
- Nuclear palisading with distinctive Verocay bodies seen in up to 90% cases
- Nuclear inclusions and intracytoplasmic vacuoles may be seen
- A cause of nondiagnostic FNA: cystic change yielding mostly fluid
- Ancient schwannoma: Pleomorphic tumor cells with marked hyperchromasia, irregular nuclear contours, large intranuclear inclusions. No mitotic figures or macronucleoli seen

Special Stains and Immunohistochemistry
- S-100 protein positivity

Modern Techniques for Diagnosis
- Noncontributory

Differential Diagnosis
- Malignant spindle cell sarcomas
  - Leiomyosarcoma or malignant peripheral nerve sheath tumor (MPNST); particularly a problem with ancient schwannomas
  - Degenerative type of nuclear atypia and large intranuclear vacuoles
  - Benign components in smears, absence of mitosis and macronucleoli and strong S-100 positivity favor a benign schwannoma
- Malignant Peripheral Nerve Sheath Tumor (MPNST)
  - Smears contain a larger number of single cells, more atypia, prominent nucleoli and mitotic figures
  - May be impossible to distinguish cellular schwannoma from MPNST
- Leiomyosarcoma
  - Spindle cells often align in parallel
  - Nuclei are often blunt ended or cigar shaped
  - Coarse chromatin and prominent nucleoli common
  - SMA and desmin positive
  - S-100 protein negative
- Spindle cell lipoma
  - Fatty and collagenous components
  - Spindle cell component is positive for CD34

PEARLS
- False-negative diagnosis is not uncommon due to hypocellularity especially in cystically degenerated tumors
- Variably cellular smears predominantly composed of tissue fragments of spindled cells with Verocay bodies and Antoni A and B areas
- Degenerative type cytologic atypia common in ancient schwannomas

LIPOMA

Clinical Features
- Most common neoplasm of mesenchymal origin
- Approximately 13% occur in the head and neck region, most commonly in the posterior cervical neck
- Slow growing tumors composed of adipose tissue

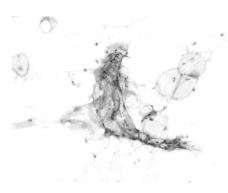

12-16. Lipoma. Mature adipose tissue fragments containing lipocytes with univacuolation and small eccentrically placed nuclei (modified Giemsa stain)

- In head and neck region, men in their seventh decade predominate
- In anterior neck can be mistaken for a thyroid nodule

Cytologic Features
- Oily material at aspiration
- Mature lipocytes in sheets or singly
- Lipocytes are univacuolated
- Adipose stromal fragments
- Adipocytes have small eccentrically placed nuclei and well-defined cell membranes

Special Stains and Immunohistochemistry
- Noncontributory

Modern Techniques for Diagnosis
- Noncontributory

Differential Diagnosis
- Thyroid nodules
  - Colloid
  - Follicular epithelium
- Lymph nodes
  - Lymphocytes
  - Tingible body macrophages

PEARLS

- True lipoblasts are absent in lipomas
- Treatment of these benign tumors is surgical excision

REFERENCES

PARATHYROID CYSTS

Absher KJ, Truong LD, Khurana KK, Ramzy I. Parathyroid cytology:avoiding diagnostic pitfalls. *Head Neck* 2002;24:157–64.

Fortson JK, Patel VG, Henderson VJ. Parathyroid cysts: a case report and review of the literature. *Laryngoscope* 2001:111:1726–8.

Katz AD, Dunkleman D. Needle aspiration of nonfunctioning parathyroid cysts. *Arch Surg* 1984;119:307–8.

Kodama T, Obara T, Fujimoto Y, Ito Y, Yashiro T, Hirayama A. Eleven cases of non-functioning parathyroid cysts – significance of needle aspiration in diagnosis and management. *Endocrinol Jpn* 1987;34:769–77.

Layfield LJ. Fine needle aspiration cytology of cystic parathyroid lesions. A cytomorphologic overlap with cystic lesions of the thyroid. *Acta Cytol* 1991;35:447–50.

Lerud KS, Tabbara SO, DelVecchio DM, Frost AR. Cytomorphology of cystic parathyroid lesions: report of four cases evaluated preoperatively by fine-needle aspiration. *Diagn Cytopathol* 1996;15:306–11.

Mevio E, Gorini E, Sbrocca M, Artesi L, Mullace M, Lecce S. Parathyroid cysts:description of two cases and review of the literature. *Acta Otorhinolaryngol Ital* 2004;24:161–4.

Silverman JF, Khazanie PG, Norris HT, Fore WW. Parathyroid hormone (PTH) assay of parathyroid cysts examined by fine needle aspiration biopsy. *Am J Clin Pathol* 1986;86:776–80.

PARATHYROID ADENOMA

Abati A, Skarulis MC, Shawker T, Solomon D. Ultrasound-guided fine-needle aspiration of parathyroid lesions: a morphological and immunocytochemical approach. *Hum Pathol* 1995;26:338–43.

Absher KJ, Truong LD, Khurana KK, Ramzy I. Parathyroid cytology: avoiding diagnostic pitfalls. *Head Neck* 2002;24:157–64.

Bondeson L, Bondeson AG, Nissborg A, Thompson NW. Cytopathological variables in parathyroid lesions: a study based on 1,600 cases of hyperparathyroidism. *Diagn Cytopathol* 1997;16:476–82.

Cavaco BM, Torrinha F, Mendonca E, Pratas S, Boavida J, Sobrinho LG, Leite V. Preoperative diagnosis of suspicious parathyroid adenomas by RT-PCR using mRNA extracted from leftover cells in a needle used for ultrasonically guided fine needle aspiration cytology. *Acta Cytol* 2003;47:5–12.

Davey DD, Giant MD, Berger EK. Parathyroid cytopathology. *Diagn Cytopathol* 1986;2:76–80.

Friedman M, Shimaoka K, Lopez CA, Shedd DP. Parathyroid adenoma diagnosed as papillary carcinoma of thyroid on needle aspiration smears. *Acta Cytol* 1983;27:337–40.

Halbauer M, Crepinko I, Brzac HT, Simonovic I. Fine needle aspiration cytology in the preoperative diagnosis of ultrasonically enlarged parathyroid glands. *Acta Cytol* 1991;35:728–35.

Layfield LJ. Fine needle aspiration cytology of cystic parathyroid lesions. A cytomorphologic overlap with cystic lesions of the thyroid. *Acta Cytol* 1991;35:447–50.

Liu F, Gnepp DR, Pisharodi LR. Fine needle aspiration of parathyroid lesions. *Acta Cytol* 2004;48:133–6.

Lori AE, Long J, Peter W, Geoffrey BT, Jon AH, Ricardo VL. Parathyroid hyperplasia, adenoma, and carcinoma: differential expression of p27 protein. *Am J Surg Pathol* 1999;23:288–95.

Mincione GP, Borrelli D, Cicchi P, et al. Fine needle aspiration cytology of parathyroid adenoma: A review of seven cases. *Acta Cytol* 1986;30:65–9.

Schachner SH, Hall A. Parathyroid adenoma and previous head-and-neck irradiation. *Ann Intern Med* 1978;88:804.

Tseng FY, Hsiao YL, Chang TC. Ultrasound-guided fine needle aspiration cytology of parathyroid lesions. A review of 72 cases. *Acta Cytol* 2002;46:1029–36.

PARATHYROID CARCINOMA

De la Garza S, Flores de la Garza E, Hernandez Batres F. Functional parathyroid carcinoma. Cytology, histology, and ultrastructure of a case. *Diagn Cytopathol* 1985;1:232–5.

Du SD, Chang TC, Chen YL, Hsiao YL, Kuo SH. Ultrasonography and needle aspiration cytology in the diagnosis and management of parathyroid lesion. *J Formos Med Assoc* 1994;93:153–9.

Guazzi A, Gabrielli M, Guadagni G. Cytologic features of a functioning parathyroid carcinoma. A case report. *Acta Cytol* 1982;26:709–13.

Ikeda K, Tate G, Suzuki T, Mitsuya T. Cytologic comparison of a primary parathyroid cancer and its metastatic lesions: A case report. *Diagn Cytopathol* 2006;34:50–5.

Spinelli C, Bonadio AG, Berti P, Materazzi G, Miccoli P. Cutaneous spreading of parathyroid carcinoma after fine needle aspiration cytology. *J Endocrinol Invest* 2000;23:255–7.

Tan MH, Morrison C, Wang P, Yang X, Haven CJ, Zhang C, Zhao P, Tretiakova MS, Korpi-Hyovalti E, Burgess JR, Soo KC, Cheah WK, Cao B, Resau J, Morreau H, Teh BT. Loss of parafibromin immunoreactivity is a distinguishing feature of parathyroid carcinoma. *Clin Cancer Res* 2004;10:6629–37.

Tseng FY, Hsiao YL, Chang TC. Ultrasound-guided fine needle aspiration cytology of parathyroid lesions. A review of 72 cases. *Acta Cytol* 2002;46:1029–36.

Wang CA, Gaz RD. Natural history of parathyroid carcinoma. Diagnosis, treatment, and results. *Am J Surg* 1985;149:522–7.

SECONDARY TUMORS

Horwitz CA, Myers WP, Foote FW, Jr. Secondary malignant tumors of the parathyroid glands. Report of two cases with associated hypoparathyroidism. *Am J Med* 1972;52:797–808.

Tang W, Kakudo K, Nakamura Y, Nakamura M, Mori I, Morita S, Miyauchi A. Parathyroid gland involvement by papillary carcinoma of the thyroid gland. *Arch Pathol Lab Med* 2002;126: 1511–14.

BRANCHIAL CLEFT CYST

Burgess KL, Hartwick RW, Bedard YC. Metastatic squamous carcinoma presenting as a neck cyst. Differential diagnosis from inflamed branchial cleft cyst in fine needle aspirates. *Acta Cytol* 1993;37:494–8.

Chandan VS, Faquin WC, Wilbur DC, Khurana KK. The utility of GLUT-1 immunolocalization in cell blocks: an adjunct to the fine needle aspiration diagnosis of cystic squamous lesions of the head and neck. *Cancer Cytopathol* 2006;25:124–8.

Daoud FS. Branchial cyst: an often forgotten diagnosis. *Asian J Surg* 2005; 28:174–8.

Glosser JW, Pires CA, Feinberg SE. Branchial cleft or cervical lymphoepithelial cysts: etiology. *J Am Dent Assoc* 2003;134:81–6.

Joseph F. Nasuti, Marian G. Braccia, Shelley Roberts, Zubair W. Baloch. Utility of cytomorphologic criteria and p53 immunolocalization in distinguishing benign from malignant cystic squamous-lined lesions of the neck on fine-needle aspiration. *Diagn Cytopathol* 2002;27:10–14.

Kadhim AL, Sheahan P, Colreavy MP, Timon CV. Pearls and pitfalls in the management of branchial cyst. *J Laryngol Otol* 2004;118:946–50.

Khurana KK, Ramzy I, Truong LD. p53 immunolocalization in cell block preparations of squamous lesions of the neck: an adjunct to fine-needle aspiration diagnosis of malignancy. *Arch Pathol Lab Med* 1999;123:421–5.

Weiner MF, Miranda RN, Bardales RH, Mukunyadzi P, Baker SJ, Korourian S, De Las Casas LE. Diagnostic value of GLUT-1 immunoreactivity to distinguish benign from malignant cystic squamous lesions of the head and neck in fine-needle aspiration biopsy material. *Diagn Cytopathol* 2004;31:294–9.

THYROGLOSSAL DUCT CYST

Dedivitis RA, Camargo DL, Peixoto GL, Weissman L, Guimaraes AV. Thyroglossal duct: a review of 55 cases. *J Am Coll Surg* 2002;194:274–7.

Falvo L, Giacomelli L, Vanni B, Marzollo A, Guerriero G, De Antoni E. Papillary thyroid carcinoma in thyroglossal duct cyst: case reports and literature review. *Int Surg* 2006;91:141–6.

Ferrer C, Ferrandez A, Dualde D, Rodriguez M, Ferrer E, Pinazo J, Sancho R. Squamous cell carcinoma of the thyroglossal duct cyst: report of a new case and literature review. *Otolaryngol* 2000;29:311–4.

Shaffer MM, Oertel YC, Oertel JE. Thyroglossal duct cysts: diagnostic criteria by fine-needle aspiration. *Arch Pathol Lab Med* 1996;120:1039–43.

Shahin A, Burroughs FH, Kirby JP, Ali SZ. Thyroglossal duct cyst: a cytopathologic study of 26 cases. *Diagn Cytopathol* 2005;33:365–9.

EPIDERMOID INCLUSION CYSTS/DERMOID CYSTS

Golden BA and Zide MF. Cutaneous cysts of the head and neck, *Head Neck* 2005;63:1613–19.

Ramzy I, Rone R, Schantz HD. Squamous cells in needle aspirates of subcutaneous lesions: a diagnostic problem. *Am J Clin Pathol* 1986;85:319–24.

Roy M, Bhattacharyya A, Sanyal S, Dasgupta S. Study of benign superficial cysts by fine needle aspiration cytology. *J Indian Med Assoc* 1995;93:8–9.

CYSTIC METASTASES
CYSTIC SQUAMOUS CELL CARCINOMA

Andrews PJ, Giddings CE, Su AP. Management of lateral cystic swellings of the neck, in the over 40s' age group. *J Laryngol Otol* 2003;117:318–20.

Chandan VS, Faquin WC, Wilbur DC, Khurana KK. The utility of GLUT-1 immunolocalization in cell blocks: an adjunct to the fine needle aspiration diagnosis of cystic squamous lesions of the head and neck. *Cancer* 2006;108:124–8.

Goldenberg D, Sciubba J, Koch WM. Cystic metastasis from head and neck squamous cell cancer: a distinct disease variant? *Head Neck* 2006;28:633–8.

Nasuti JF, Braccia MG, Roberts S, Baloch ZW. Utility of cytomorphologic criteria and p53 immunolocalization in distinguishing benign from malignant cystic squamous-lined lesions of the neck on fine needle aspiration. *Diagn Cytopathol* 2002;27:10–14.

Pisharodi LR. False-negative diagnosis in fine-needle aspirations of squamous-cell carcinoma of head and neck. *Diagn Cytopathol* 1997;17:70–3.

Sheahan P, Fitzgibbon J, O'Leary G, Lee G. Efficacy and pitfalls of fine needle aspiration in the diagnosis of neck masses. *Surgeon* 2004;2:152–6.

Thompson LD, Heffner DK. The clinical importance of cystic squamous cell carcinomas in the neck: a study of 136 cases. *Cancer* 1998;82:944–56.

Ustun M, Risberg B, Davidson B, Berner A. Cystic change in metastatic lymph nodes: a common diagnostic pitfall in fine-needle aspiration cytology. *Diagn Cytopathol* 2002;27:387–92.

CYSTIC PAPILLARY THYROID CARCINOMA METASTASIS

Cignarelli M, Ambrosi A, Marino A, Lamacchia O, Campo M, Picca G, Giorgino F. Diagnostic utility of thyroglobulin detection in fine-needle aspiration of cervical cystic metastatic lymph nodes from papillary thyroid cancer with negative cytology. *Thyroid* 2003;13:1163–67.

Domingues R, Mendonca E, Sobrinho L, Bugalho MJ. Searching for RET/PTC rearrangements and BRAF V599E mutation in thyroid aspirates might contribute to establish a pre-operative diagnosis of papillary thyroid carcinoma. *Cytopathology* 2005;16:27–31.

LiVolsi V. Thyroid papillary carcinoma in lateral neck cyst: missed primary tumour or ectopic thyroid carcinoma within a branchial cyst? (Letter to the editor with authors' reply). *Laryngol Otol* 2001;115:614–5.

Mehmood RK, Basha SI, Ghareeb E. A case of papillary carcinoma arising in ectopic thyroid tissue within a branchial cyst with neck node metastasis. *Ear Nose Throat J* 2006;85:675–6.

Sidhu S, Lioe TF, Clements B. Thyroid papillary carcinoma in lateral neck cyst: missed primary tumour or ectopic thyroid carcinoma within a branchial cyst? *Laryngol Otol* 2000;114:716–8.

Wang Z, Qiu S, Eltorky MA, Tang WW. Histopathologic and immunohistochemical characterization of a primary papillary thyroid carcinoma in the lateral cervical lymph node. *Exp Mol Pathol* 2007;82:91–4.

NASOPHARYNGEAL CARCINOMA

Jayaram G, Swain M, Khanijow V, Jalaludin MA. Fine-needle aspiration cytology of metastatic nasopharyngeal carcinoma. *Diagn Cytopathol* 1998;19:168–72.

Koller SM, El Hag IA. Fine-needle aspiration cytology of metastatic nasopharyngeal carcinoma in cervical lymph nodes: comparison with metastatic squamous-cell carcinoma, and Hodgkin's and non-Hodgkin's lymphoma. *Diagn Cytopathol* 2003;28:18–22.

Thompson L. Nasopharyngeal carcinoma. *Ear Nose Throat J* 2005;84:404–5.

Tsou MH, Wu ML, Chuang AY, Lin CY, Terng SD. Nasopharyngeal biopsy imprint cytology: a retrospective analysis of 191 cases. *Diagn Cytopathol* 2006;34:204–7.

Viguer JM, Jimenez-Heffernan JA, Lopez-Ferrer P, Banaclocha M, Vicandi B. Fine-needle aspiration cytology of metastatic nasopharyngeal carcinoma. *Diagn Cytopathol* 2005;32:233–7.

MERKEL CELL CARCINOMA

Allen PJ, Bowne WB, Jaques DP, Brennan MF, Busam K, Coit DG. Merkel cell carcinoma: prognosis and treatment of patients from a single institution. *J Clin Oncol* 2005;23:2300–9.

Brissett AE, Olsen KD, Kasperbauer JL, Lewis JE, Goellner JR, Spotts BE, Weaver AL, Strome SE. Merkel cell carcinoma of the head and neck: a retrospective case series. *Head Neck* 2002;24:982–8.

Byrd-Gloster AL, Khoor A, Glass LF, Messina JL, Whitsett JA, Livingston SK, Cagle PT. Differential expression of thyroid transcription factor 1 in small cell lung carcinoma and Merkel cell tumor. *Hum Pathol* 2000;31:58–62.

Collins BT, Elmberger PG, Tani EM, Bjornhagen V, Ramos R. Fine needle aspiration of Merkel cell Carcinoma of the skin with cytomorphology and immunocytochemical correlation. *Diagn Cytopathol* 1998;18:251–7.

Dey P, Jogai S, Amir T. Fine needle aspiration cytology of Merkel cell carcinoma. *Diagn Cytopathol* 2006;31:364–5.

Gottschalk-Sabag S, Ne'eman Z, Glick T. Merkel cell carcinoma diagnosed by fine-needle aspiration. *Am J Dermatopathol* 1996;18:269–72.

PARAGANGLIOMA (CAROTID BODY TUMOR)

Das DK, Gupta AK, Chowdhury V, Satsangi DK, Tyagi S, Mohan JC, Khan VA, Malhotra V. Fine needle aspiration diagnosis of carotid body tumor: report of a case and review of experience with cytologic features in four cases. *Diagn Cytopathol* 1997;17:143–7.

Gonzalez-Campora R, Otal-Salaverri C, Panea-Flores P, et al. Fine needle aspiration cytology of paraganglionic tumors. *Acta Cytol* 1988;32:386–90.

Gujrathi, Chetan S, Donald, Paul J. Current trends in the diagnosis and management of head and neck paragangliomas. *Curr Opin Otolaryngol Head Neck Surg* 2005;13:339–42.

Hood IC, Qizilbash AH, Young JE, et al. Fine needle aspiration biopsy cytology of paragangliomas. Cytologic, light microscopic and ultrastructural studies of three cases. *Acta Cytol* 1983;27:651–7.

Monabati A, Hodjati H, Kumar PV. Cytologic findings in carotid body tumors. *Acta Cytol* 2002;46:1101–4.

FIBROMATOSIS

Dalen BPM, Meis-Kindblom JMM, Sumathi VP, Ryd W, Kindblom LG. Fine-needle aspiration cytology and core needle biopsy in the preoperative diagnosis of desmoid tumors. *Acta Orthopaedica* 2006;77:926–31.

Dey P, Mallik MK, Gupta SK, Vasishta RK. Role of fine needle aspiration cytology in the diagnosis of soft tissue tumours and tumour-like lesions. *Cytopathology* 2004;15:32–7.

Masson J, Soule E. Desmoid tumors of the head and neck. *Am J Surg* 1966;112:615–22.

Raab SS, Silverman JF, McLeod DL, Benning TL, Geisinger KR. Fine needle aspiration biopsy of Fibromatoses. *Acta Cytol* 1993;37:323–8.

Skoog L, Pereira ST, Tani E. Fine-needle aspiration cytology and immunohistochemistry of soft-tissue tumors and osteo/chondrosarcomas of the head and neck. *Diagn Cytopathol* 1999;20:131–6.

PILOMATRIXOMA (CALCIFYING EPITHELIOMA OF MALHERBE)

El Hag IA, Kollur SM. Fine needle aspiration cytology of pilomatrixoma of the neck region: differentiation from metastatic undifferentiated nasopharyngeal carcinoma. *Acta Cytol* 2003; 47:526–7.

Lemos MM, Kindblom LG, Meis-Kindblom JM, Ryd W, Willen H. Fine needle aspiration features of pilomatrixoma. *Cancer* 2001;93:252–6.

Wang J, Cobb CJ, Martin SE, Venegas R, Wu N, Greaves TS. Pilomatrixoma: clinicopathologic study of 51 cases with emphasis on cytologic features. *Diagn Cytopathol* 2002;27:167–72.

NODULAR FASCIITIS

Azua J, Arraiza A, Delgado B, Romeo C. Nodular fasciitis initially diagnosed by aspiration cytology. *Acta Cytol* 1985:29:562–5.

Dodd LG, Martinez S. Fine needle aspiration cytology of pseudosarcomatous lesions of soft tissue. *Diagn Cytopathol* 2001;24:28–35.

Kong CS, Cha I. Nodular fasciitis. Diagnosis by fine needle aspiration biopsy. *Acta Cytol* 2004;48:473–7.

Saad RS, Talei H, Lipscomb J, Ruiz B. Nodular fasciitis of parotid region: a pitfall in the diagnosis of pleomorphic adenomas on fine needle aspiration cytology. *Diagn Cytopathol* 2005:33:191–4.

SCHWANNOMA

Domanski HA, Akerman M, Engellau J, Gustafson P, Mertens F, Rydholm A. Fine-needle aspiration of neurilemoma (schwannoma). A clinicocytopathologic study of 116 patients. *Diagn Cytopathol* 2006;34:403–12.

Klijanienko J, Caillaud JM, Lagace R. Cytohistologic correlations in schwannomas (neurilemmomas), including "ancient," cellular, and epithelioid variants. *Diagn Cytopathol* 2006;34:517–22.

Yu GH, Sack MJ, Baloch Z, Gupta PK. Difficulties in the fine needle aspiration (FNA) diagnosis of schwannoma. *Cytopathology* 1999;10:186–94.

LIPOMA

Ahuja AT, King AD, Kew J, King W, Metreweli C. Head and neck lipomas: sonographic appearance. *Am J Neuroradiol* 1998;19:505–8.

Butler SL, Oertel YC. Lipomas of the neck simulating thyroid nodules: diagnosis by fine needle aspiration. *Diagn Cytopathol* 1992;8:528–31.

El Monem MHA, Gaafar AH, Magdy EA. Lipomas of the head and neck: presentation variablility and diagnostic work-up. *J Laryngol Otol* 2006;120:47–55.

13

Salivary Glands

Pascale Levine and Joan F. Cangiarella

SIALADENOSIS (SIALOSIS, ASYMPTOMATIC PAROTID HYPERTROPHY)

Clinical Features
- Noninflammatory recurrent salivary gland enlargement
- Peak incidence in the fifth to sixth decade
- Slight female predominance
- Parotid or submandibular gland involved; usually bilateral

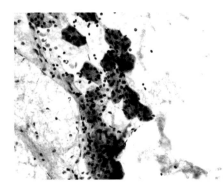

13-1. Sialadenosis. Numerous cohesive clusters of enlarged bland appearing acinar cells with polarized nuclei (Papanicolaou stain)

- Painless
- Autonomic nervous system dysregulation
- Associated with diabetes, hypothyroidism, malnutrition (including anorexia/bulimia), alcohol abuse, cirrhosis, HIV infection, hormonal variation (puberty, menopause), antihypertensive and antiepileptic drugs or idiopathic

Cytologic Features
- Acinic cell hyperplasia, followed by acinar atrophy and adipose tissue replacement
- Cellular smears
- Round clusters of plump cells with abundant vacuolated, granular, or translucent cytoplasm (hyperplastic salivary gland acini)
- Sheets of benign ductal epithelium associated with acini
- Numerous naked nuclei
- Background fat
- Background devoid of inflammation

Special Stains and Immunohistochemistry
- PAS stain highlights the cytoplasmic granules (zymogen granules)

Modern Techniques for Diagnosis
- Noncontributory

Differential Diagnosis
- Normal salivary gland
  - The size of normal acinar cells is smaller (30–40 μm)
  - Less cellularity
- Acinic cell carcinoma
  - Differentiation may be difficult
  - Hypercellular smears
  - Papillary structures and irregular clusters
  - Polygonal acinic cells that resemble normal acinar cells
  - Lack of polarization of nuclei (eccentric nuclei)
  - Ground-glass appearance of nuclei
  - Numerous naked nuclei
  - Large, dense metachromatic cytoplasmic granules on modified Giemsa stain, PAS-positive diastase-resistant
  - Absence of ductal epithelium except in less differentiated acinic cell carcinoma (ductlike cells)
  - No background fat

PEARLS

⭑ Light microscopic morphometric measurements: significant increase in mean acinar diameter in a sialadenotic gland as compared to a normal gland (average 50–70 μm vs. 30–40 μm)

⭑ Important to recognize this uncommon cytologic entity as a cause of salivary gland swelling

SIALOLITHIASIS

Clinical Features
- Major ducts are involved
- Submandibular gland and less often parotid gland

■ Peak incidence in third to fourth decade
■ No sex predilection
■ Unilateral postprandial salivary gland pain and intermittent firm enlargement
■ Possible subsequent infection resulting in squamous, mucinous or oncocytic metaplasia (acute sialadenitis) with subsequent atrophy and fibrosis (chronic sialadenitis)
■ Sonogram shows calculus and duct dilatation

Cytologic Features
■ Scanty, hypocellular aspirate
■ Sheets of benign ductal cells and metaplastic squamous cells
■ Absence of acinar cells
■ Mucoid and/or inflammatory background (lymphocytes, neutrophils)
■ Calcific material (stone fragments)

Special Stains and Immunohistochemistry
■ Noncontributory

Modern Techniques for Diagnosis
■ Noncontributory

Differential Diagnosis
■ The diagnosis is straightforward when clinical and sonographic findings are available and fragments of stones are sampled
■ Mucoepidermoid carcinoma, low grade or cystic
  ➤ Pseudohistiocytic mucus cells in loose clusters
  ➤ Intermediate cells
  ➤ Atypical squamous cells
  ➤ Absence of stone fragments
  ➤ In doubt, recommend excision
■ Mucocele
  ➤ Lower lip
  ➤ Soft and fluctuant
  ➤ Granulation tissue
  ➤ Foreign body giant cells
  ➤ Absence of stone fragments

PEARLS

★ Nontyrosine crystals identified in sialolithiasis can be found in Warthin's tumor, oncocytic papillary cystadenoma, and cellular benign mixed tumor

ACUTE SIALADENITIS

Clinical Features
■ Localized infection
■ Parotid (parotiditis) and submandibular gland most commonly affected
■ Fever, tender diffuse enlargement, warmness, erythema
■ Poor ductal drainage (sialolithiasis, dehydration, poor oral hygiene in a postoperative or postanesthesic setting, malnutrition, immunosuppression)
■ Secondary bacterial infection due to *Streptococcus viridans, Staphylococcus aureus,* Salmonella, or Gram-negative bacteria
■ Viral infections such as paramyxovirus (Mumps), coxsackie virus, Epstein–Barr virus, cytomegalovirus
■ Rare etiologies: tuberculosis and cat scratch disease

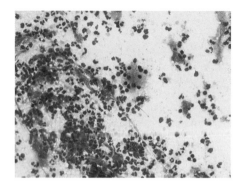

13-2. Acute sialadenitis. Cluster of acinar cells (center) surrounded by abundant acute inflammation (modified Giemsa stain)

■ Leukocytosis, elevated erythrocyte sedimentation rate (ESR), elevated serum amylase

Cytologic Features
■ Painful on aspiration
■ Numerous neutrophils
■ Foreign body giant cells
■ Normal salivary gland acini
■ Reactive ductal epithelium
■ Metaplastic squamous cells
■ Histiocytes with inflammatory atypia
■ Crystalloids and cyst debris

Special Stains and Immunohistochemistry
■ Cultures and special stains on unstained smears or cytospin preparation: acid-fast bacilli, fungal, and Gram stain

Modern Techniques for Diagnosis
■ Noncontributory

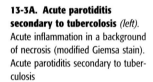

13-3A. Acute parotiditis secondary to tubercolosis *(left).* Acute inflammation in a background of necrosis (modified Giemsa stain). Acute parotiditis secondary to tuberculosis

13-3B. Acute parotiditis secondary to tubercolosis *(right).* Rare acid-fast bacilli are noted (AFB stain)

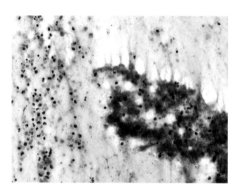 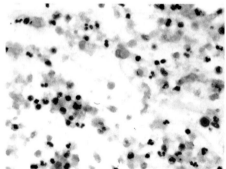

Differential Diagnosis
■ Squamous cell carcinoma
➤ Atypical to clearly malignant squamous cells
➤ Keratinaceous material
➤ Necrotic background
➤ In doubt, excise

PEARLS

★ The clinical diagnosis may be evident, however aspiration biopsy may prove useful for cultures and identification of the offending agent
★ Can be confused clinically with carcinoma

CHRONIC SCLEROSING SIALADENITIS (KUTTNER'S TUMOR, SIALOLITHIASIS OF THE SUBMANDIBULAR SALIVARY GLAND)

Clinical Features
■ Postprandial salivary gland pain and swelling
■ Palpable hard mass mimicking neoplasm clinically
■ Most common cause of sialolithiasis

- Submandibular gland most commonly affected, unilateral involvement
- Occurs in third to seventh decade, mean age forty-four years
- Slight male predominance

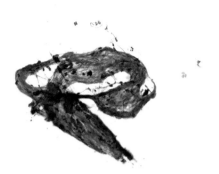

Cytologic Features
- Paucicellular smears with lymphoplasmacytic infiltrate
- Fibrous tissue
- Occasional sheets of benign ductal cells
- Acini are usually lacking
- Cytologic atypia (reactive) may affect ductal cells and lymphoid cells
- Sometimes only scant fibrous tissue and a few lymphocytes are aspirated

13-4. Chronic sclerosing sialadenitis (kuttner's tumor). Paucicellular smear with scant fragments of fibrous tissue (Ultrafast Papanicolaou stain)

Special Stains and Immunohistochemistry
- Flow cytometry with immunophenotyping is mandatory if lymphoma is suspected

Modern Techniques for Diagnosis
- Noncontributory

Differential Diagnosis
Lymphoma: cellular smears
- MALT (mucosa-associated lymphoid tissue)
  - Typically associated with lymphoepithelial sialadenitis (LESA) or myoepithelial sialadenitis (MESA) in patients with Sjögren's syndrome
  - Thick clusters of epimyoepithelial cells
  - Intermediate-sized lymphocytes with cleaved nuclei, pale chromatin, and well-defined pale cytoplasm
  - Small mature lymphocytes, monocytoid cells, plasma cells
  - Monoclonal B-cell proliferation with Kappa light chain restriction on flow cytometry (CD20+, CD23–, CD10–, CD5–)
- Follicular center lymphoma, low-grade
  - Arising from MESA or from an intraparotid lymph node
  - Monotonous population of small to intermediate-sized lymphocytes
  - Irregular small to intermediate-sized nuclei with clumped chromatin and inconspicuous nucleoli
  - Occasional larger lymphocytes, sometimes cleaved, with fine chromatin and multiple peripheral nucleoli
  - Monoclonal B-cell proliferation with light chain restriction on flow cytometry (CD20+, CD23–, CD10+, CD5–)
- Intraparotid lymph node
  - Cellular smear
  - Polymorphic lymphoid aggregates with predominance of small mature lymphocytes
  - Tingible body macrophages
  - Occasional large noncleaved lymphocytes
  - Lack of ductal epithelium
  - Flow cytometry supports a reactive process

PEARLS

★ In the appropriate setting a correct diagnosis can be made most of the time by aspiration biopsy and may alleviate surgery

GRANULOMATOUS SIALADENITIS

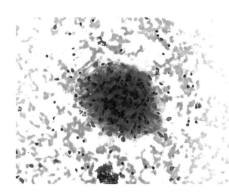

13-5. Granulomatous sialadenitis secondary to sarcoidosis. Well-formed noncaseating granuloma (epithelioid histiocytes) admixed with lymphocytes is seen (modified Giemsa stain)

Clinical Features
■ Unilateral or bilateral parotid or submandibular gland enlargement
■ Usually of the non necrotizing type and secondary to sarcoidosis
■ Duct obstruction by tumor or calculus with rupture can cause a granulomatous reaction
■ Infectious causes include tuberculosis or mycosis; rare etiologies include toxoplasmosis or brucellosis
■ No age or sex predilection

Cytologic Features
■ Cellular smears
■ Clusters of epithelioid histiocytes with carrot-shaped nuclei
■ Fibroblasts
■ Multinucleated giant cells
■ Inflammatory background
■ Necrosis
■ Asteroid bodies, calcium oxalate crystals in sarcoidosis

Special Stains and Immunohistochemistry
■ Acid-fast bacilli and fungal stains to rule out an infectious process

Modern Techniques for Diagnosis
■ Noncontributory

Differential Diagnosis
■ Nodular fasciitis
  ➤ Rapidly growing subcutaneous mass
  ➤ Reactive fibroblasts with long cytoplasmic processes and elongated nuclei
  ➤ Magenta fibrillary stroma
  ➤ Inflammatory background
  ➤ No multinucleated giant cells

PEARLS

★ Correlation with clinical diagnosis is helpful for sarcoidosis-related granulomatous sialadenitis
★ Can be mistaken for malignancy on aspiration biopsy

BENIGN LYMPHOEPITHELIAL CYST (CYSTIC BLL)

Clinical Features
■ Associated with HIV infection
■ Enlarged fluctuant multiloculated cystic intraparotid lymph nodes
■ Associated diffuse bilateral cervical lymphadenopathy
■ Often bilateral
■ Duct compression by lymphocytic infiltration
■ Basal cell hyperplasia of ducts
■ Recurrence despite aspiration or surgery

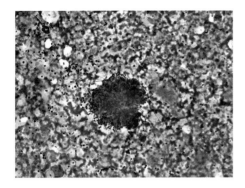 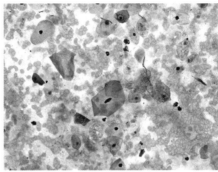

13-6A. Benign lymphoepithelial cyst *(left)*. Lymphoid aggregates and mature lymphocytes in a watery proteinaceous background (modified Giemsa stain)

13-6B. Benign lymphoepithelial cyst *(right)*. Mature squamous metaplastic cells can also be seen (modified Giemsa stain)

Cytologic Features

▓ Abundant mixed lymphoid population with predominance of small mature lymphocytes

▓ Lymphohistiocytic aggregates

▓ Sparse or abundant mature metaplastic squamous cells with small mature or pyknotic nuclei

▓ Rarely mucoepidermoid epithelium is seen

▓ Foamy macrophages

▓ Watery proteinaceous fluid

Special Stains and Immunohistochemistry

▓ Noncontributory

Modern Techniques for Diagnosis

▓ Noncontributory

Differential Diagnosis

▓ Intraparotid lymph node
  ➤ Cellular smear
  ➤ Polymorphous lymphoid population with predominance of small mature lymphocytes and tingible body macrophages
  ➤ Flow cytometry supports a reactive process
▓ Non-Hodgkin's lymphoma
▓ Large cell type
  ➤ Predominance of large lymphoid cells with round to irregular nuclei, fine to coarse chromatin, and variable number of nucleoli
  ➤ No cyst fluid
  ➤ Flow cytometry: Monoclonal B-cell population with light chain restriction, CD10+/−
▓ MALT lymphoma
  ➤ Mixed lymphoid population
  ➤ Small to medium size lymphocytes (monocytoid cells, plasmacytoid cells, large transformed lymphocytes)
  ➤ Flow cytometry: Monoclonal B-cell proliferation with Kappa light chain restriction, CD5−, CD10−, CD23−, CD20+
▓ Follicular center lymphoma
  ➤ Monotonous population of small to intermediate size lymphocytes
  ➤ Irregular small to intermediate size nuclei with clumped chromatin and inconspicuous nucleoli
  ➤ Occasional larger lymphoid cells
  ➤ Monoclonal B-cell proliferation with light chain restriction on flow cytometry (CD20+, CD23−, CD10+, CD5−)

■ Sjögren's Syndrome/ Mikulicz's disease, cystic
> ➤ Heterogeneous lymphoid population with clusters of epithelial/myoepithelial cells
> ➤ Granular background with cell debris

■ Squamous cell carcinoma
> ➤ Prominent epithelial component
> ➤ Minor or absent lymphoid component
> ➤ Keratinized and anucleated atypical to frankly malignant squamous cells with hyperchromatic large nuclei and dense cytoplasm
> ➤ Necrotic background

■ Low-grade mucoepidermoid carcinoma
> ➤ Predominant mucinous cells, intermediate cells and non keratinized squamoid cells
> ➤ Rare or absent lymphoid component
> ➤ Absence of tingible body macrophages

■ Warthin's tumor
> ➤ Cohesive clusters of oncocytes
> ➤ Dirty proteinaceous background
> ➤ Rarely oncocytes are absent making the separation with cystic BLL very difficult

■ Salivary duct cyst
> ➤ Lymphoid component is less prominent
> ➤ Goblet type mucus cells and oncocytic cells

PEARLS

⋆ The majority of salivary gland lesions of HIV patients are cystic BLL
⋆ The presence of atypia in a benign lymphoepithelial lesion warrants flow cytometry to rule out a lymphomatous process

SJÖGREN'S DISEASE/BENIGN LYMPHOEPITHELIAL LESIONS (BLL)/ MYOEPITHELIAL SIALADENITIS (MESA)/LYMPHOEPITHELIAL SIALADENITIS (LESA)

Clinical Features

■ Autoimmune myoepithelial sialadenitis with slow destruction of the salivary glands
■ Increased risk of developing marginal zone/MALT-type lymphoma
■ Most commonly affects the parotid gland, less commonly the submandibular gland
■ Ocular and oral symptoms, dry eyes, salivary gland involvement (SICCA)
■ Female to male ratio of 9:1
■ Peak incidence in the third to fourth decade and after menopause

13-7A. Sjogren's disease *(left).* Lymphohistiocytic aggregates in a background of proteinaceous debris (modified Giemsa stain)

13-7B. Sjogren's disease *(right).* The lymphoid population is heterogeneous with both small and large lymphoid cells (Papanicolaou stain)

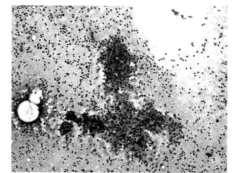 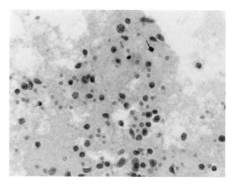

■ Serum autoantibodies (antinuclear antibodies/ANA, anti-SSA, anti-SSB, IgM rheumatoid factor) may be present
■ Suspicion of lymphoma if persistently enlarged parotid glands, regional or general lymphadenopathy, hypergammaglobulinemia

Cytologic Features
■ Hypercellular smears
■ Heterogeneous lymphoid population
■ Small mature lymphocytes, tingible body macrophages, plasma cells, germinal center lymphoid cells
■ Lymphoepithelial lesion is the hallmark
■ Clusters of epithelial/myoepithelial cells
■ Acini are not seen

Special Stains and Immunohistochemistry
■ Panel of B and T cell markers to establish polyclonality

Modern Techniques for Diagnosis
■ Flow cytometry to establish polyclonality of lymphoid cells

Differential Diagnosis
■ HIV-related lymphoepithelial cyst
  ➤ Hypocellular smears
  ➤ Mixed lymphoid infiltrate
  ➤ No epithelial/myoepithelial cells
  ➤ Squamous cells
  ➤ Cyst fluid
■ Intraparotid node
  ➤ No epimyoepithelial clusters identified
■ Lymphoma, MALT type
  ➤ Heterogenous population of lymphoid cells, cleaved (centrocytes), and plasmacytoid lymphoid cells
  ➤ Flow cytometry useful to establish clonality
Warthin's tumor
  ➤ Tight clusters of oncocytes
  ➤ Dirty granular background

PEARLS

★ The goal of aspiration biopsy is to confirm the clinical diagnosis and to rule out a lymphoproliferative disorder
★ Flow cytometry with immunophenotyping is advised if a diagnosis of lymphoma is suspected

BENIGN INTRAPAROTID LYMPH NODE

Clinical Features
■ History of prior head and neck surgery, dental work, viral infection
■ May reach 2 cm in size
■ Usually no associated cervical lymphadenopathy

Cytologic Features
■ Mixed lymphoid population
■ Predominantly small mature lymphocytes

■ Occasional tingible body macrophages
■ Lymphohistiocytic cells in clusters
■ Polyclonal by flow cytometry

Special Stains and Immunohistochemistry
■ B- and T-cell markers to establish polyclonality

Modern Techniques for Diagnosis
■ Flow cytometry to establish polyclonality

Differential Diagnosis
■ Lymphoma, CLL/SLL
  ➤ Mixed lymphoid population
  ➤ Monotonous small lymphocytes with clumped chromatin
  ➤ Larger lymphocytes with prominent nucleoli and conspicuous cytoplasm (prolymphocytes, paraimmunoblasts)
  ➤ Monoclonal B-cell proliferation with light chain restriction, CD5+, CD23+, CD10−
■ Lymphoma, MALT, described above
■ Lymphoma, follicular type, described above
■ Chronic sialadenitis
  ➤ Paucicellular aspirate
  ➤ Small lymphocytes and plasma cells
  ➤ Ductal epithelium
■ Benign lymphoepithelial lesion
  ➤ Clinical context is different (often Sjögren's syndrome)
  ➤ Epimyoepithelial islands, if present
  ➤ Ductal epithelium

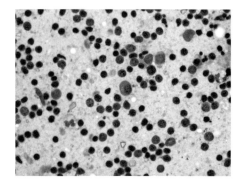

13-8. Benign intraparotid lymph node. Mixed lymphoid population with predominance of small mature lymphocytes (modified Giemsa stain)

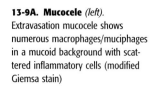

PEARLS

★ Flow cytometry is necessary, especially if persistent or enlarging

MUCOCELE

Clinical Features
■ Most common nonneoplastic lesion of the salivary glands
■ Two types: extravasation mucocele (common) and mucous retention cyst (rare)
■ Extravasation mucocele
  ➤ Affects men more often than women
  ➤ Peak incidence in the third decade
  ➤ Most commonly in the lower lip and oral cavity

13-9A. Mucocele (left). Extravasation mucocele shows numerous macrophages/muciphages in a mucoid background with scattered inflammatory cells (modified Giemsa stain)

13-9B. Mucocele (right). Mucous retention cyst shows numerous macrophages and mature metaplastic squamous cells (modified Giemsa stain)

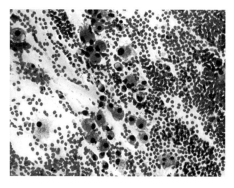
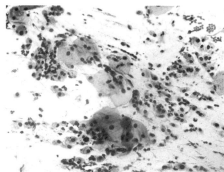

➤ Secondary to extravasation of mucus following rupture of mucus filled cyst due to microtrauma or mucus congestion
▪ Mucus retention cyst
   ➤ Affects women more than men
   ➤ Peak incidence eighth to ninth decade
   ➤ Most commonly in the cheek and palate
   ➤ Secondary to duct obstruction due to a calculus or impacted secretions

Cytologic Features
▪ Extravasation mucocele
   ➤ Clear or mucoid fluid
   ➤ Granulation tissue
   ➤ Inflammatory cells
   ➤ Foreign body giant cells and macrophages
   ➤ Collagen fibers
▪ Mucus retention cyst
   ➤ Mucoid fluid
   ➤ Cuboidal/columnar epithelial cells
   ➤ Lack of inflammation
   ➤ Oncocytic metaplasia, squamous metaplasia with and without atypia
   ➤ Tyrosine crystals

Special Stains and Immunohistochemistry
▪ Noncontributory

Modern Techniques for Diagnosis
▪ Noncontributory

Differential Diagnosis
▪ Neoplasms with cystic change
   ➤ Mucoepidermoid carcinoma
   Squamoid, mucin producing, and intermediate cells
   ➤ Squamous cell carcinoma
   Necrotic background with malignant keratinized squamous cells
▪ Warthin's tumor
   ➤ Oncocytes and prominent lymphoid population

PEARLS
★ Any mass that persists or recurs after initial drainage should be re-biopsied and/or excised

BENIGN MIXED TUMOR (BMT)/PLEOMORPHIC ADENOMA (PA)

Clinical features
▪ Most common salivary gland neoplasm
▪ Occurs most commonly in the lower pole of the superficial lobe of the parotid gland, less often submucosal nodule of lip or palate
▪ Painless, circumscribed, slow-growing, lobulated mass
▪ Peak incidence in fourth decade
▪ Recurrence if incomplete surgical excision

13-10A. Pleomorphic adenoma *(opposite, left).* Biphasic tumor with epithelial and myoepithelial cells embedded in a metachromatic fibrillary matrix (modified Giemsa stain)

13-10B. Pleomorphic adenoma *(opposite, right).* Epithelial and myoepithelial cells are embedded in fibrillary stroma (modified Giemsa stain)

13-10C. Pleomorphic adenoma *(below, left).* Polygonal epithelial cells with abundant cytoplasm are seen (modified Giemsa stain)

13-10D. Pleomorphic adenoma *(below, right).* Pleomophic adenoma with prominent fibrillary matrix and tyrosine crystals (modified Giemsa stain)

13-10E. Pleomorphic adenoma *(middle, left).* Cellular pleomorphic adenoma shows papillary aggregates with a predominance of epithelial cells (modified Giemsa stain)

13-10F. Pleomorphic adenoma *(middle, right).* Cylindromatous pattern in a pleomorphic adenoma (modified Giemsa stain)

13-10G. Pleomorphic adenoma *(bottom, left).* Cylindromatous pattern shows round hyaline globules of metachromatic stroma surrounded by epithelioid cells with fairly abundant cytoplasm (modified Giemsa stain)

13-10H. Pleomorphic adenoma *(bottom, right).* Pleomorphic adenoma with atypia shows focal clusters of atypical epithelioid cells with increased nuclear cytoplasmic ratios (modified Giemsa stain)

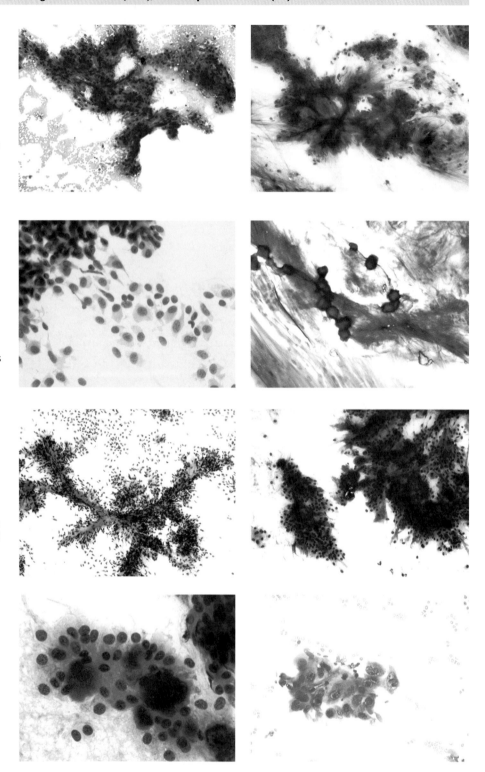

Cytologic Features

- Cellular smears
- Biphasic neoplasm with epithelial and mesenchymal components
- Abundant fibrillary chondromyxoid matrix (grey/blue in Papanicolaou stain and metachromatic/magenta in modified Giemsa stain) with irregular contours
- Fusiform, stellate or plasmacytoid stromal cells (myoepithelial cells) admixed with trabeculae, clusters, sheets or duct-like structures composed of cuboidal or polygonal epithelial cells with abundant intact cytoplasm (ductal cells)

- Ductal cells are usually bland with smooth chromatin but occasional pleomorphism can be seen
- Myoepithelial cells appear stellate or spindled with small nuclei and prominent nucleoli
- Intra- or extracellular mucin can be seen
- Histiocytes
- Tyrosine crystals (non specific)
- Metaplastic squamous cells, oncocytes, sebaceous cells may also be seen
- PA with prominent mucinous component or metaplastic squamous cells
- Cellular PA (epithelial component predominates)
- PA with oncocytic metaplasia
- PA with nuclear atypia

Special Stains and Immunohistochemistry

- Stromal (myoepithelial) cells are positive for GFAP, cytokeratin, S-100, smooth muscle actin, and calponin
- Ductal epithelial cells are positive for cytokeratin, epithelial membrane antigen, carcinoembryonic antigen, and GCDFP-15
- Ki-67 is low in pleomorphic adenomas with squamous metaplasia; high in squamous cell carcinoma and mucoepidermoid carcinoma

Modern Techniques for Diagnosis

- Noncontributory

Differential Diagnosis

- Adenoid cystic carcinoma
  - Should be differentiated from cellular and cylindromatous PA
  - Nuclear coarse chromatin
  - Tight clusters, small rosettes, cribriform pattern
  - Finger-like red bands of basement membrane-like material
  - Basaloid cells with naked slightly pleomorphic nuclei, coarse chromatin, nucleoli
  - Nuclear molding
  - Lacks myoepithelial cells
  - Metachromatic homogenous nonfibrillary acellular hyaline globules (magenta on modified Giemsa stain), isolated with smooth round borders or in sieve-like clusters hugged by balls of small cells (naked nuclei)
- Basal cell adenoma
  - Branching three-dimensional papillary structures
  - Peripheral palisading
  - Small uniform basaloid cells
  - Scant or absent cytoplasm (naked nuclei) with fine chromatin and inconspicuous nucleoli
  - Metachromatic hyaline bands (modified Giemsa stain)
  - Scant nonfibrillary and nonchondromyxoid stroma
- Monomorphic adenoma
  - Nests, cords, or islands of basaloid cells with peripheral palisading
  - Uniform oval basaloid cells
  - Smooth round scant cytoplasm
  - Angulated nuclei
- Low grade mucoepidermoid carcinoma
  - Should be differentiated from PA with prominent mucinous material and squamous metaplasia
  - Infiltrating borders, more often cystic on ultrasound
  - Goblet cells, intermediate cells

➤ Diffuse cytologic atypia
➤ No chondromyxoid fibrillary stroma
■ Oncocytoma
  ➤ Should be differentiated from PA with oncocytic metaplasia
  ➤ Lymphocytes
  ➤ Dirty background
  ➤ No chondromyxoid fibrillary stroma
■ Carcinoma ex-pleomorphic adenoma
  ➤ Should be differentiated from PA with nuclear atypia
  ➤ Rapid recent growth
  ➤ Dense cellularity with more diffuse atypia
  ➤ Increased mitotic activity
  ➤ Coarse irregularly distributed chromatin, nucleoli
  ➤ Necrosis

PEARLS

★ The use of modified Giemsa stain is helpful to identify the characteristic chondromyxoid fibrillary stroma

★ Papanicolaou and rapid Papanicolaou stains are helpful to visualize nuclear features, which may differ between benign adenoma and carcinoma

★ Cylindromatous pattern of pleomorphic adenoma can mimic adenoid cystic carcinoma

BASAL CELL ADENOMA (TUBULAR, TRABECULAR, BASALOID, MONOMORPHIC)

Clinical Features
■ Rare
■ Elderly woman
■ Single, circumscribed, solid, painless, mobile nodule
■ Parotid gland, superior aspect (70%); less commonly submandibular gland and upper lip
■ Low risk of recurrence

Cytologic Features
■ Flat branching sheets or papillary aggregates of small uniform basaloid cells
■ Bland ovoid nuclei, fine chromatin, occasional inconspicuous nucleoli
■ Naked nuclei
■ Scant barely visible cytoplasm
■ Associated nonfibrillary collagenous stroma with occasional palisading and interdigitation with basaloid cells
■ The cells may be attached to basement membrane-like material, which may show small hyaline cores or globules (cylindromatous pattern)
■ Occasional keratin debris and keratinized squamous cells (squamous whorls)

Special Stains and Immunohistochemistry
■ Can show positivity for cytokeratin, S-100 protein, smooth muscle actin, vimentin, carcinoembryonic antigen, and epithelial membrane antigen
■ Negative for GFAP

Modern Techniques for Diagnosis
■ Noncontributory

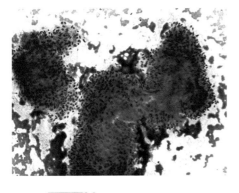
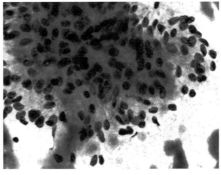
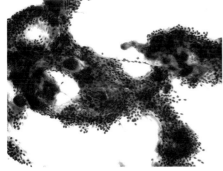
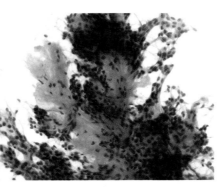

13-11A. Basal cell adenoma *(top, left)*. Sheets and large papillary aggregates of basaloid cells with interdigitating metachromatic matrix (modified Giemsa stain)

13-11B. Basal cell adenoma *(top, right)*. Higher magnification shows small uniform basaloid cells with bland ovoid nuclei (modified Giemsa stain)

13-11C. Basal cell adenoma *(bottom, left)*. Basal cell adenoma with a cylindromatous pattern shows round basement membrane globules surrounded by a proliferation of small basaloid cells with very scant cytoplasm (modified Giemsa stain)

13-11D. Basal cell adenoma *(bottom, right)*. Nuclear palisading can be seen (hematoxylin & eosin stain)

Differential Diagnosis
- Adenoid cystic carcinoma
  - Larger basement membrane globules
  - Associated multilayered clusters of larger basaloid cells
  - Irregular nuclei, mild pleomorphism
  - Nuclear molding
  - Coarse chromatin
  - No squamous differentiation
  - Lacks peripheral palisading
- Cellular pleomorphic adenoma
  - Plasmacytoid cells with greater amount of cytoplasm
  - Fibrillary chondromyxoid stroma may be scanty or absent
- Small cell carcinoma
  - Small hyperchromatic cells with pleomorphic nuclei and salt- and -pepper chromatin
  - Nuclear molding
  - Necrosis
  - Neuroendocrine differentiation by immunohistochemistry
- Basal cell adenocarcinoma
  - Pleomorphic basaloid tumor cells
  - Large three-dimensional clusters
  - Mitotic figures and necrosis are noted

PEARLS

★ May be difficult to distinguish basal cell adenoma from basal cell adenocarcinoma on cytology; mitotic figures, necrosis, and atypia favor adenocarcinoma

MYOEPITHELIOMA

Clinical Features

- Rare, majority are benign
- Equal distribution between parotid and minor salivary glands (hard and soft palate)
- Equal distribution between men and women
- Peak incidence in the third to fourth decade
- Circumscribed, asymptomatic, slow-growing, painless mass

Cytologic Features

- Myoepithelial cell–rich tumor, which can have several morphologic appearances: clear cells, spindle cells, plasmacytoid cells, epithelioid cells
- Fusiform or plasmacytoid cells (myoepithelial cells)
- Acinar or gland-like arrangement
- Ovoid nuclei with smooth textured chromatin
- Associated metachromatic fibrillary matrix
- Scant myxoid stroma
- Hyaline globules reminiscent of cylindromatous pattern

Special stains and Immunohistochemistry

- Positive for smooth muscle actin, S-100 protein, keratin, p63, calponin, GFAP
- Negative for EMA

Modern Techniques for Diagnosis

- Electron microscopy shows abundant myofilaments

Differential Diagnosis

- Pleomorphic adenoma
  - ➤ Ductal epithelial cells
  - ➤ Chondromyxoid stroma
  - ➤ Cellular PA may be very difficult to differentiate from epithelioid myoepithelioma
- Myoepithelial carcinoma
  - ➤ Tumor infiltration of adjacent tissues
  - ➤ Malignant spindle cells with pleomorphism and large nucleoli
  - ➤ Mitotic figures and necrosis are noted

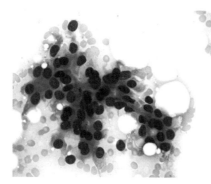
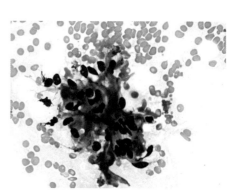

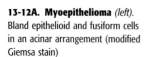

13-12A. Myoepithelioma *(left).* Bland epithelioid and fusiform cells in an acinar arrangement (modified Giemsa stain)

13-12B. Myoepithelioma *(right).* Spindle cells are intimately associated with metachromatic fibrillary matrix (modified Giemsa stain)

★ Due to the morphologic heterogeneity of myoepithelial cells, myoepitheliomas may be difficult to diagnose on fine-needle aspiration biopsy
★ Immunohistochemistry may be useful for an accurate diagnosis

ONCOCYTOMA

Clinical Features
▓ Predominantly affects the parotid gland
▓ Peak incidence in seventh to ninth decade
▓ Marked female predominance if clear cell component is present
▓ Majority are benign

Cytologic Features
▓ Cellular smears
▓ Clusters and sheets of large oncocytes
▓ Abundant granular sharply delineated cytoplasm (blue–green on Papanicolaou stain, blue–gray on modified Giemsa stain)
▓ Round, centrally placed nuclei
▓ Prominent nucleoli
▓ Variant with clear cell change

Special stains and Immunohistochemistry
▓ Phosphotungstic acid–hematoxylin (PTAH) positive

Modern Techniques for Diagnosis
▓ Electron microscopy shows numerous mitochondria in oncocytes

Differential Diagnosis
▓ Warthin's tumor
  ➤ Less cellular
  ➤ Lymphoid infiltrate
  ➤ Dirty cystic background
▓ Oncocytic carcinoma
  ➤ Infiltrating borders
  ➤ Striking nuclear atypia
  ➤ Huge nucleoli
  ➤ Mitotic activity
▓ Oncocytosis
  ➤ Aging process
  ➤ Multifocal and multinodular
  ➤ Less cellular
  ➤ Oncocytes intermixed with acinar cells
▓ Acinic cell carcinoma
  ➤ Vacuolated to glassy cytoplasm of acinar cells (purple on modified Giemsa stain)
  ➤ PAS-positive, diastase-resistant granules

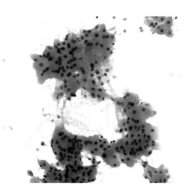

13-13. Oncocytoma. Sheets of oncocytes with abundant granular cytoplasm and prominent nucleoli. Note the clean background (hematoxylin & eosin stain)

★ Cytologic atypia in oncocytomas is not indicative of malignancy

WARTHIN'S TUMOR (PAPILLARY CYSTADENOMA LYMPHOMATOSUM)

Cytologic Features
- Almost always occurs in the parotid gland
- Male predominance
- Sixth to seventh decade
- Association with smoking
- Soft cystic mass
- Multicentric

Cytologic Features
- Small mature lymphocytes
- Flat, monolayered sheets and clusters of oncocytes (large cells with abundant granular cytoplasm, round nuclei, and conspicuous nucleoli)
- Naked nuclei
- Mast cells
- Dirty granular background due to cyst fluid
- Squamous metaplasia with occasional atypia
- Necrosis or infarction can be seen

Special stains and Immunohistochemistry
- Mucin negativity
- Keratin positivity

Modern Techniques for Diagnosis
- Noncontributory

Differential Diagnosis
- Low-grade mucoepidermoid carcinoma
  - ➤ Complex branching epithelial groups
  - ➤ Intermediate cells can be mistaken for oncocytes
  - ➤ Mucin-producing cells (goblet, clear, or vacuolated cells)
  - ➤ Mucoid stroma
  - ➤ Atypia
- Squamous cell carcinoma
  - ➤ Squamous cells are the main component
  - ➤ Cytologic atypia is marked
  - ➤ No mast cells
- Oncocytoma
  - ➤ No lymphoid component
  - ➤ No dirty background

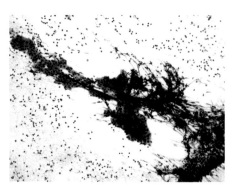
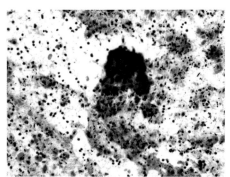

13-14A. Warthin's tumor *(left)*. Sheets of oncocytes with numerous lymphocytes and lymphoid tangles in a cystic background (hematoxylin & eosin stain)

13-14B. Warthin's tumor *(right)*. Prominent atypical squamous metaplasia can be seen in Warthin's tumor. Note the cluster of oncocytes (hematoxylin & eosin stain)

■ Benign lymphoepithelial cyst
➤ Bilateral
➤ Polymorphous lymphoid population
➤ Lacks oncocytes
➤ Tingible body macrophages

PEARLS

★ If only cyst fluid is obtained, sample the solid component under ultrasound guidance
★ Infarction following FNA can occur
★ 10% of Warthin's tumors are bilateral

MUCOEPIDERMOID CARCINOMA

Clinical features
■ Most common malignant salivary gland tumor
■ Affects parotid gland (60%) and minor salivary glands of palate, tongue
■ Slightly more prevalent in women
■ Peak incidence in the fifth decade
■ Most common malignant salivary gland neoplasm in children
■ Radiation exposure increases risk
■ Painless mass, often cystic

Cytologic Features
■ Low grade
➤ Aspiration yields clear to turbid fluid of low cellularity
➤ Overlapping epithelial groups
➤ Epithelial cells may be columnar or cuboidal mucin-secreting cells with abundant clear or vacuolated cytoplasm (goblet cells), so-called pseudohistiocytic mucous cells, polygonal squamous cells, or small intermediate cells (basaloid cells) with scant cytoplasm
➤ Foam cells
➤ Thick mucinous material
➤ Mucin stain may be useful
■ High grade
➤ Smears are dominated by malignant squamous cells
➤ Squamous pearls
➤ Prominent nucleoli
➤ Necrosis
➤ Some intermediate cells
➤ Mucinous cells are rare

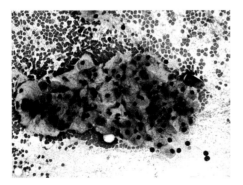
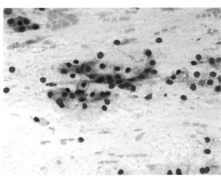

13-15A. Mucoepidermoid carcinoma, low grade *(above).* Sheets of squamoid and intermediate cells (Ultrafast Papanicolaou stain)

13-15B. Mucoepidermoid carcinoma, low grade *(left).* Clusters of pseudohistiocytic mucous cells can be noted (modified Giemsa stain)

13-15C. Mucoepidermoid carcinoma, low grade *(right).* Columnar epithelial cells with clear to vacuolated cytoplasm and background mucin (modified Giemsa stain)

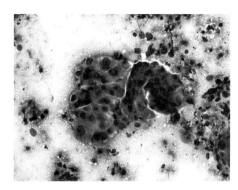

**13-16. Mucoepidermoid
carcinoma, high grade.** Cohesive
clusters of large pleomorphic epithelial
cells with high nuclear to cytoplasmic
ratios and prominent nucleoli. Squamoid
cells with pyknotic nuclei are seen
(modified Giemsa stain)

Special Stains and Immunohistochemistry
- Mucin positivity in mucous cells
- Keratin positivity in intermediate, squamous, and columnar cells

Modern Techniques for Diagnosis
- Noncontributory

Differential Diagnosis
- Mucus retention cyst
  - Background mucin
  - No intermediate cells
- Warthin's tumor with squamous metaplasia
  - Oncocytes
  - Lymphocytic infiltrate
- PA with squamous metaplasia
  - Chondromyxoid matrix
- Chronic sialadenitis with squamous metaplasia
  - Tight tubular structures
  - Lack of mucinous cells
  - No intermediate cells
- Squamous cell carcinoma, primary or metastatic
  - Keratinized dissociated tadpole squamous cells
  - Squamous pearls
  - No intermediate cells
  - Cannot be distinguished from high-grade mucoepidermoid carcinoma

PEARLS

★ Low-grade mucoepidermoid carcinoma can produce low cellularity smears that can mimic other benign conditions or can lead to a false-negative diagnosis
★ Mucoepidermoid carcinoma should be considered in the differential of any salivary gland aspirate containing mucin
★ High-grade mucoepidermoid carcinoma is difficult to distinguish from primary salivary gland high-grade carcinomas and carcinomas metastatic to the salivary gland

ADENOID CYSTIC CARCINOMA

Clinical Features
- Most common malignant salivary gland tumor of submandibular and minor salivary glands
- Fourth to sixth decade of life, slight female predilection
- Painful, slow growing malignant tumor encasing the facial nerve with local infiltration and bone erosion
- Recurrences are common

Cytologic features
- Cellular smears
- Small anaplastic (basaloid) cells (malignant epithelial–myoepithelial tumor cells) associated with stroma
- Indistinct cytoplasm
- Coarse nuclear chromatin
- Nuclear molding

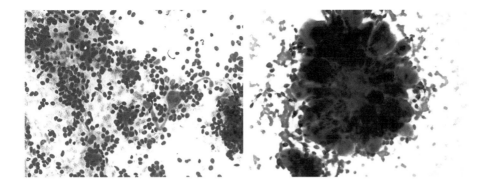

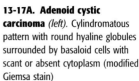

13-17A. Adenoid cystic carcinoma *(left).* Cylindromatous pattern with round hyaline globules surrounded by basaloid cells with scant or absent cytoplasm (modified Giemsa stain)

13-17B. Adenoid cystic carcinoma *(right).* Higher magnification highlights the cylindromatous arrangement (modified Giemsa stain)

13-17C. Adenoid cystic carcinoma *(below).* Tumor cells are ovoid, with coarse chromatin and indistinct cytoplasm. Dissociated tumor cells and bare nuclei are seen in the background. The stroma is acellular (Ultrafast Papanicolaou stain)

▨ The cells are aggregated in tight clusters around large round hyaline globules (rosettes or sieve-like arrangements so called cylindromatous pattern) or elongated tubules or ductules of basal lamina material

▨ Stroma is avascular and acellular (metachromatic on modified Giemsa stain, pale on Papanicolaou stain)

▨ The solid variant does not have magenta globules

▨ Dissociated tumor cells and bare oval or elongated nuclei in the background

Special Stains and Immunohistochemistry
▨ GFAP positivity
▨ Positivity for cytokeratin, vimentin, and smooth muscle actin

Modern Techniques for Diagnosis
▨ Loss of heterozygosity at 6q23-25

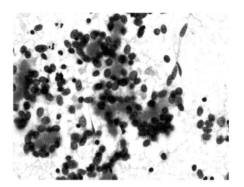

Differential Diagnosis
▨ Tumors that have a cylindromatous pattern
  ➤ Pleomorphic adenoma
  Plasmacytoid cells with conspicuous cytoplasm
  Cells embedded with fibrillar matrix
  Small hyaline globules
  ➤ Basal cell adenoma
  Same cribriform arrangement of basaloid cells
  Angular nuclei
  Smooth ovoid to round cytoplasm
  No nuclear atypia
  Smooth chromatin
  Small hyaline globules
  ➤ Low-grade polymorphous carcinoma
  Minor salivary gland
  Polygonal tumor cells with conspicuous cytoplasm
  ➤ Epithelial–myoepithelial carcinoma
  Two cell types: dark epithelial cells and vacuolated clear tumor cells
▨ Tumors with small uniform cells
  ➤ Small cell carcinoma
  Necrosis and crush artifact
  Absence of stroma

PEARLS

★ A cylindromatous pattern is not pathognomonic for adenoid cystic carcinoma but can be seen in many types of salivary gland tumors

ACINIC CELL CARCINOMA

Clinical Features
- Slow-growing circumscribed lobulated solid or microcystic mass that occurs primarily in the parotid gland
- Occurs primarily in the fourth to fifth decade with female predominance
- High recurrence rate if incompletely excised

Cytologic Features
- Highly cellular smears
- Clusters, sheets, papillary structures, and rounded acinar groups of epithelial cells
- Bland monomorphic fragile tumor cells
- Numerous round naked nuclei in the background
- Inconspicuous to prominent nucleoli
- Tumor cells have abundant granular cytoplasm (best seen on Papanicolaou stain), sometimes vacuolated (best seen on modified Giemsa stain) or ground glass in appearance
- The cytoplasmic granules are purple on Papanicolaou stain and red on modified Giemsa stain

Special Stains and Immunohistochemistry
- Cytoplasmic granules are PAS-positive, diastase-resistant
- Positivity for cytokeratin, CD15 (Leu-M1), carcinoembryonic antigen

Modern Techniques for diagnosis
- Electron microscopy shows numerous electron dense cytoplasmic secretory granules

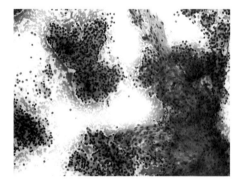
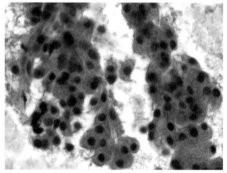
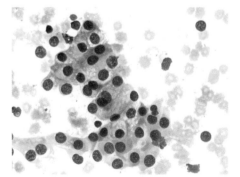
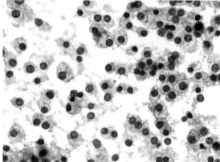

13-18A. Acinic cell carcinoma *(top, left).* Papillary groupings and irregular clusters of acinic cells with eccentric nuclei and abundant vacuolated cytoplasm. Note the lack of ductal epithelium (modified Giemsa stain)

13-18B. Acinic cell carcinoma *(top, right).* Acinar cells with granular cytoplasm (PAS stain)

13-18C. Acinic cell carcinoma *(bottom, left).* Intracytoplasmic metachromatic granules and vacuoles are seen (modified Giemsa stain)

13-18D. Acinic cell carcinoma *(bottom, right).* Cells have vacuolated cytoplasm and prominent nucleoli (rapid Papanicolaou stain)

Differential Diagnosis

- Sialadenosis
  - Less cellular smears
  - Polarization of nuclei
  - Ductal structures
- Warthin's tumor/Oncocytoma
  - Lymphocytosis
  - Dirty cystic background
- Metastatic renal cell carcinoma
  - Tumor cells have foamy to vacuolated cytoplasm with prominent nucleoli
  - Immunohistochemistry is positive for CD10 and RCC marker

PEARLS

★ Aspirates from acinic cell carcinoma can be bland and mimic normal salivary gland acinar tissue. The lack of ductal cells and fat should be a clue to the diagnosis

POLYMORPHOUS LOW-GRADE ADENOCARCINOMA

- Occurs almost exclusively in the minor salivary glands of the palate
- Peak incidence in the fifth to sixth decade with a female to male ratio of 2:1
- Encapsulated firm tumor invading surrounding soft tissue and bone
- Indolent course with local recurrences

Cytologic Features

- Polygonal/oval ductal cells arranged in pseudopapillary structures, sheets and clusters
- Purple magenta globules and tubules, reminiscent of those seen in adenoid cystic carcinoma
- Cuboidal tumor cells with fine chromatin, inconspicuous nucleoli, and minimal nuclear irregularities
- Eosinophilic stromal fragments
- Tyrosine crystals can be seen

Special Stains and Immunohistochemistry

- GFAP: negative or weakly positive
- Potential utility of c-kit and smooth muscle actin: weaker staining as compared to adenoid cystic carcinoma
- Positivity for cytokeratin, S-100 protein, vimentin, carcinoembryonic antigen, and epithelial membrane antigen

Modern Techniques for Diagnosis

- Noncontributory

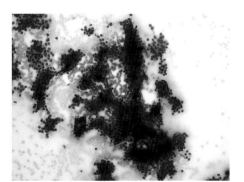
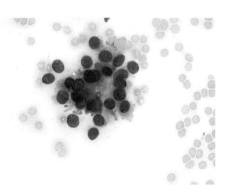

13-19A. Polymorphous low-grade adenocarcinoma *(left).* Bland basaloid cells arranged in clusters and pseudopapillary arrangements (modified Giemsa stain)

13-19B. Polymorphous low-grade adenocarcinoma *(right).* Tumor cells are cuboidal with fine chromatin and inconspicuous nucleoli (modified Giemsa stain)

Differential Diagnosis

- Papillary cystadenocarcinoma
  - ➤ Clusters of ovoid cells with stippled chromatin
  - ➤ Rare pseudopapillary configurations
  - ➤ Absence of hyaline globules
- Pleomorphic adenoma, cellular type
  - ➤ Plasmacytoid cells
  - ➤ More fibrillar chondromyxoid matrix with myoepithelial cells within the matrix
- Adenoid cystic carcinoma
  - ➤ Smaller ovoid angulated nuclei with higher nuclear to cytoplasmic ratios, necrosis, no pseudopapillary formations
- Epithelial myoepithelial carcinoma
  - ➤ Two cell populations: ductal cells with dark cytoplasm and myoepithelial cells with clear cytoplasm (Papanicolaou stain)
  - ➤ If composed of only myoepithelial cells, differentiation may be impossible

PEARLS

★ The cytologic findings of polymorphous low-grade adenocarcinoma overlaps with the more common tumors, including pleomorphic adenomas and adenoid cystic carcinoma and must be included in the differential diagnosis of a salivary gland neoplasm

EPITHELIAL-MYOEPITHELIAL CARCINOMA

Clinical Features

- Rare, indolent malignant biphasic neoplasm with tendency to recur
- Peak incidence in the sixth to seventh decade; slight female predominance
- Occurs most commonly in the parotid gland, followed by the submandibular gland
- Well-delineated mass, solid, and painful

Cytologic Features

- Appropriately diagnosed as malignant; however, often confused with adenocarcinoma NOS, low-grade epithelial malignancy, or adenoid cystic carcinoma
- Two cell populations: ductal epithelial cells and myoepithelial cells
- Pseudopapillary structures with eosinophilic cores covered by uniform cuboidal cells (ductal cells) with abundant fragile cytoplasm (rarely vacuolated) and irregular elongated nuclei, and peripheral basaloid cells with scant basophilic cytoplasm and uniform round bland nuclei (myoepithelial cells)
- Single cells and naked nuclei (myoepithelial cells) can also be noted
- Myoepithelial cells may have clear cytoplasm with mild nuclear atypia
- Hyaline stromal globules, stromal fragments, and mucoid substance can be seen

Special Stains and Immunohistochemistry

- Myoepithelial cells show positivity for S-100 protein, smooth muscle actin, and p63 and variable immunoreactivity for GFAP, myosin, vimentin, and cytokeratins
- Ductal cells show positivity for cytokeratin

Modern Techniques for Diagnosis

- Noncontributory

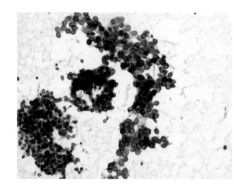

13-20. Epithelial-myoepithelial carcinoma. Pseudopapillary structures with small bland cells (myoepithelial cells) and larger epithelial cells with fragile cytoplasm (rapid Papanicolaou stain)

Differential Diagnosis
■ Adenoid cystic carcinoma
  ➤ Characteristic cylindrical and finger-like projections of magenta stroma
  ➤ Lacks clear cells
■ Polymorphous low-grade carcinoma
  ➤ Polyhedral uniform cells in clusters and singly
  ➤ Cells lack cytoplasmic vacuolation
  ➤ Absence of clear cells
■ Papillary cystadenocarcinoma
  ➤ Clusters of uniform ovoid cells with large cytoplasm and mottled chromatin
  ➤ Rare papillary structures are present

PEARLS

★ This uncommon neoplasm recurs in approximately 30% of cases and can spread to the regional lymph nodes and occasionally to distant sites

SQUAMOUS CELL CARCINOMA

Clinical Features
▦ Occurs in males more commonly than females
▦ Peak incidence in the sixth to seventh decade
▦ More often metastatic than primary
▦ When primary, develop from squamous metaplasia of the salivary gland ducts associated with sialolithiasis, or chronic sialadenitis, or history of radiation to head and neck
▦ Locally advanced disease
▦ Local failure rate is high (60%) and five-year survival is 30%

Cytologic Features
▦ Cellular smears
▦ Numerous dissociated keratinized malignant squamous cells
▦ Keratinaceous debris
▦ Sheets of malignant epidermoid cells
▦ Necrosis and inflammation
▦ If poorly differentiated, may resemble adenocarcinoma
▦ May exhibit some mucoid material if necrotic

Special Stains and Immunohistochemistry
▦ Noncontributory

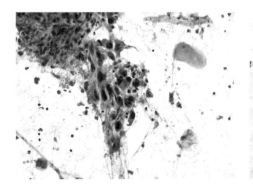
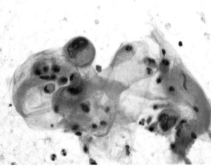

13-21A. Squamous cell carcinoma, primary *(left).* Cohesive sheets of malignant epithelial cells with hyperchromatin nuclei and squamoid cytoplasm in a cystic and necrotic background (Ultrafast Papanicolaou stain)

13-21B. Squamous cell carcinoma, primary *(right).* Atypical pseudohistiocytic cells and keratinized squamous cells in a background of inflammation (Papanicolaou stain)

Modern Techniques for Diagnosis
◼ Noncontributory

Differential Diagnosis
◼ Chronic and post irradiation sialadenitis
   ➤ Scant cellularity
   ➤ Cohesive clusters of atypical cells, sometimes bizarre
   ➤ No single dissociated keratinized malignant squamous cells
◼ Pleomorphic adenoma, Warthin's tumor, Kuttner's tumor, or adenoid cystic carcinoma
   ➤ Squamous cells that are benign or have mild atypia
◼ High-grade mucoepidermoid carcinoma
   ➤ May be impossible to differentiate from squamous cell carcinoma on aspiration biopsy
   ➤ Distinction is essential as course is much less aggressive
   ➤ Rarely mucinous background or mucin-producing cells
   ➤ Some intermediate cells
   ➤ PAS, mucicarmine, and Alcian blue stains are positive

PEARLS

★ Exclusion of a metastatic squamous cell carcinoma is critical as treatment differs

MALIGNANT MIXED TUMOR (CARCINOMA EXPLEOMORPHIC ADENOMA)

Clinical Features
◼ Malignant transformation occurs in less than 10% of pleomorphic adenomas
◼ Several types of carcinoma can arise from pleomorphic adenomas: Adenoid cystic carcinoma, salivary duct carcinoma, adenocarcinoma, NOS, mucoepidermoid carcinoma, squamous cell carcinoma, polymorphous low grade carcinoma, basal cell adenocarcinoma; poorly differentiated adenocarcinoma is the most common
◼ Most commonly involves the parotid gland
◼ Rare in young patients; predilection for women
◼ Arises in a patient with a history of long standing parotid mass or after multiple recurrences of pleomorphic adenoma
◼ Poorly circumscribed solid mass with infiltrating borders
◼ History of rapid growth
◼ Often associated with regional or distant metastases

13-22A. Carcinoma ex-pleomorphic adenoma *(left).* Clusters of large malignant pleomorphic epithelial cells with severe nuclear atypia and prominent nucleoli embedded in a fibrillary matrix (modified Giemsa stain)

13-22B. Carcinoma ex-pleomorphic adenoma *(right).* The tumor cells are pleomorphic with marked nuclear atypia and prominent nucleoli (modified Giemsa stain)

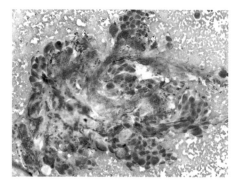
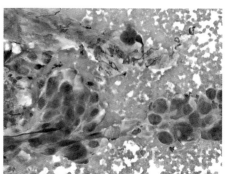

Cytologic Features
▢ According to tumor type
▢ Common features include three-dimensional clusters of malignant epithelial cells with marked nuclear atypia, high nuclear cytoplasmic ratio, and conspicuous nucleoli
▢ Dissociated keratinizing squamous cells and sheets of malignant epidermoid cells are seen in high-grade mucoepidermoid and squamous cell carcinoma
▢ Glandular or acinar structures
▢ Mitotic activity, mucoid background, and necrosis
▢ The presence of chondromyxoid stroma and plasmacytoid cells suggest association to pleomorphic adenoma

Special Stains and Immunohistochemistry
▢ Positivity for cytokeratin, epithelial membrane antigen, and carcinoembryonic antigen

Modern Techniques for Diagnosis
▢ Loss of heterozygosity at 8q and 12q

Differential Diagnosis
▢ Benign mixed tumor with atypia
  ➤ The atypia is mild and focal as opposed to the diffuse marked atypia seen in malignant mixed tumors
▢ Metastatic carcinoma
  ➤ Clinical context is different
  ➤ Lacks the characteristic matrix of a pleomorphic adenoma

PEARLS

★ The carcinomatous component in carcinoma ex-pleomorphic adenoma may be focal and thus FNA may be falsely negative

LYMPHOMA

Clinical Features
▢ Can be primary or secondary; nodal or extranodal
▢ Majority are B-cell non-Hodgkin's lymphoma
▢ MALT lymphoma and diffuse large B-cell lymphoma (DLBCL) affects predominantly the parotid gland; follicular center cell lymphomas (FCL) affects predominantly the submandibular gland
▢ MALT lymphomas arise in older MESA/LESA patients

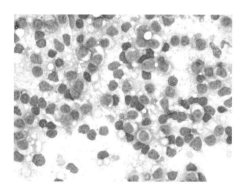 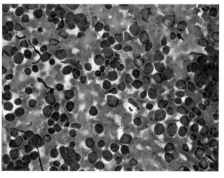

13-23A. Marginal zone lymphoma/malt *(left)*. Marginal zone lymphoma/MALT. Lymphoma mixed lymphoid population with conspicuous medium-sized, round lymphoid cells with clear cytoplasm (monocytoid B-cells) (modified Giemsa stain)

13-23B. Follicular lymphoma *(right)*. Follicular lymphoma of center cell origin (FCL). Mixed small and large lymphoid cells with irregular notched nuclei (modified Giemsa stain)

Cytologic Features
■ Depends on cell type
■ Mucosal-associated lymphoid tissue lymphoma
  ➤ Lymphoepithelial lesions
  ➤ Numerous pale monocytoid B cells with abundant clear cytoplasm
  ➤ Small lymphocytes and centrocytes
  ➤ Flow cytometric studies: CD20+, CD23 , CD10−, CD5− (variable), cyclin D1−
■ Follicular center cell lymphoma
  ➤ Mixed small and large lymphoid cells with notched grooved nuclei
  ➤ Flow cytometric studies: CD20+, CD45-, CD23- (variable), CD10+ (variable), CD5-, bcl-6+
  ➤ T(14:18) translocation by FISH
■ DLBCL
  ➤ Large malignant lymphoid cells with prominent nucleoli (immunoblasts and centroblasts) and marked atypia
  ➤ Flow cytometric studies: CD20+, CD45+

Special Stains and Immunohistochemistry
■ As above

Modern Techniques for Diagnosis
■ Flow cytometry is a useful adjunct

Differential Diagnosis
■ Intraparotid lymph node hyperplasia
  ➤ Mixed population of lymphoid cells
  ➤ Polyclonal population by flow cytometry
■ HIV- associated lymphadenopathy
  ➤ Mixed population of lymphoid cells with atypical lymphocytes and tingible body macrophages
  ➤ Flow cytometric analysis demonstrates a polyclonal population

PEARLS

★ Flow cytometry should be performed on any atypical lymphoid infiltrate on cytologic smears or in any high-risk patient (previous history of lymphoma, HIV positivity, history of lymphoepithelial lesions, persistent lymphadenopathy)

SECONDARY MALIGNANCIES

Clinical Features
■ Often affects the parotid gland parenchyma, and intraparotid or submandibular lymph nodes
■ The majority present with a solitary salivary gland metastasis
■ Knowledge of previous history is very helpful to reach a correct diagnosis
■ Interval between primary tumor diagnosis and metastasis to salivary gland varies between five months and several years
■ Most common tumors in decreasing frequency: Squamous cell carcinoma, melanoma, and carcinomas of the lung and breast
■ Uncommon tumors such as rhabdomyosarcoma and retinoblastoma have been reported
■ Prognosis is poor

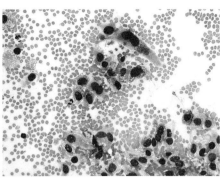

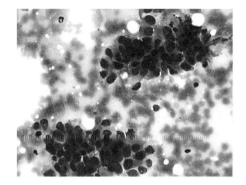

13-24. Squamous cell carcinoma, metastatic *(left).* Dissociated keratinized malignant squamous cells in a cystic background (Papanicolaou stain). Mixed small and large lymphoid cells with irregular notched nuclei (modified Giemsa stain)

13-25. Metastatic melanoma *(right).* Dissociated epithelioid and spindle cells with intracytoplasmic pigment and fine vacuoles (modified Giemsa stain)

13-26. Metastatic carcinoma of breast orign *(below).* Clusters of malignant plasmacytoid cells (modified Giemsa stain)

Cytologic Features

- Depends on site of origin
  - Squamous cell carcinoma

  Malignant-dissociated keratinized squamous cells

  Keratinaceous debris

  Necrotic and dirty background with acute inflammation
  - Melanoma

  Dissociated epithelioid and spindle cells

  Large occasionally binucleated nuclei with prominent nucleoli

  Intranuclear inclusions and intracytoplasmic melanin pigment
  - Metastatic carcinoma

  Tubules, papillae, and/or clusters of malignant epithelial cells with abundant cytoplasm and irregular, large, pleomorphic nuclei

Special Stains and Immunohistochemistry

- Mucin may be helpful in mucoepidermoid carcinoma
- Melanoma markers (HMB-45, MART-1, S-100 protein)
- Coordinate expression of CK7/20 and specific markers for breast (GCDFP15, ER), and lung (TTF-1)

Modern Techniques for Diagnosis

- Noncontributory

Differential Diagnosis

- Primary squamous cell carcinoma
  - No prior history of malignancy
- High-grade mucoepidermoid carcinoma
  - No prior history of malignancy
  - Glandular cells (mucin secreting cells)
  - Intermediate cells (smaller and basaloid)
  - Rare keratinaceous debris
- Large cell (undifferentiated) carcinoma
  - No prior history of malignancy
  - Poorly cohesive pleomorphic cells, epithelial and spindled
  - No squamous or glandular differentiation
  - Multinucleated tumor giant cells
  - Necrosis and mitotic figures are common

PEARLS

★ Pertinent clinical history and morphologic correlation with previous primary tumor are essential

REFERENCES

SIALADENOSIS (SIALOSIS, ASYMPTOMATIC PAROTID HYPERTROPHY)

Ascoli V, Albedi FM, De Blasiis R, Nardi F. Sialadenosis of the parotid gland: report of four cases diagnosed by fine-needle aspiration cytology. *Diagn Cytopathol* 1993;9:151–155.

Donath K, Seifert G. Ultrastructural studies of the parotid glands in sialadenosis. *Virchows Arch A Pathol Anat Histol* 1975;365:119–135.

Gupta S, Sodhani P. Sialadenosis of parotid gland: a cytomorphologic and morphometric study of four cases. *Anat Quant Cytol Histol* 1998;20:225–228.

Henry-Stanley MJ, Beneke J, Bardales RH, Stanley MW. Fine-needle aspiration of normal tissue from enlarged salivary glands: sialosis or missed target? *Diagn Cytopathol* 1995; 13:300–303.

Klijanienko J, Vielh P. Fine-needle sampling of salivary gland lesions V: Cytology of 22 cases of acinic cell carcinoma with histologic correlation. *Diagn Cytopathol* 1997;17:347–352.

Layfield LJ. Cytopathology of head and neck. *ASCP Theory and Practice of Cytopathology Series*, Chicago, IL, 1997.

Palma O, Torri AM, de Cristofaro JA, Fiaccavento S. Fine needle aspiration cytology in two cases of well-differentiated acinic-cell carcinoma of the parotid gland. Discussion of diagnostic criteria. *Acta Cytol* 1985;29:516–521.

SIALOLITHIASIS

Gupta PK, Fleisher SR, LiVolsi VA. Nontyrosine crystalloids in salivary gland lesions: report of seven cases with fine-needle aspiration cytology and follow-up pathology. *Diagn Cytopathol* 2000;22:167–171.

Stanley MW, Bardales RH, Beneke J, Korourian S, Stern SJ. Sialolithiasis. Differential diagnostic problems in fine-needle aspiration cytology. *Am J Clin Pathol* 1996;106:229–233.

Zajicek J, Eneroth CM, Jakobsson P. Aspiration biopsy of salivary gland tumors. VI. Morphologic studies on smears and histologic sections from mucoepidermoid carcinoma. *Acta Cytol* 1976;20:35–41.

ACUTE SIALADENITIS

Chiu CH, Lin TY. Clinical and microbiological analysis of six children with acute suppurative parotitis. *Acta Paediatr* 1996;85:106–108.

Johnson FB, Oertel YC, Ammann K. Sialadenitis with crystalloid formation: a report of six cases diagnosed by fine-needle aspiration. *Diagn Cytopathol* 1995;12:76–80.

Reyes CV, Jensen JD. Parotid abscess due to salmonella enteritidis: a case report. *Acta Cytol* 2006;50:677–679.

Wax TD, Layfield LJ, Zaleski S, Bhargara V, Cohen M, Lyerly HK, Fisher SR. Cytomegalo-virus sialadenitis in patients with the acquired immunodeficiency syndrome: a potential diagnostic pitfall with fine-needle aspiration cytology. *Diagn Cytopathol* 1994;10: 169–172.

CHRONIC SCLEROSING SIALADENITIS (KUTTNER'S TUMOR, SIALOLITHIASIS OF THE SUBMANDIBULAR SALIVARY GLAND)

Cheuk W, Chan JK. Kuttner tumor of the submandibular gland: fine-needle aspiration cytologic findings of seven cases. *Am J Clin Pathol* 2002; 117:103–108.

Kaba S, Kojima M, Matsuda H, Sugihara S, Masawa N, Kobayashi TK, Fukuda T. Kuttner's tumor of the submandibular glands: report of five cases with fine-needle aspiration cytology. *Diagn Cytopathol* 2006;34:631–635.

Kojima M, Nakamura S, Itoh H, Yamane Y, Shimizu K, Masawa N. Kuttner's tumor of salivary glands resembling marginal zone B-cell lymphoma of the MALT type: a histopathologic and immunohistochemical study of 7 cases. *Int J Surg Pathol* 2004;12:389–393.

Kojima M, Nakamura S, Itoh H, Yamane Y, Tanaka H. Sclerosing variant of follicular lymphoma arising from submandibular glands and resembling "Kuttner tumor": a report of 3 patients. *Int J Surg Pathol* 2003 11:303–307.

GRANULOMATOUS SIALADENITIS

Abendroth CS, Frauenhoffer EE. Nodular fasciitis of the parotid gland. Report of a case with presentation in an unusual location and cytologic differential diagnosis. *Acta Cytol* 1995;39:530–534.

Aggarwal AP, Jayaram G, Mandal AK. Sarcoidosis diagnosed on fine-needle aspiration cytology of salivary glands: a report of three cases. *Diagn Cytopathol* 1989;5:289–292.

Chhieng DC, Cohen JM, Cangiarella JF. Fine-needle aspiration of spindle cell and mesenchymal lesions of the salivary glands. *Diagn Cytopathol* 2000;23:253–259.

Frable MA, Frable WJ. Fine-needle aspiration biopsy: efficacy in the diagnosis of head and neck sarcoidosis. *Laryngoscope* 1984;94:1281–1283.

Hughes JH, Volk EE, Wilbur DC. Cytopathology Resource Committee, College of American Pathologists. Pitfalls in salivary gland fine-needle aspiration cytology: lessons from the College of American Pathologists Interlaboratory Comparison Program in Nongynecologic Cytology. *Arch Path Lab Med* 2005;129:26–31.

Mair S, Leiman G, Levinsohn D. Fine needle aspiration cytology of parotid sarcoidosis. *Acta Cytol* 1989;33:169–172.

Perez-Guillermo M, Perez JS, Parr FJE. Asteroid bodies and calcium oxalate crystals: two infrequent findings in fine-needle aspirates of parotid sarcoidosis. *Diagn Cytopathol* 1992;8: 248–252.

Saad RS, Takei H, Lipscomb J, Ruiz B. Nodular fasciitis of parotid region: a pitfall in the diagnosis of pleomorphic adenomas on fine-needle aspiration cytology. *Diagn Cytopathol* 2005;33: 191–194.

BENIGN LYMPHOEPITHELIAL CYST (CYSTIC BLL)

Benharrats I, Jacob L, Taulera O. Parotitis due to mycobacterium and HIV infection. *Rev Med Intern* 1998;19:676–677.

Chhieng DC, Argosino R, McKenna BJ, Cangiarella JF, Cohen JM. Utility of fine-needle aspiration in the diagnosis of salivary gland lesions in patients infected with human immunodeficiency virus. *Diagn Cytopathol* 1999, 21:260–264.

Finfer MD, Gallo L, Perchick A, Schinella RA, Burstein DE. Fine needle aspiration biopsy of cystic benign lymphoepithelial lesion of the parotid gland in patients at risk for the acquired immune deficiency syndrome. *Acta Cytol* 1990;34:821–826.

Weidner N, Geisinger KR, Sterling RT, Miller TR, Yen TS. Benign lymphoepithelial cysts of the parotid gland. A histologic, cytologic, and ultrastructural study. *Am J Clin Pathol* 1986;85: 395–401.

SJÖGREN'S DISEASE/BENIGN LYMPHOEPITHELIAL LESIONS (BLL)/MYOEPITHELIAL SIALADENITIS (MESA)/LYMPHOEPITHELIAL SIALADENITIS (LESA)

Brauneis J, Schroder M, Laskawi R, Droese M. The significance and limits of cytologic diagnosis in myoepithelial sialadenitis. *Laryngorhinootologie* 1989;68:209–211.

Chai C, Dodd LG, Glasgow BJ, Layfield LJ. Salivary gland lesions with a prominent lymphoid component: cytologic findings and differential diagnosis by fine-needle aspiration biopsy. *Diagn Cytopathol* 1997;17:183–190.

Fox RI. Sjogren's syndrome. *Lancet* 2005;366:321–331.

Ruschenburg I, Kneitz S, Brinck U, Korabiowska M, Harms H, Droese M. Myoepithelial sialadenitis versus low-grade non-Hodgkin's lymphoma of the salivary gland in FNAB: is discrimination by means of an image processing system possible? *In Vivo* 1999;13: 515–518.

BENIGN INTRAPAROTID LYMPH NODE

Allen EA, Syed ZA, Mathew S. Lymphoid lesions of the parotid. *Diagn Cytopathol* 1999;21: 170–173.

Chhieng DC, Cangiarella JF, Cohen JM. Fine-needle aspiration cytology of lymphoproliferative lesions involving the major salivary glands. *Am J Clin Pathol* 2000; 113:563–571.

Layfield LJ, Gopez E, Hirschowitz S. Cost efficiency analysis for fine-needle aspiration in the workup of parotid and submandibular gland nodules. *Diagn Cytopathol* 2006;34: 734–738.

MUCOCELE

Carson HJ, Raslan WF, Castelli MJ, Gattuso P. Tyrosine crystals in benign parotid gland cysts: report of two cases diagnosed by fine-needle aspiration biopsy with ultrastructural and histochemical evaluation. *Am J Clin Pathol* 1994; 102:699–702.

Oliveira DT, Consolaro A, Freitas FJ. Histopathological spectrum of 112 cases of mucocele. *Braz Dent J* 1993; 4:29–36.

Seifert G, Donath K, von Gumberz C. Mucoceles of the minor salivary glands. Extravasation mucoceles (mucus granulomas) and retention mucoceles (mucus retention cysts). *HNO* 1981; 29:179–191.

BENIGN MIXED TUMOR (BMT)/ PLEOMORPHIC ADENOMA (PA)

Eneroth CM, Zajicek J. Aspiration biopsy of salivary gland tumors: III. Morphologic studies on smears and histologic sections from 368 mixed tumors. *Acta Cytol* 1966;10: 440–454.

Klijanienko J, Vielh P. Fine-needle sampling of salivary gland lesions. I. Cytology and histology correlation of 412 cases of pleomorphic adenoma. *Diagn Cytopathol* 1996;14: 195–200.

Lee SS, Cho KJ, Jang JJ, Ham EK. Differential diagnosis of adenoid cystic carcinoma from pleomorphic adenoma of the salivary gland on fine needle aspiration cytology. *Acta Cytol* 1996; 40:1246–1252.

Nagel H, Hotze HJ, Laskawi R, Chilla R, Droese M. Cytologic diagnosis of adenoid cystic carcinoma of salivary glands. *Diagn Cytopathol* 1999;20:358–366.

Stanley MW, Horwitz CA, Rollins SD, Powers CN, Bardales RH, Korourain S, Stern SJ. Basal cell (monomorphic) and minimally pleomorphic adenomas of the salivary glands. Distinction from the solid (anaplastic) type of adenoid cystic carcinoma in fine-needle aspiration. *Am J Clin Pathol* 1996;106:35–41.

Stanley MW, Lowhagen T. Mucin production by pleomorphic adenomas of the parotid gland: a cytologic spectrum. *Diagn Cytopathol* 1990;6:49–52.

Swanson PE, Pettinato G, Lillemoe TJ, Wick MR. Gross cystic disease fluid protein-15 in salivary gland tumors. *Arch Pathol Lab Med* 1991;115:158–163.

Viguer JM, Vicandi B, Jimenez-Heffernan JA, Lopez-Ferrer P, Limeres MA. Fine needle aspiration cytology of pleomorphic adenoma. An analysis of 212 cases. *Acta Cytol* 1997;41: 786–794.

Yang GC, Waisman J. Distinguishing adenoid cystic carcinoma from cylindromatous adenomas in salivary fine-needle aspirates: the cytologic clues and their ultrastructural basis. *Diagn Cytopathol* 2006; 34:284–288.

BASAL CELL ADENOMA (TUBULAR, TRABECULAR, BASALOID, MONOMORPHIC)

Chhieng DC, Paulino A. Basaloid tumors of the salivary glands. *Ann Diagn Pathol* 2002;6: 363–372.

Hood IC, Qizilbash AH, Salama SS, Alexopoulou I. Basal cell adenoma of parotid. Difficulty of differentiation from adenoid cystic carcinoma on aspiration biopsy. *Acta Cytol* 1983;27: 515–520.

Klijanienko J, El-Naggar AK, Vielh P. Comparative cytologic and histologic study of fifteen basal cell tumors: differential diagnostic considerations. *Diagn Cytopathol* 1999;21: 30–34.

Stanley MW, Horwitz CA, Henry MJ, Burton LG, Lowhagen T. Basal cell adenoma of the salivary gland: a benign adenoma that cytologically mimics adenoid cystic carcinoma. *Diagn Cytopathol* 1988;4:342–346.

MYOEPITHELIOMA

Chhieng DC, Paulino A. Cytology of myoepithelial carcinoma of the salivary gland. A study of 4 cases. *Cancer Cytopathol* 2002;96:32–36.

Darvishian F, Lin O. Myoepithelial cell-rich neoplasms. Cytologic features of benign and malignant lesions. *Cancer Cytopathol* 2004;102:355–61.

Das DK, Haji BE, Ahmed MS, Hossain MN. Myoepithelioma of the parotid gland initially diagnosed by fine needle aspiration cytology and immunocytochemistry: a case report. *Acta Cytol* 2005;49:65–70.

DiPalma S, Alasio L, Pilotti S. Fine needle aspiration (FNA) appearances of malignant myoepithelioma of the parotid gland. *Cytopathology* 1996;7:357–365.

Dodd LG, Caraway NP, Luna MA, Byers RM. Myoepithelioma of the parotid. Report of a case initially examined by fine needle aspiration biopsy. *Acta Cytol* 1994;38: 417–421.

Kumar PV, Sobhani SA, Monabati A, Hashemi SB, Eghtadari F, Hamidi SA. Myoepithelioma of the salivary glands, fine-needle aspiration findings. *Acta Cytol* 2004;48:302–308.

Miliauskas JR, Orell SV. Fine-needle aspiration cytological findings in five cases of epithelial myoepithelial carcinoma of salivary glands. *Diagn Cytopathol* 2003;28:163–167.

Ramdall RB, Cai G, Levine P, Bhanote M, Garcia R, Cangiarella J. Fine-needle aspiration biopsy findings in epithelioid myoepithelioma of the parotid gland: a case report. *Diagn Cytopathol* 2006;34:776–779.

ONCOCYTOMA

Eneroth CM, Zajicek J. Aspiration biopsy of salivary gland tumors II. Morphologic studies on smears and histologic sections from oncocytic tumors (45 cases of papillary cystadenoma lymphomatosum and 4 cases of oncocytoma). *Acta Cytol* 1965;9:355–361.

Layfield LJ. Cytopathology of head and neck, *ASCP Theory and Practice of Cytopathology Series*, Chicago, IL, 1997.

WARTHIN'S TUMOR (PAPILLARY CYSTADENOMA LYMPHOMATOSUM)

Ballo MS, Shin HJC, Sneige N. Sources of diagnostic error in fine-needle aspiration diagnosis of Warthin's tumor and clues to a correct diagnosis. *Diagn Cytopathol* 1997;17: 230–234.

Klijanicnko J, Vielh P. Fine-needle sampling of salivary gland lesions II. Cytology and histology correlation of 71 cases of Warthin's tumor. *Diagn Cytopathol* 1997;16:221–225.

Laucirica R, Farnum JB, Leopold SK, Kalin GB, Youngberg GA. False-positive diagnosis in fine-needle aspiration of an atypical Warthin's tumor: histochemical differential stains for cyto-diagnosis. *Diagn Cytopathol* 1989;5:412–415.

Mandel L-Tomkoria A. Differentiating HIV-1 parotid cysts from papillary cystadenoma lympho-matosum. *J Am Dent Assoc* 2000;131:772–776.

Verma K, Kapila K. Salivary gland tumors with a prominent oncocytic component. Cytologic findings and differential diagnosis of oncocytomas and Warthin's tumor on fine needle aspi-rates. *Acta Cytol* 2003;47:221–226.

MUCOEPIDERMOID CARCINOMA

Cohen MB, Fisher PE, Holly EA, Ljung BM, Lowhagen T, Bottles K. Fine-needle aspira-tion biopsy of mucoepidermoid carcinoma. Statistical analysis. *Acta Cytol* 1990:34: 43–49.

Goode RK, Auclair PL, Ellis GL. Mucoepidermoid carcinoma of the major salivary glands. Clinical and histopathologic analysis of 234 cases with evaluation of grading criteria. *Cancer* 1998;82:1217–1224.

Klijanienko J, Vielh P. Fine-needle sampling of salivary gland lesions IV. Review of 50 cases of mucoepidermoid carcinoma with histologic correlation. *Diagn Cytopathol* 1997;17: 92–98.

Zajicek J, Eneroth CM, Jakobsson P. Aspiration biopsy of salivary gland tumors VI. Morphologic studies on smears and histologic sections from mucoepidermoid carcinoma. *Acta Cytol* 1976;20:35–41.

ADENOID CYSTIC CARCINOMA

Eneroth CM, Zajicek J. Aspiration biopsy of salivary gland tumors IV. Morphologic studies on smears and histologic sections from 45 cases of adenoid cystic carcinoma. *Acta Cytol* 1969;19:59–63.

Klijanienko J, Vielh P. Fine-needle aspiration sampling of salivary gland lesions III. Cytologic and histologic correlations of 75 cases of adenoid cystic carcinoma: review and experience at the Institut Curie with emphasis on cytologic pitfalls. *Diagn Cytopathol* 1997;17:36–41.

Layfield LJ, Glasgow BJ. Diagnosis of salivary gland tumors by fine-needle aspiration cytology: a review of clinical utility and pitfalls. *Diagn Cytopathol* 1991;7:267–272.

Layfield LJ, Tan P, Glasgow BJ. Fine-needle aspiration of salivary gland lesions. Comparison with frozen sections and histologic findings. *Arch Pathol Lab Med* 1987;111:346–353.

Lee SS, Cho KJ, Jang JJ, Ham EK. Differential diagnosis of adenoid cystic carcinoma from pleo-morphic adenoma of the salivary gland on fine needle aspiration cytology. *Acta Cytol* 1996;40:1246–1252.

Nagel H, Hotze HJ, Laskawi R, Chilla R, Droese M. Cytologic diagnosis of adenoid cystic carci-noma of salivary glands. *Diagn Cytopathol* 1999;20:358–366.

Stallmach I, Zenklusen P, Komminoth P, Schmid S, Perren A, Roos M, Jianming Z, Heutz PU, Pfaltz M. Loss of heterozygosity at chromosome 6q23-35 correlates with clinical and histologic parameters in salivary gland adenoid cystic carcinoma. *Virchows Archiv* 2002;440:77–84.

Stanley MW, Horwitz CA, Rollins SD, Powers CN, Bardales RH, Korourain S, Stern SJ. Basal cell (monomorphic) and minimally pleomorphic adenomas of the salivary glands. Distinction from the solid (anaplastic) type of adenoid cystic carcinoma in fine-needle aspiration. *Am J Clin Pathol* 1996;106:35–41.

Yang GC, Waisman J. Distinguishing adenoid cystic carcinoma from cylindromatous adenomas in salivary fine-needle aspirates: the cytologic clues and their ultrastructural basis. *Diagn Cytopathol* 2006;34:284–288.

ACINIC CELL CARCINOMA

Klijanienko J, Vielh P. Fine-needle sampling of salivary gland lesions V. Cytology of 22 cases of acinic cell carcinoma with histologic correlation. *Diagn Cytopathol* 1997;17: 347–352.

Nagel H, Laskawi R, Buter JJ, Schroder M, Chilla R, Droesse M. Cytologic diagnosis of acinic cell carcinoma of salivary glands. *Diagn Cytopathol* 1997;16: 402–412.

Palma O, Torri AM, de Cristofaro JA, Fiaccavento S. Fine-needle aspiration of two cases of well differentiated acinic cell carcinoma of the parotid gland. Discussion of diagnostic criteria. *Acta Cytol* 1985;29:516–521.

Takahashi H, Fujita S, Okabe H, Tsuda N, Tezuka F. Distribution of tissue markers in acinic cell carcinomas of salivary gland. *Pathol Res Pract* 1992;188:692–700.

POLYMORPHOUS LOW-GRADE ADENOCARCINOMA

Beltran D, Faquin WC, Gallagher G, August M. Selective immunohistochemical comparison of polymorphous low-grade adenocarcinoma and adenoid cystic carcinoma. *J Oral Maxillofac Surg* 2006;64:415–423.

Frierson HF, Covell JL, Mills SE. Fine-needle aspiration cytology of terminal duct carcinoma of minor salivary gland. *Diagn Cytopathol* 1987;3:159–162.

Gibbons D, Saboorian MH, Vuitch F, Gokaslan ST, Ashfaq R. Fine-needle aspiration findings in patients with polymorphous low grade adenocarcinoma of the salivary glands. *Cancer (Cytopathol)* 1999;87:31–36.

Klijanienko J, Viehl P. Salivary carcinomas with papillae: cytology and histology analysis of polymorphous low-grade adenocarcinoma and papillary cystadenocarcinoma. *Diagn Cytopathol* 1998;19:244–249.

EPITHELIAL-MYOEPITHELIAL CARCINOMA

Carillo R, Poblet E, Rocanora E, Rodriguez-Peralto JL. Epithelial myoepithelial cell carcinoma of the salivary glands: Fine-needle aspiration cytologic findings. *Acta Cytol* 1990;34: 243–247.

Kawahara A, Harada H, Yokoyama T, Kage M. p63 expression of clear myoepithelial cells in epithelial-myoepithelial carcinoma of the salivary gland: a useful marker for naked myoepithelial cells in cytology. *Cancer* 2005;105:240–245.

Klijanienko J, Vielh P. Fine needle sampling of salivary gland lesions VII. Cytology and histology correlation of 5 cases of epithelial myopeithelial carcinoma. *Diagn Cytopathol* 1998;19: 405–409.

Kocjan G, Milroy C, Fisher EW, Eveson JW. Cytologic features of Epithelial myoepithelial cell carcinoma of the salivary gland: potential pitfalls in diagnosis. *Cytopathology* 1993;4: 173–180.

Miliauskas JR, Orell SR. Fine-needle aspiration cytologic findings in 5 cases of epithelial myoepithelial carcinoma of salivary glands. *Diagn Cytopathol* 2003;28:163–167.

Wax T, Layfield LJ. Epithelial myoepithelial cell carcinoma of the parotid gland. A case report and comparison of cytologic features with other stromal, epithelial, and myoepithelial cell containing lesions of the salivary glands. *Diagn Cytopathol* 1996;14: 298–304.

SQUAMOUS CELL CARCINOMA

Bonneau H, Sommer D. L'orientation du diagnostic des tumeurs salivaires par la ponction a l'aiguille fine. *Pathol Biol* 1959; 7: 785–791.

Klijanienko J, Vielh P. Fine needle sampling of salivary gland lesions VI. Cytologic review of 44 cases of primary salivary squamous cell carcinoma with histological correlation. *Diagn Cytopathol* 1998;18:174–178.

Lee S, Kim GE, Park CS, Choi EC, Yang WI, Lee CG, Keum KC, Kim YB, Suh CO. Primary squamous cell carcinoma of the parotid gland. *Am J Otolaryngol* 2001;22:400–406.

MALIGNANT MIXED TUMOR (CARCINOMA EXPLEOMORPHIC ADENOMA)

El-Naggar AK, Callender D, Coombes MM, Hurr K, Luna MA, Batsakis JG. Molecular genetic alterations in carcinoma ex-pleomorphic adenoma: a putative progression model? *Genes Chromosomes Cancer* 2000;27:162–168.

Eneroth CM, Franzen S, Zajicek J. Cytologic diagnosis on aspirate from 1000 salivary gland tumours. *Acta Otolaryngol* 1967; 24:168–171.

Klijanienko J, El-Naggar AK, Vielh P. Fine-needle sampling findings in 26 carcinoma ex pleomorphic adenomas: diagnostic pitfalls and clinical considerations. *Diagn Cytopathol* 1999;21: 163–166.

Klitz B, Pitman MB. Carcinoma ex-pleomorphic adenoma of the parotid gland: pitfalls in fine-needle aspiration biopsy diagnosis. *Acta Cytol* 1994;38:855(abstract).

Layfield LJ, Glasgow BJ. Diagnosis of salivary gland tumors by fine-needle aspiration cytology: a review of clinical utility and pitfalls. *Diagn Cytopathol* 1991;7:267–272.

Orell SR. Diagnostic difficulties in the interpretation of fine needle aspirates of salivary gland lesions: the problem revisited. *Cytopathology* 1995;6:285–300.

Stanley MW, Bardales RH, Farmer CE, Frierson HF, Surhland M, Powers CN, Rollins SD. Primary and metastatic high grade carcinomas of the salivary glands. A cytologic-histologic correlation study of 20 cases. *Diagn Cytopathol* 1995;13:37–43.

LYMPHOMA

Brauneis J, Schroder M, Laskawi R, Droese M. The significance and limits of cytologic diagnosis in myoepithelial sialadenitis. *Laryngorhinootologie* 1989;68:209–211.

Chai C, Dodd LG, Glasgow BJ, Layfield LJ. Salivary gland lesions with a prominent lymphoid component: cytologic findings and differential diagnosis by fine-needle aspiration biopsy. *Diagn Cytopathol* 1997;17:183–190.

Kojima M, Nakamura S, Ichimura K, Shimizu K, Itoh H, Masawa N. Follicular lymphoma of the salivary gland: a clinicopathological and molecular study of six cases. *Int J Surg Pathol* 2001;9:287–293.

Kojima M, Nakamura S, Itoh H, Yamane Y, Shimizu K, Masawa N. Kuttner's tumor of salivary glands resembling marginal zone B-cell lymphoma of the MALT type: a histopathologic and immunohistochemical study of 7 cases. *Int J Surg Pathol* 2004;12:389–393.

Kojima M, Nakamura S, Itoh H, Yamane Y, Tanaka H. Sclerosing variant of follicular lymphoma arising from submandibular glands and resembling "Kuttner tumor": a report of 3 patients. *Int J Surg Pathol* 2003 11:303–307.

Nakamura S, Ichimura K, Sato Y, Nakamura S, Nakamine H, Inagaki H, Sadahira Y, Ohshima K, Sakugawa S, Kondo E, Yanai H, Ohara N, Yoshino T. Follicular lymphoma frequently originates in the salivary gland. *Pathol Int* 2006;56:576–583.

Ochoa ER, Harris NL, Pilch BZ. Marginal zone B-cell lymphoma of the salivary gland arising in chronic sclerosing sialadenitis (Kuttner's tumor). *Am J Surg Pathol* 2001; 25: 1546–1550.

Ruschenburg I, Kneitz S, Brinck U, Korabiowska M, Harms H, Droese M. Myoepithelial sialadenitis versus low-grade non-Hodgkin's lymphoma of the salivary gland in FNAB: is discrimination by means of an image processing system possible? *In Vivo* 1999;13: 515–518.

Wolvius EB, van der Valk P, van der Wal JE, van Diest PJ, Huijgens PC, van der Waal I, Snow GB. Primary non-Hodgkin's lymphoma of the salivary glands. An analysis of 22 cases. *J Oral Pathol Med* 1996;25:177–181.

SECONDARY MALIGNANCIES

Lussier C, Klijanienko J, Vielh P. Fine-needle aspiration of metastatic nonlymphomatous tumors to the major salivary glands. A clinicopathologic study of 40 cases cytologically diagnosed and histologically correlated. *Cancer (Cytopathol)* 2000;90:350–356.

Moore JG, Bocklage T. Fine-needle aspiration biopsy of large-cell undifferentiated carcinoma of the salivary glands: presentation of two cases, literature review, and differential cytodiagnosis of high-grade salivary gland malignancies. *Diagn Cytopathol* 1998;19: 44–50.

Stanley MW, Bardales RH, Farmer CE, Friersin HF Jr, Suhrland M, Powers CN, Rollins SD. Primary and metastatic high-grade carcinomas of the salivary glands: a cytologic-histologic correlation study of twenty cases. *Diagn Cytopathol* 1995;13:37–43.

Zhang C, Cohen JM, Cangiarella JF, Waisman J, McKenna BJ, Chhineg DC. Fine-needle aspiration of secondary neoplasms involving the salivary glands. A report of 36 cases. *Am J Clin Pathol* 2000;113:21–28.

14

Lung, Pleura, and Mediastinum

Jing Zhai

LUNG

ABSCESS

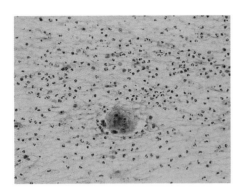

14-1. Abscess. Abundant neutrophils, necrotic debris, scattered histiocytes and rare multinucleated giant cell (Papanicalaou stain)

Clinical Features
▦ Common in immunocompromised, alcoholic, and diabetic patients
▦ Location: right lower lobe
▦ Main cause: aspiration
▦ Other causes: airway obstruction by malignancy, primary bacterial infection, and infected thromboemboli
▦ Most common microorganisms: aerobic and anaerobic bacteria
▦ Clinical symptom: Fever, cough, and purulent sputum

Cytologic Features
▦ Purulent aspirate material
▦ Abundant neutrophils
▦ Abundant amorphous necrotic debris
▦ Macrophages and lymphoid cells may be seen
▦ Microorganisms, such as bacteria and fungi, may be seen
▦ Vegetable material is associated with aspiration

Special Stains and Immunohistochemistry
▦ Culture for bacteria and fungi
▦ Gram stain for bacteria
▦ GMS stain for fungi

Modern Techniques for Diagnosis
▦ Noncontributory

Differential Diagnosis
■ Cavitating carcinoma
➤ Most are squamous cell carcinoma
➤ Abundant necrotic debris
➤ Abundant degenerated cells
➤ Scattered malignant cells with orangeophilic cytoplasm and pyknotic nuclei
■ Caseating granuloma
➤ Granular amorphous necrotic debris
➤ Granuloma: Cohesive clusters of epithelioid histiocytes
➤ Scattered multinucleated giant cells
➤ Microorganisms: Mycobacteria and fungi
■ Wegener's granulomatosis
➤ Necrotic debris
➤ Mixed neutrophils and lymphocytes
➤ Granuloma: Clusters of epithelioid histiocytes
➤ C-ANCA: Positive

PEARLS
★ Immunocompromised patients
★ Location: Right lower lobe
★ Most common microorganisms: Aerobic and anaerobic bacteria
★ Abundant neutrophils and necrotic debris
★ Culture for definitive microorganism identification

GRANULOMATOUS INFLAMMATION

Clinical Features
- Common in immunocompromised patients
- Common microorganisms: Fungi and mycobacteria
- Clinical symptom: Fever, cough, and night sweat

Cytologic Features
- Granuloma: Cohesive clusters of epithelioid histiocytes
- Epithelioid histiocyte: Elongated twisted bland nuclei, small distinct nucleoli, and abundant pale cytoplasm with indistinct border
- Scattered multinucleated giant cells
- Granular amorphous necrotic debris
- Small mature lymphocytes and neutrophils
- Fungal microorganisms may be seen
  - Aspergillus: Regular septate hyphae and 45 degree angle branching
  - Mucor: Irregular ribbon-like broad nonseptate hyphae, and wide-angle branching
  - Cryptococcus: Narrow-based unequal budding yeast with capsule (highlighted by mucin stain) (5–10 μm)
  - Blastomyces: Broad-based budding yeast with thick double-contoured wall (8–20 μm)
  - Histoplasma: Intracellular small budding yeast (1–5 μm)

Special Stains and Immunohistochemistry
- Culture for fungi and mycobacteria
- AFB and Fite stains for mycobacteria and atypical mycobacteria
- GMS stain for fungi

Modern Techniques for Diagnosis
- PCR for mycobacteria diagnosis and drug-resistant strain identification

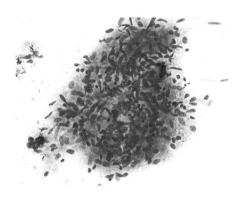
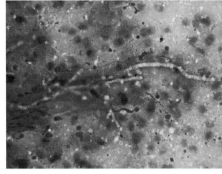
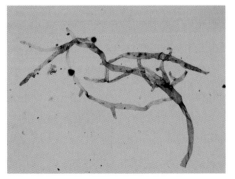
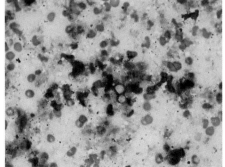

14-2A. Granuloma *(top, left)*. A cohesive cluster of epithelioid histiocytes with intermixed lymphocytes. The epithelioid histiocytes have elongated twisted bland nuclei that resemble footprints, small distinct nucleoli, and abundant pale cytoplasm with indistinct border (modified Giemsa stain)

14-2B. Aspergillus *(top, right)*. Septate hyphae and 45 degree angle branching (modified Giemsa stain)

14-2C. Mucor *(bottom, left)*. Broad nonseptate hyphae and wide-angle branching (GMS stain)

14-2D. Blastomyces *(bottom, right)*. Broad-based budding yeast with thick double-contoured wall (modified Giemsa stain)

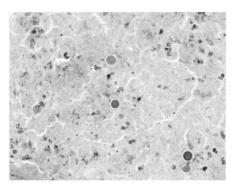
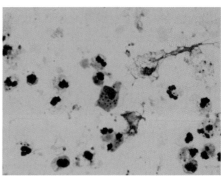

14-2E. Cryptococcus *(left)*. Yeast forms with mucin positive capsule (mucin stain)

14-2F. Histoplasma *(right)*. Intracellular yeast forms (modified Giemsa stain)

14-2G. Histoplasma *(below)*. Small unequal budding yeasts (GMS stain)

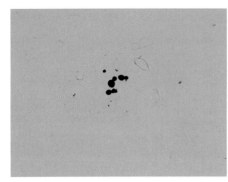

Differential Diagnosis

- Sarcoidosis
  - Granuloma
  - Langerhan's multinucleated giant cells
  - No necrosis
  - A diagnosis of exclusion
- Cavitating carcinoma
  - Most are keratinizing squamous cell carcinoma
  - Scattered malignant cells with orangeophilic cytoplasm and pyknotic nuclei
  - Abundant degenerated squamous cells
  - Foreign body–type multinucleated giant cells
  - Abundant necrotic debris
- Wegener's granulomatosis
  - Granuloma
  - Necrotic debris
  - Mixed neutrophils and lymphocytes
  - C-ANCA: positive

PEARLS

- Immunocompromised patients
- Granuloma: cohesive clusters of epithelioid histiocytes
- Necrotic debris
- Culture for definitive microorganism identification

HAMARTOMA

Clinical Features

- The most common benign lung neoplasm
- An incidental finding on routine chest radiograph
- Peripherally located coin lesion
- Small (<4 cm), round and oval shape with sharp border

Cytologic Features

- Immature fibromyxoid matrix with fibrillary appearance
- Embedded bland fibroblastic spindle cells
- Mature cartilage
- Sheets of bland bronchial epithelial cells
- Mature adipocytes

Special Stains and Immunohistochemistry

- S-100: Positive in the spindle cells

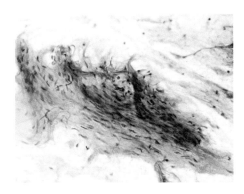 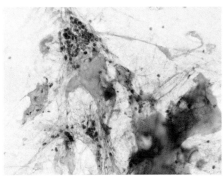

14-3A. Hamartoma *(left).* Fibrillary fibromyxoid stroma with embedded bland spindle cells (Papanicalaou stain)

14-3B. Hamartoma *(right).* Mature cartilage and sheets of bland bronchial epithelial cells (Papanicalaou stain)

Modern Techniques for Diagnosis
- Activation of HMGI(Y) gene on chromosome 6p21 by gene rearrangement

Differential Diagnosis
- Pleomorphic adenoma of bronchial salivary gland tissue
  - Fibromyxoid stroma with embedded myoepithelial cells
  - Isolated bland myoepithelial cells
  - Myoepithelial cells: epithelioid, plasmacytoid, and spindle shaped
  - Sheets of bland epithelial cells
- Pulmonary blastoma
  - Columnar epithelial cells with abundant glycogen-rich cytoplasm
  - Mesenchymal cells with spindle to oval nuclei
  - Myxoid stroma
- Chest wall "contaminant"
  - Accidentally sampled cartilage
  - Accidentally sampled fibrous tissue with stroma and bland spindle cells
  - Accidentally sampled mature fat

PEARLS
- Characteristic radiograph image: Peripherally located coin lesion
- Fibromyxoid matrix with embedded bland spindle cells
- Mature cartilage
- Bland bronchial epithelial cells

CARCINOID

Clinical Features
- Affect patients in their forties with equal sex distribution
- 20% to 40% patients are nonsmokers
- A small (<4 cm) and centrally located endobronchial lesion
- An incidental finding on radiograph
- Rarely associated with multiple endocrine neoplasia type (MEN) I
- Most are nonfunctional lesions
- Clinical symptom: Cough and hemoptysis

Cytologic Features
- Loosely cohesive clusters and singly dispersed cells
- Monotonous small to intermediate cells
- Round, plasmacytoid, or spindle shaped cells
- Fine granular salt-and-pepper chromatin

14-4A. Carcinoid *(left)*. Singly dispersed and loose clusters of monotonous round and plasmacytoid cells with salt-and pepper chromatin, small nucleoli, binucleation and moderate amount granular cytoplasm (Papanicalaou stain)

14-4B. Carcinoid *(right)*. A loose cluster of uniform, round to spindle-shaped cells (modified Giemsa stain)

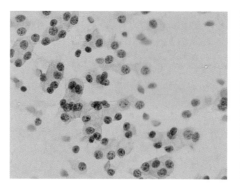
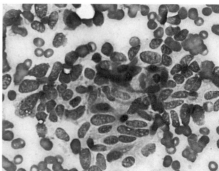

- Small distinct nucleoli
- Moderate amount of granular cytoplasm
- Atypical carcinoid
  - Necrosis
  - Mitosis
  - Nuclear pleomorphism

Special Stains and Immunohistochemistry
- Neuroendocrine markers (chromogranin, synaptophysin, CD56, and CD57): Positive
- Thyroid transcription factor 1 (TTF-1): Positive (~70%)
- CD99: Positive in 50% of typical carcinoid
- K-i67: Low-level staining in atypical carcinoid

Modern Techniques for Diagnosis
- Electron microscopy: Dense core neurosecretory granules

Differential Diagnosis
- Reserve cell hyperplasia
  - Low cellularity
  - Tight clusters of small uniform cells
  - Lack of single cells
  - Scant cytoplasm with high N/C ratio
  - Frequently attached to benign bronchial columnar cells with cilia or terminal bar
- Bronchioloalveolar carcinoma
  - Large cohesive sheets of monotonous cells
  - Lack of single cells
  - Fine and open chromatin
- Small cell carcinoma
  - Differential diagnosis of atypical carcinoid
  - Prominent nuclear molding and chromatin crush artifact
  - Abundant necrosis, apoptosis, and mitosis

PEARLS

- Loosely cohesive clusters and abundant single cells
- Uniform round, plasmacytoid and spindle cells
- Fine granular salt–pepper chromatin
- Moderate amount of granular cytoplasm
- Neuroendocrine markers (chromogranin, synaptophysin, CD56, and CD57): Positive

SQUAMOUS CELL CARCINOMA

Clinical Features
- 25–40% of lung cancers
- Most patients are male
- Closely related to smoking
- Most are centrally located lesions
- Cavitation is common
- Clinical symptom: Cough, weight loss, sputum production, chest pain, and dyspnea

Cytologic Features
- Well-differentiated squamous cell carcinoma
  - ➤ Abundant isolated round or polygonal cells
  - ➤ Scattered bizarre-shaped, tad pole–shaped and fiber-like cells
  - ➤ Marked hyperchromatic and pyknotic nuclei
  - ➤ Cytoplasmic keratinization: dense orangeophilia on Pap stain and robin's egg blue on modified Giemsa stain
  - ➤ Necrosis and neutrophils are common
  - ➤ Multinucleated giant cell reaction may occur
- Poorly differentiated squamous cell carcinoma
  - ➤ Predominant three-dimensional groups of cells
  - ➤ Dense cytoplasm without cytoplasmic keratinization
  - ➤ Enlarged nuclei
  - ➤ Coarsely granular chromatin
  - ➤ Prominent nucleoli may be seen
- Basaloid squamous cell carcinoma
  - ➤ Tight clusters and irregular cell fragments
  - ➤ Peripheral nuclear palisading
  - ➤ Relatively small cells with scant cytoplasm

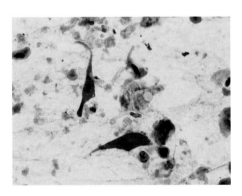
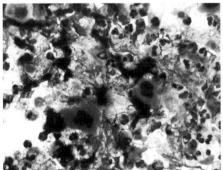
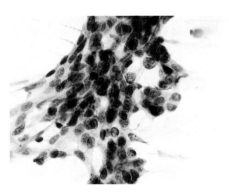
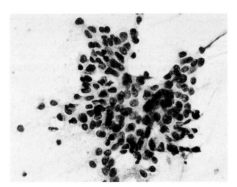

14-5A. Well-differentiated squamous cell carcinoma *(top, left).* Spindle-shaped fiber-like cells with pyknotic nuclei and dense orangeophilic cytoplasm (Papanicalaou stain)

14-5B. Well-differentiated squamous cell carcinoma *(top, right).* Malignant squamous cells with pyknotic nuclei, irregular nuclear contour and Robin's egg blue cytoplasm, in the background of abundant neutrophils (modified Giemsa stain)

14-5C. Poorly differentiated squamous cell carcinoma *(bottom, left).* A three-dimensional group of cells with enlarged nuclei, nuclear pleomorphism, and coarsely granular chromatin (Papanicalaou stain)

14-5D. Basaloid squamous cell carcinoma *(bottom, right).* A cluster of relatively small malignant cells with dense chromatin and peripheral nuclear palisading (Papanicalaou stain)

➤ Dense chromatin
➤ Small distinct nucleoli

Special Stains and Immunohistochemistry
▨ High-molecular-weight keratin (34βE12): Positive
▨ p63: Positive
▨ Thyroid transcription factor 1 (TTF-1): Negative
▨ Cytokeratin 7: Negative
▨ Cytokeratin 20: Negative

Modern Techniques for Diagnosis
▨ p53 mutation

Differential Diagnosis
■ Abscess
  ➤ Abundant neutrophils
  ➤ Abundant necrotic debris
  ➤ Degenerated cells
  ➤ Lack of malignant cells
■ Poorly differentiated adenocarcinoma
  ➤ Three-dimensional groups or acinar structures
  ➤ Irregular nuclear membrane contour
  ➤ Prominent nucleoli
  ➤ Abundant delicate cytoplasm
■ Large cell undifferentiated carcinoma
  ➤ Abundant small clusters and isolated cells
  ➤ Markedly enlarged nuclei
  ➤ Multinucleated tumor giant cells
■ Small cell carcinoma
  ➤ Differential diagnosis of basaloid squamous cell carcinoma
  ➤ Loosely cohesive clusters and abundant isolated cells
  ➤ Finely granular salt-and-pepper chromatin
  ➤ Abundant necrosis and apoptosis
  ➤ Nuclear molding and crush
  ➤ Neuroendocrine markers: Positive

PEARLS

✶ Most are centrally located lesions
✶ Cavitation is common
✶ Isolated cells with hyperchromatic and pyknotic nuclei
✶ Scattered bizarre-shaped, tadpole–shaped and fiber-like cells
✶ Cytoplasmic keratinization: Dense orangeophilia on Pap stain and robin's egg blue on modified Giemsa stain
✶ p63: Positive

ADENOCARCINOMA

Clinical Features
▨ 25–40% of lung cancers
▨ The most common lung cancer in women and nonsmokers
▨ Most are peripherally located lesions
▨ Less frequently related to smoking (>75%)

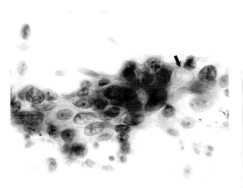 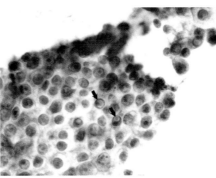

14-6A. Adenocarcinoma *(left).* A crowded group of malignant cells with overlapping nuclei, nuclear pleomorphism, open chromatin, prominent nucleoli, and delicate cytoplasm. Note the intracytoplasmic vacuole (arrow) (Papanicalaou stain)

14-6B. Bronchioloalveolar carcinoma *(right).* A large monolayer sheet of uniform cells with round nuclei, fine chromatin, prominent nucleoli, and intranuclear cytoplasmic inclusions (arrow) (Papanicalaou stain)

- Clinical symptom: Cough, weight loss, chest pain, and dyspnea
- Bronchioloalveolar carcinoma
  - Multiple diffuse nodules in the peripheral lung
  - Better biologic behavior

Cytologic Features
- Flat sheets with nuclear overlapping and crowding
- Three-dimensional clusters
- Acinar structures
- Eccentrically located nuclei
- Prominent nucleoli
- Abundant delicate foamy cytoplasm with indistinct border
- Cytoplasmic or extracellular mucin
- Poorly differentiated tumor shows more isolated cells and necrosis
- Bronchioloalveolar carcinoma:
  - Three-dimensional groups and large monolayer sheets
  - Uniform cells
  - Nuclear membrane groove
  - Intranuclear cytoplasmic inclusion
  - Definitive diagnosis requires histological confirmation of the lack of invasion

Special Stains and Immunohistochemistry
- Thyroid transcription factor 1 (TTF-1): Positive
- Cytokeratin 7 (CK7): Positive
- Cytokeratin 20 (CK20): Negative
- Mucin stain: Positive intracytoplasmic mucin droplet

Modern Techniques for Diagnosis
- EGFR mutation: favorable response to tyrosine kinase inhibitor
- K-Ras oncogene mutation in one-third of tumors: resistance to tyrosine kinase inhibitor

Differential Diagnosis
- Reactive/reparative bronchial epithelial cells
  - Cohesive two-dimensional honeycombing sheets
  - Most cells are small and bland
  - Scattered cells show nuclear enlargement, hyperchromasia, and nucleoli
  - The presence of cilia or terminal bar
- Poorly differentiated squamous cell carcinoma
  - More isolated cells
  - Dense cytoplasm with distinct cell border
  - Marked hyperchromasia with indiscernible nucleoli
- Large-cell undifferentiated carcinoma
  - Abundant small clusters and isolated cells

➤ Markedly enlarged nuclei
➤ Multinucleated tumor giant cells
➤ Marked nuclear pleomorphism
■ Small cell carcinoma
➤ Poorly cohesive clusters and abundant isolated cells
➤ Scant cytoplasm with high N/C ratio
➤ Finely granular salt-and-pepper chromatin
➤ Inconspicuous nucleoli
➤ Abundant necrosis, mitosis, and apoptosis
➤ Nuclear molding and crush
➤ Neuroendocrine markers: Positive
■ Metastatic adenocarcinoma
➤ Clinical history of previous malignancy
➤ Comparison with previous malignancy is critical
➤ Immunostains: Organ-specific markers and CK7/CK20 pattern

PEARLS

★ Crowded sheets and three dimensional clusters
★ Eccentric nuclei
★ Abundant delicate and foamy cytoplasm
★ Prominent nucleoli
★ TTF-1: Positive

LARGE CELL UNDIFFERENTIATED CARCINOMA

Clinical Features
■ 10–15% of lung cancers
■ Most are related to smoking
■ Peripherally located large lesions with cavitation
■ Lack of light microscopic features of small cell carcinoma, glandular and squamous differentiation
■ Clinical symptom: Cough, weight loss, chest pain, and dyspnea

Cytologic Features
■ Abundant isolated cells
■ Poorly cohesive clusters
■ Markedly enlarged cells
■ Hyperchromatic and pleomorphic nuclei
■ Prominent single or multiple nucleoli
■ Giant cell carcinoma: Numerous multinucleated tumor giant cells
■ Spindle cell carcinoma: Malignant spindle cells

Special Stains and Immunohistochemistry
■ Cytokeratin: Positive
■ TTF-1: Positive (>50%)

Modern Techniques for Diagnosis
■ Electron microscopy: Most show glandular and squamous differentiation

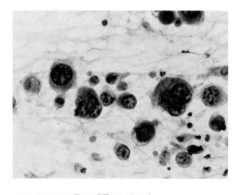

14-7. Large cell undifferentiated carcinoma. Singly dispersed malignant cells with markedly enlarged nuclei, marked nuclear pleomorphism, clumpy chromatin, and prominent nucleoli. Scattered multinucleated tumor giant cells (Papanicalaou stain)

Differential Diagnosis
■ Poorly differentiated squamous cell carcinoma
➤ Focal and minimal cytoplasmic keratinization

➤ Indiscernible nucleoli due to marked hyperchromasia
➤ More cell cohesion
■ Poorly differentiated adenocarcinoma
➤ Focal and minimal glandular differentiation: eccentrically located nuclei, abundant foamy cytoplasm, and cytoplasmic vacuoles
➤ More cell cohesion
■ Large cell malignant lymphoma
➤ Monotonous population of dyshesive lymphoid cells
➤ Lack of cell cohesion
➤ Lymphoglandular bodies on Romanowsky-type stain
➤ CD45: Positive
■ Melanoma
➤ Abundant isolated cells
➤ Plasmacytoid cells with abundant cytoplasm and eccentric nuclei
➤ Intranuclear inclusion
➤ Binucleation and multinucleation
➤ Cytoplasmic melanin pigmentation may be seen
➤ HMB-45 and melan A: Positive
■ Metastatic poorly differentiated malignancy
➤ Clinical history of previous large cell malignancy, especially in pancreas, thyroid, and liver
➤ Comparison with primary malignancy is the key
➤ Immunostains: Organ-specific markers and CK7/CK20 pattern

PEARLS

✶ Abundant isolated cells
✶ Marked enlarged cells with pleomorphic nuclei and prominent nucleoli
✶ Tumor giant cells and malignant spindle cells may be seen
✶ Cytokeratin: Positive

SMALL CELL CARCINOMA

Clinical Features
■ 20–25% of lung cancers
■ Strongly related to smoking
■ Centrally located lesions
■ Initial presentation at an advanced stage
■ Surgical resection is ineffective due to advanced stage
■ Sensitive to radiation and chemotherapy
■ Clinical symptom: related to local spread and distant metastasis

Cytologic Features
■ Poorly cohesive clusters
■ Abundant isolated cells
■ Nuclear size: 1.5 times the size of small lymphocyte
■ Scant basophilic cytoplasm
■ High N/C ratio
■ Finely granular chromatin with salt-and-pepper appearance
■ Inconspicuous nucleoli
■ Nuclear molding
■ Abundant necrosis, mitosis, and apoptosis
■ Nuclear crush artifact

14-8A. Small cell carcinoma
(left). Poorly cohesive clusters of cells with nuclear crushing artifact. Abundant cellular necrotic debris and pyknotic nuclei (Papanicalaou stain)

14-8B. Small cell carcinoma
(right). A poorly cohesive cluster of cells with scant cytoplasm, high N/C ratio, finely granular salt-and-pepper chromatin, and inconspicuous nucleoli (Papanicalaou stain)

14-8C. Small cell carcinoma
(below). A cluster of cells with very scant cytoplasm, high N/C ratio and nuclear molding (modified Giemsa stain)

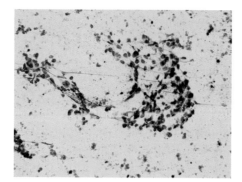
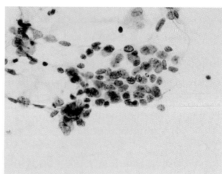

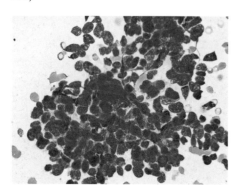

Special Stains and Immunohistochemistry

■ Cytokeratin: Paranuclear dotlike stain pattern
■ Neuroendocrine markers (chromogranin, synaptophysin, and CD56): Positive in 70% of cases
■ Thyroid transcription factor 1 (TTF-1): Positive
■ Cytokeratin 7: Negative
■ Cytokeratin 20: Negative
■ c-kit overexpression: 70%

Modern Techniques for Diagnosis

■ Electron microscopy: Dense-core neuroendocrine granules, 100 nm in diameter
■ p53 mutation
■ RB oncogene mutation
■ Bcl-2 (pro-apoptotic molecule) upregulation

Differential Diagnosis

■ Malignant lymphoma
  ➤ Monotonous population of dyshesive lymphoid cells
  ➤ Dense or clumpy chromatin
  ➤ Lack of nuclear molding
  ➤ Lymphoglandular bodies on Romanowsky-type stain
  ➤ CD45: Positive
■ Basaloid squamous cell carcinoma
  ➤ Tight clusters with greater cell cohesion
  ➤ Hyperchromatic and coarse chromatin
  ➤ Focal squamous differentiation
  ➤ Lack of nuclear molding and chromatin crush artifact
■ Small round cell neoplasm
  ➤ Younger age group of patients
  ➤ Clusters and isolated cells with high N/C ratio
  ➤ Nuclear chromatin crush artifact
  ➤ Immunostains
■ Atypical carcinoid
  ➤ Nuclear molding, chromatin crush artifact, and necrosis to a lesser degree
  ➤ Occasional prominent nucleoli
  ➤ Peripherally located in the lung
■ Carcinoid
  ➤ Plasmacytoid or spindle-shaped uniform cells
  ➤ Moderate amount of granular cytoplasm
  ➤ Lack of nuclear molding
  ➤ Lack of necrosis, mitosis, and apoptosis

★ Strongly related to smoking
★ Centrally located lesions
★ Loosely cohesive clusters and isolated cells
★ Scant cytoplasm with high N/C ratio
★ Finely granular and salt-and-pepper chromatin
★ Inconspicuous nucleoli
★ Nuclear molding and chromatin crush artifact
★ Prominent necrosis, mitosis and apoptosis
★ Neuroendocrine markers: Positive in 70% of cases
★ Cytokeratin: Paranuclear dotlike stain pattern
★ TTF-1: Positive

LARGE CELL NEUROENDOCRINE CARCINOMA

Clinical Features
▦ 3% of lung cancers
▦ A variant of large cell undifferentiated carcinoma with poor prognosis

Cytologic Features
▦ Flattened three-dimensional clusters with peripheral palisading
▦ Abundant isolated cells
▦ Enlarged nuclei: three times the size of small lymphocytes
▦ Moderate amount of cytoplasm leads to moderate N/C ratio
▦ Coarsely granular chromatin
▦ Thickened nuclear membrane
▦ Conspicuous nucleoli
▦ Occasional nuclear molding and crushing artifact
▦ Abundant necrosis and mitosis

Special Stains and Immunohistochemistry
▦ Neuroendocrine markers (chromogranin and synaptophysin): Positive
▦ Thyroid transcription factor 1 (TTF-1): Positive (50%)

Modern Techniques for Diagnosis
▦ Electron microscopy: Dense-core neuroendocrine granules

Differential Diagnosis
▦ Large cell undifferentiated carcinoma
  ➤ More isolated cells
  ➤ Marked enlarged nuclei with nuclear pleomorphism
  ➤ Lack of peripheral palisading
  ➤ Lack of chromatin crush artifact and nuclear molding
▦ Basaloid squamous cell carcinoma
  ➤ More cell cohesion
  ➤ Intermediate-sized nuclei with scant cytoplasm
  ➤ Dense chromatin
  ➤ Lack of chromatin crush artifact and nuclear molding
▦ Small cell carcinoma
  ➤ Small and intermediate-sized nuclei (1.5 times the size of lymphocyte)

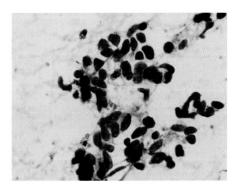

14-9. Large cell neuro endocrine carcinoma. A group of malignant cells with nuclear enlargement, coarsely granular chromatin, and moderate amount cytoplasm (Papanicalaou stain)

➤ Scant cytoplasm leads to high N/C ratio
➤ Finely granular salt-and-pepper chromatin
➤ Inconspicuous nucleoli
➤ Lack of peripheral palisading
■ Atypical carcinoid
➤ Moderate-sized nuclei
➤ Finely granular salt-and-pepper chromatin
➤ Moderate amount of cytoplasm
➤ Nuclear molding, chromatin crush artifact, and necrosis may be seen
➤ Lack of peripheral palisading

PEARLS

★ Flattened groups of large cells with peripheral palisading
★ Abundant isolated cells
★ Nuclear enlargement: three times the size of lymphocytes
★ Coarsely granular chromatin
★ Conspicuous nucleoli
★ Moderate amount of cytoplasm
★ Abundant necrosis and mitosis
★ Neuroendocrine markers (chromogranin and synaptophysin): Positive

ADENOID CYSTIC CARCINOMA – BRONCHIAL GLAND TUMOR

Clinical Features
■ 1% of lung cancers
■ Affects patients in their forties with equal sex distribution
■ No association with smoking
■ An endobronchial lesion within trachea, main stem, and lobar bronchi
■ Prognosis: indolent with local recurrence
■ Clinical symptom: shortness of breath, cough, wheezing, and hemoptysis

Cytologic Features
■ Cohesive clusters
■ Small uniform basaloid cells with scant cytoplasm and dark nuclei
■ Extracellular basement membrane-like stroma forming hyaline globules
➤ Pap stain: Pale and translucent
➤ Romanowsky-type stain: Metachromatic and homogeneous
■ Sharp interface between hyaline globules and tumor cells

14-10A. Adenoid cystic carcinoma *(left)*. Cohesive clusters of small uniform basaloid cells with scant cytoplasm and dark nuclei, surrounding pale and translucent hyaline globules (Papanicalaou stain)

14-10B. Adenoid cystic carcinoma *(right)*. Cohesive clusters of small uniform basaloid cells, surrounding metachromatic and homogeneous hyaline globules. Note the sharp interface between tumor cells and hyaline globules (modified Giemsa stain)

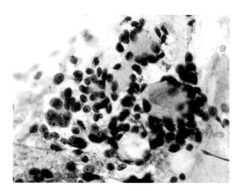
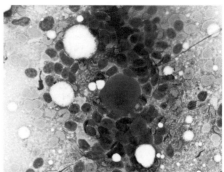

Special Stains and Immunohistochemistry

- S-100: Positive
- Type IV collagen: Positive in hyaline globule

Modern Techniques for Diagnosis

- Rearrangement of 9p13

Differential Diagnosis

- Pleomorphic adenoma
  - ➤ Sheets and clusters epithelial cells with delicate cytoplasm
  - ➤ Isolated spindle or plasmacytoid myoepithelial cells
  - ➤ Fibromyxoid and chondroid stroma with fibrillary appearance and embedded myoepithelial cells
  - ➤ Irregular and jagged interface between stroma and tumor cells
- Metastatic adenoid cystic carcinoma
  - ➤ Clinical history of primary malignancy
  - ➤ Radiology: Multiple lung parenchyma lesions
  - ➤ Cytomorphology is the same

PEARLS

- ✶ An endobronchial lesion
- ✶ Cohesive clusters of small uniform basaloid cells
- ✶ Hyaline globule formed by basement membrane like material
- ✶ Sharp interface between tumor cells and hyaline globule

MUCOEPIDERMOID CARCINOMA – BRONCHIAL GLAND TUMOR

Clinical Features

- 1% of lung cancers
- An endobronchial lesion
- Affects patients in thirties and forties with equal sex distribution
- Also occurs in children
- No association with smoking
- Clinical symptom: Shortness of breath, cough, wheezing, hemoptysis, and pneumonia

Cytologic Features

- Low grade tumor
  - ➤ Mucinous/glandular cells: Round to columnar cells with abundant vacuolated cytoplasm and mucin production
  - ➤ Squamous cells: Immature metaplastic cells to mature squamous cells
  - ➤ Intermediated cells: Small cells with high N/C ratio
  - ➤ Cystic contents: Histiocytes and debris
- High grade tumor
  - ➤ Predominant malignant squamous cells
  - ➤ Scattered to rare glandular cells
  - ➤ Abundant necrosis and mitosis

Special Stains and Immunohistochemistry

- Mucin stain: Positive
- Thyroid transcription factor (TTF-1): Negative

Modern Techniques for Diagnosis
■ Noncontributory

Differential Diagnosis
■ Mucinous bronchioloalveolar carcinoma
➤ Differential diagnosis of low-grade tumor
➤ Large sheets of uniform cells with abundant mucin containing cytoplasm
➤ Lack of intermediate cells and squamous cells
■ Squamous cell carcinoma
➤ Differential diagnosis of high grade tumor
➤ Lack of scattered glandular cells
➤ The distinction may be difficult
■ Metastatic mucoepidermoid carcinoma
➤ Clinical history of primary malignancy
➤ Radiology: Multiple lung parenchyma lesions
➤ Cytomorphology is the same

PEARLS

★ An endobronchial lesion
★ Mixture of mucinous cells, squamous cells and intermediate cells
★ High-grade tumor: Predominant malignant squamous cells

MALIGNANT LYMPHOMA

Clinical Features
■ Less than 0.5% of primary lung cancers
■ 0.4% of all malignant lymphomas
■ Favorable prognosis compared to lung cancers
■ Marginal zone B-cell lymphoma of the mucosa-associated lymphoid tissue (MALT)
➤ 70–90% of primary lung lymphomas
➤ Preexisting inflammatory or autoimmune processes
➤ Low-grade lymphoma with an indolent course
■ Diffuse large B-cell lymphoma
➤ 5–20% of primary lung lymphomas
➤ Preexisting immunodeficiency

14-11A. Malt lymphoma.
A polymorphous population of dispersed lymphoid cells, including predominant small lymphoid cells, scattered intermediate cells, and monocytoid cells with moderate amount pale cytoplasm (arrow). Note the lymphoglandular bodies in the background (arrow) (modified Giemsa stain)

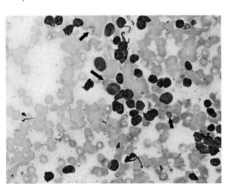

Cytologic Features
■ MALT lymphoma
➤ Polymorphous population of dispersed lymphoid cells
➤ Predominant small lymphoid cells with round nuclei and clumpy chromatin
➤ Scattered monocytoid cells with moderate amount pale cytoplasm
➤ Scattered plasmacytoid cells and immunoblast-like large cells
➤ Lymphoglandular bodies
■ Diffuse large B-cell lymphoma
➤ Monotonous population of large atypical lymphoid cells
➤ Irregular nuclear membrane contour, coarse chromatin, multiple small nucleoli, or single prominent nucleoli
➤ Lymphoglandular bodies

Special Stains and Immunohistochemistry
- CD45 (LCA): Positive
- CD20: Positive
- Flow cytometry is essential to establish clonality and immunophenotype

Modern Techniques for Diagnosis
- Demonstration of clonal rearrangement of immunoglobulin gene

Differential Diagnosis
- Inflammatory/reactive process
  - Polymorphous population of lymphoid cells
  - Predominant small lymphoid cells with smooth nuclear contour and coarse chromatin
  - Scattered intermediate cells, large immunoblast-like cells, plasma cells, histiocytes, and tangible body macrophages
- Small cell carcinoma
  - Poorly cohesive clusters and abundant isolated cells
  - Salt-and-pepper chromatin
  - Inconspicuous nucleoli
  - Nuclear molding
  - Lack of lymphoglandular bodies
  - Neuroendocrine markers: Positive
- Large cell undifferentiated carcinoma
  - Poorly cohesive clusters and abundant single cells
  - Hyperchromatic and pleomorphic nuclei
  - Moderate amount of cytoplasm
  - Lack of lymphoglandular bodies
  - Cytokeratin: Positive
- Involvement by systemic malignant lymphoma
  - History of systemic malignant lymphoma
  - Cytomorphology is the same

14-11B. Diffuse large B-cell lymphoma. A monotonous population of dispersed large atypical lymphoid cells with irregular nuclear contour, coarse chromatin, and prominent multiple or single nucleoli (Papanicalaou stain)

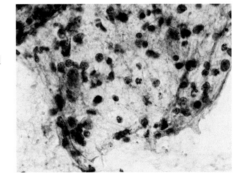

PEARLS

- Very rare primary lung cancer
- Polymorphous or monotonous population of dispersed lymphoid cells
- Variable nuclear atypia
- Lymphoglandular bodies
- CD45: Positive
- Flow cytometry is essential for diagnosis

INFLAMMATORY MYOFIBROBLASTIC TUMOR

Clinical Features
- Most common in children
- Peripherally located solitary mass on radiograph
- Complete excision leads to excellent survival in most cases
- Recurrence and metastasis rarely occur
- Clinical symptom: Fever, cough, and chest pain

Cytologic Features
- Loose aggregates and isolated cells
- Plump spindle-shaped fibroblasts

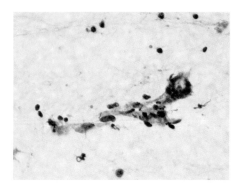

14-12. Inflammatory myofibroblastic tumor. A loose aggregate of bland plump spindle cells and scattered small lymphoid cells. Some spindle cells have reactive atypia, including slightly enlarged nuclei and distinct nucleoli (Papanicalaou stain)

- Mixed inflammatory cells: Neutrophils, histiocytes, lymphocytes, and plasma cells
- Reactive atypia: Nuclear enlargement and prominent nucleoli

Special Stains and Immunohistochemistry
- ALK: Positive (40%)
- p80: Positive (40%)
- Vimentin: Positive
- Smooth muscle actin: Positive

Modern Techniques for Diagnosis
- Rearrangement of ALK gene located on chromosome 2p23

Differential Diagnosis
- Sclerosing hemangioma
  - ➤ Stromal-like cells: Oval to spindle shaped
  - ➤ Epithelial cells: Polygonal shaped
  - ➤ Hemorrhagic background
  - ➤ TTF-1: Positive in both types of cells
- Sarcoma
  - ➤ Malignant spindle cells
  - ➤ Markedly enlarged nuclei
  - ➤ Increased N/C ratio
  - ➤ Necrosis

PEARLS
- ★ Plump spindle cells
- ★ Mixed inflammatory cells
- ★ ALK: Positive (40%)
- ★ p80: Positive (40%)

SARCOMA

Clinical Features
- Primary lung sarcoma is extremely rare
- Most are metastatic sarcomas

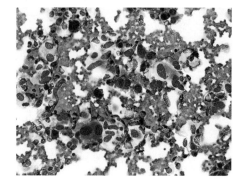

14-13. Sarcoma. Spindle cells with marked nuclear pleomorphism, irregular nuclear membrane contour, and binucleation (modified Giemsa stain)

Cytologic Features
- Poorly cohesive flat sheets
- Numerous isolated spindle cells
- Cellular pleomorphism and multinucleated giant cells are common
- Fragile cytoplasm with ill-defined border
- Different types of sarcoma may show some distinct features
- Further classification may not be possible based on cytomorphology

Special Stains and Immunohistochemistry
- A panel of immunostains are useful
- Immunoprofile is determined by the type of sarcoma

Modern Techniques for Diagnosis
- Electron microscopy: Useful for certain sarcomas
- Gene translocation: Useful for certain sarcomas

Differential Diagnosis
- Sarcomatoid carcinoma
  - Pleomorphic malignant spindle cells
  - Cytokeratin: Positive
- Inflammatory myofibroblastic tumor
  - Bland plump spindle cells, singly and in loose aggregates
  - Mixed inflammatory cells
  - ALK: Positive
- Hamartoma
  - Bland spindle cells
  - Fibromyxoid matrix with fibrillary appearance
  - Mature cartilage, benign epithelial cells, and adipocytes
- Spindle cell carcinoid
  - Monotonous spindle-shaped cells, singly and in loose aggregates
  - Fine granular salt-and-pepper chromatin
  - Neuroendocrine markers: positive
- Granulomatous inflammation
  - Granuloma: Aggregates of epithelioid histiocytes
  - Elongated spindle shaped nuclei with fine chromatin
  - Lack of nuclear atypia
- Benign mesenchymal tumor (leiomyoma and peripheral nerve sheath tumor)
  - Tissue fragments with low cellularity
  - Abundant isolated cells
  - Bland spindle cells
- Metastatic sarcoma
  - Clinical history of previous sarcoma
  - Comparison with previous sarcoma is the key

PEARLS

- Primary lung sarcoma is extremely rare
- Most are metastatic sarcoma
- Poorly cohesive flat sheets and isolated spindle cells
- Cellular pleomorphism and multinucleated giant tumor cells are common

METASTATIC MALIGNANCY

Clinical Features
- Lung is the most common site for metastasis
- Radiography: peripheral, multiple, and bilateral discrete nodules
- The most common primary sites: breast, colon, pancreas, and stomach
- History of other primary malignancy

Cytologic Features
- Comparison with diagnostic material from primary malignancy
- Metastatic colon adenocarcinoma
  - Strips of columnar cells with palisading
  - Well-formed glands
  - Elongated and hyperchromatic nuclei
  - Dirty necrosis
- Metastatic melanoma
  - Isolated neoplastic cells
  - Moderate to abundant cytoplasm
  - Plasmacytoid cells are common

14-14A. Metastatic colon adenocarcinoma *(left)*. A strip of columnar cells with elongated, hyperchromatic nuclei and nuclear palisading, in the background of cellular necrosis (Papanicalaou stain)

14-14B. Metastatic melanoma *(right)*. Singly dispersed round and plasmacytoid cells with macronucleoli, intranuclear cytoplasmic invagination (arrow), and moderate amount of cytoplasm (modified Giemsa stain)

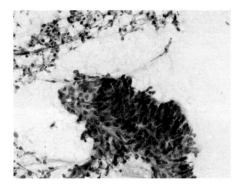
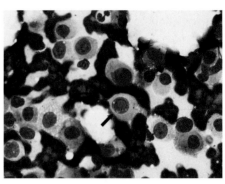

> Macronucleoli and intranuclear cytoplasmic invagination
> Binucleation and multinucleation
> Cytoplasmic melanin pigmentation in 60% of cases

Special Stains and Immunohistochemistry
■ TTF-1: Positive in the majority of primary lung tumors
■ CK7 and CK20 immunoprofile
■ Organ specific markers: Prostate-specific antigen, thyroglobulin, gross cystic disease protein 15 (breast), HMB-45 and melan A (melanoma)

Modern Techniques for Diagnosis
■ Noncontributory

Differential Diagnosis
■ Primary lung malignancy
> Solitary nodule
> The majority of lung primary tumors are carcinoma
> Primary lung lymphoma, melanoma, and sarcoma are rare
> The majority are TTF-1 positive
> The majority are positive for CK7 and negative for CK20
> The distinction is difficult or impossible on cytomorphology

PEARLS
★ Lung is the most common site for metastasis
★ Multiple and bilateral discrete nodules
★ History of other primary malignancy
★ Comparison with diagnostic material from primary malignancy is the key

PLEURA

MALIGNANT MESOTHELIOMA

Clinical Features
■ A rare neoplasm
■ Affects elders in their fifties and sixties with male predominance
■ Major risk factor: asbestos exposure
■ Simian virus-40 viral sequences are detected by PCR (cocarcinogenic effect)
■ Prognosis: median survival ~1 year
■ Radiology: Diffuse (75% of the cases) and localized growth
■ Clinical symptom: Dyspnea, chest wall pain, and pleural effusion or incidental finding

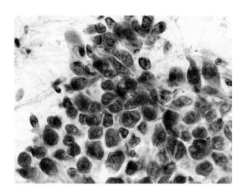
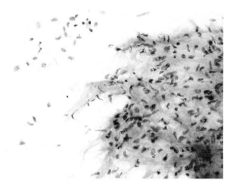

14-15A. Malignant mesothelioma epithelioid type *(left)*. A large sheet of polygonal cells with enlarged nuclei, high N/C ratio, nuclear pleomorphism, dense cytoplasm with well-defined border and intercellular "window" (Papanicalaou stain)

14-15B. Malignant mesothelioma sarcomatoid type *(right)*. Isolated and sheet of spindle-shaped cells with elongated and pleomorphic nuclei, hyperchromasia and ill-defined cytoplasm (Papanicalaou stain)

14-15C. Malignant mesothelioma mixed type *(below)*. A cluster of crowded malignant epithelial cells and a microfragment of pleomorphic spindle cells (Papanicalaou stain)

■ Variants: Epithelioid (65%), sarcomatoid (10%), mixed (20%), and desmoplastic (rare)

Cytologic Features
■ Epithelioid type
➤ Large sheets, three-dimensional clusters, papillary clusters, and isolated cells
➤ Polygonal cells with enlarged oval nuclei, hyperchromasia, high N/C ratio, and prominent nucleoli
➤ Dense cytoplasm with well-defined border
➤ Intercellular "window" in cell groups
➤ Occasional intracytoplasmic vacuoles
■ Sarcomatoid type
➤ Isolated cells, loose clusters, and sheets
➤ Spindle shaped cells with elongated nuclei, hyperchromasia, small to prominent nucleoli, scant and ill-defined cytoplasm
■ Mixed type
➤ Mixtures of malignant spindle and epithelial cells

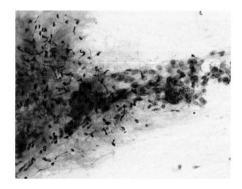

Special Stains and Immunohistochemistry
■ Alcian blue stain: Positive and hyaluronidase sensitive
■ Mucin stain: Negative
■ Positive markers: Calretinin, CK5/6 and WT-1
■ Negative markers: CEA, Ber-EP4, Leu M1 (CD15), MOC31 and B72.3

Modern Techniques for Diagnosis
■ Electron microscopy: Long, slender, and branching microvilli
■ Chromosomal abnormalities: Deletion of 1p, 3p, 9p, and 6q and loss of Ch22

Differential Diagnosis
■ Well-differentiated adenocarcinoma
➤ Differential diagnosis of epithelioid malignant mesothelioma
➤ Malignant epithelial cells with fluffy and ill-defined cytoplasm
➤ Lack of intercellular "window"
➤ Immunostains are necessary: Positive for CEA, Ber-EP4, Leu M1, MOC31 and B72.3
➤ Electron microscopy: Short and stubby microvilli with rootlet and terminal webs
■ Mesothelial hyperplasia and reactive mesothelial cells
➤ Differential diagnosis of epithelioid malignant mesothelioma
➤ The distinction can be very difficult on cytomorphology
➤ Small cell groups without isolated cells
➤ Reactive atypia: Mild nuclear enlargement, hyperchromasia, and prominent nucleoli
➤ Radiology: Lack of a dominant mass

■ Solitary fibrous tumor
  ➤ Differential diagnosis of sarcomatoid malignant mesothelioma
  ➤ Isolated, loose clusters, or stripped short spindle cells
  ➤ Irregular ropy collagen fragments
  ➤ CD34 and Bcl-2: Positive
■ Sarcomatoid carcinoma
  ➤ Differential diagnosis of sarcomatoid malignant mesothelioma
  ➤ Malignant spindle cells
  ➤ Cytokeratin: Positive
  ➤ Calretinin: Negative
■ Spindle cell sarcoma
  ➤ Differential diagnosis of sarcomatoid malignant mesothelioma
  ➤ Malignant spindle cells
  ➤ Calretinin and cytokeratin: Negative
■ Carcinosarcoma of the lung
  ➤ Differential diagnosis of mixed malignant mesothelioma
  ➤ Mixed malignant epithelial and spindle cells
  ➤ Calretinin: Negative

PEARLS

★ Clinical history of asbestos exposure
★ Radiology: Most are diffuse growth
★ Dense cytoplasm with well-defined border
★ Intercellular "window" in cell groups
★ Positive markers: Calretinin, CK5/6 and WT-1
★ Negative markers: CEA, Ber-EP4, Leu M1 (CD15), MOC31 and B72.3
★ Electron microscopy: Long, slender, and branching microvilli

SOLITARY FIBROUS TUMOR

Clinical Features
■ Affects patients in their sixties with equal gender distribution
■ No association with asbestos exposure
■ Radiology: pleural-based well-defined mass
■ Most have a benign clinical behavior with complete resection
■ Clinical symptom: dyspnea, cough, chest pain- or asymptomatic

Cytologic Features
■ Loose cell clusters and isolated single cells
■ Stripped nuclei

14-16A. Solitary fibrous tumor
(left). Singly dispersed uniform short spindle cells with oval to spindle nuclei, fine granular chromatin and ill-defined thin cytoplasm (Papanicalaou stain)

14-16B. Solitary fibrous tumor
(right). A loose cluster of uniform short spindle cells embedded in loose collagen fibers (Papanicalaou stain)

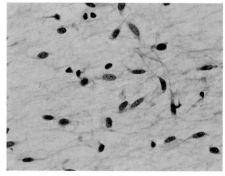
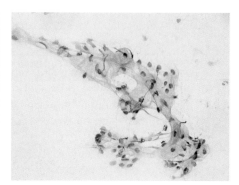

▦ Uniform short spindle cells with oval to spindle nuclei, fine granular chromatin, and thin and ill-defined cytoplasm
▦ Irregular ropy collagen fragment with trapped loose cell clusters
▦ Rare malignant solitary fibrous tumor: Greater cellularity, less cell cohesion, and nuclear pleomorphism

Special Stains and Immunohistochemistry
▦ CD34: Positive
▦ Bcl-2: Positive
▦ Cytokeratin and EMA: Negative

Modern Techniques for Diagnosis
▦ Noncontributory

Differential Diagnosis
■ Sarcomatoid malignant mesothelioma
   ➤ Malignant spindle cells with nuclear pleomorphism and hyperchromasia
   ➤ Lack of collagen fragments
   ➤ Calretinin: Positive
■ Hemangiopericytoma
   ➤ Spindle cells with more oval and round nuclei
   ➤ Less collagen fragments
   ➤ CD34: Positive
   ➤ The distinction is very difficult
■ Synovial sarcoma
   ➤ Biphasic tumor
   ➤ Short spindle cells clusters and epithelioid cell clusters
   ➤ Lack of collagen fragments
   ➤ Cytokeratin and EMA: Focally positive
■ Peripheral nerve sheath tumor
   ➤ Short oval to spindle cells with wavy nuclei
   ➤ Lack of collagen fragments
   ➤ S-100: Positive
■ Smooth muscle tumor
   ➤ Short oval to spindle cells with cigar-shaped nuclei
   ➤ Lack of collagen fragments
   ➤ Actin and desmin: Positive

PEARLS

★ No association with asbestos exposure
★ Pleural-based well-defined mass
★ Singly dispersed and loose clusters of short spindle cells
★ Irregular ropy collagen fragments
★ CD34 and Bcl-2: Positive

MEDIASTINUM

CYST

Clinical Features
▦ 15–20% of mediastinal masses
▦ Located in mid-mediastinum
▦ Nonneoplastic congenital cysts in children

14-17A. Cyst *(left)*. Abundant macrophages and amorphous cyst fluid (modified Giemsa stain)

14-17B. Cyst *(right)*. A cluster of benign columnar cells and amorphous cyst fluid (modified Giemsa stain)

14-17C. Cyst *(below)*. Scattered benign columnar cells with cilia and detached cilia, as seen in a bronchogenic cyst (modified Giemsa stain)

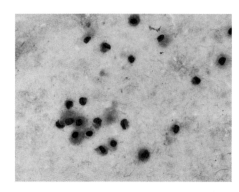
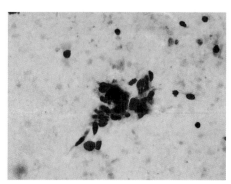
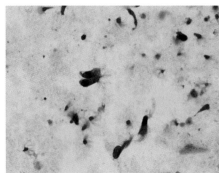

- Radiology: Unilocular or multilocular cyst
- Location: bronchogenic cyst – trachea, enteric cyst – esophagus, pericardial cyst – pericardium, and thymic cyst – thymus
- Clinical symptom: most are asymptomatic; may have chest pain and dysphagia

Cytologic Features
- Clear cyst fluid
- Paucicellular
- Cellular component; abundant macrophages and histiocytes
- Bronchogenic cyst
  - ➤ Pseudostratified columnar epithelial cells with cilia and scattered goblet cells
- Enteric cyst
  - ➤ Squamous or glandular epithelial cells
- Pericardial cyst
  - ➤ Mesothelial cells
- Thymic cyst
  - ➤ Squamous or glandular epithelial cells

Special Stains and Immunohistochemistry
- Noncontributory

Modern Techniques for Diagnosis
- Noncontributory

Differential Diagnosis
- Neoplastic cysts
  - ➤ Cystic degeneration is known in thymoma, lymphoma, and germ cell tumors
  - ➤ Extensive sampling of the solid component is critical for diagnosis

PEARLS

★ Congenital cysts in pediatric population
★ Located in mid-mediastinum
★ Paucicellular cystic fluid
★ Abundant macrophages and histiocytes
★ Cellular components vary from benign squamous, glandular, mesothelial cells to ciliated columnar epithelial cells
★ Neoplastic cysts need to be ruled out by extensive sampling

THYMOMA

Clinical Features
- The most common anterosuperior mediastinal neoplasms (20%)
- Affect patients >40 years with equal sex distribution
- Radiology: Well-defined lobulated mass; may have cyst formation
- The majority are encapsulated benign thymoma
- 20–25% are invasive malignant thymoma
- Clinical symptom: Typically an incidental finding on chest radiograph; may have chest pain, cough, dyspnea, or superior vena cava syndrome
- Paraneoplastic syndromes, such as myasthenia gravis (30–50%), hypogammaglobulinemia (10%), and pure red blood cell aplasia (5%) may occur

Cytologic Features
- Dual population of epithelial cells and lymphocytes
- Neoplastic epithelial cells
  - ➤ Cohesive aggregates or isolated cells
  - ➤ Polygonal cells with bland round to oval nuclei, fine granular chromatin, small nucleoli, and abundant cytoplasm
  - ➤ Dispersed lymphocytes in epithelial aggregates
- Thymic lymphocytes
  - ➤ Predominant small mature lymphocytes
  - ➤ Scattered large transformed lymphocytes
- Spindle cell thymoma
  - ➤ cohesive fragments of bland spindle-shaped epithelial cells
- Cystic thymoma
  - ➤ Paucicellular
  - ➤ Extensive sampling is critical
- Cytomorphology cannot distinguish benign from invasive malignant thymoma

Special Stains and Immunohistochemistry
- Epithelial cells: Cytokeratin positive; CD5 negative
- Thymic T cells (mature and immature): CD3, CD5, CD1a, and Tdt positive; CD20 negative

Modern Techniques for Diagnosis
- Noncontributory

Differential Diagnosis
- Thymic hyperplasia
  - ➤ Predominant small mature B cells
  - ➤ Lack of epithelial cells
  - ➤ CD20: Positive

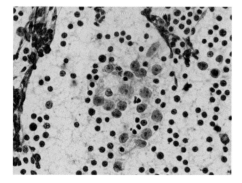 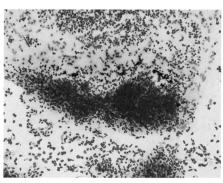

14-18A. Thymoma *(left)*. A loose cluster of epithelial cells with intermixed lymphocytes. The bland epithelial cells have finely granular chromatin, small nucleoli, and abundant cytoplasm. The background shows predominant small mature lymphocytes (Papanicalaou stain)

14-18B. Spindle cell thymoma *(right)*. Tight clusters of bland spindle-shaped epithelial cells in a background of small mature lymphocytes (modified Giemsa stain)

■ Precursor T-cell lymphoblastic lymphoma
  ➤ Affect male children and young adults
  ➤ Monotonous population of intermediate blasts
  ➤ Finely granular chromatin and small nucleoli
  ➤ Frequent mitosis and necrosis
  ➤ Lack of epithelial cells
  ➤ Immunophenotyping: Immature T cells (CD4, CD5, CD8, and Tdt positive); cannot be distinguished from the thymic lymphocytes in thymoma
■ Seminoma
  ➤ Affect adult male
  ➤ Isolated and loose groups of large germ cells: Prominent nucleoli and glycogen-filled cytoplasmic vacuoles
  ➤ Polymorphous lymphocytic background
  ➤ PLAP: Positive in germ cells
■ Large B-cell lymphoma
  ➤ Monotonous population of large atypical lymphoid cells
  ➤ Irregular nuclear contour, single or multiple nucleoli
  ➤ Lack of epithelial cells
  ➤ CD20: Positive
  ➤ Demonstration of B-cell clonality
■ Hodgkin lymphoma
  ➤ Isolated Reed–Sternberg cell and its variants: Marked enlarged nuclei and macronucleoli
  ➤ Polymorphous lymphocytic background
  ➤ Lack of epithelial cells
  ➤ CD15 and CD30: Positive in Reed–Sternberg cell and its variants
■ Nonneoplastic cysts
  ➤ Differential diagnosis of cystic thymoma
  ➤ Cellular components vary from benign squamous, glandular, mesothelial cells to ciliated columnar epithelial cells
  ➤ No lymphoid component
■ Mesenchymal lesions/neoplasm of smooth muscle, peripheral nerve sheath, and fibroblasts
  ➤ Differential diagnosis of spindle cell thymoma
  ➤ Bland spindle cell fragments
  ➤ No lymphoid cells
  ➤ Immunostains for actin, desmin, S-100, and vimentin

PEARLS

★ The most common anterior mediastinal neoplasm
★ Paraneoplastic syndromes may occur
★ Dual population of epithelial cells and lymphocytes
  • Bland neoplastic epithelial cells
  • Small mature thymic lymphocytes
★ Epithelial cells: Cytokeratin positive
★ Thymic T cells: CD3, CD5, CD1a, and TdT positive

THYMIC CARCINOMA

Clinical Features
■ A rare malignancy
■ Occurs predominantly in middle-aged men

▨ Radiology: heterogeneous mass with necrosis and calcification
▨ Squamous cell carcinoma is the most common histological type
▨ Other histological variants: lymphoepithelioma-like carcinoma, basaloid carcinoma, mucoepidermoid carcinoma, sarcomatoid carcinoma, and neuroendocrine carcinoma
▨ Clinical symptom: Cough, chest pain, and shortness of breath

Cytologic Features
▨ Clearly malignant epithelial cells
▨ Squamous cell carcinoma
  ➤ Poorly cohesive groups and isolated cells with enlarged, hyperchromatic, and pyknotic nuclei, and dense keratinized cytoplasm
▨ Basaloid carcinoma
  ➤ Tight clusters of small to intermediate-sized cells with dense chromatin and peripheral palisading
▨ Mucoepidermoid carcinoma
  ➤ Squamous, glandular, and intermediate neoplastic cells

Special Stains and Immunohistochemistry
▨ CD5: Positive

Modern Techniques for Diagnosis
▨ Noncontributory

Differential Diagnosis
▨ Metastatic carcinoma
  ➤ The most common mediastinal mass
  ➤ Lung small cell carcinoma is the most common primary malignancy
  ➤ Comparison with material from the primary malignancy is the key
  ➤ Immunostains: Organ-specific markers
▨ Nonseminomatous germ cell tumor
  ➤ Three-dimensional clusters, papillary and glandular
  ➤ Large malignant cells with prominent nucleoli
  ➤ Moderate amount of finely vacuolated cytoplasm
  ➤ Mucoid background or metachromatic extracellular material may be seen
  ➤ Mainly affect children and young adult
  ➤ CD30, AFP, and hCG may be positive
▨ Thymic carcinoid
  ➤ Poorly cohesive groups and isolated cells
  ➤ Monotonous round, plasmacytoid, and spindle cells
  ➤ Characteristic salt-and-pepper chromatin
  ➤ Neuroendocrine markers: Positive

PEARLS

★ Squamous cell carcinoma is the most common histological type
★ Clearly malignant epithelial cells
★ Cytomorphology mimics their counterparts in other organs
★ CD5: Positive

THYMIC CARCINOID

Clinical Features
▨ The incidence is rare
▨ Cushing syndrome is common

- 25% of patients have associated MEN-1 syndrome
- Metastasis and local invasion are common
- Clinical symptom: Cough, chest pain, and dyspnea

Cytologic Features

- Loosely cohesive clusters and isolated cells
- Monotonous small to intermediate cells
- Round to oval nuclei
- Salt-and-pepper chromatin
- Moderate amount of granular cytoplasm

Special Stains and Immunohistochemistry

- Neuroendocrine markers (synaptophysin and chromogranin): Positive

Modern Techniques for Diagnosis

- Electron microscopy: Dense core neurosecretory granules

Differential Diagnosis

- Metastatic carcinoid
  - More frequent compared to primary thymic carcinoid
  - Clinical history and imaging studies are the key
  - TTF-1: Variably positive in pulmonary carcinoid
- Paraganglioma
  - Located in posterior mediastinum
  - Hemorrhagic background
  - Cytomorphology is similar
  - Cytokeratin: Negative
- Ectopic mediastinal parathyroid adenoma
  - Clinical presentation of hypercalcemia
  - Loosely cohesive and dispersed cells
  - Parathyroid hormone immunostain: positive

PEARLS

- The incidence is rare
- Commonly associated with Cushing's syndrome and MEN-1
- Loosely cohesive and isolated monotonous cells
- Salt-and-pepper chromatin
- Neuroendocrine markers: Positive
- Metastatic pulmonary carcinoid need to be ruled out

PRIMARY MEDIASTINAL LARGE B-CELL LYMPHOMA

Clinical Features

- A subtype type of diffuse large B-cell lymphoma
- Putative origin: Thymic B cell
- Primarily affecting young adult with a female predominance
- Anterior and superior mediastinal infiltrating mass without superficial lymphadenopathy or hepatosplenomegaly
- Clinical symptom: Dyspnea, tracheal compression, and superior vena cava syndrome

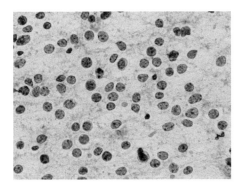 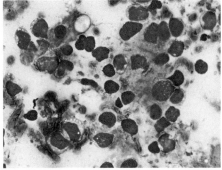

14-19A. Large cell lymphoma *(left)*. A monotonous population of large atypical lymphocytes with irregular nuclear contour, coarsely granular chromatin, and some with prominent nucleoli (Papanicalaou stain)

14-19B. Large cell lymphoma *(right)*. Monotonous population of large atypical lymphocytes with irregular nuclear contour, scant to moderate pale cytoplasm with fine vacuolization, and background lymphoglandular bodies (modified Giemsa stain)

Cytologic Features
▨ Monotonous population of large atypical lymphocytes (two to five times of mature lymphocytes)
▨ Irregular nuclear contour
▨ Coarsely granular chromatin
▨ Prominent nucleoli
▨ Scant to moderate pale cytoplasm with fine vacuolization
▨ Background lymphoglandular bodies
▨ Connective tissue microfragments may be seen

Special Stains and Immunohistochemistry
▨ CD45: Positive
▨ B-cell surface markers (CD20 and CD79a): Positive

Modern Techniques for Diagnosis
▨ Flow cytometry: A population of large cells marked exclusively with pan B-cell markers (CD19 and CD20)
▨ Usually lack of surface expression of immunoglobulin light chain

Differential Diagnosis
▨ Mediastinal involvement by peripheral nodal-based diffuse large B-cell lymphoma
  ➤ Clinical and radiological evidence of peripheral lymphadenopathy and/or hepato-splenomegaly is the key
  ➤ Surface expression of immunoglobulin light chain
  ➤ Flow cytometry: Surface immunoglobulin light chain restricted clonal B-cell population
▨ Precursor T-cell lymphoblastic lymphoma
  ➤ Affect male children or young adults
  ➤ Monotonous population of intermediate blasts
  ➤ Finely granular chromatin and small nucleoli
  ➤ Immunophenotyping: Immature T cells (CD4, CD5, CD8, and Tdt positive)
▨ Small cell carcinoma
  ➤ Isolated and poorly cohesive clusters of intermediate cells
  ➤ Salt-and-pepper chromatin and inconspicuous nucleoli
  ➤ Nuclear molding
  ➤ Neuroendocrine markers: Positive
▨ Thymoma
  ➤ Predominant small thymic lymphocytes
  ➤ Clusters of epithelial cells
  ➤ Thymic T-cell markers: CD3, CD5, CD1a, and Tdt positive

★ Affect young adult with a female predominance
★ Monotonous population of large atypical lymphocytes
★ Irregular nuclear contour with prominent nucleoli
★ Scant to moderate pale cytoplasm with fine vacuolization
★ B-cell surface markers (CD20 and CD79a): Positive
★ Usually lack of surface expression of immunoglobulin light chain

PRECURSOR T-CELL LYMPHOBLASTIC LYMPHOMA

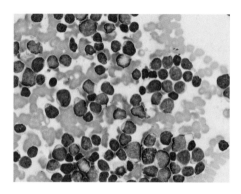

14-20. T-cell lymphoblastic lymphoma. A monotonous population of intermediate-sized blasts with fine chromatin and a thin rim of basophilic cytoplasm (modified Giemsa stain)

Clinical Features
■ Represent 90% of lymphoblastic lymphoma
■ An anterior mediastinal mass
■ Predominantly affect male adolescents and young adults
■ Clinical symptom: Cough, tracheal compression, superior vena cava syndrome, pleural and pericardial effusions

Cytologic Features
■ Monotonous population of isolated intermediate-sized blasts (two times of small lymphocytes)
■ Irregular nuclear contour
■ Finely granular chromatin
■ Small nucleoli
■ A thin rim of basophilic cytoplasm
■ Frequent mitosis, tangible body macrophages, and necrosis

Special Stains and Immunohistochemistry
■ Terminal deoxynucleotidyl transferase (Tdt): Positive (nuclear stain)
■ T-cell markers (CD4, CD5 and CD8): Positive

Modern Techniques for Diagnosis
■ Flow cytometry: Expression of Tdt and T-cell markers (CD4, CD5, and CD8)
■ Both T-cell receptor and immunoglobulin gene rearrangement are identified, and they may not be lineage specific

Differential Diagnosis
■ Thymoma
  ➤ Dual population of epithelial cells and lymphocytes
  ➤ Small mature thymic lymphocytes without blast features
  ➤ Bland neoplastic epithelial cells
  ➤ Thymic T-cells are immunophenotypically identical to T-cell lymphoblasts
  ➤ Gene rearrangement reveals no clonal lymphoid cells
■ Small cell carcinoma
  ➤ Isolated and poorly cohesive clusters of intermediate cells
  ➤ Salt-and-pepper chromatin and inconspicuous nucleoli
  ➤ Nuclear molding
  ➤ Neuroendocrine markers: Positive
■ Neuroblastoma
  ➤ A posterior mediastinal mass in younger patients
  ➤ Isolated cells with high N/C ratio
  ➤ Pseudorosettes
  ➤ Delicate fibrillary neuropil stroma
  ➤ Neuron-specific enolase: Positive

■ Large B-cell lymphoma
    ➤ Monotonous population of large atypical lymphocytes
    ➤ Coarsely granular chromatin and prominent nucleoli
    ➤ B-cell surface markers (CD20 and CD79a): Positive

PEARLS

✶ An anterior mediastinal mass of male adolescents and young adults
✶ Monotonous population of isolated intermediate-sized blasts
✶ Fine chromatin and small nucleoli
✶ Immunophenotype: Expression of Tdt and T-cell markers (CD4, CD5, and CD8)

HODGKIN LYMPHOMA

Clinical Features

■ Primary mediastinal Hodgkin lymphoma is rare (10%) compared to involvement by systemic disease
■ Represent 50–70% of primary mediastinal lymphoma
■ The commonest type: Nodular sclerosing subtype of the classic Hodgkin lymphoma
■ An anterior mediastinal mass
■ Predilection for young women in their thirties
■ Clinical symptom: Cough, chest pain, dyspnea, and superior vena cava syndrome
■ Constitutional symptom (B symptom): Fever, night sweat, and weight loss

Cytologic Features

■ Classic Reeds-Sternberg (RS) cells: Mirror-imaged binucleation
■ Mononuclear variant: Irregular and multilobated nuclei
■ Macronucleoli
■ Moderate amount of basophilic cytoplasm
■ Characteristic polymorphous lymphoid background, including mainly small mature lymphocytes and scattered eosinophils, plasma cells, neutrophils, and histiocytes
■ Metachromatic extracellular stroma
■ Necrosis
■ The diagnosis is challenging due the scarcity of RS cells
■ Cannot be acutely subtyped by cytomorphology alone

Special Stains and Immunohistochemistry

■ CD15 and CD30: Positive in RS cells
■ CD45 and CD20: Negative in RS cells
■ CD45 and CD3: Positive in background lymphoid cells

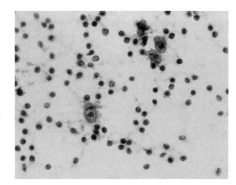

14-21A. Hodgkin lymphoma
(above). The classic RS cell has mirror-imaged binucleation and macronucleoli. The mononuclear variant shows irregular nuclei and macronucleoli. The background exhibits polymorphous lymphocytes (Papanicalaou stain)

14-21B. Hodgkin lymphoma
(left). The mononuclear RS cell is markedly enlarged with large, irregular, and multilobated nuclei, macronucleoli, and moderate amount of basophilic cytoplasm (modified Giemsa stain)

14-21C. Hodgkin lymphoma
(right). Characteristic polymorphous lymphoid background, including predominant small mature lymphocytes, intermediate lymphocytes, scattered eosinophils, and neutrophils (modified Giemsa stain)

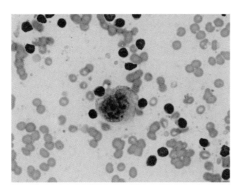
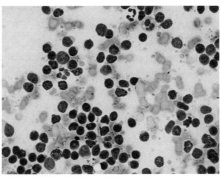

Modern Techniques for Diagnosis

▦ Rearrangement of immunoglobulin genes in RS cells, indicating a clonal B-cell process

▦ Epstein–Barr virus: Identified in ~20% of cases

Differential Diagnosis

▦ Mediastinal involvement by systemic nodal-based Hodgkin lymphoma
  ➤ Clinical and radiological evidence of lymphadenopathy and/or hepatosplenomegaly is the key
▦ Thymoma
  ➤ Groups and isolated bland polygonal epithelial cells without marked cytomegaly
  ➤ Small mature thymic T-lymphocytes
  ➤ Epithelial cells: Cytokeratin positive
▦ Seminoma
  ➤ Isolated and loose groups of large malignant germ cells with prominent nucleoli and moderate amount of vacuolated cytoplasm
  ➤ Heterogeneous population of lymphocytes
  ➤ PLAP: Positive in malignant germ cells
▦ T-cell–rich B-cell lymphoma
  ➤ Predominant small mature lymphocytes
  ➤ Scattered large atypical lymphoid cells with pleomorphic nuclei and prominent nucleoli
  ➤ CD45 and CD20: Positive
▦ T-cell lymphoma
  ➤ A spectrum of small to large to bizarre lymphocytes with convoluted and irregular nuclear membrane
  ➤ Reactive polymorphous lymphoid background
  ➤ CD3: Positive
▦ Anaplastic large cell lymphoma
  ➤ Single and poorly cohesive groups of large cells
  ➤ Pleomorphic nuclei, some resembling horseshoe and "doughnut"
  ➤ Many binucleated and multinucleated Reed–Sternberg–like tumor cells
  ➤ CD30, EMA, and ALK: Positive
  ➤ T (2:5) translocation

PEARLS

★ An anterior mediastinal mass
★ Predilection for young women in their thirties
★ Scattered classic Reeds–Sternberg (RS) cell and its mononuclear variant
★ Characteristic polymorphous lymphoid background, including scattered eosinophils
★ CD15 and CD30: Positive

MEDIASTINAL TERATOMA

Clinical Features

▦ Mediastinum is the most common site for extragonadal germ cell tumors
▦ Germ cell tumor accounts for ~20% of mediastinal neoplasms
▦ Mixed germ cell tumor represents ~20% of all mediastinal germ cell tumors
▦ Teratoma is most common mediastinal germ cell tumor (~ 50%)
▦ Affect children with equal sex distribution
▦ An anterior mediastinal multilocular cystic mass
▦ Clinical symptoms: Cough, chest pain, and dyspnea

Cytologic Features

- Depend on the components of the tumor
- The most common component are skin and its appendages, represented by squamous and sebaceous epithelium
- Bronchial pseudostratified columnar epithelium with terminal bar and cilia
- Gastrointestinal epithelium with goblet cells
- Other components: pancreas, neural tissue, muscle, adipose tissue, and cartilage
- The background may be mucoid
- Immature teratoma
    - ➤ Immature neuroepithelium: Poorly differentiated round cells forming rosettes
- Malignant teratoma
    - ➤ Non-germ cell malignancy: Carcinoma and/or sarcoma

Special Stains and Immunohistochemistry

- S-100 and NSE: Positive in the immature neural component

Modern Techniques for Diagnosis

- Noncontributory

Differential Diagnosis

- Mixed germ cell tumor
    - ➤ Features of other germ cell tumors
    - ➤ Extensive sampling is extremely important
- Mediastinal congenital cyst
    - ➤ Paucicellular
    - ➤ Rare to scattered glandular, squamous, and/or bronchial epithelium
    - ➤ Cystic component: Histiocytes and clear fluid
    - ➤ A mid-mediastinal cyst

PEARLS

- ★ The most common mediastinal germ cell tumor
- ★ Affects children
- ★ An anterior mediastinal multilocular cystic mass
- ★ Squamous, bronchial, and gastrointestinal epithelium are the most common components

MEDIASTINAL SEMINOMA

Clinical Features

- The second most common mediastinal germ cell tumor
- Almost exclusively affects men in their thirties and forties
- An anterior mediastinal mass
- Clinical symptom: Cough, chest pain, and dyspnea

Cytologic Features

- Dual population of germ cells and lymphoid cells
- Malignant germ cells
    - ➤ Isolated and loose groups of large polygonal cells
    - ➤ Round to oval nuclei, vesicular chromatin, and prominent nucleoli
    - ➤ Moderate amount of fragile and pale cytoplasm with glycogen-filled vacuoles
    - ➤ Stripped nuclei are common
- Heterogeneous population of lymphocytes
- Frequent mitosis
- Frothy tigroid background may be seen

14-22A. Seminoma *(left).*
A poorly cohesive cluster of large malignant germ cells with vesicular chromatin, prominent nucleoli and moderate amount of fragile and pale cytoplasm. Scattered small mature lymphocytes (Papanicalaou stain)

14-22B. Seminoma *(right).*
A poorly cohesive cluster of large malignant germ cells with prominent nucleoli. The fragile and vacuolated cytoplasm is easily disrupted, leading to stripped nuclei and frothy background (modified Giemsa stain)

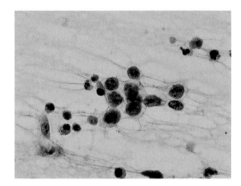 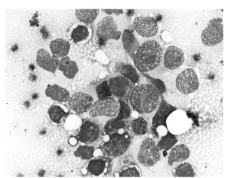

Special Stains and Immunohistochemistry
- Placenta like alkaline phosphatase (PLAP): Positive (diffuse and strong membrane and cytoplasmic staining pattern)
- c-kit (CD117): Positive
- OCT-4: Positive (nuclear stain)
- Cytokeratin: Negative; may show focal and weak stain

Modern Techniques for Diagnosis
- Isochromosome 12p with loss of long arm

Differential Diagnosis
- Metastatic gonadal or other extragonadal seminoma
  - ➤ Cytomorphology is indistinguishable
  - ➤ Clinical history is the key
- Thymoma
  - ➤ Groups and isolated bland epithelial cells without marked cytomegaly
  - ➤ Small mature thymic T-lymphocytes
  - ➤ Epithelial cells: Cytokeratin positive
- Hodgkin lymphoma
  - ➤ Scattered isolated Reed–Sternberg cells and its variants
  - ➤ Lack of cell cohesion
  - ➤ Polymorphic lymphoid cells
  - ➤ CD15 and CD30: Positive
- Anaplastic large cell lymphoma
  - ➤ Single and poorly cohesive groups of large cells
  - ➤ Pleomorphic nuclei, some resembling horseshoe and "doghnut"
  - ➤ CD30, EMA, and ALK: Positive
  - ➤ T (2:5) translocation
- Mixed germ cell tumor
  - ➤ Extensive sampling is extremely important
  - ➤ Features of other germ cell tumors

PEARLS
- ★ An anterior mediastinal mass
- ★ Predominantly affect males in their thirties and forties
- ★ Dual population of malignant germ cells and heterogeneous lymphoid cells
- ★ Malignant germ cells with prominent nucleoli and fragile, vacuolated cytoplasm
- ★ Tigroid background
- ★ PLAP: Positive

MEDIASTINAL NONSEMINOMATOUS GERM CELL TUMORS

Clinical Features

▧ Subtypes: Embryonic carcinoma, yolk sac tumor, and choriocarcinoma

▧ An anterior mediastinal mass

▧ Embryonic carcinoma and choriocarcinoma: Affects young males in their twenties and thirties

▧ Yolk sac tumor: Affects prepubertal girls

▧ Serologic tumor marker

➢ Choriocarcinoma: β-human chorionic gonadotropin (hCG)

➢ Yolk sac tumor: α-fetal protein (AFP)

▧ Clinical symptom: Cough, chest pain, and dyspnea

Cytologic Features

▧ Cohesive groups and isolated epithelial cells

▧ Acinar and papillary structures

▧ Large pleomorphic malignant cells with prominent nucleoli

▧ Necrosis

▧ Yolk sac tumor

➢ Abundant vacuolated cytoplasm

➢ PAS-positive intracellular and extracellular hyaline globules

➢ Metachromatic basement membrane-like extracellular material

➢ Mucoid background

▧ Choriocarcinoma. dual population of cells

➢ Cytotrophoblasts: sheets of pleomorphic epithelial cells

➢ Syncytiotrophoblasts: multinucleated tumor giant cells

Special Stains and Immunohistochemistry

▧ Cytokeratin: Positive

▧ Embryonic carcinoma: CD30 and OCT-4 positive; PLAP positive in half of the cases

▧ Yolk sac tumor: AFP positive

▧ Choriocarcinoma: HCG positive

Modern Techniques for Diagnosis

▧ Isochromosome 12p with loss of long arm

Differential Diagnosis

▧ Metastatic gonadal or other extragonadal nonseminomatous germ cell tumor

➢ Cytomorphology is indistinguishable

➢ Clinical history is the key

▧ Metastatic large cell undifferentiated carcinoma

➢ Cytomorphology shows great similarity

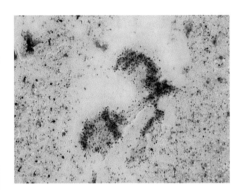

14-23A. Yolk sac tumor (above). Poorly cohesive aggregates of malignant epithelial cells form papillary structures, which is the cytological features of disrupted glomeruloid Schiller–Duval bodies seen on histology. Note abundant necrosis in the background (Papanicalaou stain)

14-23B. Yolk sac tumor (left). Loose clusters and isolated malignant epithelial cells with abundant vacuolated cytoplasm and basement membrane-like extracellular material (modified Giemsa stain)

14-23C. Choriocarcinoma (right). Dual population of cells, including clusters of pleomorphic cytotrophoblasts and single multinucleated syncytiotrophoblasts (arrow) (Papanicalaou stain)

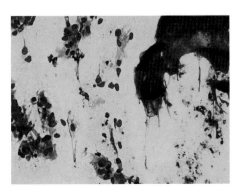 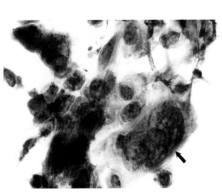

➤ Radiology: pulmonary mass
➤ Affect elder patients
■ Mixed germ cell tumor
➤ Extensive sampling is extremely important
➤ Features of other germ cell tumors

PEARLS

★ An anterior mediastinal mass
★ Mainly affects children and young adults
★ Cohesive groups and isolated large pleomorphic malignant cells with prominent nucleoli
★ Cytokeratin: Positive
★ Embryonic carcinoma: CD30 and OCT-4 positive
★ Yolk sac tumor: AFP positive
★ Choriocarcinoma: HCG positive

BENIGN PERIPHERAL NERVE SHEATH TUMOR (SCHWANNOMA AND NEUROFIBROMA)

Clinical Features
■ Neurogenic tumor accounts for 12–21% of all mediastinal masses
■ Benign peripheral nerve sheath tumor accounts for 40–65% of all mediastinal neurogenic tumors
■ Schwannoma accounts for 75% of mediastinal benign nerve sheath tumors
■ Affects young adults in their twenties to forties with equal sex distribution
■ A posterior mediastinal mass
■ Neurofibroma may be associated with Von Recklinghausen disease
■ Clinical symptom: asymptomatic

Cytologic Features
■ Variable cellularity
■ Microfragments of haphazardly arranged or parallel arranged spindle cells
■ Singly dispersed spindle cells
■ Spindle to oval nuclei with wavy nuclear contour and blunt end, fine chromatin, and small nucleoli
■ Indistinct cytoplasm
■ Fibrillary and myxoid matrix background
■ No mitosis
■ Schwannoma
➤ Verocay body with nuclear palisading

14-24A. Benign peripheral nerve sheath tumor *(left)*. A large microfragment of parallel arranged bland spindle cells with slightly wavy nuclear contour and blunt end (Papanicalaou stain)

14-24B. Benign peripheral nerve sheath tumor *(right)*. Bland spindle cells with oval to spindle nuclei and indistinct cytoplasm, embedded in the fibrillary extracellular matrix material (Papanicalaou stain)

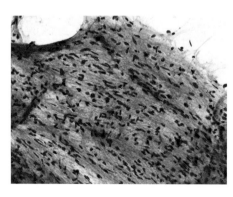
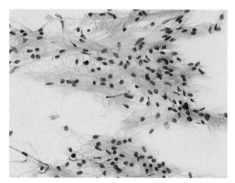

- Ancient schwannoma
  - ➤ Focal nuclear pleomorphism
- Melanocytic schwannoma
  - ➤ Nonrefractile granular cytoplasmic pigment
- The cytomorphology between schwannoma and neurofibroma is indistinguishable

Special Stains and Immunohistochemistry
- S-100: Strongly positive

Modern Techniques for Diagnosis
- Noncontributory

Differential Diagnosis
- Solitary fibrous tumor
  - ➤ Monotonous spindle cells with pointed ends
  - ➤ An anterior and superior mediastinal mass
  - ➤ CD34: Positive
- Spindle cell thymoma
  - ➤ Syncytial groups and singly dispersed bland spindle cells
  - ➤ Small mature thymic lymphocytes
  - ➤ An anterior mediastinal mass
  - ➤ Cytokeratin: Positive in spindle cells
- Reactive spindle cell lesions
  - ➤ Include fibromatosis, idiopathic fibrosing mediastinitis, and fibrous cyst wall
  - ➤ Microfragments and isolated bland spindle cells with pointed ends
  - ➤ Vimentin and smooth muscle actin: Positive
- Malignant peripheral nerve sheath tumor
  - ➤ Differential diagnosis of ancient schwannoma
  - ➤ Marked cellularity
  - ➤ Diffuse marked nuclear pleomorphism
  - ➤ Necrosis and mitosis
  - ➤ S-100: Focal and weak positivity

PEARLS
- ✶ A posterior mediastinal mass
- ✶ Microfragments and isolated bland spindle cells
- ✶ Wavy nuclear contour with blunt ends
- ✶ Fibrillary and myxoid background
- ✶ S-100: Positive

MALIGNANT PERIPHERAL NERVE SHEATH TUMOR

Clinical Features
- A rare posterior mediastinal mass
- Affects adults in their thirties to fifties with equal sex distribution
- Closely associated with Von Recklinghausen disease (neurofibromatosis)
- Clinical symptom: pain and nerve deficits

Cytologic Features
- Moderate to high cellularity
- Microfragments of parallelly arranged spindle cells
- Abundant singly dispersed spindle cells
- Marked nuclear pleomorphism

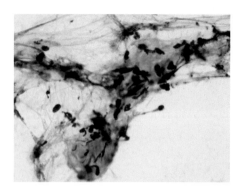

■ Spindle to oval nuclei with blunt ends, hyperchromasia, and prominent nucleoli
■ Fibrillary and myxoid matrix background
■ Frequent mitosis

Special Stains and Immunohistochemistry
■ S-100: Focal and weak positivity

Modern Techniques for Diagnosis
■ Noncontributory

14-25. Malignant peripheral nerve sheath tumor. A microfragment of spindle cells with nuclear pleomorphism and hyperchromasia (Papanicalaou stain)

Differential Diagnosis
■ Benign peripheral nerve sheath tumor
  ➤ Microfragments and isolated spindle cells
  ➤ Lack of nuclear pleomorphism
  ➤ No mitosis
  ➤ S-100: Strongly positive
■ Ancient schwannoma
  ➤ Focal nuclear pleomorphism
  ➤ No mitosis
  ➤ S-100: Strongly positive
■ Sarcomatoid carcinoma
  ➤ Isolated and poorly cohesive groups spindle cells
  ➤ Malignant nuclear features
  ➤ Cytokeratin: Positive
■ Spindle cell sarcoma
  ➤ Include synovial sarcoma, fibrosarcoma, and leiomyosarcoma
  ➤ Isolated and poorly cohesive groups spindle cells
  ➤ Malignant nuclear features
  ➤ Immunohistochemistry is the key: Cytokeratin, vimentin, CEA, and desmin
  ➤ Molecular diagnosis may be helpful
■ Spindle cell melanoma
  ➤ Singly dispersed malignant spindle cells
  ➤ Melanin pigment may be seen
  ➤ Melanocyte markers (melan A and HMB-45): Positive
  ➤ S-100: Strongly positive

PEARLS
★ A rare posterior mediastinal mass
★ Closely associated with Von Recklinghausen disease (neurofibromatosis)
★ Isolated and microfragments of spindle cells with blunt ends
★ Nuclear pleomorphism
★ Frequent mitosis
★ S-100: Focal and weak positivity

PARAGANGLIOMA

Clinical Features
■ A rare mediastinal tumor
■ Affects adults in their fifties
■ An anterior–superior mediastinal mass if arising from aorticopulmonary body
■ A posterior mediastinal mass if arising from paravertebral sympathetic chain

- Most are nonfunctional
- Clinical symptom: Chest pain, hoarseness, and dysphagia

Cytologic Features
- Hemorrhagic smears
- Poorly cohesive groups, isolated cells, and occasional acinar structures
- Abundant plasmacytoid cells with eccentrically located round to oval nuclei
- Moderate to abundant ill-defined cytoplasm
- Focal mild to marked pleomorphism
- Binucleation and multinucleation
- Intranuclear pseudoinclusion
- Occasional fine reddish intracytoplasmic granules on Romanowsky-type stain

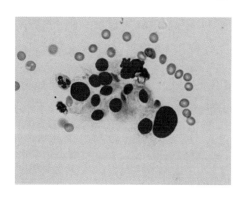

14-26. Paraganglioma. A loose cluster of cells with round to oval nuclei, slight nuclear pleomorphism, smooth nuclear contour, and moderate to abundant granular cytoplasm (modified Giemsa stain)

Special Stains and Immunohistochemistry
- Neuroendocrine markers (synaptophysin and chromogranin): Positive
- S-100: Positive in sustentacular cells
- Cytokeratin: Negative

Modern Techniques for Diagnosis
- Electron microscopy: Dense core neurosecretory granules

Differential Diagnosis
- Carcinoid
  - ➤ Similar cytomorphology
  - ➤ Cytokeratin: Positive
- Metastatic adenocarcinoma
  - ➤ Crowded groups
  - ➤ More isolated malignant cells in poorly differentiated malignancy
  - ➤ Nuclear pleomorphism
  - ➤ Neuroendocrine markers: Negative
  - ➤ Cytokeratin: Positive

PEARLS
- ★ A rare anterior–superior or posterior mediastinal mass
- ★ Hemorrhagic smears
- ★ Poorly cohesive groups and isolated plasmacytoid cells with ill-defined cytoplasm
- ★ Focal nuclear pleomorphism
- ★ Neuroendocrine markers: Positive
- ★ Cytokeratin: Negative
- ★ Electron microscopy: Dense-core neurosecretory granules

GANGLIONEUROMA

Clinical Features
- Affects elder adolescents and young adults
- A posterior mediastinal mass
- Clinical symptom: asymptomatic

Cytologic Features

■ Hypocellular smears
■ Ganglion cells: Large polygonal cells with eccentric nuclei, prominent nucleoli, and abundant granular cytoplasm
■ Spindle cells: Microfragments of uniform spindle cells with wavy nuclei

Special Stains and Immunohistochemistry

■ Neuron-specific enolase (NSE): Positive in ganglion cells
■ S-100: Positive in spindle cells

Modern Techniques for Diagnosis

■ Noncontributory

Differential Diagnosis

■ Benign peripheral nerve sheath tumor
　➤ Microfragments of uniform spindle cells with wavy nuclei
　➤ No ganglion cells
■ Ganglioneuroblastoma
　➤ Rich cellularity
　➤ Ganglion cells
　➤ Neuroblasts: Small blue round cells forming rosettes
　➤ Necrosis and mitosis

PEARLS

✶ A posterior mediastinal mass
✶ Large polygonal ganglion cells with eccentric nuclei, prominent nucleoli, and abundant granular cytoplasm
✶ Microfragments of uniform spindle cells with wavy nuclei
✶ NSE: Positive in ganglion cells
✶ S-100: Positive in spindle cells

NEUROBLASTOMA AND GANGLIONEUROBLASTOMA

Clinical Features

■ Affects children younger than five years
■ A posterior mediastinal mass
■ Radiology: 80% have calcification
■ Clinical symptom: Pain, neurologic deficits, Horner syndrome, respiratory distress, and ataxia

Cytologic Features

■ Rich cellularity
■ Loose clusters and dispersed uniform neuroblasts
■ Blue round cells (two to three times of small lymphocytes) with scant cytoplasm, high N/C ratio, coarsely granular chromatin and inconspicuous nucleoli
■ Homer-Wright rosettes: neuroblasts around fibrillary material
■ Abundant mitosis and necrosis
■ Ganglioneuroblastoma: Adequate sampling is the key
　➤ Neuroblasts
　➤ Ganglion cells: large polygonal cells with eccentric nuclei, prominent nucleoli and abundant granular cytoplasm
　➤ Intermediate cells: abundant cytoplasm without prominent nucleoli

Special Stains and Immunohistochemistry
▨ Neuroendocrine markers (NSE, chromogranin, and synaptophysin): Positive

Modern Techniques for Diagnosis
▨ N-myc oncogene amplification
▨ Del 1p
▨ Electron microscopy: Cytoplasmic neurosecretory granules

Differential Diagnosis
■ Malignant small blue round cell tumors of childhood
➤ Non-Hodgkin lymphoma
Monotonous population of dispersed cells
Lymphoglandular bodies
CD45: positive
➤ Rhabdomyosarcoma
Cytomorphology shows great similarity
Desmin and myoglobulin: positive
➤ Peripheral neuroectodermal tumor
The "dark" cells: small blue round cells
The "light" cells: larger pale nuclei
Cytoplasmic glycogen vacuoles
CD99: Positive

PEARLS

✶ A posterior mediastinal mass
✶ Mainly affect young children less than five years old
✶ Loose clusters and dispersed uniform neuroblasts
✶ Homer-Wright rosettes
✶ Ganglioneuroblastoma shows mixture of neuroblasts and ganglion cells
✶ Neuroendocrine markers: Positive
✶ Electron microscopy: Neurosecretory granule

REFERENCES

LUNG
ABSCESS
Cagle PT, Kovach M, Ramzy I. Causes of false results in transthoracic fine needle lung abscesses: US examination and US-guided transthoracic aspiration. *Radiology* 1991;180(1):17–1–5.

Dominguez S, Florez Alia C. Yield of percutaneous needle lung aspiration in lung aspirates. *Acta Cytol* 1993;37(1):16–20.

Kaneishi NK, Howell LP, Russell LA, Vogt PJ, Lie JT. Fine needle aspiration cytology of pulmonary Wegener's granulomatosis with biopsy correlation. A report of three cases. *Acta Cytol* 1995;39(6):1094–100.

Pena Grinan N, Munoz Lucena F, Vargas Romero J, Alfageme Michavila I, Umbria Yang PC, Luh KT, Lee YC, Chang DB, Yu CJ, Wu HD, Lee LN, Kuo SH. Lung abscess. *Chest* 1990;97(1):69–74.

GRANULOMATOUS INFLAMMATION
Carrafiello G, Lagana D, Nosari AM, Guffanti C, Morra E, Recaldini C, D'Alba MJ Das DK, Pant CS, Pant JN, Sodhani P. Transthoracic (percutaneous) fine needle aspiration cytology diagnosis of pulmonary tuberculosis. *Tuber Lung Dis* 1995;76(1):84–9.

Ferreiros J, Bustos A, Merino S, Castro E, Dorao M, Crespo C. Transthoracic needle aspiration biopsy: value in the diagnosis of mycobacterial lung opacities. *J Thorac Imaging* 1999;14(3):194–200.

Gong G, Lee H, Kang GH, Shim YH, Huh J, Khang SK. Nested PCR for diagnosis of tuberculous lymphadenitis and PCR-SSCP for identification of rifampicin resistance in fine-needle aspirates. *Diagn Cytopathol* 2002;26(4):228–31.

Morales CF, Patefield AJ, Strollo PJ, Jr., Schenk DA. Flexible transbronchial needle aspiration in the diagnosis of sarcoidosis. *Chest* 1994;106(3):709–11.

Silverman JF, Johnsrude IS. Fine needle aspiration cytology of granulomatous cryptococcosis of the lung. *Acta Cytol* 1985;29(2):157–61.

Sonvico U, Vanzulli A, Fugazz ola C. Utility of computed tomography (CT) and of fine needle aspiration biopsy (FNAB) in early diagnosis of fungal pulmonary infections. *Radiol Med (Torino)* 2006;111(1):33–41.

HAMARTOMA

Cosgrove MM, Chandrasoma PT, Martin SE. Diagnosis of pulmonary blastoma by fine needle aspiration biopsy: cytologic and immunocytochemical findings. *Diagn Cytopathol* 1991;7(1):83–7.

Dunbar F, Leiman G. The aspiration cytology of pulmonary hamartomas. *Diagn Cytopathol* 1989;5(2):174–80.

Kazmierczak B, Meyer-Bolte K, Tran KH, Wockel W, Breightman I, Rosigkeit J, Bartnitzke S, Bullerdiek J. A high frequency of tumors with rearrangements of genes of the HMGI(Y) family in a series of 191 pulmonary chondroid hamartomas. *Genes Chromosomes Cancer* 1999;26(2):125–33.

Xiao S, Lux ML, Reeves R, Hudson TJ, Fletcher JA. HMGI(Y) activation by chromosome 6p21 rearrangements in multilineage mesenchymal cells from pulmonary hamartoma. *Am J Pathol* 1997;150(3):901–10.

Wiatrowska BA, Yazdi HM, Matzinger FR, MacDonald LL. Fine needle aspiration biopsy of pulmonary hamartomas. Radiologic, cytologic and immunocytochemical study of 15 cases. *Acta Cytol* 1995;39(6):1167–74.

CARCINOID

Brambilla E, Negoescu A, Gazzeri S, Lantuejoul S, Moro D, Brambilla C, Coll JL. Apoptosis-related factors p53, Bcl2, and Bax in neuroendocrine lung tumors. *Am J Pathol* 1996;149(6):1941–52.

Costes V, Marty-Ane C, Picot MC, Serre I, Pujol JL, Mary H, Baldet P. Typical and atypical bronchopulmonary carcinoid tumors: a clinicopathologic and KI-67-labeling study. *Hum Pathol* 1995;26(7):740–5.

Cai YC, Banner B, Glickman J, Odze RD. Cytokeratin 7 and 20 and thyroid transcription factor 1 can help distinguish pulmonary from gastrointestinal carcinoid and pancreatic endocrine tumors. *Hum Pathol* 2001;32(10):1087–93.

Nicholson SA, Ryan MR. A review of cytologic findings in neuroendocrine carcinomas including carcinoid tumors with histologic correlation. *Cancer* 2000;90(3):148–61.

Pelosi G, Fraggetta F, Sonzogni A, Fazio N, Cavallon A, Viale G. CD99 immunoreactivity in gastrointestinal and pulmonary neuroendocrine tumours. *Virchows Arch* 2000;437(3):270–4.

Renshaw AA, Haja J, Lozano RL, Wilbur DC. Distinguishing carcinoid tumor from small cell carcinoma of the lung: correlating cytologic features and performance in the College of American Pathologists Non-Gynecologic Cytology Program. *Arch Pathol Lab Med* 2005;129(5):614–8.

Sachithanandan N, Harle RA, Burgess JR. Bronchopulmonary carcinoid in multiple endocrine neoplasia type 1. *Cancer* 2005;103(3):509–15.

Wick MR. Immunohistology of neuroendocrine and neuroectodermal tumors. *Semin Diagn Pathol* 2000;17(3):194–203.

Yang YJ, Steele CT, Ou XL, Snyder KP, Kohman LJ. Diagnosis of high-grade pulmonary neuroendocrine carcinoma by fine-needle aspiration biopsy: nonsmall-cell or small-cell type? *Diagn Cytopathol* 2001;25(5):292–300.

SQUAMOUS CELL CARCINOMA

Franklin WA, Veve R, Hirsch FR, Helfrich BA, Bunn PA, Jr. Epidermal growth factor receptor family in lung cancer and premalignancy. *Semin Oncol* 2002;29(1 Suppl 4):3–14.

Kamiya M, Uei Y, Shimosato Y. Cytologic features of peripheral squamous cell carcinoma of the lung. *Acta Cytol* 1995;39(1):61–8.

Mooney EE, Dodd LG, Vollmer RT, Bossen EH. Fine-needle aspiration biopsy diagnosis of primary bronchial basaloid-squamous carcinoma. *Diagn Cytopathol* 1997;16(2):187–8.

Nhung NV, Mirejovsky P, Mirejovsky T, Melinova L. Cytokeratins and lung carcinomas. *Cesk Patol* 1999;35(3):80–4.

Wu M, Szporn AH, Zhang D, Wasserman P, Gan L, Miller L, Burstein DE. Cytology applications of p63 and TTF-1 immunostaining in differential diagnosis of lung cancers. *Diagn Cytopathol* 2005;33(4):223–7.

Zusman-Harach SB, Harach HR, Gibbs AR. Cytological features of non-small cell carcinomas of the lung in fine needle aspirates. *J Clin Pathol* 1991;44(12):997–1002.

ADENOCARCINOMA

MacDonald LL, Yazdi HM. Fine-needle aspiration biopsy of bronchioloalveolar carcinomas. *Cancer* 2001;93(1):29–34.

Nhung NV, Mirejovsky P, Mirejovsky T, Melinova L. Cytokeratins and lung carcinomas. *Cesk Patol* 1999;35(3):80–4.

Ohori NP, Santa Maria EL. Cytopathologic diagnosis of bronchioloalveolar carcinoma: does it correlate with the 1999 World Health Organization definition? *Am J Clin Pathol* 2004;122(1): 44–50.

Saleh HA, Haapaniemi J, Khatib G, Sakr W. Bronchioloalveolar carcinoma: diagnostic pitfalls and immunocytochemical contribution. *Diagn Cytopathol* 1998;18(4):301–6.

Slebos RJ, Kibbelaar RE, Dalesio O, Kooistra A, Stam J, Meijer CJ, Wagenaar SS, Vanderschueren RG, van Zandwijk N, Mooi WJ and others. K-ras oncogene activation as a prognostic marker in adenocarcinoma of the lung. *N Engl J Med* 1990;323(9):561–5.

Wu M, Szporn AH, Zhang D, Wasserman P, Gan L, Miller L, Burstein DE. Cytology applications of p63 and TTF-1 immunostaining in differential diagnosis of lung cancers. *Diagn Cytopathol* 2005;33(4):223–7.

Zusman-Harach SB, Harach HR, Gibbs AR. Cytological features of non-small cell carcinomas of the lung in fine needle aspirates. *J Clin Pathol* 1991;44(12):997–1002.

LARGE CELL UNDIFFERENTIATED CARCINOMA

Craig ID, Desrosiers P, Lefcoe MS. Giant-cell carcinoma of the lung. A cytologic study. *Acta Cytol* 1983;27(3):293–8.

Haque AK. Pathology of carcinoma of lung: an update on current concepts. *J Thorac Imaging* 1991;7(1):9–20.

Johansson L. Histopathologic classification of lung cancer: Relevance of cytokeratin and TTF-1 immunophenotyping. *Ann Diagn Pathol* 2004;8(5):259–67.

Kodama T, Shimosato Y, Koide T, Watanabe S, Teshima S. Large cell carcinoma of the lung – ultrastructural and immunohistochemical studies. *Jpn J Clin Oncol* 1985;15(2):431–41.

Zusman-Harach SB, Harach HR, Gibbs AR. Cytological features of non-small cell carcinomas of the lung in fine needle aspirates. *J Clin Pathol* 1991;44(12):997–1002.

SMALL CELL CARCINOMA

Arora VK, Singh N, Chaturvedi S, Bhatia A. Significance of cytologic criteria in distinguishing small cell from non-small cell carcinoma of the lung. *Acta Cytol* 2003;47(2):216–20.

Brambilla E, Negoescu A, Gazzeri S, Lantuejoul S, Moro D, Brambilla C, Coll JL. Apoptosis-related factors p53, Bcl2, and Bax in neuroendocrine lung tumors. *Am J Pathol* 1996;149(6):1941–52.

Campbell AM, Campling BG, Algazy KM, el-Deiry WS. Clinical and molecular features of small cell lung cancer. *Cancer Biol Ther* 2002;1(2):105–12.

Delgado PI, Jorda M, Ganjei-Azar P. Small cell carcinoma versus other lung malignancies: diagnosis by fine-needle aspiration cytology. *Cancer* 2000;90(5):279–85.

Nicholson SA, Beasley MB, Brambilla E, Hasleton PS, Colby TV, Sheppard MN, Falk R, Travis WD. Small cell lung carcinoma (SCLC): a clinicopathologic study of 100 cases with surgical specimens. *Am J Surg Pathol* 2002;26(9):1184–97.

Nicholson SA, Ryan MR. A review of cytologic findings in neuroendocrine carcinomas including carcinoid tumors with histologic correlation. *Cancer* 2000;90(3):148–61.

Renshaw AA, Voytek TM, Haja J, Wilbur DC. Distinguishing small cell carcinoma from non-small cell carcinoma of the lung: correlating cytologic features and performance in the College of American Pathologists Non-Gynecologic Cytology Program. *Arch Pathol Lab Med* 2005;129(5):619–23.

Szyfelbein WM, Ross JS. Carcinoids, atypical carcinoids, and small-cell carcinomas of the lung: differential diagnosis of fine-needle aspiration biopsy specimens. *Diagn Cytopathol* 1988;4(1):1–8.

LARGE CELL NEUROENDOCRINE CARCINOMA

Arora VK, Singh N, Chaturvedi S, Bhatia A. Significance of cytologic criteria in distinguishing small cell from non-small cell carcinoma of the lung. *Acta Cytol* 2003;47(2):216–20.

Campbell AM, Campling BG, Algazy KM, el-Deiry WS. Clinical and molecular features of small cell lung cancer. *Cancer Biol Ther* 2002;1(2):105–12.

Delgado PI, Jorda M, Ganjei-Azar P. Small cell carcinoma versus other lung malignancies: diagnosis by fine-needle aspiration cytology. *Cancer* 2000;90(5):279–85.

Nicholson SA, Beasley MB, Brambilla E, Hasleton PS, Colby TV, Sheppard MN, Falk R, Travis WD. Small cell lung carcinoma (SCLC): a clinicopathologic study of 100 cases with surgical specimens. *Am J Surg Pathol* 2002;26(9):1184–97.

Nicholson SA, Ryan MR. A review of cytologic findings in neuroendocrine carcinomas including carcinoid tumors with histologic correlation. *Cancer* 2000;90(3):148–61.

Renshaw AA, Haja J, Lozano RL, Wilbur DC. Distinguishing carcinoid tumor from small cell carcinoma of the lung: correlating cytologic features and performance in the College of American Pathologists Non-Gynecologic Cytology Program. *Arch Pathol Lab Med* 2005;129(5): 614–8.

ADENOID CYSTIC CARCINOMA – BRONCHIAL GLAND TUMOR

Higashi K, Jin Y, Johansson M, Heim S, Mandahl N, Biorklund A, Wennerberg J, Hambraeus G, Johansson L, Mitelman F. Rearrangement of 9p13 as the primary chromosomal aberration in adenoid cystic carcinoma of the respiratory tract. *Genes Chromosomes Cancer* 1991;3(1):21–3.

Moran CA, Suster S, Koss MN. Primary adenoid cystic carcinoma of the lung. A clinicopathologic and immunohistochemical study of 16 cases. *Cancer* 1994;73(5):1390–7.

Qiu S, Nampoothiri MM, Zaharopoulos P, Logrono R. Primary pulmonary adenoid cystic carcinoma: report of a case diagnosed by fine-needle aspiration cytology. *Diagn Cytopathol* 2004;30(1):51–6.

Segletes LA, Steffee CH, Geisinger KR. Cytology of primary pulmonary mucoepidermoid and adenoid cystic carcinoma. A report of four cases. *Acta Cytol* 1999;43(6):1091–7.

MUCOEPIDERMOID CARCINOMA – BRONCHIAL GLAND TUMOR

Shilo K, Foss RD, Franks TJ, DePeralta-Venturina M, Travis WD. Pulmonary mucoepidermoid carcinoma with prominent tumor-associated lymphoid proliferation. *Am J Surg Pathol* 2005, 29:407–11.

Segletes LA, Steffee CH, Geisinger KR. Cytology of primary pulmonary mucoepidermoid and adenoid cystic carcinoma. A report of four cases. *Acta Cytol* 1999; 43:1091–7.

MALIGNANT LYMPHOMA

Crapanzano JP, Lin O. Cytologic findings of marginal zone lymphoma. *Cancer* 2003;99(5):301–9.

Kim JH, Lee SH, Park J, Kim HY, Lee SI, Park JO, Kim K, Kim WS, Jung CW, Park YS, et al. Primary pulmonary non-Hodgkin's lymphoma. *Jpn J Clin Oncol* 2004;34(9):510–4.

Reyes CV, Jensen JA, Chinoy M. Pulmonary lymphoma in cardiac transplant patients treated with OKT3 for rejection: diagnosis by fine-needle aspiration. *Diagn Cytopathol* 1995;12(1): 32–6.

INFLAMMATORY MYOFIBROBLASTIC TUMOR

Cessna MH, Zhou H, Sanger WG, Perkins SL, Tripp S, Pickering D, Daines C, Coffin CM. Expression of ALK1 and p80 in inflammatory myofibroblastic tumor and its mesenchymal mimics: a study of 135 cases. *Mod Pathol* 2002;15(9):931–8.

Gal AA, Nassar VH, Miller JI. Cytopathologic diagnosis of pulmonary sclerosing hemangioma. *Diagn Cytopathol* 2002;26(3):163–6.

Machicao CN, Sorensen K, Abdul-Karim FW, Somrak TM. Transthoracic needle aspiration biopsy in inflammatory pseudotumors of the lung. *Diagn Cytopathol* 1989;5(4):400–3.

Thunnissen FB, Arends JW, Buchholtz RT, ten Velde G. Fine needle aspiration cytology of inflammatory pseudotumor of the lung (plasma cell granuloma). Report of four cases. *Acta Cytol* 1989;33(6):917–21.

Yousem SA, Shaw H, Cieply K. Involvement of 2p23 in pulmonary inflammatory pseudotumors. *Hum Pathol* 2001;32(4):428–33.

SARCOMA

Crosby JH, Hooeg K, Hager B. Transthoracic fine needle aspiration of primary and metastatic sarcomas. *Diagn Cytopathol* 1985;1(3):221–7.

Hummel P, Cangiarella JF, Cohen JM, Yang G, Waisman J, Chhieng DC. Transthoracic fine-needle aspiration biopsy of pulmonary spindle cell and mesenchymal lesions: a study of 61 cases. *Cancer* 2001;93(3):187–98.

Kim K, Naylor B, Han IH. Fine needle aspiration cytology of sarcomas metastatic to the lung. *Acta Cytol* 1986;30(6):688–94.

METASTATIC MALIGNANCY

Flint A, Lloyd RV. Colon carcinoma metastatic to the lung. Cytologic manifestations and distinction from primary pulmonary adenocarcinoma. *Acta Cytol* 1992;36(2):230–5.

Perry MD, Gore M, Seigler HF, Johnston WW. Fine needle aspiration biopsy of metastatic melanoma. A morphologic analysis of 174 cases. *Acta Cytol* 986;30(4):385–96.

Zaman MB, Hajdu SI, Melamed MR, Watson RC. Transthoracic aspiration cytology of pulmonary lesions. *Semin Diagn Pathol* 1986;3(3):176–87.

PLEURA MALIGNANT MESOTHELIOMA

Nguyen GK, Akin MR, Villanueva RR, Slatnik J. Cytopathology of malignant mesothelioma of the pleura in fine-needle aspiration biopsy. *Diagn Cytopathol* 1999;21(4):253–9.

Nguyen GK. Cytopathology of pleural mesotheliomas. *Am J Clin Pathol* 2000;114 Suppl:S68–81.

Ordonez NG. Immunohistochemical diagnosis of epithelioid mesotheliomas: a critical review of old markers, new markers. *Hum Pathol* 2002;33(10):953–67.

Pistolesi M, Rusthoven J. Malignant pleural mesothelioma: update, current management, and newer therapeutic strategies. *Chest* 2004;126(4):1318–29.

SOLITARY FIBROUS TUMOR

Ali SZ, Hoon V, Hoda S, Heelan R, Zakowski MF. Solitary fibrous tumor. A cytologic histologic study with clinical, radiologic, and immunohistochemical correlations. *Cancer* 1997;81(2):116–21.

Clayton AC, Salomao DR, Keeney GL, Nascimento AG. Solitary fibrous tumor: a study of cytologic features of six cases diagnosed by fine-needle aspiration. *Diagn Cytopathol* 2001;25(3):172–6.

Hasegawa T, Matsuno Y, Shimoda T, Hirohashi S, Hirose T, Sano T. Frequent expression of bcl-2 protein in solitary fibrous tumors. *Jpn J Clin Oncol* 1998;28(2):86–91.

MEDIASTINUM

CYST

Panelli F, Erickson RA, Prasad VM. Evaluation of mediastinal masses by endoscopic ultrasound and endoscopic ultrasound-guided fine needle aspiration. *Am J Gastroenterol* 2001;96(2):401–8.

Powers CN, Geisinger, K. R. Fine needle aspiration biopsy of the mediastinum: an overview. *Pathol Case Rev* 2001;6(2):49–58.

Suster S, Rosai J. Cystic thymomas. A clinicopathologic study of ten cases. *Cancer* 1992;69(1):92–7.

Wakely PE, Jr. Thymic cysts: an association with thymic neoplasia. *Pathol Case Rev* 2001;6(2):59–63.

THYMOMA

Duwe BV, Sterman DH, Musani AI. Tumors of the mediastinum. *Chest* 2005;128(4):2893–909.

Pantidou A, Kiziridou A, Antoniadis T, Tsilikas C, Destouni C. Mediastinum thymoma diagnosed by FNA and ThinPrep technique: a case report. *Diagn Cytopathol* 2006;34(1):37–40.

Powers CN, Geisinger KR. Fine needle aspiration biopsy of the mediastinum: an overview. *Pathology Case Rev* 2001;6(2):49–58.

Shabb NS, Fahl M, Shabb B, Haswani P, Zaatari G. Fine-needle aspiration of the mediastinum: a clinical, radiologic, cytologic, and histologic study of 42 cases. *Diagn Cytopathol* 1998;19(6):428–36.

Shin HJ, Katz RL. Thymic neoplasia as represented by fine needle aspiration biopsy of anterior mediastinal masses. A practical approach to the differential diagnosis. *Acta Cytol* 1998;42(4):855–64.

Wakely PE, Jr. Cytopathology-histopathology of the mediastinum: epithelial, lymphoproliferative, and germ cell neoplasms. *Ann Diagn Pathol* 2002;6(1):30–43.

THYMIC CARCINOMA

Dorfman DM, Shahsafaei A, Chan JK. Thymic carcinomas, but not thymomas and carcinomas of other sites, show CD5 immunoreactivity. *Am J Surg Pathol* 1997;21(8):936–40.

Duwe BV, Sterman DH, Musani AI. Tumors of the mediastinum. *Chest* 2005;128(4):2893–909.

Kaw YT, Esparza AR. Fine needle aspiration cytology of primary squamous cell carcinoma of the thymus. A case report. *Acta Cytol* 1993;37(5):735–9.

Posligua L, Ylagan L. Fine-needle aspiration cytology of thymic basaloid carcinoma: case studies and review of the literature. *Diagn Cytopathol* 2006;34(5):358–66.

Tanaka T, Morishita Y, Mori Y, Shimonaka E. Fine needle aspiration cytology of mucoepidermoid carcinoma of the thymus. *Cytopathology* 1990;1(1):49–53.

Wakely PE, Jr. Cytopathology-histopathology of the mediastinum: epithelial, lymphoproliferative, and germ cell neoplasms. *Ann Diagn Pathol* 2002;6(1):30–43.

THYMIC CARCINOID

Duwe BV, Sterman DH, Musani AI. Tumors of the mediastinum. *Chest* 2005;128(4):2893–909.

Gherardi G, Marveggio C, Placidi A. Neuroendocrine carcinoma of the thymus: aspiration biopsy, immunocytochemistry, and clinicopathologic correlates. *Diagn Cytopathol* 1995;12(2):158–64.

Gonzalez-Campora R, Otal-Salaverri C, Panea-Flores P, Lerma-Puertas E, Galera Davidson, H. Fine needle aspiration cytology of paraganglionic tumors. *Acta Cytol* 1988;32(3):386–90.

Tseng FY, Hsiao YL, Chang TC. Ultrasound-guided fine needle aspiration cytology of parathyroid lesions. A review of 72 cases. *Acta Cytol* 2002;46(6):1029–36.

Wang DY, Kuo SH, Chang DB, Yang PC, Lee YC, Hsu HC, Luh KT. Fine needle aspiration cytology of thymic carcinoid tumor. *Acta Cytol* 1995;39(3):423–7.

PRIMARY MEDIASTINAL LARGE B-CELL LYMPHOMA

Glaser SL, Lin RJ, Stewart SL, Ambinder RF, Jarrett RF, Brousset P, Pallesen G, Gulley ML, Khan G, O'Grady J and others. Epstein-Barr virus-associated Hodgkin's disease: epidemiologic characteristics in international data. *Int J Cancer* 1997;70(4):375–82.

Kardos TF, Vinson JH, Behm FG, Frable WJ, O'Dowd GJ. Hodgkin's disease: diagnosis by fine-needle aspiration biopsy. Analysis of cytologic criteria from a selected series. *Am J Clin Pathol* 1986;86(3):286–91.

Kuppers R. Molecular biology of Hodgkin's lymphoma. *Adv Cancer Res* 2002;84:277–312.

Powers CN, Geisinger KR. Fine needle aspiration biopsy of the mediastinum: an overview. *Pathology Case Rev* 2001;6(2):49–58.

Wakely PE, Jr. Cytopathology-histopathology of the mediastinum: epithelial, lymphoproliferative, and germ cell neoplasms. *Ann Diagn Pathol* 2002;6(1):30–43.

PRECURSOR T-CELL LYMPHOBLASTIC LYMPHOMA

Friedman HD, Hutchison RE, Kohman LJ, Powers CN. Thymoma mimicking lymphoblastic lymphoma: a pitfall in fine-needle aspiration biopsy interpretation. *Diagn Cytopathol* 1996;14(2):165–9; discussion 169–71.

Jacobs JC, Katz RL, Shabb N, el-Naggar A, Ordonez NG, Pugh W. Fine needle aspiration of lymphoblastic lymphoma. A multiparameter diagnostic approach. *Acta Cytol* 1992;36(6):887–94.

Kardos TF, Sprague RI, Wakely PE, Jr., Frable WJ. Fine-needle aspiration biopsy of lymphoblastic lymphoma and leukemia. A clinical, cytologic, and immunologic study. *Cancer* 1987;60(10):2448–53.

Powers CN, Geisinger KR. Fine needle aspiration biopsy of the mediastinum: an overview. *Pathology Case Rev* 2001;6(2):49–58.

Szczepanski T, Pongers-Willemse MJ, Langerak AW, Harts WA, Wijkhuijs AJ, van Wakely PE, Jr. Cytopathology-histopathology of the mediastinum: epithelial, lymphoproliferative, and germ cell neoplasms. *Ann Diagn Pathol* 2002;6(1):30–43.

Wering ER, van Dongen JJ. Ig heavy chain gene rearrangements in T-cell acute lymphoblastic leukemia exhibit predominant DH6-19 and DH7-27 gene usage, can result in complete V-D-J rearrangements, and are rare in T-cell receptor alpha beta lineage. *Blood* 1999;93(12):4079–85.

HODGKIN LYMPHOMA

Glaser SL, Lin RJ, Stewart SL, Ambinder RF, Jarrett RF, Brousset P, Pallesen G, Gulley ML, Khan G, O'Grady J and others. Epstein-Barr virus-associated Hodgkin's disease: epidemiologic characteristics in international data. *Int J Cancer* 1997;70(4):375–82.

Kardos TF, Vinson JH, Behm FG, Frable WJ, O'Dowd GJ. Hodgkin's disease: diagnosis by fine-needle aspiration biopsy. Analysis of cytologic criteria from a selected series. *Am J Clin Pathol* 1986;86(3):286–91.

Kuppers R. Molecular biology of Hodgkin's lymphoma. *Adv Cancer Res* 2002;84:277–312.

Powers CN, Geisinger KR Fine needle aspiration biopsy of the mediastinum: an overview. *Pathology Case Rev* 2001;6(2):49–58.

Wakely PE, Jr. Cytopathology–histopathology of the mediastinum: epithelial, lymphoproliferative, and germ cell neoplasms. *Ann Diagn Pathol* 2002;6(1):30–43.

MEDIASTINAL TERATOMA

Dominguez Malagon H, Perez Montiel D. Mediastinal germ cell tumors. *Semin Diagn Pathol* 2005;22(3):230–40.

Motoyama T, Yamamoto O, Iwamoto H, Watanabe H. Fine needle aspiration cytology of primary mediastinal germ cell tumors. *Acta Cytol* 1995;39(4):725–32.

Powers CN, Geisinger, K. R. Fine needle aspiration biopsy of the mediastinum: an overview. *Patholgy Case Rev* 2001;6(2):49–58.

MEDIASTINAL SEMINOMA

Chhieng DC, Lin O, Moran CA, Eltoum IA, Jhala NC, Jhala DN, Simsir A. Fine-needle aspiration biopsy of nonteratomatous germ cell tumors of the mediastinum. *Am J Clin Pathol* 2002;118(3):418–24.

Dominguez Malagon H, Perez Montiel D. Mediastinal germ cell tumors. *Semin Diagn Pathol* 2005;22(3):230–40.

Kwon MS. Aspiration cytology of mediastinal seminoma: report of a case with emphasis on the diagnostic role of aspiration cytology, cell block and immunocytochemistry. *Acta Cytol* 2005;49(6):669–72.

Wakely PE, Jr. Cytopathology-histopathology of the mediastinum: epithelial, lymphoproliferative, and germ cell neoplasms. *Ann Diagn Pathol* 2002;6(1):30–43.

Powers CN, Geisinger, K. R. Fine needle aspiration biopsy of the mediastinum: an overview. *Patholgy Case Rev* 2001;6(2):49–58.

MEDIASTINAL NONSEMINOMATOUS GERM CELL TUMORS

Chhieng DC, Lin O, Moran CA, Eltoum IA, Jhala NC, Jhala DN, Simsir A. Fine-needle aspiration biopsy of nonteratomatous germ cell tumors of the mediastinum. *Am J Clin Pathol* 2002;118(3):418–24.

Dominguez Malagon H, Perez Montiel D. Mediastinal germ cell tumors. *Semin Diagn Pathol* 2005;22(3):230–40.

Powers CN, Geisinger, K. R. Fine needle aspiration biopsy of the mediastinum: an overview. *Patholgy Case Rev* 2001;6(2):49–58.

Wakely PE, Jr. Cytopathology-histopathology of the mediastinum: epithelial, lymphoproliferative, and germ cell neoplasms. *Ann Diagn Pathol* 2002;6(1):30–43.

BENIGN PERIPHERAL NERVE SHEATH TUMOR (SCHWANNOMA AND NEUROFIBROMA)

Duwe BV, Sterman DH, Musani AI. Tumors of the mediastinum. *Chest* 2005;128(4):2893–909.

Mooney EE, Layfield LJ, Dodd LG. Fine-needle aspiration of neural lesions. *Diagn Cytopathol* 1999;20(1):1–5.

Powers CN, Geisinger KR. Fine needle aspiration biopsy of the mediastinum: an overview. *Patholgy Case Rev* 2001;6(2):49–58.

Resnick JM, Fanning CV, Caraway NP, Varma DG, Johnson M. Percutaneous needle biopsy diagnosis of benign neurogenic neoplasms. *Diagn Cytopathol* 1997;16(1):17–25.

Slagel DD, Powers CN, Melaragno MJ, Geisinger KR, Frable WJ, Silverman JF. Spindle cell lesions of the mediastinum: diagnosis by fine-needle aspiration biopsy. *Diagn Cytopathol* 1997;17(3):167–76.

Wakely PE, Jr. Cytopathology-histopathology of the mediastinum II. Mesenchymal, neural, and neuroendocrine neoplasms. *Ann Diagn Pathol* 2005;9(1):24–32.

MALIGNANT PERIPHERAL NERVE SHEATH TUMOR

Das DK, Gupta AK, Chowdhury V, Satsangi DK, Tyagi S, Mohan JC, Khan VA, Malhotra V. Fine-needle aspiration diagnosis of carotid body tumor: report of a case and review of experience with cytologic features in four cases. *Diagn Cytopathol* 1997;17(2):143–7.

Duwe BV, Sterman DH, Musani AI. Tumors of the mediastinum. *Chest* 2005;128(4):2893–909.

Mooney EE, Layfield LJ, Dodd LG. Fine-needle aspiration of neural lesions. *Diagn Cytopathol* 1999;20(1):1–5.

Slagel DD, Powers CN, Melaragno MJ, Geisinger KR, Frable WJ, Silverman JF. Spindle cell lesions of the mediastinum: diagnosis by fine-needle aspiration biopsy. *Diagn Cytopathol* 1997;17(3):167–76.

Wakely PE, Jr. Cytopathology-histopathology of the mediastinum II. Mesenchymal, neural, and neuroendocrine neoplasms. *Ann Diagn Pathol* 2005;9(1):24–32.

PARAGANGLIOMA

Das DK, Gupta AK, Chowdhury V, Satsangi DK, Tyagi S, Mohan JC, Khan VA, Malhotra V. Fine-needle aspiration diagnosis of carotid body tumor: report of a case and review of experience with cytologic features in four cases. *Diagn Cytopathol* 1997;17(2):143–7.

Rana RS, Dey P, Das A. Fine needle aspiration (FNA) cytology of extra-adrenal paragangliomas. *Cytopathology* 1997;8(2):108–13.

Wakely PE, Jr. Cytopathology-histopathology of the mediastinum II. Mesenchymal, neural, and neuroendocrine neoplasms. *Ann Diagn Pathol* 2005;9(1):24–32.

GANGLIONEUROMA

Domanski HA. Fine-needle aspiration of ganglioneuroma. *Diagn Cytopathol* 2005;32(6):363–6

Powers CN, Gelslnger KR. Fine needle aspiration biopsy of the mediastinum: an overview. *Patholgy Case Rev* 2001;6(2):49–58.

Wakely PE, Jr. Cytopathology-histopathology of the mediastinum II. Mesenchymal, neural, and neuroendocrine neoplasms. *Ann Diagn Pathol* 2005;9(1):24–32.

NEUROBLASTOMA AND GANGLIONEUROBLASTOMA

Duwe BV, Sterman DH, Musani AI. Tumors of the mediastinum. *Chest* 2005;128(4):2893–909.

Frostad B, Tani E, Kogner P, Maeda S, Bjork O, Skoog L. The clinical use of fine needle aspiration cytology for diagnosis and management of children with neuroblastic tumours. *Eur J Cancer* 1998;34(4):529–36.

Mooney EE, Layfield LJ, Dodd LG. Fine-needle aspiration of neural lesions. *Diagn Cytopathol* 1999;20(1):1–5.

Powers CN, Geisinger KR. Fine needle aspiration biopsy of the mediastinum: an overview. *Patholgy Case Rev* 2001;6(2):49–58.

Wakely PE, Jr. Cytopathology-histopathology of the mediastinum II. Mesenchymal, neural, and neuroendocrine neoplasms. *Ann Diagn Pathol* 2005;9(1):24–32.

15

Liver

Shriram Jakate, Antonino Di Certo, and Paolo Gattuso

CONGENITAL CYSTS

Clinical Features
▪ May present at any age including adulthood and more common in females
▪ Congenital dilatations of parts of the bile duct system or peribiliary glands. Rarely these cysts may represent intestinal duplications (ciliated hepatic foregut cysts)
▪ Classified by size, number, and location (intra- or extrahepatic choledochal cyst)
▪ Rarely cause symptoms when small but when large (>8 cm) symptoms may include abdominal pain, RUQ mass, nausea, and jaundice
▪ May be associated with autosomal dominant or recessive polycystic kidney disease

Cytologic Features
▪ Usually the FNA material contains clear, straw-colored fluid

- Sparse bile duct epithelium and macrophages are present in the aspirated material
- Hepatocytes rarely seen
- Squamous metaplasia of the bile ducts can be seen
- Bile pigments and calcific debris can be present

Special Stains and Immunohistochemistry
- The lining of the cyst is usually composed of biliary epithelium, which is stainable by cytokeratins 7 and 19, CEA (cytoplasmic), and EMA

Modern Techniques for Diagnosis
- Noncontributory

Differential Diagnosis
- Noncontributory

PEARLS

* Squamous cell carcinoma or adenocarcinoma may complicate the course
* Polycystic disease of the kidney and lung is associated with congenital liver cysts

HYDATID CYST

Clinical Features
- Caused by larval forms of Helminth Cestode tapeworm, most frequently *Echinococcus granulosus* (adult worm is about 5 mm long and the scolex has 4 suckers and double row of twenty-eight to fifty hooklets)
- Dogs and sheep are the commonest definitive and intermediate hosts respectively
- Most patients are adults (mean age of diagnosis: forty-five years)
- Most cases are asymptomatic and cysts are discovered incidentally by imaging
- Cyst grows slowly (about 1 cm per year) and becomes symptomatic when large (>10 cm) due to growth and compression causing hepatomegaly, portal hypertension, and jaundice
- Rupture of cysts may result in anaphylaxis and seeding of abdomen and other organs

Cytologic Features
- The diagnostic cytologic material is the presence of scolices or hooklets

Special Stains and Immunohistochemistry
- The scolices are highlighted by PAS and GMS
- The suckers within the scolices contains hooklets stainable by acid-fast (Ziel–Neelson) and trichrome stains

Modern Techniques for Diagnosis
- Noncontributory

Differential Diagnosis
- Noncontributory

PEARLS

* Spillage of the cystic fluid content may cause anaphylactic reaction; FNA should be avoided if an ecchynococcal cyst is clinical suspected

ABSCESS

Clinical Features
▇ Acute hepatitis caused by several infectious agents may result in microabscess or pyogenic abscess formation
▇ Infectious agents include bacteria, mycobacteria, actinomycosis, spirochetes, fungi, parasites, and viruses
▇ Infections may reach the liver via portal vein from organs such as appendix, intestine, and pancreas, by way of hepatic artery in septicemia and through biliary tree in suppurative obstructive and nonobstructive cholangitis
▇ Right upper quadrant pain and tenderness and fever are consistent clinical finding
▇ Prognosis varies depending upon the size and multiplicity of lesions, infectious agent, immune status, and underlying disease

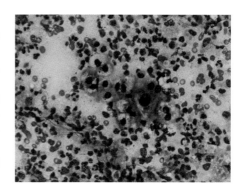

15-1. Abscess. The center of the microphotograph shows a cluster of hepatocytes surrounded by a neutrophilic exudate and macrophages (modified Giemsa stain)

Cytologic Features
▇ The cytologic material aspirated consists of neutrophils, macrophages, and reactive epithelial cells
▇ Amebic abscess, lacks significant inflammation. However, necrotic hepatocytes and macrophages are present

Special Stains and Immunohistochemistry
▇ Clinically and/or cytologically suspected infectious agent can be examined directly (parasites), by special stains such as Gram, PAS, GMS, AFB, or immunohistochemistry for suspected organism

Modern Techniques for Diagnosis
▇ Culture studies and detection of specific microbial DNA or RNA

Differential Diagnosis
▇ Metastatic tumors with marked inflammatory response a necrosis may obscure the neoplastic cells

PEARLS
★ Aspiration of the wall should be attempted to demonstrate possible amebic organisms

GRANULOMAS

Clinical Features
▇ Granulomas occur commonly (about 10%) in the liver in a broad variety of conditions including specific liver diseases, as incidental finding, and as a part of systemic granulomatous process
▇ Causes of granulomas are numerous and include infections, immunological diseases, foreign materials, neoplasia, hypersensitivity, and miscellaneous conditions
▇ Most common causes are sarcoidosis, primary biliary cirrhosis, lipogranuloma, and foreign materials
▇ Patients may be asymptomatic or have vague abdominal pain, weight loss, and fever

Cytologic Features

■ Collections of epitheliod histiocytes arc diagnostics of granumatous inflammation
■ Multinucleated giant cells may be present
■ If necrosis is present you may consider tuberculosis

Special Stains and Immunohistochemistry

■ Foreign material may be demonstrated by polarizing microscopy and infectious agents by special stains (Gram, PAS, GMS, AFB)

Modern Techniques for Diagnosis

■ Noncontributory

Differential Diagnosis

■ Noncontributory

PEARLS

★ Many clinical entities can produce morphologically similar granulomas, and the cause is not clear from the FNA material

HEMANGIOMA

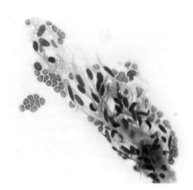

15-2. Hemangioma. Cluster of uniform spindle cells, some of which show classic nuclear envelope notch (modified Giemsa stain)

Clinical Features

■ The most common benign lesion in the liver (incidence ranges from 0.4% to 20% of the population) and the most common location for visceral cavernous hemangioma
■ Occurs in all ages but more commonly found in adults
■ More frequent in females and may enlarge or rupture during pregnancy or estrogen therapy
■ Usually single, small (less than 5 cm) and flat subcapsular lesions but occasionally may be quite large (>10 cm "giant hemangioma")
■ Often incidentally detected but symptoms may occur in relation to large size (pain or swelling), rupture (hemoperitoneum) and consumption coagulopathy

Cytologic Features

■ Aspiration of fresh blood
■ Endothelial cells, usually single or in small groups
■ The nuclei have fine chromatin pattern with longitudinal nuclear groove
■ Binucleation may be seen
■ Fibrovascular connective tissue or smooth muscle can be present

Special Stains and Immunohistochemistry

■ Vimentin and endothelial markers such as CD31, CD34, and Factor VIII are positive

Modern Technique for Diagnosis

■ Noncontributory

Differential Diagnosis

■ Angiomyolipoma
 ➤ Adipose tissue
 ➤ Smooth muscle cells
 ➤ Endothelial cells

★ Cell block material may be useful to increase the sensitivity
★ Bleeding can be a complication to the FNA procedure. However, it is not a contra-indication

FOCAL NODULAR HYPERPLASIA

Clinical Features

▪ Nonneoplastic lesion is composed of central stellate fibrous scar with thick-walled arteries, proliferating periseptal cholangioles, and surrounding hyperplastic nodular parenchyma
▪ Most common in females (90%) and adults but may occur in males and children
▪ Often liver function tests are normal and the mass is incidentally detected in an asymptomatic patient. Rarely, there may be abdominal discomfort or pain
▪ Often the mass is single (85%) and circumscribed and varies from 1 to 10 cm (generally less than 5 cm). Multiplicity may be associated with other vascular malformations
▪ Thought to be hyperplastic response to localized anomalous angio-genesis. Unlike hepatocellular adenoma, etiological relationship with oral contraceptives is not determined

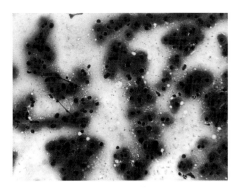

15-3. Focal nodular hyperplasia. Population of small uniform hepatocytes lacking nuclear enlargement or atypia (modified Giemsa stain)

Cytologic Features

▪ Cellular cytologic smears composed mainly of small to normal hep-atocytes
▪ Minimal nuclear enlargement or atypia
▪ Reactive bile duct epithelium is usually present
▪ Spindle-shaped Kupffer cells, chronic inflammation, and fibrous tissue can be also present
▪ Hemorrhage, necrosis, and mitoses are not usually present in focal nodular hyperplasia
▪ Bile stasis may be seen, but is not prominent

Special Stains and Immunohistochemistry

▪ Cytokeratin 7 is helpful in highlighting the periseptal proliferating cholangioles
▪ Stromal and vascular components from the scar show vimentin and smooth muscle actin positivity
▪ Markers such as CD10, Hep Par-1, CEA-P, and CD34 are useful to differentiate from metastatic tumors but are not helpful when trying to differentiate from hepatocellular carcinoma

Modern Technique for Diagnosis

▪ Noncontributory

Differential Diagnosis

▪ Liver cell adenoma
  ➤ Lack of bile duct epithelium
  ➤ Three-dimensional groups of hepatocytes
  ➤ Bile stasis uncommon
  ➤ Hemorrhage and necrosis can be prominent
▪ Hepatocellular carcinoma
  ➤ Lack of bile duct epithelium
  ➤ Lack of benign hepatocytes

> ➤ Trabecular pattern
> ➤ Nuclear pleomorphism is common
> ➤ Binucleation and multinucleation
> ➤ Prominent nucleoli
> ➤ Dense cytoplasm
> ➤ Bile production by malignant cells (in the cytoplasm of the hepatocytes or the canaliculi between the malignant cells)

PEARLS

★ The diagnosis of focal nodular hyperplasia on FNA material requires to be correlated with x-ray findings and clinical setting

HEPATOCELLULAR ADENOMA (LIVER CELL ADENOMA)

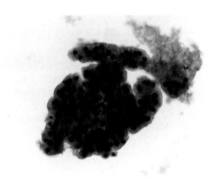

15-4. Hepatocellular adenoma (liver cell adenoma). Cluster of hepatocytes with mild nuclear enlargement and low nuclear/cytoplasmic ratio (Papanicolaou stain)

Clinical Features

▧ Benign neoplasm composed of cells resembling normal hepatocytes
▧ Strongly associated with long-term use of oral contraceptive and anabolic steroids and thus overwhelmingly common in females in the reproductive years (mean age thirty years)
▧ Usually solitary, between 5 and 15 cm and may bulge from the surface. Occasional multiplicity is seen and more commonly related to anabolic steroid use and rarely glycogenoses. When several nodules are present (>10), the term "adenomatosis" is recommended
▧ Unlike focal nodular hyperplasia more patients are symptomatic (90–95%) than asymptomatic and present with abdominal discomfort, palpable mass, episodic mild abdominal pain, or acute abdominal pain often related to intratumoral or intraperitoneal hemorrhage
▧ Risk of hemorrhage increases with pregnancy, large size and pedunculation and necessitates resection. Tumor rupture and intraperitoneal hemorrhage may cause mortality in up to 20% patients

Cytologic Features

▧ Lack of bile duct epithelium
▧ Hemorrhage and necrosis may be prominent
▧ Low nuclear/cytoplasmic ratio
▧ Benign-appearing hepatocytes with mild nuclear enlargement
▧ Smooth nuclear membranes
▧ Fat or glycogen accumulation in the cytoplasm can be marked
▧ Granulomas may be present

Special Stains and Immunohistochemistry

▧ Absence of cytokeratin 7 is helpful in demonstrating lack of biliary channels
▧ Markers such as CD10, Hep Par-1, CEA-P, and CD34 are useful to differentiate from metastatic tumors but are not helpful when trying to differentiate from hepatocellular carcinoma

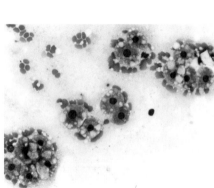

15-5. Hepatocellular adenoma (liver cell adenoma). Liver cell adenoma showing marked fatty metamorphosis (modified Giemsa stain)

Modern Technique for Diagnosis

▧ Noncontributory

Differential Diagnosis

▧ Well-differentiated hepatocellular carcinoma
  ➤ Almost impossible to differentiate from an adenoma

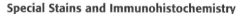

■ Focal nodular hyperplasia
➤ Is not possible at times on FNA material to differentiate an adenoma from FNH
➤ Hemorrhage and necrosis very uncommon
➤ Presence of bile ducts

★ Clinical and radiographic correlations are crucial in the interpretation of a benign hepatocellular neoplasm: adenoma/focal nodular hyperplasia

BILE DUCT HAMARTOMA (BILE DUCT ADENOMA)

Clinical Features
■ Always incidentally discovered at laparotomy or autopsy
■ Excised locally for concern about metastatic tumor in patients with known primary
■ Most are solitary, subcapsular, and small (<2 cm)
■ Benign behavior
■ It is a reactive growth of peribiliary glands (appropriately called peribiliary gland hamartoma) rather than adenoma

Cytologic Features
■ Usually hypocellular specimen due to fibrotic background
■ Uniform, two-dimensional monolayered ductal epithelium
■ Columnar appearance not unusual

Special Stains and Immunohistochemistry
■ Immunophenotype is that of biliary epithelium (cytokeratins 7 and 19, cytoplasmic CEA, EMA positive)

Modern Technique for Diagnosis
■ Noncontributory

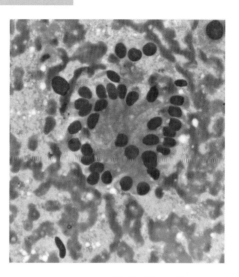

15-6. Bile duct hamartoma.
Cluster of uniform bile duct epithelium showing columnar arrangement (modified Giemsa stain)

Differential Diagnosis
■ Cholangiocarcinoma
➤ Atypical columnar cells with lost nuclear polarity
➤ Bile stasis

★ Not to be confused with cholangiocarcinoma

CIRRHOTIC NODULES, ADENOMATOUS HYPERPLASIA, AND DYSPLASIA

Clinical Features
■ Tumor-like 1–3 cm nodules within cirrhotic liver
■ These are referred to by various names roughly corresponding with presence or absence of atypia, dysplasia or carcinoma: macroregenerative nodule, adenomatous hyperplasia, dysplastic nodule (low and high grades and large cell and small cell), and well-differentiated hepatocellular carcinoma
■ The dysplastic nodules are considered precancerous or early hepatocellular carcinomas

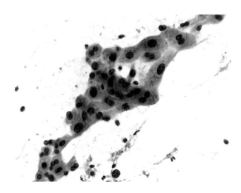

15-7. Adenomatous hyperplasia with associate dysplasia. Cluster of hepatocytes showing nuclear enlargement, binucleation, and presence of nucleoli. Cholestasis is also appreciated (Papanicolaou stain)

▥ Clinical findings correspond to underlying cirrhosis and these nodules are identified mainly by imaging studies

Cytologic Features
▥ Hepatocytes usually show reactive atypia
▥ Dysplatic changes of the hepatocytes can be seen, which include nuclear pleomorphism, coarse chromatin pattern, irregular nuclear membranes, binucleation, and large macronucleoli
▥ Bile duct proliferation is quite common cytologic finding
▥ Connective tissue also can be present
▥ Mature lymphoid cells are commonly seen in the background of the smear
▥ Necrosis and mitosis may occur

Special Stains and Immunohistochemistry
▥ Reticulin stain helps in assessing stratified cell plates and CD34 in activated sinusoidal endothelium
▥ Markers such as Hep Par-1, and pericanalicular CEA-P, CD10 highlight the hepatocytic origin but do not provide any marker for dysplasia

Modern Technique for Diagnosis
▥ Noncontributory

Differential Diagnosis
▥ Hepatocellular carcinoma
  ➤ Lack of bile duct cells
  ➤ Trabecular growth partially lined by sinusoidal endothelial cells
  ➤ Dense granular cytoplasm
  ➤ Atypical stripped nuclei and tumor giant cells

PEARLS

★ Reactive atypia and nuclear dysplasia should not be confused with a neoplastic process (hepatocellular carcinoma)

HEPATOCELLULAR CARCINOMA

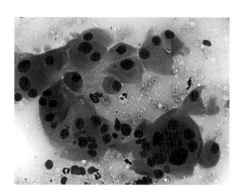

15-8. Hepatocellular carcinoma. Neoplastic hepatocytes with polygonal dense cytoplasm. Binucleation and multinucleation is evident (modified Giemsa stain)

Clinical Features
▥ The commonest primary malignant tumor of the liver and one of the commonest cancers worldwide. Wide geographic variation in incidence based upon variations in common etiological factors such as hepatitis viruses B and C, alcohol abuse, and diet including aflatoxin
▥ Strong association with underlying cirrhosis (75–90%) independent of its etiology
▥ More common in males in the ratio of 2:1 to 5:1. The majority of patients are older than fifty years of age presumably related to increasing likelihood of exposure to etiological factors and latency period for development of cirrhosis
▥ Clinical presentation commonly includes features of underlying cirrhosis with decompensation and ascites, hepatomegaly, abdominal pain, hemorrhage and weight loss. Surveillance of patients with cirrhosis based upon imaging studies and serum AFP (significant increase: >500 ng/ml in 70–90% cases) may lead to early detection

▦ Tumor invasion in the portal and hepatic veins with resultant obstructive syndromes may occur and rarely paraneoplastic syndromes such as hypoglycemia, erythrocytosis, and hypercalcemia are described

▦ Tumor may be of any size and present as a solitary mass, multiple nodules, or massive involvement of liver with large mass or numerous "cirrhosis-like" nodules

▦ A variety of cytoarchitectural patterns are described (trabecular, pseudoglandular, pleomorphic, sarcomatous, clear cell, combined hepatocellular- cholangiocarcinoma), but fibrolamellar carcinoma is the only variant distinctively different clinically, radiologically, and cytologically

▦ The prognosis of unresectable hepatocellular carcinoma in symptomatic patients is generally poor (<5% five-year survival). Asymptomatic patients with treatable tumors (resection or transplantation) are likely to show long-term survival

▦ Fibrolamellar carcinoma occurs in noncirrhotic livers, younger patients (mean age 23), nearly equally in both genders, more commonly in the left lobe (two-thirds of the cases), and shows central stellate scar reminiscent of FNH and normal levels of AFP. Prognosis is better (56% five-year survival) owing to better respectability and lack of underlying chronic liver disease

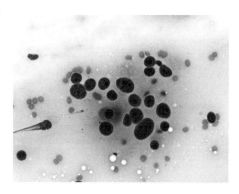

15-9. Hepatocellular carcinoma.
Characteristic naked nuclei seen in the background of a hepatocellular (modified Giemsa stain)

Cytologic Features

▦ Lack of bile duct cells

▦ Lack of benign hepatocytes

▦ Polygonal cells with dense cytoplasm, centrally located nuclei, and prominent nucleoi

▦ Single cells or in three-dimensional groups

▦ Trabecular growth is characteristic

▦ Sinusoidal endothelial cells partially lining balls of tumor cells

▦ Acinar pattern is relatively common

▦ Binucleation/multinucleation

▦ The background shows atypical naked nuclei, at times can be a large amount

▦ Nuclear membrane irregularity

▦ Intranuclear cytoplasmic inclusions

▦ Bile production can be considered pathognomonic

▦ Cytoplasmic hyaline inclusions (α1-antitrypsin, α-fetoprotein) are the most commonly seen

▦ Fatty changes can be seen in the cytoplasm mimicking liposarcoma

▦ Fibrolamellar variant of hepatocellular carcinoma

  ➤ The cytologic features similar to the ordinary hepatocellular carcinoma

  ➤ Bile duct cells can be seen

  ➤ Oncocytic dense granular cytoplasm

  ➤ Dense fibrous connective tissue

  ➤ Intracytoplasmic pale bodies characteristic of fibrolamellar hepatocellular carcinoma (intracellular lumina lined by microvilli)

▦ Acinar or adenoid HCC

  ➤ Pseudoglandular patter, usually focal

  ➤ Dense granular cytoplasm

  ➤ Intranuclear cytoplasmic invagination

  ➤ Hyaline cytoplasmuc inclusions

▦ Clear cell type HCC

  ➤ Significant proportion of clear cells

  ➤ Classic HCC is usually present in the smears

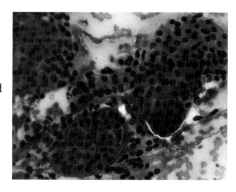

15-10. Hepatocellular carcinoma.
Sinusoidal endothelial cells partially lining balls of tumor cells (modified Giemsa stain)

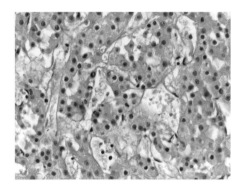

15-11. Hepatocellular carcinoma.
Cell block material of the
aspirated material from Figure 15-10
showing prominent sinusoidal
endothelial cells (H&E stain)

➤ The cytoplasm is foamy and bubbly
➤ Can be confused with other clear cell carcinoma, for example, renal,
cortical and ovary
▦ Giant cell HC
  ➤ Many giant cells have to be present
  ➤ Giant cells usually are large and polygonal and the nuclei contain prominent nucleoli
▦ Sarcomatoid HCC
  ➤ Rarely seen in his pure form, usually associated with classic HCC
  ➤ Metaplastic bone and cartilage can be present
  ➤ Can be confused with primary and/or metastatic sarcoma
  ➤ Increased connective tissue
▦ Sclerotic HCC
  ➤ Seen in noncirrhotic liver
  ➤ The cytologic features are similar to the classic HCC
  ➤ Marked increase stromal connective tissue

Special Stains and Immunohistochemistry
▦ CEA-Polyclonal and CD10 show pericanalicular staining typical of hepatocellular origin
▦ Hep Par-1 positivity is useful in less differentiated tumors
▦ CD34 marks activated sinusoidal endothelium and thickened cell plates
▦ Reticulin stain helps in assessing stratified hepatocytic cell plates
▦ Cytokeratin 8/18 is positive and CK7, 20 and AE1/AE3 are generally negative
▦ AFP is positive in a minority of cases (<25%), even when there is serological positivity

Modern Technique for Diagnosis
▦ In undifferentiated tumors ultrastructural demonstration of bile canaliculi is diagnostic
▦ In some studies P53 mutation is suggestive of progression

Differential Diagnosis
▦ Metastatic adenocarcinoma
  ➤ Common acinar formation
  ➤ Lack of trabecular pattern
  ➤ Often vacuolated cytoplasm
  ➤ Necrosis often present
  ➤ Hyline globules, Mallory bodies rarely seen
  ➤ Mucin material often present
  ➤ Bile production absent
  ➤ CEA diffuse positivity
  ➤ AFP negative
▦ Cholangiocarcinoma
  ➤ Columnar cells
  ➤ Bile stasis
  ➤ Delicate, squamoid cytoplasm
  ➤ May show signet ring features
  ➤ Wide range of differentiation (bland to frankly malignant)
▦ Mixed hepatocellular/cholangiocarcinoma
  ➤ Rarely seen
  ➤ Both components are present
▦ Nodular regeneration
  ➤ Mixed cell types

> Bile duct cells present
> Smooth nuclear membranes
> Scattered atypical cells
> Thin trabecular structures
- Melanoma
  > Granular cytoplasm
  > Intranuclear cytoplasmic inclusions
  > Binucleation
  > Prominent nucleoli
  > Melanin pigments
  > Single cells with eccentric located nuclei
- Renal cell carcinoma
  > Oncocytic and clear cell variant may mimic hepatocellular carcinoma

⋆ Mimics of hepatocellular carcinoma are metastatic melanoma and renal cell carcinoma
⋆ Scattered atypical hepatocellular nuclei, trabecular pattern, and peripherally arranged endothelium around the trabeculae are quite characteristic of hepatocellular carcinoma
⋆ High nuclear/cytoplasmic ratio

HEPATOBLASTOMA

Clinical Features
- Most common liver neoplasm in children and a malignant tumor simulating divergent embryonal patterns of differentiation ranging from undifferentiated embryonal cells, immature or fetal hepatocytes, to differentiated mesenchymal tissue such as skeletal muscle and osteoid
- Most cases (90%) occur under five years of age with male predominance of 1.5–2:1
- Associated with numerous clinical syndromes (such as familial polyposis, Beckwith–Wiedemann syndrome, low birth weight), congenital anomalies (such as trisomy 18, type 1a glycogen storage disease), and multiple other pediatric tumors (such as Wilms', gonadoblastoma)
- Commonest clinical finding is abdominal enlargement. Less commonly there may be weight loss, nausea, abdominal pain, vomiting, jaundice, anemia, and thrombocytopenia. Rarely tumor may produce HCG and other sex hormones leading to sexual precocity
- Usually single (80% cases) mass, more often in the right lobe with size varying from 5 to 22 cm
- Most cases (90%) have elevated AFP, which can be used to verify complete tumor resection and monitor for tumor recurrence

Cytologic Features
- Epithelial hepatoblastoma component may have anaplastic cells
  > Small blue cells similar to those of "neuroblastoma, Ewing sarcoma and Wilm's tumor"
- Embryonal cells
  > Small, oval to spindle-shaped cells with round to oval nuclei with scanty cytoplasm
  > Coarse, hyperchromatic nuclear chromatin, and prominent nucleoli
  > Frequent mitoses

■ Fetal cells
  ➤ Minimal pleomorphism
  ➤ Small round to oval nuclei with abundant cytoplasm resembling a normal fetal hepatocytes
  ➤ Hematopoietic cells
■ Mesenchymal component cells may have osteoid, squamous, muscle, and cartilage differentiation

Special Stains and Immunohistochemistry
■ The staining pattern matches the microscopic component:
■ Fetal – diffuse staining of sinusoidal endothelial cells by CD34, variable cytoplasmic glycogen (PAS positive, diastase sensitive) and lipid (Oil red O)
■ Embryonal – lack of fetal type staining
■ Mixed epithelial and mesenchymal – cytokeratin, EMA, vimentin, A1AT, AFP, CEA and chromogranin may be positive even in the mesenchymal cells suggestive of an epithelial origin of all cells

Modern Technique for Diagnosis
■ DNA ploidy – usually diploid in fetal type and aneuploid in embryonal and anaplastic types
■ Cytogenetic abnormalities such as trisomy for chromosomes 2 and 20 and LOH of 11p
■ P53 overexpression less frequent than other childhood tumors

Differential Diagnosis
■ Hepatocellular carcinoma
  ➤ Marked pleomorphism
  ➤ Giant tumor cells
  ➤ Usually seen in the pediatric group
  ➤ Dense granular cytoplasm
  ➤ Prominent nucleoli
  ➤ Complex branching and anastomosing thick trabeculae
  ➤ Naked nuclei can be numerous

PEARLS

★ Usually effects children younger than three years old
★ Presence of metaplastic epithelium favor the diagnosis of hepatoblastoma
★ Presence of extramedullary hematopoiesis

MESENCHYMAL HAMARTOMA

Clinical Features
■ Benign variably cystic lesion occurring in young children (under two years) with slight male predominance
■ Usually a single mass that can be very large (up to 30 cm), more commonly in the right lobe (75%)
■ Usual presentation is enlarging abdominal mass
■ May be associated with other findings of ductal plate malformation such as biliary hamartoma, polycystic liver disease, and congenital hepatic fibrosis
■ Prognosis is excellent after resection. Behavior of unresected lesions is not known and there is no firm evidence of malignant transformation

Cytologic Features
■ Mucoid background

■ Loose clusters of epithelial and mesenchymal spindle-shaped cells
■ Fragments of connective tissue

Special Stains and Immunohistochemistry
■ Vimentin is positive in mesenchymal cells
■ The bile duct epithelium is positive for the usual biliary markers (cytokeratins 7 and 19, CEA, and EMA)

Modern Technique for Diagnosis
■ Noncontributory

Differential Diagnosis
■ Hepatoblastoma, mixed type (epithelial/mesenchymal)
➤ Epithelial (small blue cells)
➤ Mesenchymal (embryonal, fetal, and mesenchymal component)

PEARLS

★ Pathologist should be aware of patient's age and cytologic features to reach the right diagnosis

CHOLANGIOCARCINOMA

Clinical Features
■ Cholangiocarcinoma may be intrahepatic (or peripheral) or extrahepatic (bile duct carcinoma) including hilar (Klatskin tumor)
■ Rare overall with marked geographical variation (high incidence in Southeastern Asia) but second most common (15%) among primary malignant liver tumors
■ In North America, mean age is sixty-two years with male predominance
■ Cause is unknown in many cases but parasitic liver flukes in Southeast Asia (clonorchiasis and opisthorchiasis), fibrocystic congenital biliary malformations (diffuse von Meyenburg complexes, congenital hepatic fibrosis, polycystic liver disease, Caroli disease), hepatolithiasis (oriental cholangiohepatitis), and primary sclerosing cholangitis (PSC) in IBD are known risk factors. PSC is also a risk factor for extrahepatic cholangiocarcinoma
■ Symptoms depend upon the location within the liver; peripheral tumor may be asymptomatic until it is large when there may be abdominal pain, weight loss, and fatigue; hilar and extrahepatic tumors cause jaundice more commonly
■ Majority of tumors show no underlying cirrhosis, but a variant associated with cirrhosis and/or hepatocellular carcinoma is known to occur
■ The intrahepatic tumor may be a solitary mass, a large mass with satellite smaller nodules, or multiple tumor nodules throughout the liver. Extrahepatic tumor may be diffuse bile duct thickening, stricture, or luminal growth
■ Prognosis is worse than hepatocellular carcinoma with five-year survival of 39% in mass-forming tumors

Cytologic Features
■ Columnar cells have granular bubbly amphophilic cytoplasm
■ Bile stasis
■ It may resemble signet ring carcinoma adenosquamous and squamous cell carcinoma

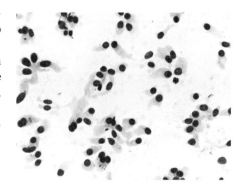

15-12. Cholangiocarcinoma.
Columnar cells with amphophilic cytoplasm and cholestasis (modified Giemsa stain)

- Microacinar formation
- Loss nuclear polarity
- Irregular nuclear membranes
- Sclerotic stroma

Special Stains and Immunohistochemistry
- Immunohistochemical stains such as cytokeratins 7 and 19, cytoplasmic CEA, EMA are useful for differentiation from HCC but not some metastatic tumors
- Mucin stains – mucicarmine, PAS, MUC (mucous core proteins) are positive

Modern Technique for Diagnosis
- KRAS and P53 mutations are most common

Differential Diagnosis
- Reactive atypia of bile duct epithelium
  - Reparative changes
  - Two-dimensional, monolayered bile duct epithelium
  - Less prominent nucleoi
  - Nuclear/cytoplasmic ratio not increased
  - No nuclear membrane irregularities
  - Benign squamous metaplasia
- Metastatic adenocarcinoma
  - Colon, pancreas, and stomach adenocarcinomas should be considered in the differential diagnosis

PEARLS

- Coexpression of cytokeratins 7 and 20 in cholangiocarcinoma it may help differentiate from hepatocellular carcinoma and metastatic colonic cancer
- Aspiration of single liver mass yielding a poor cellularity resulting from a high content of stromal tissue may suggest the diagnosis of cholangiocarcinoma

SARCOMAS

EMBRYONAL SARCOMA (UNDIFFERENTIATED SARCOMA)

Clinical Features
- Malignant mesenchymal tumor comprising about 6% of all childhood tumors
- Usually occurs between the ages of five and twenty years with equal sex incidence
- Common presentation is with abdominal pain and swelling. Rarely, the tumor invades the vena cava and grows into the right atrium mimicking primary cardiac tumor
- Prognosis has improved with modern therapy but is still poor at about 15% after five years

Special Stains and Immunohistochemistry
- The pleomorphic undifferentiated tumor cells are consistently positive for vimentin and variably positive for CD10 and keratins suggestive of undifferentiated (mesenchymal and epithelial) cell lineage
- The hyaline globules are positive for PAS with diastase and generally positive for alpha-1-antitrypsin, desmin, and muscle-specific actin

Modern Technique for Diagnosis
- Cell lineage determination can be attempted ultrastructurally. Consistent findings are secondary lysosomes with dense precipitates and dilated RERs (contributing to hyaline globules). Other multiple findings are variable and include fibroblastic,

rhabdomyoblastic and leiomyoblastic differentiation (hence 'embryonal' rather than 'undifferentiated' sarcoma)

ANGIOSARCOMA

Clinical Features
- A rare (1% of primary liver cancers) high-grade malignant neoplasm of endothelial cells but the commonest sarcoma arising in the liver
- Male predominance (3:1) and peak age in the sixth and seventh decade
- Most (75%) have no known etiology but the rest may have exposure to agents such as Thorotrast, vinyl chloride, arsenic, steroids, pesticides, and radiation
- Presentation varies and may be related to liver disease (hepatomegaly, ascites, nausea, splenomegaly), hemoperitoneum or distant metastases
- Typically the tumor involves the entire liver with ill-defined hemorrhagic nodules
- Prognosis is very poor

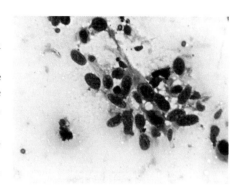

15-13. Angiosarcoma. Loosely cohesive cluster of pleomorphic cells with oval to spindle nuclei with coarse chromatin pattern (modified Giemsa stain)

Special Stains and Immunohistochemistry
- Vimentin and endothelial markers CD31 and CD34 are positive; factor VIII may or may not be positive
- Keratins are negative
- Perithelial cells are demonstrated by smooth muscle actin
- Vinyl chloride related tumors may expresses P53

Modern Technique for Diagnosis
- In Thorotrast related tumors, thorium particles are visualized by scanning electron microscopy
- High rate of KRAS-2 mutation

EPITHELIOID HEMANGIOENDOTHELIOMA

Clinical Features
- A rare low-grade malignant neoplasm of endothelial cells most commonly occurring in the liver (also seen in lung, soft tissue, and head and neck)
- Wide age range (average about fifty) and more common in females (2:1)
- Multiple variably sized nodules often throughout the liver
- Presentation varies from incidental detection in an asymptomatic patient to any or multiple signs and symptoms including weight loss, weakness, anorexia, upper abdominal discomfort or pain, jaundice, and rarely Budd–Chiari syndrome and liver failure
- Synchronous, metachronous, or metastatic lesions may occur in the lungs
- Prognosis is unpredictable and long survival is well known even with metastasis

Special Stains and Immunohistochemistry
- Vimentin and endothelial markers such as CD31, CD34, and Factor VIII are positive
- Keratins may be infrequently positive (epithelioid)
- Basement membrane around tumor cells can be demonstrated by PAS and laminin

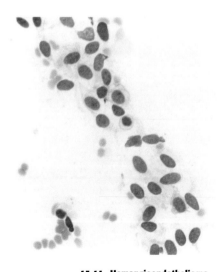

15-14. Hemangioendothelioma. The neoplastic cells have abundant pale cytoplasm with focal vacuolization. The nuclei are enlarged and some of which are lobulated (modified Giemsa stain)

Modern Technique for Diagnosis

- Ultrastructurally the tumor cells show endothelial features such as Weibel–Palade bodies and pinocytic vesicles
- Ultrastructurally, unlike usual endothelial cells, the tumor cells also contain intermediate filaments consistent with their epithelioid appearance

SARCOMAS

Cytologic Features

- Embryonal undifferentiated sarcoma
  - Sparse tumor cells in an abundant myxoid material
  - Oval, lobulated nuclei with fine chromatin pattern and small nucleoli
  - Large amount of pale cytoplasm, often vacuolated
  - Sparse multinucleated tumor giant cells can be seen
- Angiosarcoma
  - Bloody aspirates
  - Necrosis is common
  - Single pleomorphic malignant endothelium cells
  - Intracytoplasmic hemosiderin is common
  - Erythrophagocytosis by tumor cells is suggestive of angiosarcoma
  - Solid aggregates, papillary and tubular structures may be present
- Epitheloid hemangioendothelioma
  - Sparse cellularity due to fibrotic background
  - Single tumor cells with large nuclei often lobulated to convoluted nuclei
  - Adundant, pale, and vacuolated cytoplasm

Differential Diagnosis

- Metastatic adenocarcinoma
  - The presence of intracytoplasmic vacuoles may mimic epitheloid hemangioendothelioma
  - The presence of pseudoacinar and papillary groups may mimic angiosaroma
- Hemangiopericytoma
  - The cytologic features of hemangiopericytoma can be similar to that of other highly vascular tumors

PEARLS

- Bloody aspirates
- Erythrophagocytosis seen in angiosarcoma
- Cytoplasmic vacuoles seen in epitheliod hemangioendothelioma
- Abundant myxoid material seen in embryonal (undifferentiated) sarcoma

HEPATIC METASTASES

Clinical Features

- A prime location for metastases due to rich systemic and portal vascular perfusion
- Portal-systemic shunting in cirrhosis provides relative protection against metastases
- Most of liver secondary tumors are carcinomas from gastrointestinal tract, lung, breast, and genitourinary tract. Lymphoma and sarcoma are less common
- While most liver metastases are sign of disseminated malignancy some carcinomas such as renal cell, neuroendocrine, and colorectal may be isolated

■ Metastases predominate over primary hepatic cancers 40:1 in Western countries

■ Majority (two-thirds) of patients are symptomatic with RUQ pain, hepatomegaly, anorexia, weight loss, and sometimes biliary obstruction

■ Prognosis is variable depending upon dissemination or isolation of tumor and curative resectability

Cytologic Features

■ Majority of metastatic adenocarcinoma tumors to the liver do not have specific cytologic features to suggest the primary site

■ Colonic adenocarcinoma, clusters of tumors cells showing peripheral palisading of elongated cigar-shaped nuclei with central luminal granular "dirty" necrosis

■ Gastric and breast carcinomas can be suggested if the cytologic material shows signet ring cells

■ Melanoma should be considered, if the aspirated material shows pleomorphic cells, spindle cells, multinucleation, and binucleation

■ Sarcoma usually the aspirate will show spindle cells

■ Small round blue cell tumors, the aspirate usually will be composed of uniform small round blue cells (Ewing's sarcoma, lymphoma, small variant of melanoma)

■ Undifferentiated small cell carcinoma, small cells with scanty cytoplasm, nuclear molding, usually inconspicuous nucleoli and crush-artifact

■ Lymphoma, single cell population of small to large cells with round or cleaved nuclei. Lymphoglandular bodies are usually seen in the background

Special Stains and Immunohistochemistry

■ Immunohistochemical stains such as PSA, TTF-1, ER, CDX-2, WT-1, HMB-45 may be very helpful in relative site specificity in known or unknown primaries

■ Cytokeratins 7 and 20 (one, both, or neither positive) may be helpful in confirmation of known primaries or narrowing down the list of potential sites for exploration of unknown primaries

■ Pan-neuroendocrine markers such as synaptophysin and chromogranin A are useful in relative site restriction, potential for isolated metastasis, further exploration for selective neuroendocrine marker (such as insulin, gastric, or glucagon) and therapy

Modern Technique for Diagnosis

■ EM may be helpful in unknown primary, when IHC fails to illuminate the origin of a poorly differentiated tumor

Differential Diagnosis

■ Hepatocellular carcinoma

➤ Hepatocellular carcinoma should be differentiated from metastatic adenocarcinoma and melanoma. Hepatocellular carcinoma usually have polygonal cells with central nuclei, trabecular arrangement with endothelium lining, bile production, numerous naked nuclei, lack of mucous material, and usually absence of benign liver cells

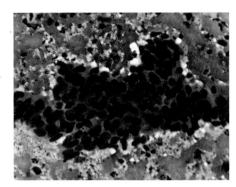

15-15. Metastatic colonic adenocarcinoma. Cluster of metastatic colonic adenocarcinoma showing peripheral nuclear stratification in a background of granular necrotic debris material

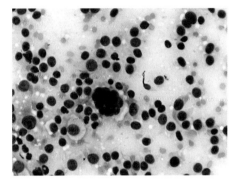

15-16. Metastatic melanoma. Mostly single cells with abundant cytoplasm and enlarged nuclei with prominent nucleoli. Binucleation and multinucleation is evident

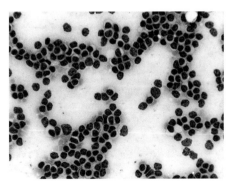

15-17. Malignant lymphoma, large cell type. Uniform population of single cells with small amount of cytoplasm

★ Metastatic melanoma may closely mimic hepatocellular carcinoma
★ The most common metastases are from the gastrointestinal tract
★ Immunodiagnostic studies and clinical history may play a big role in reaching the right diagnosis

REFERENCES

CONGENITAL CYSTS

Blonski WC, Campbell MS, Faust T, Metz DC. Successful aspiration and ethanol sclerosis of a large, symptomatic, simple liver cyst: case presentation and review of the literature. *World J Gastroenterol.* 2006 May 14;12(18):2949–54.

Bose SM, Lobo DN, Singh G, Wig JD. Bile duct cysts: presentation in adults. *Aust N Z J Surg.* 1993 Nov;63(11):853–7.

Pinto MM, Kaye AD. Fine needle aspiration of cystic liver lesions. Cytologic examination and carcinoembryonic antigen assay of cyst contents. *Acta Cytol.* 1989 Nov–Dec;33(6):852–6.

Stringer MD, Dhawan A, Davenport M, Mieli-Vergani G, Mowat AP, Howard ER. Choledochal cysts: lessons from a 20 year experience. *Arch Dis Child.* 1995 Dec;73(6):528–31.

Stringer MD, Jones MO, Woodley H, Wyatt J. Ciliated hepatic foregut cyst. *J Pediatr Surg.* 2006 Jun;41(6):1180–3.

Vick DJ, Goodman ZD, Deavers MT, Cain J, Ishak KG. Ciliated hepatic foregut cyst: a study of six cases and review of the literature. *Am J Surg Pathol.* 1999 Jun;23(6):671–7.

HYDATID CYST

Das DK, Bhambhani S, Pant CS. Ultrasound guided fine-needle aspiration cytology: diagnosis of hydatid disease of the abdomen and thorax. *Diagn Cytopathol.* 1995 Mar;12(2):173–6.

Firpi RJ, Lozada LR, Torres EA, Villamarzo G, Lobera A. Fine-needle aspiration diagnosis of hydatid cyst. *P R Health Sci J.* 1999 Jun;18(2):129–31.

Kapila K, Verma K. Aspiration cytology diagnosis of echinococcosis. *Diagn Cytopathol.* 1990;6(5):301–3.

Niscigorska J, Sluzar T, Marczewska M, Karpinska E, Boron-Kaczmarska A, Moranska I, Daniel B. Parasitic cysts of the liver – practical approach to diagnosis and differentiation. *Med Sci Monit.* 2001 Jul–Aug;7(4):737–41.

Parwani AV, Burroughs FH, Ali SZ. Echinococcal cyst of the liver. *Diagn Cytopathol.* 2004 Aug;31(2):111–2.

von Sinner WN, Nyman R, Linjawi T, Ali AM. Fine needle aspiration biopsy of hydatid cysts. *Acta Radiol.* 1995 Mar;36(2):168–72.

ABSCESS

Bhambhani S, Kashyap V. Amoebiasis: diagnosis by aspiration and exfoliative cytology. *Cytopathology.* 2001 Oct;12(5):329–33.

Pinto MM, Kaye AD. Fine needle aspiration of cystic liver lesions. Cytologic examination and carcinoembryonic antigen assay of cyst contents. *Acta Cytol.* 1989 Nov–Dec;33(6):852–6.

Vairani G, Rebeschini R, Barbazza R. Hepatic and subcutaneous abscesses due to aspergillosis. Initial diagnosis of a case by intraoperative fine needle aspiration cytology. *Acta Cytol.* 1990 Nov–Dec;34(6):891–4.

Wee A, Nilsson B, Yap I, Chong SM. Aspiration cytology of liver abscesses. With an emphasis on diagnostic pitfalls. *Acta Cytol.* 1995 May–Jun;39(3):453–62.

GRANULOMAS

Karagiannidis A, Karavalaki M, Koulaouzidis A. Hepatic sarcoidosis. *Ann Hepatol.* 2006 Oct–Dec;5(4):251–6.

Radhika S, Rajwanshi A, Kochhar R, Kochhar S, Dey P, Roy P. Abdominal tuberculosis. Diagnosis by fine needle aspiration cytology. *Acta Cytol.* 1993 Sep–Oct;37(5):673–8.

Stastny JF, Wakely PE, Frable WJ. Cytologic features of necrotizing granulomatous inflammation consistent with cat-scratch disease. *Diagn Cytopathol.* 1996 Aug;15(2):108–15.

Stormby N, Akerman M. Aspiration cytology in the diagnosis of granulomatous liver lesions. *Acta Cytol*. 1973 May–Jun;17(3):200–4.

HEMANGIOMA

Glinkova V, Shevah O, Boaz M, Levine A, Shirin H. Hepatic haemangiomas: possible association with female sex hormones. *Gut*. 2004 Sep;53(9):1352–5.

Guy CD, Yuan S, Ballo MS. Spindle-cell lesions of the liver: diagnosis by fine-needle aspiration biopsy. *Diagn Cytopathol*. 2001 Aug;25(2):94–100.

Kaw YT, Esparza AR. Cytologic diagnosis of cavernous hemangioma of the liver with fine-needle biopsy. *Diagn Cytopathol*. 1991;7(6):628–30.

Layfield LJ, Mooney EE, Dodd LG. Not by blood alone: diagnosis of hemangiomas by fine-needle aspiration. *Diagn Cytopathol*. 1998 Oct;19(4):250–4.

Mortele KJ, Ros PR. Benign liver neoplasms. *Clin Liver Dis*. 2002 Feb;6(1):119–45.

FOCAL NODULAR HYPERPLASIA

Kong CS, Appenzeller M, Ferrell LD. Utility of CD34 reactivity in evaluating focal nodular hepatocellular lesions sampled by fine needle aspiration biopsy. *Acta Cytol*. 2000 Mar–Apr;44(2):218–22.

Krishnamurthy S, Nerurkar AY. Spindle cell fragments in focal nodular hyperplasia of the liver. A case report. *Acta Cytol*. 2002 May–Jun;46(3):582–4.

Ruschenburg I, Droese M. Fine needle aspiration cytology of focal nodular hyperplasia of the liver. *Acta Cytol*. 1989 Nov–Dec;33(6):857–60.

Russack V, Vass L, Gupta PK. Comparison of morphologic features of benign hepatocytes associated with nonmalignant and malignant liver lesions. *Acta Cytol*. 1993 Mar–Apr;37(2): 153–7.

Suen KC. Diagnosis of primary hepatic neoplasms by fine-needle aspiration cytology. *Diagn Cytopathol*. 1986 Apr–Jun;2(2):99–109.

Wanless IR. The use of morphometry in the study of nodular and vascular lesions of the liver. *Anal Quant Cytol Histol*. 1987 Mar;9(1):39–41.

HEPATOCELLULAR ADENOMA (LIVER CELL ADENOMA)

Bottles K, Cohen MB. An approach to fine-needle aspiration biopsy diagnosis of hepatic masses. *Diagn Cytopathol*. 1991;7(2):204–10.

Gonzalez F, Marks C. Hepatic tumors and oral contraceptives: surgical management. *J Surg Oncol*. 1985 Jul;29(3):193–7.

Suen KC. Diagnosis of primary hepatic neoplasms by fine-needle aspiration cytology. *Diagn Cytopathol*. 1986 Apr–Jun;2(2):99–109.

Tao LC. Are oral contraceptive-associated liver cell adenomas premalignant? *Acta Cytol*. 1992 May–Jun;36(3):338–44.

Yang GC, Yang GY, Tao LC. Distinguishing well-differentiated hepatocellular carcinoma from benign liver by the physical features of fine-needle aspirates. *Mod Pathol*. 2004 Jul;17(7):798–802.

BILE DUCT HAMARTOMA (BILE DUCT ADENOMA)

Bhathal PS, Hughes NR, Goodman ZD. The so-called bile duct adenoma is a peribiliary gland hamartoma. *Am J Surg Pathol*. 1996 Jul;20(7):858–64.

Brunt EM. Benign tumors of the liver. *Clin Liver Dis*. 2001 Feb;5(1):1–15, v.

Hornick JL, Lauwers GY, Odze RD. Immunohistochemistry can help distinguish metastatic pancreatic adenocarcinomas from bile duct adenomas and hamartomas of the liver. *Am J Surg Pathol*. 2005 Mar;29(3):381–9.

Mortele KJ, Ros PR. Benign liver neoplasms. *Clin Liver Dis*. 2002 Feb;6(1):119–45.

Principe A, Lugaresi ML, Lords RC, D'Errico A, Polito E, Gallö MC, Bicchierri I, Cavallari A. Bile duct hamartomas: diagnostic problems and treatment. *Hepatogastroenterology*. 1997 Jul–Aug;44(16):994–7.

CIRRHOTIC NODULES, ADENOMATOUS HYPERPLASIA, AND DYPLASIA

Hill KA, Nayar R, DeFrias DV. Cytohistologic correlation of cirrhosis and hepatocellular carcinoma. Pitfall in diagnosis? *Acta Cytol*. 2004 Mar–Apr;48(2):127–32.

Hollerbach S, Reiser M, Topalidis T, König M, Schmiegel W. Diagnosis of hepatocellular carcinoma (HCC) in a high-risk patient by using transgastric EUS-guided fine-needle biopsy (EUS-FNA). *Z Gastroenterol*. 2003 Oct;41(10):995–8.

Lin CC, Lin CJ, Hsu CW, Chen YC, Chen WT, Lin SM. Fine-needle aspiration cytology to distinguish dysplasia from hepatocellular carcinoma with different grades. *J Gastroenterol Hepatol.* 2007 May 27; [Epub ahead of print].

Yang GC, Yang GY, Tao LC. Distinguishing well-differentiated hepatocellular carcinoma from benign liver by the physical features of fine-needle aspirates. *Mod Pathol.* 2004 Jul;17(7):798–802.

HEPATOCELLULAR CARCINOMA

Bottles K, Cohen MB. An approach to fine-needle aspiration biopsy diagnosis of hepatic masses. *Diagn Cytopathol.* 1991;7(2):204–10.

Kong CS, Appenzeller M, Ferrell LD. Utility of CD34 reactivity in evaluating focal nodular hepatocellular lesions sampled by fine needle aspiration biopsy. *Acta Cytol.* 2000 Mar–Apr;44(2):218–22.

Kuo FY, Chen WJ, Lu SN, Wang JH, Eng HL. Fine needle aspiration cytodiagnosis of liver tumors. *Acta Cytol.* 2004 Mar–Apr;48(2):142–8.

Lin F, Abdallah H, Meschter S. Diagnostic utility of CD10 in differentiating hepatocellular carcinoma from metastatic carcinoma in fine-needle aspiration biopsy (FNAB) of the liver. *Diagn Cytopathol.* 2004 Feb;30(2):92–7.

Suen KC. Diagnosis of primary hepatic neoplasms by fine-needle aspiration cytology. *Diagn Cytopathol.* 1986 Apr–Jun;2(2):99–109.

Wang L, Vuolo M, Suhrland MJ, Schlesinger K. HepPar1, MOC-31, pCEA, mCEA and CD10 for distinguishing hepatocellular carcinoma vs. metastatic adenocarcinoma in liver fine needle aspirates. *Acta Cytol.* 2006 May–Jun;50(3):257–62.

Wee A, Nilsson B. Highly well differentiated hepatocellular carcinoma and benign hepatocellular lesions. Can they be distinguished on fine needle aspiration biopsy? *Acta Cytol.* 2003 Jan–Feb;47(1):16–26.

Yang GC, Yang GY, Tao LC. Cytologic features and histologic correlations of microacinar and microtrabecular types of well-differentiated hepatocellular carcinoma in fine-needle aspiration biopsy. *Cancer.* 2004 Feb 25;102(1):27–33.

Yang GC, Yang GY, Tao LC. Distinguishing well-differentiated hepatocellular carcinoma from benign liver by the physical features of fine-needle aspirates. *Mod Pathol.* 2004 Jul;17(7):798–802.

Zimmerman RL, Logani S, Baloch Z. Evaluation of the CD34 and CD10 immunostains using a two-color staining protocol in liver fine-needle aspiration biopsies. *Diagn Cytopathol.* 2005 Feb;32(2):88–91.

HEPATOBLASTOMA

Bakshi P, Srinivasan R, Rao KL, Marwaha RK, Gupta N, Das A, Nijhawan R, Cangiarella J, Greco MA, Waisman J. Hepatoblastoma. Report of a case with cytologic, histologic and ultrastructural findings. *Acta Cytol.* 1994 May–Jun;38(3):455–8.

Dekmezian R, Sneige N, Popok S, Ordonez NG. Fine-needle aspiration cytology of pediatric patients with primary hepatic tumors: a comparative study of two hepatoblastomas and a liver-cell carcinoma. *Diagn Cytopathol.* 1988;4(2):162–8.

Ersoz C, Zorludemir U, Tanyeli A, Gumurdulu D, Celiktas M. Fine needle aspiration cytology of hepatoblastoma. A report of two cases. *Acta Cytol.* 1998 May–Jun;42(3):799–802.

Gupta RK, Naran S, Alansari AG. Fine needle aspiration cytodiagnosis in a case of hepatoblastoma. *Cytopathology.* 1994 Apr;5(2):114–7.

Iyer VK, Kapila K, Agarwala S, Verma K. Fine needle aspiration cytology of hepatoblastoma. Recognition of subtypes on cytomorphology. *Acta Cytol.* 2005 Jul–Aug;49(4):355–64.

Jain R, Jain M. Mixed hepatoblastoma diagnosed by fine-needle aspiration biopsy cytology: a case report. *Diagn Cytopathol.* 1998 Oct;19(4):306–8.

Kaw YT, Hansen K. Fine needle aspiration cytology of undifferentiated small cell ("anaplastic") hepatoblastoma. A case report. *Acta Cytol.* 1993 Mar–Apr;37(2):216–20.

Rajwanshi A. Fine needle aspiration biopsy in pediatric space-occupying lesions of liver: a retrospective study evaluating its role and diagnostic efficacy. *J Pediatr Surg.* 2006 Nov;41(11):1903–8.

Sola Perez J, Perez-Guillermo M, Bas Bernal AB, Mercader JM. Hepatoblastoma. An attempt to apply histologic classification to aspirates obtained by fine needle aspiration cytology. *Acta Cytol.* 1994 Mar–Apr;38(2):175–82.

Us-Krasovec M, Pohar-Marinsek Z, Golouh R, Jereb B, Ferlan-Marolt V, Cerar A. Hepatoblastoma in fine needle aspirates. *Acta Cytol.* 1996 May–Jun;40(3):450–6.

MESENCHYMAL HAMARTOMA

al-Rikabi AC, Buckai A, al-Sumayer S, al-Damegh S, al-Bassam AR. Fine needle aspiration cytology of mesenchymal hamartoma of the liver. A case report. *Acta Cytol.* 2000 May–Jun;44(3):449–53.

Bakshi P, Srinivasan R, Rao KL, Marwaha RK, Gupta N, Das A, Nijhawan R, Rajwanshi A. Fine needle aspiration biopsy in pediatric space-occupying lesions of liver: a retrospective study evaluating its role and diagnostic efficacy. *J Pediatr Surg.* 2006 Nov;41(11):1903–8.

Jiménez-Heffernan JA, Vicandi B, López-Ferrer P, Lamas M, Viguer JM. Fine-needle aspiration cytology of mesenchymal hamartoma of the liver. *Diagn Cytopathol.* 2000 Apr;22(4):250–3.

Siddiqui MA, McKenna BJ. Hepatic mesenchymal hamartoma: a short review. *Arch Pathol Lab Med.* 2006 Oct;130(10):1567–9.

Stringer MD, Alizai NK. Mesenchymal hamartoma of the liver: a systematic review. *J Pediatr Surg.* 2005 Nov;40(11):1681–90.

von Schweinitz D, Dammeier BG, Glüer S. Mesenchymal hamartoma of the liver – new insight into histogenesis. *J Pediatr Surg.* 1999 Aug;34(8):1269–71.

CHOLANGIOCARCINOMA

Dusenbery D. Combined hepatocellular-cholangiocarcinoma. Cytologic findings in four cases. *Acta Cytol.* 1997 May–Jun;41(3):903–9.

Hertz G, Reddy VB, Green L, Spitz D, Massarani-Wafai R, Selvaggi SM, Kluskens L, Gattuso P. Fine-needle aspiration biopsy of the liver: a multicenter study of 602 radiologically guided FNA. *Diagn Cytopathol.* 2000 Nov;23(5):326–8.

Lal A, Okonkwo A, Schindler S, De Frias D, Nayar R. Role of biliary brush cytology in primary sclerosing cholangitis. *Acta Cytol.* 2004 Jan–Feb;48(1):9–12.

Meara RS, Jhala D, Eloubeidi MA, Eltoum I, Chhieng DC, Crowe DR, Varadarajulu S, Jhala N. Endoscopic ultrasound-guided FNA biopsy of bile duct and gallbladder: analysis of 53 cases. *Cytopathology.* 2006 Feb;17(1):42–9.

Papillo JL, Leslie KO, Dean RA. Cytologic diagnosis of liver fluke infestation in a patient with subsequently documented cholangiocarcinoma. *Acta Cytol.* 1989 Nov–Dec;33(6):865–9.

Sampatanukul P, Leong AS, Kosolbhand P, Tangkijvanich P. Proliferating ductules are a diagnostic discriminator for intrahepatic cholangiocarcinoma in FNA biopsies. *Diagn Cytopathol.* 2000 Jun;22(6):359–63.

Wee A, Nilsson B. Combined hepatocellular-cholangiocarcinoma. Diagnostic challenge in hepatic fine needle aspiration biopsy. *Acta Cytol.* 1999 Mar–Apr;43(2):131–8.

Wight CO, Zaitoun AM, Boulton-Jones JR, Dunkley C, Beckingham IJ, Ryder SD. Improving diagnostic yield of biliary brushings cytology for pancreatic cancer and cholangiocarcinoma. *Cytopathology.* 2004 Apr;15(2):87–92.

Wolber RA, Greene CA, Dupuis BA. Polyclonal carcinoembryonic antigen staining in the cytologic differential diagnosis of primary and metastatic hepatic malignancies. *Acta Cytol.* 1991 Mar–Apr;35(2):215–20.

SARCOMAS

Aalaei S, Jakate S. Right upper quadrant pain and fever in a 41-year-old man. Epithelioid hemangioendothelioma of the liver with metastasis to porta hepatis lymph nodes and lung. *Arch Pathol Lab Med.* 2005 May;129(5):e134–5.

Agaram NP, Baren A, Antonescu CR. Pediatric and adult hepatic embryonal sarcoma: a comparative ultrastructural study with morphologic correlations. *Ultrastruct Pathol.* 2006 Nov–Dec;30(6):403–8.

Bakshi P, Srinivasan R, Rao KL, Marwaha RK, Gupta N, Das A, Nijhawan R, Rajwanshi A. Fine needle aspiration biopsy in pediatric space-occupying lesions of liver: a retrospective study evaluating its role and diagnostic efficacy. *J Pediatr Surg.* 2006 Nov;41(11):1903–8.

Boucher LD, Swanson PE, Stanley MW, Silverman JF, Raab SS, Geisinger KR. Cytology of angiosarcoma. Findings in fourteen fine-needle aspiration biopsy specimens and one pleural fluid specimen. *Am J Clin Pathol.* 2000 Aug;114(2):210–9.

Chen KT. Cytology of epithelioid hemangioendothelioma. *Diagn Cytopathol.* 1996 Mar;14(2):187–8.

Cho NH, Lee KG, Jeong MG. Cytologic evaluation of primary malignant vascular tumors of the liver. One case each of angiosarcoma and epithelioid hemangioendothelioma. *Acta Cytol.* 1997 Sep–Oct;41(5):1468–76.

Cho NH, Lee KG, Jeong MG. Cytologic evaluation of primary malignant vascular tumors of the liver. One case each of angiosarcoma and epithelioid hemangioendothelioma. *Acta Cytol.* 1997 Sep–Oct;41(5):1468–76.

Gambacorta M, Bonacina E. Epithelioid hemangioendothelioma: report of a case diagnosed by fine-needle aspiration. *Diagn Cytopathol.* 1989;5(2):207–10.

García-Bonafé M, Allende H, Fantova MJ, Tarragona J. Fine needle aspiration cytology of undifferentiated (embryonal) sarcoma of the liver. A case report. *Acta Cytol.* 1997 Jul–Aug;41 (4 Suppl):1273–8.

Iyer VK, Bandhu S, Verma K. An unusual mass lesion of the liver with distinctive cytology. *Cytopathology.* 2004 Aug;15(4):233–6.

Kiani B, Ferrell LD, Qualman S, Frankel WL. Immunohistochemical analysis of embryonal sarcoma of the liver. *Appl Immunohistochem Mol Morphol.* 2006 Jun;14(2):193–7.

Krishnamurthy SC, Datta S, Jambhekar NA. Fine needle aspiration cytology of undifferentiated (embryonal) sarcoma of the liver: a case report. *Acta Cytol.* 1996 May–Jun;40(3):567–70.

Liu K, Layfield LJ. Cytomorphologic features of angiosarcoma on fine needle aspiration biopsy. *Acta Cytol.* 1999 May–Jun;43(3):407–15.

Nguyen GK, Husain M. Fine-needle aspiration biopsy cytology of angiosarcoma. *Diagn Cytopathol.* 2000 Aug;23(2):143–5.

Nicol K, Savell V, Moore J, Teot L, Spunt SL, Qualman S. Distinguishing undifferentiated embryonal sarcoma of the liver from biliary tract rhabdomyosarcoma: a Children's Oncology Group study. *Pediatr Dev Pathol.* 2007 Mar–Apr;10(2):89–97.

Pollono DG, Drut R. Undifferentiated (embryonal) sarcoma of the liver: fine-needle aspiration cytology and preoperative chemotherapy as an approach to diagnosis and initial treatment. A case report. *Diagn Cytopathol.* 1998 Aug;19(2):102–6.

Saleh HA, Tao LC. Hepatic angiosarcoma: aspiration biopsy cytology and immunocytochemical contribution. *Diagn Cytopathol.* 1998 Mar;18(3):208–11.

Soslow RA, Yin P, Steinberg CR, Yang GC. Cytopathologic features of hepatic epithelioid hemangioendothelioma. *Diagn Cytopathol.* 1997 Jul;17(1):50–3.

Wong JW, Bedard YC. Fine-needle aspiration biopsy of hepatic angiosarcoma: report of a case with immunocytochemical findings. *Diagn Cytopathol.* 1992;8(4):380–3.

HEPATIC METASTASES

Das DK. Cytodiagnosis of hepatocellular carcinoma in fine-needle aspirates of the liver: its differentiation from reactive hepatocytes and metastatic adenocarcinoma. *Diagn Cytopathol.* 1999 Dec;21(6):370–7.

Gokden M, Shinde A. Recent immunohistochemical markers in the differential diagnosis of primary and metastatic carcinomas of the liver. *Diagn Cytopathol.* 2005 Sep;33(3):166–72.

Granados R, Aramburu JA, Murillo N, Camarmo E, de la Cal MA, Fernandez-Segoviano P. Fine-needle aspiration biopsy of liver masses: diagnostic value and reproducibility of cytological criteria. *Diagn Cytopathol.* 2001 Dec;25(6):365–75.

Khalbuss WE, Grigorian S, Bui MM, Elhosseiny A. Small-cell tumors of the liver: a cytological study of 91 cases and a review of the literature. *Diagn Cytopathol.* 2005 Jul;33(1):8–14.

Parwani AV, Chan TY, Mathew S, Ali SZ. Metastatic malignant melanoma in liver aspirate: cytomorphologic distinction from hepatocellular carcinoma. *Diagn Cytopathol.* 2004 Apr;30(4):247–50.

Reyes CV, Thompson KS, Jensen JD, Choudhury AM. Metastasis of unknown origin: the role of fine-needle aspiration cytology. *Diagn Cytopathol.* 1998 May;18(5):319–22.

Saad RS, Luckasevic TM, Noga CM, Johnson DR, Silverman JF, Liu YL. Diagnostic value of HepPar1, pCEA, CD10, and CD34 expression in separating hepatocellular carcinoma from metastatic carcinoma in fine-needle aspiration cytology. *Diagn Cytopathol.* 2004 Jan;30(1):1–6.

Wu M, Szporn AH, Zhang D, Wasserman P, Gan L, Miller L, Burstein DE. Cytology applications of p63 and TTF-1 immunostaining in differential diagnosis of lung cancers. *Diagn Cytopathol.* 2005 Oct;33(4):223–7.

16

Pancreas

Shriram Jakate and Paolo Gattuso

ACUTE PANCREATITIS

Clinical Features
- Wide range of severity from mild undetectable disease to severe hemorrhagic and necrotizing pancreatitis
- Incidence is difficult to estimate as mild cases may remain undiagnosed
- More common in older (>40 years) adults
- Most common underlying and associated conditions are cholelithiasis and alcoholism
- Other less common etiological factors include hypercalcemic conditions, drugs, complication of FNA, and rarely hereditary predisposition due to mutations in cationic trypsinogen and serine protease inhibitor genes
- Severe pancreatitis is an extreme medical emergency presenting with acute abdomen and systemic noninfectious toxemia

Cytologic Features
- FNA is performed rarely in clinical practice
- Amorphous material
- Cellular debris
- Acute inflammatory cells (neutrophils)
- Histiocytes are usually present
- Fat necrosis

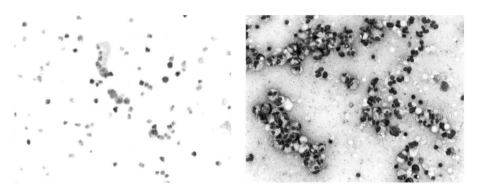

16-1A. Acute pancreatitis *(left)*. Cellular debris, amorphous material, and mixed inflammatory cells (Papanicolaou stain)

16-1B. Acute pancreatitis *(right)*. Numerous inflammatory cells (modified Giemsa stain)

- Reactive acinar and ductal cells
- Granulation tissue
- Reactive mesothelial cells can be prominent

Special Stains and Immunohistochemistry
- Noncontributory

Modern Technique for Diagnosis
- Noncontributory

Differential Diagnosis
- Pseudocyst
  - ➤ Rarely epithelial cells are present
  - ➤ Fluid material usually aspirated may vary in color from yellow to hemorrhagic to dark brown
  - ➤ Histiocytes are usually present
  - ➤ Mesenchymal repair

PEARLS

- ★ Safe, reliable procedure to confirm the diagnosis
- ★ Reactive atypical mesothelial cells should not be confused with adenocarcinoma

CHRONIC PANCREATITIS

Clinical Features
- Persistent inflammation and fibrosis of pancreas, often associated with calcifications that may affect any part of the pancreas

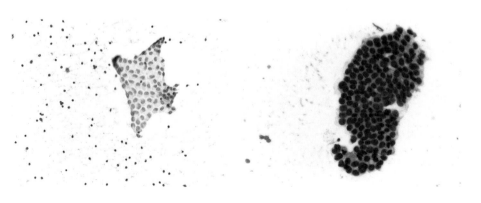

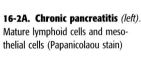

16-2A. Chronic pancreatitis *(left)*. Mature lymphoid cells and mesothelial cells (Papanicolaou stain)

16-2B. Chronic pancreatitis *(right)*. Cluster of ductal epithelium and sparse mature lymphoid cells (modified Giemsa stain)

- Common causes include alcoholism, obstructive conditions, smoking, autoimmunity, nutritional, and hereditary any conditions including cystic fibrosis
- More common in males and most frequent in fourth to sixth decades
- Clinical features include continuous or intermittent abdominal pain, nausea, jaundice, malabsorption, and eventually endocrine insufficiency leading to diabetes
- Often diagnosed late clinically and may mimic tumor mass, cause ascites, fat necrosis, pseudocyst formation, and gastrointestinal bleeding

Cytologic Features

- Fragments of connective tissue
- Mostly ductal cells, usually occurring in uniform sheets; they may show mild atypical changes
- Sparse acinar cells, which may look atypical with coarse chromatin pattern, and prominent nucleoli
- Lymphocytes and plasma cells in the background and debris material
- Reactive mesothelial cells
- Islet cells are seen only rarely

Special Stains and Immunohistochemistry

- Noncontributory

Modern Technique for Diagnosis

- Noncontributory

Differential Diagnosis

- Adenocarcinoma
  - Cellular FNA material
  - Cell crowding
  - High nuclear/cytoplasmic ratio
  - Marked pleomorphism
  - Irregular nuclear membranes
  - Microacinar pattern

PEARLS

- ★ Sparse or absent acinar and islet cells
- ★ Mesenchymal repair
- ★ Microacinar pattern rarely seen
- ★ Reactive mesothelial cells should not be confused with adenocarcinoma

PANCREATIC PSEUDOCYST

Clinical Features

- Most common cystic lesion (about 75%) of the pancreas lined by inflammatory and fibrous tissue but no epithelium
- More frequently extrapancreatic and attached to pancreas rather than within the pancreas
- Resulting from autodigestive tissue necrosis from acute, chronic, surgical, traumatic, or obstructive pancreatitis
- Size may vary from small to large (2–20 cm)
- Usually uniloculated, filled with hemorrhagic and fibrinous debris, and may or may not communicate with the pancreatic duct

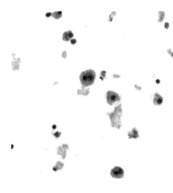

16-3. Pancreatic pseudocyst.
Necrotic debris, mixed inflammatory cells, and hemosiderin–laden macrophages (Papanicolaou stain)

Cytologic Features
- Yellow, hemorrhagic, or dark brown fluid
- Histiocytes
- Necrotic debris
- Calcifications, cholesterol crystals
- Sparse or no epithelial cells
- Atypical mesenchymal cells may be present

Special Stains and Immunohistochemistry
- Noncontributory

Modern Technique for Diagnosis
- Noncontributory

Differential Diagnosis
- Congenital cysts
  ➤ Fluid can be clear, serous, turbid, or mucoid
  ➤ Small clusters of small uniform cuboidal cells can be present
- Lymphoepithelial cysts
  ➤ Keratinous debris material
  ➤ Small mature lymphocytes and histiocytes
  ➤ Cholesterol crystals may also be seen

PEARLS

★ Rare or no epithelial cells
★ The cytologic changes are not specific for pseudocysts

DUCTAL ADENOCARCINOMA

Clinical Features
- The most common pancreatic neoplasm (85–90% of all pancreatic tumors), when all variants are included (well-differentiated adenocarcinoma, pleomorphic giant cell, spindle cell or sarcomatoid, osteoclastic giant cell, small cell (anaplastic carcinoma) adenosquamous, oncocytic tumors, clear cell tumors, and signet ring carcinoma)
- Occurs almost exclusively in older adults (usually between sixty and eighty years) and slightly more commonly in males than females
- Risk factors include smoking, pancreatitis, diabetes, prior gastrectomy, chemical and radiation exposure and hereditary conditions (hereditary pancreatitis, Peutz–Jeghers, familial cancers)
- Commonest location is upper pancreatic head (70%), the rest occurring in the body or tail
- Clinical presentation may include abdominal pain, weight loss, jaundice (often painless), diabetes, pancreatitis, migratory thromophlebitis, and ascites (with peritoneal spread)
- Very poor prognosis

Cytologic Features
- Cellular smears
- Usually one single cell type, that is, ductal
- Neoplastic cells usually form groups, sheets, clusters, or three-dimensional cell balls
- Crowded, poorly cohesive, and increased number of single cells
- Enlarged pleomorphic nuclei, irregular nuclear membranes, prominent nucleoli
- High nuclear/cytoplasmic ratio, coarse chromatin pattern, mitosis, necrosis

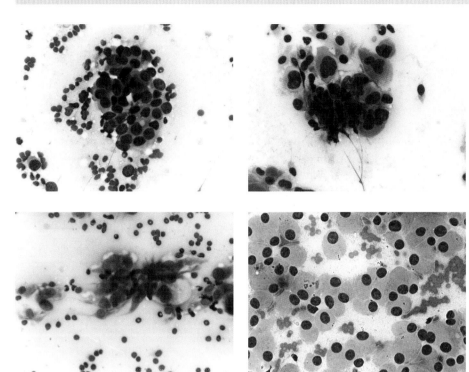

16-4A. Adenocarcinoma
(top, left). Three-dimensional cluster of adenocarcinoma cells some of which show intracytoplasmic mucin material (modified Giemsa stain)

16-4B. Pleomorphic giant cell carcinoma *(top, right)*. Large pleomorphic cells, binucleation and multinucleation is apparent (modified Giemsa stain)

16-4C. Spindle cell or sarcomatoid variant of carcinoma *(bottom, left)*. Clusters of adenocarcinoma cells showing spindle-shaped nuclei (modified Giemsa stain)

16-4D. Oncocytic variant of adenocarcinoma *(bottom, right)*. Single adenocarcinoma cells showing eosinophilic granular cytoplasm (modified Giemsa stain)

- Squamoid cytoplasm
- Well-differentiated adenocarcinoma
  - Cellular aspirate, predominantly ductal cells
  - Numerous large sheets of ductal cells with bland cytologic features
  - Absence of acinar, islet, and inflammatory cells
  - Irregular nuclear membrane contours
  - Nuclear enlargement
  - Cytoplasmic vacuolization
- Pleomorphic giant cell carcinoma
  - Pleomorphic, bizarre, multinucleated giant cells
  - The tumor giant cells are obviously malignant
  - Atypical mitotic figures are commonly seen
  - Phagocytosis of inflammatory cells by tumor cells is a common finding
- Spindle cell or sarcomatoid variant of carcinoma
  - Composed of a predominance of pleomorphic spindle-shaped neoplastic cells
- Osteoclastic giant cell tumor
  - Osteoclastic giant cells with multiple uniform, small, bland nuclei with prominent nucleoli
  - The background cellularity may include conventional adenocarcinoma
- Small cell (anaplastic) carcinoma
  - Before making a diagnosis of primary small cell carcinoma of the pancreas, a metastatic lung cancer should be excluded
- Adenosquamous carcinoma
  - Cells with squamoid cytoplasm is a common finding
  - Neoplastic glandular component is also present
- Oncocytic tumors
  - Oncocytic changes may be seen in ductal, acinar, and islet cell neoplasms
  - Electron microscopy and immunohistochemistry may be necessary to classify these lesions

▦ Clear cell tumors
> Clear cell changes may be seen in ductal carcinoma and islet cell neoplasms
> Metastatic renal cell carcinoma, clear cell type, should be considered in the differential diagnosis
▦ Signet ring carcinoma
> Pure signet ring adenocarcinoma of the pancreas is uncommon

Special Stains and Immunohistochemistry
▦ Strongly positive for CK7, positive for CK8/18, and generally negative for CK20 (similar to normal pancreatic ductal cells)
▦ Generally positive for CA19-9, Du-Pan 2, Span-1, CA 125, and TAG 72
▦ CEA strongly positive, typically along luminal borders
▦ Generally negative for vimentin, endocrine markers, and pancreatic acinar enzymes (trypsin, chymotrypsin, and lipase)
▦ Mucin stains (PAS, mucicarmine, MUC 1, and not MUC 2) are generally positive

Modern Techniques for Diagnosis
▦ Aneuploidy is associated with higher stage
▦ High K-ras point mutation rate (75–90% of cases) at codon 12
▦ P53 mutation in 50–70% of cases
▦ Her-2-Neu overexpression in 70% of cases

Differential Diagnosis
▦ Benign inflammatory atypia and repair
> Low to moderate cellularity
> Flat monolayer of two-dimensional glandular cells
> Mild nuclear enlargement
> Nuclear membranes are smooth
> Macronucleoli, rarely present
> Necrotic debris, rarely seen

PEARLS

★ Well-differentiated mucus producing adenocarcinoma could be confused with benign ductal cells
★ Subtypes of carcinoma, for example, sarcomatoid and small cell can mimic metastatic tumors
★ Chronic and acute pancreatitis can be confused with adenocarcinoma

INTRADUCTAL PAPILLARY MUCINOUS TUMOR OF THE PANCREAS (IPMT)

Clinical Features
▦ Unlike cystic mucinous neoplasm, IPMT arises in the main pancreatic duct or its branches and is more common in males, but like cystic mucinous neoplasm, it shares a spectrum of benign, borderline, in situ or invasive malignant neoplasms
▦ Typical but variable components include papillary epithelial hyperplasia, mucin secretion and duct ectasia, reflected in the synonyms mucin-hypersecreting duct-ectatic tumor, intraductal papillary adenoma, and endoluminal tumor of the main pancreatic duct
▦ Rare tumors (1% of pancreatic tumors) that are seen in the sixth decade (mean age sixty-two years) with a male:female ratio 2:1
▦ Majority occur in the main pancreatic duct and its branches in the head of pancreas, but localized, diffuse, and multifocal pancreatic involvement is known to occur
▦ Size varies from 1 to 8 cm

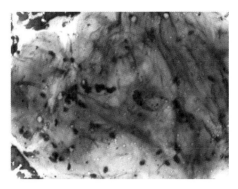 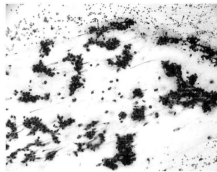

16-5A. Intraductal papillary mucinous tumor *(left)*. Lake of mucinous material (modified Giemsa stain)

16-5B. Intraductal papillary mucinous tumor *(right)*. Low-power view shows a micropapillary pattern (modified Giemsa stain)

16-5C. Intraductal papillary mucinous tumor *(below)*. Papillary configuration with some nuclear overlapping (modified Giemsa stain)

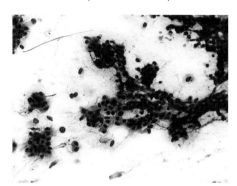

▩ Thick viscous mucin may protrude from the dilated ampullary opening aiding both endoscopic recognition and cytological sampling
▩ May be incidentally detected but symptoms may include abdominal pain, weight loss, obstructive pancreatitis, jaundice, and diabetes

Cytologic Features
▩ Thick mucinous material usually present
▩ Mucinous epithelium usually present
▩ True papillae with fibrovascular cores
▩ Small three-dimensional micropapillary clusters
▩ Nuclear grooves
▩ Monolayered sheets of epithelium is predominant in benign cases
▩ Nonmucinous epithelium, marked atypia, single atypical cells speak in favor of malignancy
▩ Pancreatobiliary, intestinal, or oncocytic epithelium has been described

Special Stains and Immunohistochemistry
▩ Positive for cytokeratins and epithelial membrane antigens (EMA)
▩ May be focally positive for neuroendocrine markers
▩ Positive for mucin stains (PAS, mucicarmine)

Modern Technique for Diagnosis
▩ Cell proliferation markers such as Ki-67 show progressive increase from benign to borderline to invasive carcinoma
▩ K-ras and P53 mutations are potential markers of progression
▩ MUC2 (intestinal type mucin) marker is expressed particularly when IPMN is associated with extrapancreatic cancers

Differential Diagnosis
▩ Mucinous cystic neoplasms
　➤ Benign muciphages are usually present
　➤ Mucus material in the background
　➤ Intracellular mucin material
　➤ Papillae rarely seen
　➤ Spectrum of maturation of the glandular cells
　➤ Presence of goblet or signet ring cells if present facilitate the diagnosis

PEARLS

★ Contamination by gastrointestinal epithelium and mucus that often occurs in EUS-FNAB samples, should be taken into consideration in every case examined
★ At times the papillary nature of the lesion is not obvious

★ The distinction on FNA material between IPMT and a mucinous adenocarcinoma or a cystic mucinous neoplasm is a matter of correlation with clinical and radiologic data

SEROUS CYSTADENOMA

Clinical Features

▓ Also known as serous microcystic adenoma and glycogen-rich cystadenoma

▓ Uncommon tumor (1% of all pancreatic tumors and 4–10% of pancreatic cystic tumors), which is almost always benign

▓ Exceptional cases show locally aggressive or malignant behavior (serous cystadenocarcinoma)

▓ Occurs more often in women (70%) and in older age (median age sixty-six years)

▓ The microcystic adenoma variant is far more common than oligocystic or macrocystic adenoma variant, which has fewer and larger cysts

▓ Association with von Hippel–Lindau syndrome is described in younger patients and without sex predilection

▓ Found incidentally in one-third patients (autopsy, imaging, or physical examination) or due to local pressure of mass (abdominal pain, nausea)

▓ More often located in body or tail than the head, often solitary with average size 6–10 cm, sponge-like with numerous tiny cysts and sometimes containing central stellate scar

Cytologic Features

▓ Clear, watery fluid

▓ Sparse cellularity

▓ The cells can be single or arranged in a honeycombed pattern

▓ The nuclei are small, usually round, uniform, and lack nucleoli

▓ Nuclear grooves, intranuclear cytoplasmic inclusions and irregular nuclear membranes have been sporadically described

▓ The cytoplasm is usually clear and finely granular

▓ The cytoplasm contains glycogen

▓ Foamy cells, papillary structures, and islet cells may be seen

▓ No mitosis

▓ No mucin material in the background

Special Stains and Immunohistochemistry

▓ PAS without diastase digestion is strongly positive. PAS with diastase is negative confirming the presence of intracytoplasmic glycogen

▓ Mucin stains are negative

▓ Cytokeratins 7, 8, 18, and 19, and CA19-9 are positive

▓ Vimentin, neuroendocrine markers, CEA, and muscle markers are negative

16-6A. Serous cystadenoma *(left).* Cluster of cells with uniform, round nuclei and fine indistinct granular cytoplasm (modified Giemsa stain)

16-6B. Serous cystadenoma *(right).* Monolayered cluster of cells with round nuclei and indistinct cytoplasmic borders (modified Giemsa stain)

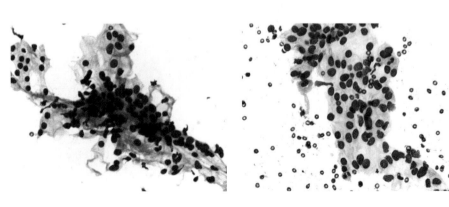

Modern Technique for Diagnosis
▦ Electron microscopy demonstrates numerous cytoplasmic glycogen granules

Differential Diagnosis
▦ Mucinous cystic neoplasms
  ➤ Mucous material in the background
  ➤ Columnar cells with varying degree of pleomorphism
  ➤ Goblet or signet ring cells can be present
▦ Solid and papillary epithelial neoplasm
  ➤ Papillary structures
  ➤ Nuclear grooves
  ➤ Metachromatic hyaline globules
▦ Pseudocyst
  ➤ Macrophages
  ➤ Rare or no epithelial cells
  ➤ Calcifications, cholesterol crystals
  ➤ Mesenchymal repair can be present

PEARLS

★ More often seen in elderly females
★ Usually benign tumors with a few reported cases of malignant serous cystadeno-carcinoma
★ Features causing diagnostic difficulty include: scanty cellularity, papillary groups, and nuclear atypia
★ Contaminating gastrointestinal epithelium and mucin material should not be confused with a cystic mucinous neoplasm

MUCINOUS CYSTIC NEOPLASMS

Clinical Features
▦ Uncommon cystic tumors (2% of pancreatic tumors) occurring almost exclusively in women and often between thirty and sixty years of age
▦ Most tumors occur in the tail or body of pancreas (>80%) and markedly vary in size (2–35 cm)
▦ Smaller tumor is found incidentally, but larger tumor may cause palpable mass, abdominal pain, nausea, and weight loss. Jaundice is uncommon even in tumors that occur in the pancreatic head
▦ Association with diabetes is frequent
▦ Smaller cysts tend to be unilocular and benign (mucinous cystadenoma), while larger cysts tend to multilocular and borderline or malignant (mucinous cystadenocarcinoma)
▦ Mucinous cysts typically show ovarian-like stroma and show no communication with the pancreatic ductal system

Cytologic Features
▦ Mucoid material in the background
▦ Cellularity can be variable, depending on the amount of mucus aspirated
▦ The neoplastic cells usually are arranged in sheets or in groups showing nuclear overlapping, atypia, and lost polarity
▦ Papillary clusters may be present
▦ Intracellular mucin material is quite characteristic
▦ Benign muciphages are usually present
▦ Spectrum of maturation of glandular cells from benign to malignant is often observed

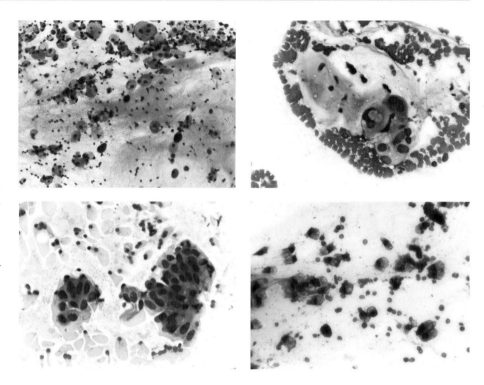

16-7A. Mucinous cystic neoplasm *(top, left).* Abundant mucous material with numerous mucophages in the background (modified Giemsa stain)

16-7B. Mucinous cystic neoplasm *(top, right).* Cluster of mature ductal epithelium with intra-cytoplasmic mucous material (modified Giemsa stain)

16-7C. Mucinous cystic neoplasm *(bottom, left).* Cluster of neoplastic epithelium showing strati-fication and loss of polarity (border-line mucinous tumor) (modified Giemsa stain)

16-7D. Adenocarcinoma *(bottom, right).* Isolated adenocarci-noma cells showing signet ring con-figuration (modified Giemsa stain)

- Single cells with obvious malignant cytologic features (mucinous cystadenocarci-noma) can be present
- Presence of goblet or signet rings cells help in making the diagnosis
- Papillae may also be present

Special Stains and Immunohistochemistry
- Cytokeratins, EMA and CEA positive
- Most cases show positive staining for neuroendocrine markers
- Histochemical (PAS, mucicarmine) stains for mucin as well as immunohistochem-ical stain for pancreatic mucin (CA19-9) are positive

Modern Technique for Diagnosis
- P53 nuclear positivity in most tumor cells correlates with mucinous cystadenocar-cinoma
- Mutations and/or deletions of K-ras are more common in mucinous cystadenocar-cinoma

Differential Diagnosis
- Intraductal papillary mucinous tumors of the pancreas
  - ➤ True papillae with fibrovascular cores
  - ➤ Small three-dimensional micropillary clusters
  - ➤ Psammoma bodies
  - ➤ Nuclear grooves
  - ➤ Mucinous epithelium, in most cases

PEARLS

- ★ Well-differentiated tumors may resemble endocervical cells
- ★ Distinction between intraductal papillary mucinous tumors of the pancreas (IPMT) and mucinous cystic lesions of FNA material is a matter of correlation with clinical and image data

SOLID PSEUDOPAPILLARY NEOPLASM

Clinical Features
▨ Also known as solid-cystic tumor, papillary-cystic tumor, and solid and papillary epithelial neoplasm
▨ Most common in young women (mean age: three years) and rare in men; however, gender or hormonal pathogenesis is not definitely identified
▨ Often incidentally detected, solitary, encapsulated, often cystic appearing with internal hemorrhage and found anywhere in the pancreas
▨ Size varies widely from small to very large (2–20 cm, mean 8 cm)
▨ Mostly benign with aggressive or malignant behavior seen in less than 5% of cases
▨ Malignant forms are low-grade and slow growing, with long disease-free periods of several years

Cytologic Features
▨ Delicate branching papillary fragments with central capillaries covered with several layers of bland tumor cells
▨ Acinar/rosette-like pattern
▨ Fine chromatin pattern with inconspicuous nucleoli
▨ Folded nuclear membranes
▨ Nuclear grooves can be seen
▨ Single uniform cells
▨ Metachromatic hyaline globules often present in the background
▨ Cytoplasmic processes can be seen
▨ Mitotic activity is virtually absent
▨ Necrosis, histiocytes can be present if cystic changes occur

Special Stains and Immunohistochemistry
▨ Consistently positive for vimentin, progesterone receptor (PR), and NSE
▨ When cytoplasmic eosinophilic globules are present, these are positive for PAS-D and alpha-1-antitrypsin (focal positivity)
▨ Generally negative for keratin and neuroendocrine markers

Modern Technique for Diagnosis
▨ Most benign-behaving tumors are diploid

Differential Diagnosis
▨ Islet cell tumor
  ➤ Monotomous population of small to medium-sized cells
  ➤ Round to oval nuclei with smooth nuclear membranes
  ➤ Small amount of cytoplasm
  ➤ Salt-and-pepper chromatin pattern is characteristic
  ➤ Multinucleated tumor giant cells and spindle cells may be seen in malignant cases

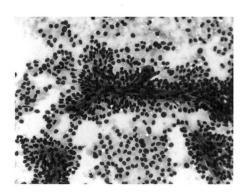

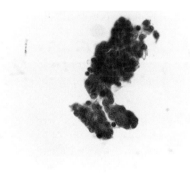

16-8A. Solid-pseudopapillary neoplasm *(left)*. Branching papillary fragments. Acinar/rosette-like pattern is seen in the background (modified Giemsa stain)

16-8B. Solid-pseudopapillary neoplasm *(right)*. Papillary cluster of cells showing nuclear grooving (Papanicolaou stain)

■ Acinar cell carcinoma
➤ Loosely cohesive clusters of cells
➤ Acinar formation
➤ Large polygonal cells with moderate amount of finely vacuolated cytoplasm
➤ Clumped chromatin pattern with prominent nucleoli

PEARLS

✶ Young women in their twenties, body/tail, low-grade pancreatic malignancy
✶ Branching papillae with myxoid stroma are best seen in cell block material
✶ Metachromatic hyaline globules
✶ Metastatic tumors may show cytologic atypia (pleomorphic tumor cells and mitotic activity)

PANCREATOBLASTOMA

Clinical Features
■ Extremely rare malignant epithelial tumor but commonest pancreatic tumor in young children (median age: four years)
■ Rare cases are described in older children, adults, and newborns
■ Slight male predominance (1.3:1)
■ Clinical findings include incidentally detected abdominal mass, abdominal pain, weight loss, and diarrhea
■ Usually lobulated, solitary, and encapsulated solid fleshy mass markedly varying in size (1.5–20 cm) and presenting anywhere in the pancreas

Cytologic Features
■ Oval to cuboidal cells with vesicular chromatin pattern, small nucleoli, and a moderate amount of granular cytoplasm
■ Primitive spindled mesenchymal tissue
■ Cartilage may be present
■ Stromal fragments, some of which are surrounded by epithelial cells
■ Solid sheets, three-dimensional, loosely cohesive epithelial groups
■ Acinar formation and squamoid corpuscles best appreciated in cell block preparations

Special Stains and Immunohistochemistry
■ Most cases show PAS-D-positive acinar-type cytoplasmic granules
■ Positive for cytokeratins, EMA, and CEA
■ Pancreatic acinar enzyme immunostains such as trypsin, chymotrypasin, and lipase are generally positive
■ Neuroendocrine markers may be positive but cells showing acinar markers are greater in numbers
■ AFP is positive in some cases

Modern Technique for Diagnosis
■ Ultrastructural findings include acinar-type electron-dense zymogen granules and a potential minor component of smaller endocrine type granules

Differential Diagnosis
■ Acinar-cell carcinoma
➤ Presence of squamous corpuscles and/or heterologous elements such as cartilage support the diagnosis of pancreatoblastoma

✷ Pancreatoblastoma is the most difficult neoplasm to differentiate from acinar cell carcinoma clinically and cytogically, especially in young children

ACINIC CELL CARCINOMA

Clinical Features
▨ Uncommon tumor (1–2% of all pancreatic tumors) affecting older adults (mean age sixty-two years) and frequently males (M:F ratio 2:1)
▨ Most patients present with nonspecific symptoms related to either local mass or metastasis
▨ About 15% of patients present with a syndrome of disseminated fat necrosis, eosinophilia, and polyarthralgia related to hypersecretion of lipase
▨ Most tumors are large (mean size: 10 cm), nodular, soft, and solid and arise in any part of pancreas
▨ Rare cystic variants and mixed acinar–endocrine variants are described

Cytologic Features
▨ Highly cellular cytologic smears
▨ Numerous single cells
▨ Prominent acinar formation
▨ Abundant delicate cytoplasm containing small granules (zymogen)
▨ Round to oval eccentrically located nucleus
▨ Prominent nucleoli, single or multiple
▨ Numerous stripped round nuclei in the background of the smear

Special Stains and Immunohistochemistry
▨ Positive for cytokeratins (8/18 and AE1/AE3)
▨ Most (95%) tumors are positive for pancreatic enzymes trypsin and chymotrypsin and also often positive for lipase (70%)
▨ One-third of cases may be positive for neuroendocrine markers synaptophysin and chromogranin

Modern Technique for Diagnosis
▨ Ultrastructurally apical electron dense granules (125–1000 nm) tend to be larger than nonneoplastic acinar cells
▨ In contrast to ductal adenocarcinoma, K-ras mutation, and P53 immunoreactivity is rare in acinic cell carcinoma

Differential Diagnosis
▨ Islet cell tumor
  ➤ Aspirates are often highly cellular

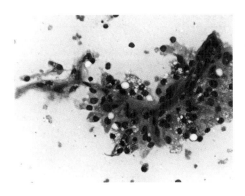 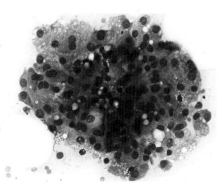

16-9A. Acinic cell carcinoma
(left). Cluster of neoplastic cells with large amount of vacuolated cytoplasm, some of which contain small red granules (Zymogen). Stripped round nuclei in the background are seen (modified Giemsa stain)

16-9B. Acinic cell carcinoma
(right). High-power view showing red granular cytoplasm (modified Giemsa stain)

> ➤ Small to medium-sized loose clusters and numerous single cells
> ➤ Acinar pseudorosette formation is often present
> ➤ Prominent vascularity can be present
> ➤ Uniform round to oval nuclei
> ➤ Fine granular chromatin pattern
> ➤ Prominent nucleoli may be seen
- ▪ Solid and papillary epithelial neoplasm
  - ➤ Highly cellular aspirates with branching papillae
  - ➤ Small uniform cells with bland round to oval nuclei that can be clefted
  - ➤ Fine chromatin pattern
  - ➤ Background often contains metachromatic hyaline material

PEARLS

✶ The cytologic features of acinar cell carcinoma show significant overlap with those of pancreatic endocrine tumors

✶ Abundant granular cytoplasm (zymogen granules) and prominent nucleoli may help to differentiate acinic cell carcinoma from pancreatic endocrine tumors

ISLET CELL TUMOR

Clinical Features

▪ Uncommon (1–2% of all pancreatic tumors), heterogeneous, and generally low-grade neuroendocrine tumors

▪ May occur at any age but common in adults (between thirty and sixty years)

▪ May secrete a variety of native pancreatic (insulin, glucagon, somatostatin, and PP) or other gastroenteropancreatic (gastrin, VIP, serotonin, calcitonin, etc.) hormones

▪ Hyperfunction of hormone may produce characteristic hormone-related syndrome (65–75% cases). The secretion may be nonfunctional (25–35% cases)

▪ Nonfunctional tumors cause nonspecific symptoms related to their location within pancreas such as biliary obstruction and jaundice in the head of pancreas

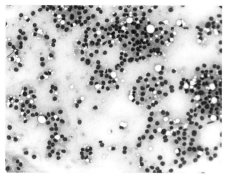
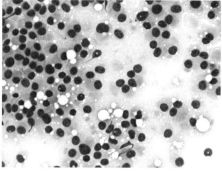
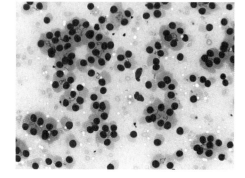

16-10A. Islet cell tumor *(top, left)*. Microacinar pattern is evident (modified Giemsa stain)

16-10B. Islet cell tumor *(top, right)*. High-power-view shows abundant cytoplasm and eccentric located nuclei (modified Giemsa stain)

16-10C. Islet cell tumor *(opposite)*. Oncocytic cytoplasm is evident (modified Giemsa stain)

▥ Identification of the hormone and associated clinical syndrome and prediction of prognosis are the most challenging aspects of this tumor

▥ Indolent behavior is associated with small size (<2 cm), insulin secretion, lower grade, and lack of necrosis, mitoses, and vascular or extrapancreatic invasion

▥ Most are sporadic but some occur as a component of multiple endocrine neoplasia 1 (MEN-1) syndrome and von Hipple–Lindau syndrome

Cytologic Features

▥ Prominent cellular dissociation with many single cells and small, poorly cohesive groups

▥ Variable nuclear pleomorphism with fine granular chromatin pattern

▥ Most tumor cells have abundant cytoplasm and eccentrically located nuclei

▥ Rarely the cytoplasm can be oncocytic, clear, or lipid rich

▥ Binucleation, multinucleation, intranuclear inclusions, mitotic figures, and necrosis may be present

▥ Amyloid material deposits may occur

▥ Psammoma bodies can be also seen

Special Stains and Immunohistochemistry

▥ All islet cell tumors are positive for cytokeratins (8/18 and AE1/AE3, and generally negative for cytokeratin 7), and positive for NSE, synaptophysin, and chromogranin

▥ Depending on the clinical syndrome immunohistochemistry may be positive for specific hormone such as insulin, somatostatin, glucagon, gastrin, and PP

▥ There may be discrepancy between antigenically positive but functionally inactive components of a hormone

▥ Some tumors contain amyloid demonstrated by congo red stain with apple-green birefringence on polarized light

Modern Technique for Diagnosis

▥ Ultrastructural studies for detection of membrane-bound 100–400 nm dense-core neurosectretory granules is now less popular due to availability and specificity of immunohistochemical stains

▥ A crystalline ultrastructural appearance of neurosecretory granules is often associated with insulinoma

Differential Diagnosis

▪ Solid and papillary epithelial neoplasm
  ➤ Metachromatic hyaline globules may be seen
  ➤ Folded nuclear membranes
  ➤ Nucleoli absent or inconspicuous
  ➤ Delicate branching papillary fragments
  ➤ Acinar/rosette-like pattern
  ➤ Lack of mitotic activity
  ➤ Cystic changes may be present, for example, necrosis and histiocytes
▪ Well-differentiated adenocarcinoma
  ➤ Cellular aspirates dominated by ductal cells
  ➤ Numerous large sheets of bland ductal cells
  ➤ Rare isolated neoplastic cells with obvious malignant features are usually present
  ➤ Nuclear membrane irregularities
  ➤ Single, multiple nucleoli
  ➤ Irregular chromatin distribution
▪ Metastatic small cell carcinoma
  ➤ Small clusters, Indian files, and many single cells
  ➤ Scanty cytoplasm
  ➤ Hyperchromatic nuclear chromatin
  ➤ Nuclear molding

➤ Crush artifact
➤ Necrosis
➤ Small and inconspicuous nucleoli
■ Malignant lymphoma
➤ Majority of lymphomas involving the pancreas are secondary and are mostly of large cell type, B-phenotype
➤ Homogenous neoplastic proliferation of tumor cells
➤ Round to oval nuclei, fine chromatin pattern, and multiple nucleoli are usually present
➤ Variable amount of cytoplasm, usually moderate amount and basophilic on modified Giemsa stain
■ Multiple myeloma/plasmacytoma
➤ Plasmacytoid cells with mature nuclei showing typical coarse "clock face" chromatin
➤ Plasmacytoid cells with immature nuclei showing fine chromatin pattern and prominent nucleoli
➤ Binucleation, multinucleation and bizarre plasma cells can be seen
➤ Cytoplasm is dense blue on (modified Giemsa stain) or amphophilic on (papanicolaou) with a perinuclear clearing

PEARLS

✷ The islet cell tumor may be confused on FNA material with solid and papillary epithelial neoplasm

METASTATIC TUMORS

Clinical Features
■ Direct extension of adenocarcinoma may occur in the pancreas from adjacent organs such as stomach, intestine, and biliary tract

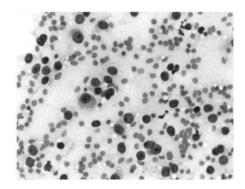
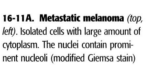
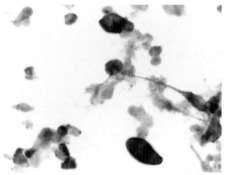
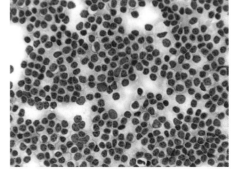

16-11A. Metastatic melanoma *(top, left)*. Isolated cells with large amount of cytoplasm. The nuclei contain prominent nucleoli (modified Giemsa stain)

16-11B. Metastatic melanoma *(top, right)*. S-100 protein positive in melanoma cells

16-11C. Metastatic malignant lymphoma *(opposite)*. Uniform population of lymphoid cells (modified Giemsa stain)

Secondary tumors of the pancreas are uncommon (4–11% of all pancreatic tumors), occur through lymphatic or hematogenous spread and are usually part of widely metastatic disease

Affect males and females equally with highest incidence in the sixth decade

Common primary sites include lung, breast, kidney, and skin (melanoma)

Metastatic lesions may be solitary or multiple and any part of pancreas may be involved

Clinically and radiologically metastatic tumors may mimic primary pancreatic tumors

Pancreatic metastasis from renal cell carcinoma may be late and solitary

Cytologic Features

Unusual cytomorphologic appearance that is not typical of a primary pancreatic neoplasm such as: a population of single cells with lymphoglandular bodies in the background, should raise the possibility of a malignant lymphoma

Presence of single cells, binucleation, multinucleation, and intranuclear cytoplasmic inclusions, may raise the possibility of a metastatic melanoma

Special Stains and Immunohistochemistry

Choice of stains depends upon suspected primary

Lung, non–small cell carcinoma: Cytokeratin 7 and TTF-1: Often positive

Breast ductal carcinoma: Cytokeratin 7, GCDFP-15, ER and PR: Often positive

Renal cell carcinoma: Cytokeratin 7 and 20: Negative and PAX-2: Positive

Melanoma: Cytokeratin: Negative and S-100 and HMB-45: Positive

Modern Technique for Diagnosis

Noncontributory

Differential Diagnosis

Consider metastatic neoplasm if the cytologic features are not typical for a pancreatic tumor

PEARLS

☆ Clinical, radiographic, and cytologic findings should be correlated before rendering a diagnosis of a metastatic tumor to the pancreas

☆ Immunocytochemistry, when possible, may help to confirm a suspected diagnosis

REFERENCES

ACUTE PANCREATITIS

Banks PA. Pro: computerized tomographic fine needle aspiration (CT-FNA) is valuable in the management of infected pancreatic necrosis. *Am J Gastroenterol.* 2005 Nov;100(11):2371–2.

Eloubeidi MA, Gress FG, Savides TJ, Wiersema MJ, Kochman ML, Ahmad NA, Ginsberg GG, Erickson RA, Dewitt J, Van Dam J, Nickl NJ, Levy MJ, Clain JE, Chak A, Sivak MV Jr, Wong R, Isenberg G, Scheiman JM, Bounds B, Kimmey MB, Saunders MD, Chang KJ, Sharma A, Nguyen P, Lee JG, Edmundowicz SA, Early D, Azar R, Etemad B, Chen YK, Waxman I, Shami V, Catalano MF, Wilcox CM. Acute pancreatitis after EUS-guided FNA of solid pancreatic masses: a pooled analysis from EUS centers in the United States. *Gastrointest Endosc.* 2004 Sep;60(3):385–9.

Eloubeidi MA, Tamhane A, Varadarajulu S, Wilcox CM. Frequency of major complications after EUS-guided FNA of solid pancreatic masses: a prospective evaluation. *Gastrointest Endosc.* 2006 Apr;63(4):622–9.

Mayer J, Rau B, Grewe M, Schoenberg MH, Nevalainen TJ, Beger HG. Secretory phospholipase A2 in patients with infected pancreatic necroses in acute pancreatitis. *Pancreas.* 1998 Oct;17(3):272–7.

Moulton JS. The radiologic assessment of acute pancreatitis and its complications. *Pancreas.* 1991;6 Suppl 1:S13–22.

Olah A, Belagyi T, Issekutz A, Makay R, Zaborszky A. Value of procalcitonin quick test in the differentiation between sterile and infected forms of acute pancreatitis. *Hepatogastroenterology.* 2005 Jan–Feb;52(61):243–5.

O'Toole D, Palazzo L, Arotcarena R, Dancour A, Aubert A, Hammel P, Amaris J, Ruszniewski P. Assessment of complications of EUS-guided fine-needle aspiration. *Gastrointest Endosc.* 2001 Apr;53(4):470–4.

Weynand B, Deprez P.Endoscopic ultrasound guided fine needle aspiration in biliary and pancreatic diseases: pitfalls and performances. *Acta Gastroenterol Belg.* 2004 Jul–Sep;67(3):294–300.

CHRONIC PANCREATITIS

Farrell JJ, Garber J, Sahani D, Brugge WR. EUS findings in patients with autoimmune pancreatitis. *Gastrointest Endosc.* 2004 Dec;60(6):927–36.

Ho S, Bonasera RJ, Pollack BJ, Grendell J, Feuerman M, Gress F. A single-center experience of endoscopic ultrasonography for enlarged pancreas on computed tomography. *Clin Gastroenterol Hepatol.* 2006 Jan;4(1):98–103.

Iglesias-Garcia J, Abdulkader I, Larino-Noia J, Forteza J, Dominguez-Munoz JE. Histological evaluation of chronic pancreatitis by endoscopic ultrasound-guided fine needle biopsy. *Gut.* 2006 Nov;55(11):1661–2.

Khalid A, Nodit L, Zahid M, Bauer K, Brody D, Finkelstein SD, McGrath KM. Endoscopic ultrasound fine needle aspirate DNA analysis to differentiate malignant and benign pancreatic masses. *Am J Gastroenterol.* 2006 Nov;101(11):2493–500.

Lerma E, Musulen E, Cuatrecasas M, Martinez A, Montserrat E, Prat J. Fine needle aspiration cytology in pancreatic pathology. *Acta Cytol.* 1996 Jul–Aug;40(4):683–6.

Levy MJ, Wiersema MJ, Chari ST. Chronic pancreatitis: focal pancreatitis or cancer? Is there a role for FNA/biopsy? Autoimmune pancreatitis. *Endoscopy.* 2006 Jun;38 Suppl. 1:S30–5.

Marchevsky AM, Nelson V, Martin SE, Greaves TS, Raza AS, Zeineh J, Cobb CJ. Telecytology of fine-needle aspiration biopsies of the pancreas: a study of well-differentiated adenocarcinoma and chronic pancreatitis with atypical epithelial repair changes. *Diagn Cytopathol.* 2003 Mar;28(3):147–52.

Stelow EB, Bardales RH, Lai R, Mallery S, Linzie BM, Crary GS, Stanley MW. The cytological spectrum of chronic pancreatitis. *Diagn Cytopathol.* 2005 Feb;32(2):65–9.

Varadarajulu S, Tamhane A, Eloubeidi MA. Yield of EUS-guided FNA of pancreatic masses in the presence or the absence of chronic pancreatitis. *Gastrointest Endosc.* 2005 Nov;62(5):728–36; quiz 751, 753.

PANCREATIC PSEUDOCYST

Centeno BA, Warshaw AL, Mayo-Smith W, Southern JF, Lewandrowski K. Cytologic diagnosis of pancreatic cystic lesions. A prospective study of 28 percutaneous aspirates. *Acta Cytol.* 1997 Jul–Aug;41(4):972–80.

Jorda M, Essenfeld H, Garcia E, Ganjei P. The value of fine-needle aspiration cytology in the diagnosis of inflammatory pancreatic masses. *Diagn Cytopathol.* 1992;8(1):65–7.

Kloppel G. Pseudocysts and other non-neoplastic cysts of the pancreas. *Semin Diagn Pathol.* 2000 Feb;17(1):7–15.

Levy MJ, Clain JE. Evaluation and management of cystic pancreatic tumors: emphasis on the role of EUS FNA. *Clin Gastroenterol Hepatol.* 2004 Aug;2(8):639–53.

Liu J, Shin HJ, Rubenchik I, Lang E, Lahoti S, Staerkel GA. Cytologic features of lymphoepithelial cyst of the pancreas: two preoperatively diagnosed cases based on fine-needle aspiration. *Diagn Cytopathol.* 1999 Nov;21(5):34650.

Nguyen GK, Suen KC, Villanueva RR. Needle aspiration cytology of pancreatic cystic lesions. *Diagn Cytopathol.* 1997 Sep;17(3):177–82.

Pinto MM, Meriano FV. Diagnosis of cystic pancreatic lesions by cytologic examination and carcinoembryonic antigen and amylase assays of cyst contents. *Acta Cytol.* 1991 Jul–Aug; 35(4):456–63.

Sperti C, Pasquali C, Di Prima F, Rugge M, Petrin P, Costantino V, Canton A, Pedrazzoli S. Percutaneous CT-guided fine needle aspiration cytology in the differential diagnosis of pancreatic lesions. *Ital J Gastroenterol.* 1994 Apr;26(3):126–31.

DUCTAL ADENOCARCINOMA

Basir Z, Pello N, Dayer AM, Shidham VB, Komorowski RA. Accuracy of cytologic interpretation of pancreatic neoplasms by fine needle aspiration and pancreatic duct brushings. *Acta Cytol.* 2003 Sep–Oct;47(5):733–8.

David O, Green L, Reddy V, Kluskens L, Bitterman P, Attal H, Prinz R, Gattuso P. Pancreatic masses: a multi-institutional study of 364 fine-needle aspiration biopsies with histopathologic correlation. *Diagn Cytopathol.* 1998 Dec;19(6):423–7.

Fekete PS, Nunez C, Pitlik DA. Fine-needle aspiration biopsy of the pancreas: a study of 61 cases. *Diagn Cytopathol.* 1986 Dec;2(4):301–6.

Fujita N, Noda Y, Kobayashi G, Kimura K, Ito K. Endoscopic approach to early diagnosis of pancreatic cancer. *Pancreas.* 2004 Apr;28(3):279–81.

Silverman JF, Finley JL, Berns L, Unverferth M. Significance of giant cells in fine-needle aspiration biopsies of benign and malignant lesions of the pancreas. *Diagn Cytopathol.* 1989;5(4):388–91.

Silverman JF, Finley JL, MacDonald KG, Jr. Fine-needle aspiration cytology of osteoclastic giant-cell tumor of the pancreas. *Diagn Cytopathol.* 1990;6(5):336–40.

Suits J, Frazee R, Erickson RA. Endoscopic ultrasound and fine needle aspiration for the evaluation of pancreatic masses. *Arch Surg.* 1999 Jun;134(6):639–42; discussion 642–3.

Thompson K, Castelli MJ, Gattuso P. Metastatic papillary oncocytic carcinoma of the pancreas to the liver diagnosed by fine-needle aspiration. *Diagn Cytopathol.* 1998 Apr;18(4):291–6.

INTRADUCTAL PAPILLARY MUCINOUS TUMOR OF THE PANCREAS

Emerson RE, Randolph ML, Cramer HM. Endoscopic ultrasound-guided fine-needle aspiration cytology diagnosis of intraductal papillary mucinous neoplasm of the pancreas is highly predictive of pancreatic neoplasia. *Diagn Cytopathol.* 2006 Jul;34(7):457–62.

Layfield LJ, Cramer H. Fine-needle aspiration cytology of intraductal papillary-mucinous tumors: a retrospective analysis. *Diagn Cytopathol.* 2005 Jan;32(1):16–20.

Lee SY, Choi DW, Jang KT, Lee KT, Choi SH, Heo JS, Lee JK, Paik SW, Rhee JC. High expression of intestinal-type mucin (MUC2) in intraductal papillary mucinous neoplasms coexisting with extrapancreatic gastrointestinal cancers. *Pancreas.* 2006 Mar;32(2):186–9.

Michaels PJ, Brachtel EF, Bounds BC, Brugge WR, Pitman MB. Intraductal papillary mucinous neoplasm of the pancreas: cytologic features predict histologic grade. *Cancer.* 2006 Jun 25;108(3):163–73.

Schoedel KE, Finkelstein SD, Ohori NP. K-Ras and microsatellite marker analysis of fine-needle aspirates from intraductal papillary mucinous neoplasms of the pancreas. *Diagn Cytopathol.* 2006 Sep;34(9):605–8.

Sole M, Iglesias C, Fernandez-Esparrach G, Colomo L, Pellise M, Gines A. Fine-needle aspiration cytology of intraductal papillary mucinous tumors of the pancreas. *Cancer.* 2005 Oct 25;105(5):298–303.

Yamaguchi K, Nakamura M, Shirahane K, Kawamoto M, Konomi H, Ohta M, Tanaka M. Pancreatic juice cytology in IPMN of the pancreas. *Pancreatology.* 2005;5(4-5):416–21; discussion 421. Epub 2005 Jun 28.

Yamaguchi T, Shirai Y, Ishihara T, Sudo K, Nakagawa A, Ito H, Miyazaki M, Nomura F, Saisho H. Pancreatic juice cytology in the diagnosis of intraductal papillary mucinous neoplasm of the pancreas: significance of sampling by peroral pancreatoscopy. *Cancer.* 2005 Dec 15;104(12):2830–6.

Zhai J, Sarkar R, Ylagan L. Pancreatic mucinous lesions: a retrospective analysis with cytohistological correlation. *Diagn Cytopathol.* 2006 Nov;34(11):724–30.

SEROUS CYSTADENOMA

Basir Z, Pello N, Dayer AM, Shidham VB, Komorowski RA. Accuracy of cytologic interpretation of pancreatic neoplasms by fine needle aspiration and pancreatic duct brushings. *Acta Cytol.* 2003 Sep–Oct;47(5):733–8.

Carlson SK, Johnson CD, Brandt KR, Batts KP, Salomao DR. Pancreatic cystic neoplasms: the role and sensitivity of needle aspiration and biopsy. *Abdom Imaging.* 1998 Jul–Aug;23(4):387–93.

Huang P, Staerkel G, Sneige N, Gong Y. Fine-needle aspiration of pancreatic serous cystadenoma: cytologic features and diagnostic pitfalls. *Cancer.* 2006 Aug 25;108(4):239–49.

Jones EC, Suen KC, Grant DR, Chan NH. Fine-needle aspiration cytology of neoplastic cysts of the pancreas. *Diagn Cytopathol.* 1987 Sep;3(3):238–43.

Kloppel G, Kosmahl M. Cystic lesions and neoplasms of the pancreas. The features are becoming clearer. *Pancreatology.* 2001;1(6):648–55.

Lal A, Bourtsos EP, DeFrias DV, Nemcek AA, Nayar R. Microcystic adenoma of the pancreas: clinical, radiologic, and cytologic features. *Cancer.* 2004 Oct 25;102(5):288–94.

Linder JD, Geenen JE, Catalano MF. Cyst fluid analysis obtained by EUS-guided FNA in the evaluation of discrete cystic neoplasms of the pancreas: a prospective single-center experience. *Gastrointest Endosc.* 2006 Nov;64(5):697–702.

Rampy BA, Waxman I, Xiao SY, Logrono R. Serous cystadenoma of the pancreas with papillary features: a diagnostic pitfall on fine-needle aspiration biopsy. *Arch Pathol Lab Med.* 2001 Dec;125(12):1591–4.

Recine M, Kaw M, Evans DB, Krishnamurthy S. Fine-needle aspiration cytology of mucinous tumors of the pancreas. *Cancer.* 2004 Apr 25;102(2):92–9.

Sand JA, Hyoty MK, Mattila J, Dagorn JC, Nordback IH. Clinical assessment compared with cyst fluid analysis in the differential diagnosis of cystic lesions in the pancreas. *Surgery.* 1996 Mar;119(3):275–80.

Sperti C, Pasquali C, Perasole A, Liessi G, Pedrazzoli S. Macrocystic serous cystadenoma of the pancreas: clinicopathologic features in seven cases. *Int J Pancreatol.* 2000 Aug;28(1):1–7.

MUCINOUS CYSTIC NEOPLASMS

Basir Z, Pello N, Dayer AM, Shidham VB, Komorowski RA. Accuracy of cytologic interpretation of pancreatic neoplasms by fine needle aspiration and pancreatic duct brushings. *Acta Cytol.* 2003 Sep–Oct;47(5):733–8.

Centeno BA, Warshaw AL, Mayo-Smith W, Southern JF, Lewandrowski K. Cytologic diagnosis of pancreatic cystic lesions. A prospective study of 28 percutaneous aspirates. *Acta Cytol.* 1997 Jul–Aug;41(4):972–80.

Emerson RE, Randolph ML, Cramer HM. Endoscopic ultrasound-guided fine-needle aspiration cytology diagnosis of intraductal papillary mucinous neoplasm of the pancreas is highly predictive of pancreatic neoplasia. *Diagn Cytopathol.* 2006 Jul;34(7):457–62.

Fernandez-del Castillo C, Warshaw AL. Cystic neoplasms of the pancreas. *Pancreatology.* 2001;1(6):641–7.

Kloppel G, Kosmahl M. Cystic lesions and neoplasms of the pancreas. The features are becoming clearer. *Pancreatology.* 2001;1(6):648–55.

Lai R, Stanley MW, Bardales R, Linzie B, Mallery S. Endoscopic ultrasound-guided pancreatic duct aspiration: diagnostic yield and safety. *Endoscopy.* 2002 Sep;34(9):715–20.

Linder JD, Geenen JE, Catalano MF. Cyst fluid analysis obtained by EUS-guided FNA in the evaluation of discrete cystic neoplasms of the pancreas: a prospective single-center experience. *Gastrointest Endosc.* 2006 Nov;64(5):697–702.

Maire F, Couvelard A, Hammel P, Ponsot P, Palazzo L, Aubert A, Degott C, Dancour A, Felce-Dachez M, O'toole D, Levy P, Ruszniewski P. Intraductal papillary mucinous tumors of the pancreas: the preoperative value of cytologic and histopathologic diagnosis. *Gastrointest Endosc.* 2003 Nov;58(5):701–6.

O'Toole D, Palazzo L, Hammel P, Ben Yaghlene L, Couvelard A, Felce-Dachez M, Fabre M, Dancour A, Aubert A, Sauvanet A, Maire F, Levy P, Ruszniewski P. Macrocystic pancreatic cystadenoma: The role of EUS and cyst fluid analysis in distinguishing mucinous and serous lesions. *Gastrointest Endosc.* 2004 Jun;59(7):823–9.

Recine M, Kaw M, Evans DB, Krishnamurthy S. Fine-needle aspiration cytology of mucinous tumors of the pancreas. *Cancer.* 2004 Apr 25;102(2):92–9.

Zhai J, Sarkar R, Ylagan L. Pancreatic mucinous lesions: a retrospective analysis with cytohistological correlation. *Diagn Cytopathol.* 2006 Nov;34(11):724–30.

SOLID PSEUDOPAPILLARY NEOPLASM

Bardales RH, Centeno B, Mallery JS, Lai R, Pochapin M, Guiter G, Stanley MW. Endoscopic ultrasound-guided fine-needle aspiration cytology diagnosis of solid-pseudopapillary tumor of the pancreas: a rare neoplasm of elusive origin but characteristic cytomorphologic features. *Am J Clin Pathol.* 2004 May;121(5):654–62.

Bhanot P, Nealon WH, Walser EM, Bhutani MS, Tang WW, Logrono R. Clinical, imaging, and cytopathological features of solid pseudopapillary tumor of the pancreas: a clinicopathologic study of three cases and review of the literature. *Diagn Cytopathol.* 2005 Dec;33(6):421–8.

Mariappan MR, Fadare O, Jain D, Chacho MS. Diagnostic intraoperative imprint cytology of a solid pseudopapillary tumor of the pancreas. *Diagn Cytopathol.* 2005 Jun;32(6):351–2.

Master SS, Savides TJ. Diagnosis of solid-pseudopapillary neoplasm of the pancreas by EUS-guided FNA. *Gastrointest Endosc.* 2003 Jun;57(7):965–8.

Mergener K, Detweiler SE, Traverso LW. Solid pseudopapillary tumor of the pancreas: diagnosis by EUS-guided fine-needle aspiration. *Endoscopy.* 2003 Dec;35(12):1083–4.

Nadler EP, Novikov A, Landzberg BR, Pochapin MB, Centeno B, Fahey TJ, Spigland N. The use of endoscopic ultrasound in the diagnosis of solid pseudopapillary tumors of the pancreas in children. *J Pediatr Surg.* 2002 Sep;37(9):1370–3.

Nguyen GK, Suen KC, Villaneuva RR. Needle aspiration cytology of pancreatic cystic lesions. *Diagn Cytopathol.* 1997 Sep;17(3):177–82.

Pettinato G, Di Vizio D, Manivel JC, Pambuccian SE, Somma P, Insabato L. Solid-pseudopapillary tumor of the pancreas: a neoplasm with distinct and highly characteristic cytological features. *Diagn Cytopathol*. 2002 Dec;27(6):325–34.

Tiemann K, Kosmahl M, Ohlendorf J, Krams M, Kloppel G. Solid pseudopapillary neoplasms of the pancreas are associated with FLI-1 expression, but not with EWS/FLI-1 translocation. *Mod Pathol*. 2006 Nov;19(11):1409–13. Epub 2006 Aug 25.

Tien YW, Ser KH, Hu RH, Lee CY, Jeng YM, Lee PH. Solid pseudopapillary neoplasms of the pancreas: is there a pathologic basis for the observed gender differences in incidence? *Surgery*. 2005 Jun;137(6):591–6.

Tomsova M, Ryska A, Podhola M, Pohnetalova D. Solid and papillary epithelial tumor of the pancreas: cytologic and histologic features. *Cesk Patol*. 2002 Oct;38(4):178–82. Czech.

PANCREATOBLASTOMA

Hasegawa Y, Ishida Y, Kato K, Ijiri R, Miyake T, Nishimata S, Watanabe T, Namba I, Hayabuchi Y, Kigasawa H, Tanaka Y. Pancreatoblastoma. A case report with special emphasis on squamoid corpuscles with optically clear nuclei rich in biotin. *Acta Cytol*. 2003 Jul–Aug;47(4):679–84.

Henke AC, Kelley CM, Jensen CS, Timmerman TG. Fine-needle aspiration cytology of pancreatoblastoma. *Diagn Cytopathol*. 2001 Aug;25(2):118–21.

Pitman MB, Faquin WC. The fine-needle aspiration biopsy cytology of pancreatoblastoma. *Diagn Cytopathol*. 2004 Dec;31(6):402–6.

Silverman JF, Holbrook CT, Pories WJ, Kodroff MB, Joshi VV. Fine needle aspiration cytology of pancreatoblastoma with immunocytochemical and ultrastructural studies. *Acta Cytol*. 1990 Sep–Oct;34(5):632–40.

Zhu LC, Sidhu GS, Cassai ND, Yang GC. Fine-needle aspiration cytology of pancreatoblastoma in a young woman: report of a case and review of the literature. *Diagn Cytopathol*. 2005 Oct;33(4):258–62.

ACINIC CELL CARCINOMA

al-Kaisi N, Weaver MG, Abdul-Karim FW, Siegler E. Fine needle aspiration cytology of neuroendocrine tumors of the pancreas. A cytologic, immunocytochemical and electron microscopic study. *Acta Cytol*. 1992 Sep–Oct;36(5):655–60.

Das DK, Bhambhani S, Kumar N, Chachra KL, Prakash S, Gupta RK, Tripathi RP.

Ishihara A, Sanda T, Takanari H, Yatani R, Liu PI. Elastase-1-secreting acinar cell carcinoma of the pancreas. A cytologic, electron microscopic and histochemical study. *Acta Cytol*. 1989 Mar–Apr;33(2):157–63.

Labate AM, Klimstra DL, Zakowski MF. Comparative cytologic features of pancreatic acinar cell carcinoma and islet cell tumor. *Diagn Cytopathol*. 1997 Feb;16(2):112–6.

Ohori NP, Khalid A, Etemad B, Finkelstein SD. Multiple loss of heterozygosity without K-ras mutation identified by molecular analysis on fine-needle aspiration cytology specimen of acinar cell carcinoma of pancreas. *Diagn Cytopathol*. 2002 Jul;27(1):42–6.

Qizilbash AH. The pathological features of carcinoma of the pancreas. *Can J Surg*. 1981 Mar;24(2):168–70, 175.

Roldo C, Missiaglia E, Hagan JP, Falconi M, Capelli P, Bersani S, Calin GA, Ultrasound guided percutaneous fine needle aspiration cytology of pancreas: a review of 61 cases. *Trop Gastroenterol*. 1995 Apr–Jun;16(2):101–9.

Rouleau C, Serre I, Roger P, Guibal MP, Galifer RB, Bonardet A, Baldet P. Acinar cell carcinoma of the pancreas in a young patient with cells immunoreactive for somatostatin. *Histopathology*. 2006 Feb;48(3):307–9.

Samuel LH, Frierson HF Jr. Fine needle aspiration cytology of acinar cell carcinoma of the pancreas: a report of two cases. *Acta Cytol*. 1996 May–Jun;40(3):585–91.

Stelow EB, Bardales RH, Shami VM, Woon C, Presley A, Mallery S, Lai R, Stanley MW. Cytology of pancreatic acinar cell carcinoma. *Diagn Cytopathol*. 2006 May;34(5):367–72.

Villanueva RR, Nguyen-Ho P, Nguyen GK. Needle aspiration cytology of acinar-cell carcinoma of the pancreas: report of a case with diagnostic pitfalls and unusual ultrastructural findings. *Diagn Cytopathol*. 1994;10(4):362–4.

Volinia S, Liu CG, Scarpa A, Croce CM. MicroRNA expression abnormalities in pancreatic endocrine and acinar tumors are associated with distinctive pathologic features and clinical behavior. *J Clin Oncol*. 2006 Oct 10;24(29):4677–84. Epub 2006 Sep 11.

ISLET CELL TUMOR

Akosa AB, Desa LA, Phillips I, Benjamin IS, Polak JM, Krausz T. Aspiration cytodiagnosis of pancreatic endocrine tumours. *Cytopathology*. 1994 Dec;5(6):369–79.

al-Kaisi N, Weaver MG, Abdul-Karim FW, Siegler E. Fine needle aspiration cytology of neuro-endocrine tumors of the pancreas. A cytologic, immunocytochemical and electron micro-scopic study. *Acta Cytol.* 1992 Sep–Oct;36(5):655–60.

Bell DA. Cytologic features of islet-cell tumors. *Acta Cytol.* 1987 Jul–Aug;31(4):485–92.

Chang F, Vu C, Chandra A, Meenan J, Herbert A. Endoscopic ultrasound-guided fine needle aspiration cytology of pancreatic neuroendocrine tumours: cytomorphological and immuno-cytochemical evaluation. *Cytopathology.* 2006 Feb;17(1):10–7.

Collins BT, Cramer HM. Fine-needle aspiration cytology of islet cell tumors. *Diagn Cytopathol.* 1996 Jul;15(1):37–45.

Gu M, Ghafari S, Lin F, Ramzy I. Cytological diagnosis of endocrine tumors of the pancreas by endoscopic ultrasound-guided fine-needle aspiration biopsy. *Diagn Cytopathol.* 2005 Apr;32(4):204–10.

Hsiu JG, D'Amato NA, Sperling MH, Greenspan M, Jaffe AH, Smith R, 3rd, DeLaTorre R. Malig-nant islet-cell tumor of the pancreas diagnosed by fine needle aspiration biopsy. A case report. *Acta Cytol.* 1985 Jul–Aug;29(4):576–9.

Saleh HA, Masood S, Khatib G. Percutaneous and intraoperative aspiration biopsy cytology of pancreatic neuroendocrine tumors: cytomorphologic study with an immunocytochemical contribution. *Acta Cytol.* 1996 Mar–Apr;40(2):182–90.

Shaw JA, Vance RP, Geisinger KR, Marshall RB. Islet cell neoplasms. A fine-needle aspiration cytology study with immunocytochemical correlations. *Am J Clin Pathol.* 1990 Aug;94(2):142–9.

Sneige N, Ordonez NG, Veanattukalathil S, Samaan NA. Fine-needle aspiration cytology in pan-creatic endocrine tumors. *Diagn Cytopathol.* 1987 Mar;3(1):35–40.

Stelow EB, Woon C, Pambuccian SE, Thrall M, Stanley MW, Lai R, Mallery S, Gulbahce HE. Fine-needle aspiration cytology of pancreatic somatostatinoma: the importance of immunohisto-chemistry for the cytologic diagnosis of pancreatic endocrine neoplasms. *Diagn Cytopathol.* 2005 Aug;33(2):100–5.

Wick MR, Graeme-Cook FM. Pancreatic neuroendocrine neoplasms: a current summary of diagnostic, prognostic, and differential diagnostic information. *Am J Clin Pathol.* 2001 Jun;115 Suppl:S28–45.

METASTATIC TUMORS

Bechade D, Palazzo L, Fabre M, Algayres JP. EUS-guided FNA of pancreatic metastasis from renal cell carcinoma. *Gastrointest Endosc.* 2003 Nov;58(5):784–8.

Carson HJ, Green LK, Castelli MJ, Reyes CV, Prinz RA, Gattuso P. Utilization of fine-needle aspiration biopsy in the diagnosis of metastatic tumors to the pancreas. *Diagn Cytopathol.* 1995 Feb;12(1):8–13.

David O, Green L, Reddy V, Kluskens L, Bitterman P, Attal H, Prinz R, Gattuso P. Pancreatic masses: a multi-institutional study of 364 fine-needle aspiration biopsies with histopathologic correlation. *Diagn Cytopathol.* 1998 Dec;19(6):423–7.

DeWitt J, Jowell P, Leblanc J, McHenry L, McGreevy K, Cramer H, Volmar K, Sherman S, Gress F. EUS-guided FNA of pancreatic metastases: a multicenter experience. *Gastrointest Endosc.* 2005 May;61(6):689–96.

Eloubeidi MA, Jhala D, Chhieng DC, Jhala N, Eltoum I, Wilcox CM. Multiple late asymptomatic pancreatic metastases from renal cell carcinoma: diagnosis by endoscopic ultrasound-guided fine needle aspiration biopsy with immunocytochemical correlation. *Dig Dis Sci.* 2002 Aug; 47(8):1839–42.

Gupta RK, Lallu S, Delahunt B. Fine-needle aspiration cytology of metastatic clear-cell renal carcinoma presenting as a solitary mass in the head of the pancreas. *Diagn Cytopathol.* 1998 Sep;19(3):194–7.

Mesa H, Stelow EB, Stanley MW, Mallery S, Lai R, Bardales RH. Diagnosis of nonprimary pan-creatic neoplasms by endoscopic ultrasound-guided fine-needle aspiration. *Diagn Cytopathol.* 2004 Nov;31(5):313–8.

Sherman S, Gress F. EUS-guided FNA of pancreatic metastases: a multicenter experience. *Gastro-intest Endosc.* 2005 May;61(6):689–96.

Siddiqui AA, Olansky L, Sawh RN, Tierney WM. Pancreatic metastasis of tall cell variant of papillary thyroid carcinoma: diagnosis by endoscopic ultrasound-guided fine needle aspira-tion. *JOP.* 2006 Jul 10;7(4):417–22.

Silva RG, Dahmoush L, Gerke H. Pancreatic metastasis of an ovarian malignant mixed mullerian tumor identified by EUS-guided fine needle aspiration and Trucut needle biopsy. *JOP.* 2006 Jan 11;7(1):66–9.

Volmar KE, Jones CK, Xie HB. Metastases in the pancreas from nonhematologic neoplasms: report of 20 cases evaluated by fine-needle aspiration. *Diagn Cytopathol.* 2004 Oct; 31(4):216–20.

17

FNA of the Prostate Gland

Umesh Kapur, Güliz A. Barkan, and Eva M. Wojcik

Although fine-needle aspiration has been mostly displaced by core biopsy gun approach in diagnosing prostatic lesions in certain parts of the world, up till recently, it is still considered a useful diagnostic tool.

ATROPHIC PROSTATIC EPITHELIUM

Clinical features
- Hard prostate on palpation

Cytologic Features
- Large to medium-sized mono- or bilayered cohesive sheets made up of ductal and acinar prostatic cells with hyperchromatic deeply stained and closely packed nuclei
- Nuclei are smaller in size than those observed in normal prostatic epithelium
- Chromatin may be very dense and patternless

▓ Occasionally, atrophic sheets are deep blue in color on modified Giemsa staining and may be mistaken for an artifact

Special Stains and Immunohistochemistry
▓ Noncontributory

Modern Techniques for Diagnosis
▓ Noncontributory

Differential Diagnosis
▓ Squamous metaplasia and urothelial cells
➤ Squamous metaplasia appears as monolayered and cohesive sheets
➤ Nuclei are round, large, and monomorphic with a clear chromatin pattern compared to normal ductal/acinar prostatic epithelium
➤ Both squamous metaplastic cells and urothelial cells may be seen and a continuum between them and normal acinar epithelium may occasionally be observed
➤ Urothelial cells form smaller clusters and the nuclei are ovoid and eccentric

PEARLS

★ Nuclear monomorphism
★ Distinctly prominent nucleoli are never seen in atrophy

BENIGN PROSTATIC HYPERPLASIA

Clinical Features
▓ Increased hesitancy, sensation of incomplete bladder emptying, straining to urinate with postvoid dribbling
▓ Urgency, increased frequency, and nocturia
▓ Digital rectal examination shows a smooth, firm, and elastic enlargement of the prostate gland, induration suggests possibility of malignancy

Cytologic Features
▓ Large, two-dimensional, honeycomb-like sheets of prostatic ductal cells
▓ Well-defined cell membranes
▓ Low nuclear/cytoplasmic (N:C) ratio
▓ Uniform round to oval nucleus, with fine chromatin, inconspicuous nucleoli
▓ Coarse intracytoplasmic granules (modified Giemsa stain)

Special Stains and Immunohistochemistry
▓ Noncontributory

17-1. Benign prostate *(left)*. Sheet of columnar cells with centrally placed nuclei, inconspicuous nucleoli (Papanicolaou stain)

17-2. Benign prostate *(middle)*. Benign prostatic glands and corpora amylecea showing concentric laminations (Papanicolaou stain)

17-3. Benign prostate *(right)*. Benign prostatic glands and spindles stromal cells (Papanicolaou stain)

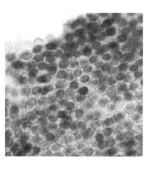
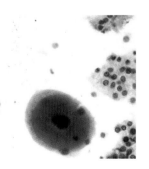
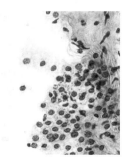

Modern Techniques for Diagnosis
- Noncontributory

Differential Diagnosis
- Prostatic adenocarcinoma
  - ➤ Cellular aspirates
  - ➤ High N:C ratio
  - ➤ Prominent nucleoli
  - ➤ Absent cytoplasmic granules

PEARLS

★ Single benign cells may be seen but are similar to the cells forming sheets
★ Cytoplasmic granules are better seen in modified Giemsa stain versus Papanicolaou stain
★ Squamous cells aspirated from region adjacent to an area of infarction are cytologically benign and should not raise suspicion of malignancy

PROSTATITIS

Clinical Features
- Fever
- Irritative voiding symptoms
- Pain on rectal examination

Cytological Features
- Many inflammatory cells including neutrophils, lymphocytes, monocytes, and histiocytes
- Benign glandular epithelial cells with degenerative changes and mild cytological atypia including presence of nucleoli and slight nuclear membrane irregularities

Special Stains and Immunohistochemistry
- Noncontributory

Modern Techniques for Diagnosis
- Noncontributory

Differential Diagnosis
- Prostatic adenocarcinoma
  - ➤ Microacinar groups
  - ➤ Absent or rare inflammatory cells
  - ➤ Absent cytoplasmic granules

PEARLS

★ Do not make a diagnosis of malignancy based on few atypical cells especially in an inflammatory background

GRANULOMATOUS PROSTATITIS

Clinical Features
- Could be seen in different clinical settings: Tuberculosis, mycotic infection, postsurgical, and idiopathic

Cytologic Features

■ Numerous epithelioid cells forming loose cohesive aggregates (granulomas)

■ Other inflammatory cells: lymphocytes, plasma cells, polymorphonuclear leucocytes, and multinucleated giant cells

■ Prostatic epithelium may display certain atypical features: Increased nuclear size, hyperchromasia, polymorphism, nucleoli, and diminished intercellular cohesion

■ Cytoplasm is basophilic; honeycomb pattern and red cytoplasmic granules are not seen

Special stains and Immunohistochemistry

■ Periodic acid–Schiff (PAS), Gomori methenamine silver (GMS), and acid-fast bacilli (AFB) stains performed to exclude fungal and mycobacterial infections

■ CD68 immunohistochemical stain is useful in identifying the histiocytes

Differential Diagnosis

■ Prostatic adenocarcinoma
   ➤ Microacinar groups
   ➤ Absent inflammatory cells or granulomas
   ➤ Absent cytoplasmic granules

PEARLS

★ Histiocytes have a single kidney-shaped/oval nucleus, which is mostly eccentrically placed, and finely vacuolated cytoplasm

★ The chromatin is fine with small inconspicuous nucleoli

★ Histiocytes occur as single cells but sometimes may cluster causing diagnostic difficulties

★ CD68 stain is useful in identifying them correctly

OTHER BENIGN ENTITIES INCLUDING NORMAL COMPONENTS

SEMINAL VESICLE EPITHELIUM

■ Loosely arranged epithelial- cell clusters are made up of ten to twelve cells with large, hyperchromatic, and polymorphic nuclei; with a single small nucleolus

■ Binucleation can be observed

■ Dense cytoplasm

■ Some cells may contain a yellow-brown cytoplasmic pigment (Papanicolaou stain) or black to greenish cytoplasmic pigment (modified Giemsa stain)

■ Seminal vesicle cells could be seen associated to spermatozoa and seminal vesicle secretions (dense basophilic amorphous material)

GANGLION CELLS

■ Large and display a round, bluish cytoplasm with ill-defined borders

■ The nucleus is large and round, and sometimes eccentric

■ Smooth chromatin prominent nucleolus

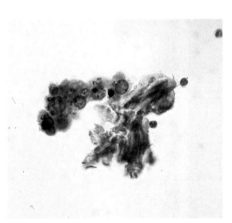

17-4. Seminal vesicle cells. Cells with high N:C ratio, prominent nucleoli, and cytoplasmic golden-brown pigmentation (Papanicolaou stain)

TREATMENT EFFECTS OF ESTROGEN COMPOUNDS

■ Squamous metaplasia

■ Atrophic acinar cells

■ Large cells with broad transparent cytoplasm resembling a fried egg – "glycogen cells"
■ Nuclear pyknosis
■ Loss of nucleoli and nuclear shrinking
■ Most common effects on malignant cells are reduction in the amount of cytoplasm, cytoplasmic vacuolization, nuclear pyknosis, and loss of nucleolar prominence

PROSTATIC (ACINAR) ADENOCARCINOMA

Clinical Features
■ Most common cancer of males and second leading cause of cancer-related death
■ The incidence of prostate cancer increases with age; it is higher in African-Americans, patients with family history of prostate cancer, and with a high dietary fat intake
■ Digital rectal examination reveals an indurated nodular prostate
■ Prostatic specific antigen (PSA) is usually elevated
■ Most common site of metastases is the axial skeleton

Cytological Features
■ Cellular aspirate
■ Loosely cohesive three-dimensional cells aggregates with nuclear overlapping, poorly defined cell borders, microacinar pattern
■ As the Gleason score increases more sheets of cells and fused microacinar groups are seen as opposed to separate acinar structures

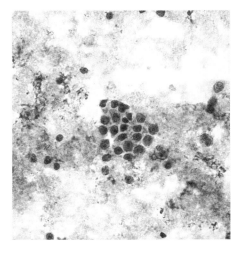
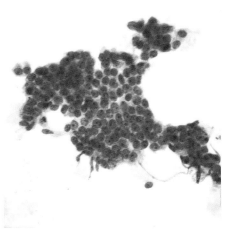
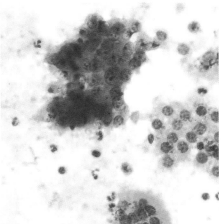
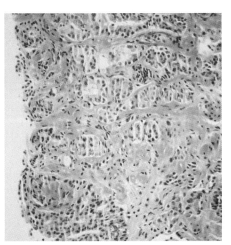

17-5. Prostatic adenocarcinoma *(top, left)*. Loose cluster of adenocarcinoma cells with enlarged nuclei, high nuclear/cytoplasmic ratio and prominent nucleoli (Papanicolaou stain)

17-6. Prostatic adenocarcinoma *(top, right)*. Sheets of adenocarcinoma cells with high nuclear/cytoplasmic ratio and prominent nucleoli (Papanicolaou stain)

17-7. Prostatic adenocarcinoma *(bottom, left)*. Fused acinar structure showing prominent nucleoli (Papanicolaou stain)

17-8. Prostatic adenocarcinoma *(bottom, right)*. Core biopsy section showing Gleason score of 4+3=7, with a predominant pattern of fused acinar structures (hematoxylin and eosin stain)

- Many single cells, naked nuclei
- Vacuolated cytoplasm
- High N:C ratio with prominent nucleoli
- Absent intracytoplasmic granules

Special Stains and Immunohistochemistry

- Prostatic-specific antigen (PSA) and prostatic-specific acid phosphatase (PSAP) immunostains are useful specially in cases of FNA of metastatic prostatic adenocarcinoma
- Alpha-methylacyl-CoA racemase (AMACR) stain is positive in prostatic adenocarcinoma
- High molecular weight cytokeratin and p63 highlight the basal layer in benign acini

Modern Techniques for Diagnosis

- DNA ploidy studies (patients with aneuploid tumors are at higher risk for local recurrence and distant metastases than patients with diploid tumors)

Differential Diagnosis

- Basal cell hyperplasia
  - Cohesive cluster of cells with increased N:C ratio
  - Absent acinar pattern
  - Nucleoli may be seen in atypical hyperplasia
- High-grade PIN
  - Few small clusters of atypical cells
  - High cellularity with pronounced atypia excludes diagnosis of PIN
  - Cytoplasmic granules and crystalloids do not distinguish between PIN and adenocarcinoma
- Urothelial carcinoma
  - Many single cells, loose clusters or papillary fragments
  - Cells with dense cytoplasm, eccentric nuclei with a high N:C ratio
  - Hyperchromatic, pleomorphic nuclei with irregular nuclear membranes
  - Cercarial cells (urothelial cells showing nucleated globular body and a variable thin cytoplasmic process with non tapered and flattened end)
  - CK7 and CK20 positive
  - PSA and PSAP negative
- Seminal vesicle epithelium
  - Highly atypical cells with bizarre, hyperchromatic nuclei
  - Coarse cytoplasmic pigment, golden brown on Papanicolaou and blue–green on modified Giemsa stain
  - Background usually shows spermatozoa
- Rectal epithelium
  - Tall columnar cells
  - Goblet cells
  - Background of amorphous colonic content

PEARLS

★ Two-cell population is usually seen with prostatic adenocarcinoma, benign epithelial cells forming two-dimensional, honeycomb sheets along with the second population of malignant cells forming crowded clusters with microacinar pattern

★ Prostatic epithelial cells are negative for CK7 and CK20

DUCTAL (ENDOMETRIOID) ADENOCARCINOMA

Clinical Features
- Accounts for less than 1% of prostatic adenocarcinomas
- Arises in the periurethral prostatic ducts

Cytological Features
- Papillary fragments, monolayered, folded sheets
- Variable degree of cytological atypia
- Abundant clear cytoplasm
- Fine granular chromatin with inconspicuous nucleoli
- Nuclear grooves

Special stains and Immunohistochemistry
- Tumor cells are positive for PSA, PSAP, and AMACR
- Highland-molecular-weight cytokeratin (HMWK) will highlight the basal cells in benign ducts

Modern Techniques for Diagnosis
- Noncontributory

Differential Diagnosis
- Metastatic poorly differentiated carcinoma
  - ➤ Tumor cells are not positive for PSA, PSAP, and AMACR
- Acinar carcinoma
  - ➤ It is impossible to differentiate between a poorly differentiated acinar carcinoma and ductal carcinoma based on cytology alone

PEARLS
★ Because of the rarity of this tumor and the nonspecific cytologic features, this tumor may mimic adenocarcinomas from other sites

SMALL CELL CARCINOMA

Clinical Features
- History of hormonally treated acinar cell carcinoma
- PSA levels may be undetectable as the small cell component predominates
- May produce ACTH and ADH

Cytologic features
- Cellular smears
- Single cells as well as cells in tight cohesive clusters
- Nuclear molding, smearing artifact
- Very high N:C ratio
- Inconspicuous nucleoli
- Typical salt- and -pepper chromatin pattern
- Many apoptotic cells
- Acinar type of adenocarcinoma coexists in many of the cases

Special Stains and Immunohistochemistry
- Small cell component is negative for PSA and PSAP
- Small cells are positive for cytokeratins, chromogranin, synaptophysin as well as CD56
- Small cell carcinoma of the prostate may be positive for TTF-1

Modern Techniques for Diagnosis
▪ Noncontributory

Differential Diagnosis
▪ Poorly differentiated adenocarcinoma
  ➤ Cytological features are similar to small cell carcinoma
  ➤ PSA and PSAP are positive in most cases
  ➤ Chromogranin could be focally positive
▪ Lymphoma
  ➤ Cytologically may be difficult to distinguish
  ➤ Mostly single discohesive cells
  ➤ Absent nuclear molding
  ➤ CD45 stain is positive; lymphoma cells are negative for keratin and chromogranin
  ➤ Flow cytometric evaluation aids in the differential diagnosis

PEARLS

★ Tumors could have both components of small cell carcinoma and adenocarcinoma, hence composite tumors

OTHER TUMORS THAT MAY RARELY BE ENCOUNTERED IN THE PROSTATE INCLUDE

Squamous Cell Carcinoma of the Prostate
▪ Sheets and small clusters of squamous cells with hyperchromatic elongated nuclei
▪ Abundant blue cytoplasm in modified Giemsa–stained smears
▪ The squamous lineage is better seen in isolated cells, particularly if stained with Papanicolaou: eosinophilic, dense polygonal cytoplasm, crisp cytoplasmic boundaries, and squamous pearls
▪ Rare isolated cells with nuclear pleomorphism

Foamy Gland Carcinoma
▪ Mono- and multilayered sheets, with occasionally microacini can be seen
▪ Abundant clear to bubbly cytoplasm
▪ Microvacuoles are most evident with modified Giemsa stain
▪ Nuclei are bland, round, small, dark, and centrally located, although mild atypia may be seen
▪ Nucleoli are usually conspicuous
▪ The background is made up of abundant amorphous foamy material similar to that seen in the cytoplasm; foamy cells are also seen

Leiomyosarcoma
▪ Cohesive spindle cells with ill-defined cytoplasmic borders and pleomorphic oval nuclei
▪ Spindle cells are positive for vimentin, h-caldesmon, and smooth muscle actin

Embryonal Rhabdomyosarcoma
▪ Highly cellular aspirate composed predominantly of single cells
▪ Pleomorphic, polygonal to spindled malignant cells with basophilic cytoplasm
▪ Intracytoplasmic cross-striations or cytoplasmic condensation could be seen
▪ Hyperchromatic nuclei, dense chromatin, and irregular nuclear membranes
▪ A tigroid background could be seen
▪ Tumor cells are positive for desmin, muscle-specific actin, Myo-D1, and myogenin

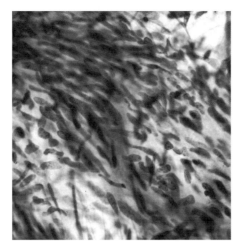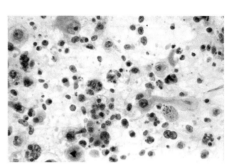

17-9. Leiomyosarcoma *(left).* Cohesive spindle cells with ill-defined cytoplasmic borders and oval nuclei (Papanicolaou stain)

17-10. Rhabdomyosarcoma *(right).* Pleomorphic, polygonal to spindled malignant cells with basophilic cytoplasm, coarse chromatin, and prominent nucleoli (Papanicolaou stain)

Sarcomatoid Carcinoma

- Pleomorphic spindle cells found singly or in clusters
- Spindle cells are pancytokeratin positive

REFERENCES

ATROPHIC PROSTATIC EPITHELIUM

Perez-Guillermo M, Acosta-Ortega J, Garcia-Solano J. Pitfalls and infrequent findings in fine-needle aspiration of the prostate gland. *Diagn Cytopathol* 2005 Aug;33(2):126–137.

BENIGN PROSTATIC HYPERPLASIA

Perez-Guillermo M, Acosta-Ortega J, Garcia-Solano J. Pitfalls and infrequent findings in fine-needle aspiration of the prostate gland. *Diagn Cytopathol* 2005 Aug;33(2):126–137.

PROSTATITIS

Perez-Guillermo M, Acosta-Ortega J, Garcia-Solano J. Pitfalls and infrequent findings in fine-needle aspiration of the prostate gland. *Diagn Cytopathol* 2005 Aug;33(2):126–137.

GRANULOMATOUS PROSTATITIS

Perez-Guillermo M, Acosta-Ortega J, Garcia-Solano J. Pitfalls and infrequent findings in fine-needle aspiration of the prostate gland. *Diagn Cytopathol* 2005 Aug;33(2):126–137.

Stanley MW, Horwitz CA, Sharer W, et al. Granulomatous prostatitis: a spectrum including nonspecific, infectious, and spindle cell lesions. *Diagn Cytopathol.* 2006 Jul. 7(5): 508–512.

PROSTATIC (ACINAR) ADENOCARCINOMA

Bardales RH. *Practical Urologic Cytopathology.* Oxford University Press, Oxford, 2002, p. 144.

Ibarrola de Andres C, Castellano Megias VM, Perez Barrios A, et al. Seminal vesicle epithelium as a potential pitfall in the cytodiagnosis of presacral masses. A report of two cases. *Acta Cytol* 2000 May–Jun; 44(3):399–402.

Kaufman JJ, Ljung BM, Walther P, et al. Aspiration biopsy of prostate. *Urology.* 1982 Jun;19(6): 587–591.

Koss LG, Woyke S, Schreiber K, et al. Thin-needle aspiration biopsy of the prostate. *Urol Clin North Am* 1984 May;11(2):237–251.

Paz-Bouza JI, Orafao A, Abad M, et al. Transrectal fine needle aspiration biopsy of the prostate combining cytomorphologic, DNA ploidy status and cell cycle distribution studies. *Pathol Res Pract* 1994 Aug;190(7):682–689.

Perez-Guillermo M, Acosta-Ortega J, Garcia-Solano J. Pitfalls and Infrequent findings in fine-needle aspiration of the prostate gland. *Diagn Cytopathol* 2005;33(2):126–137.

Schowinsky JT, Epstein JI. Distorted rectal tissue on prostate needle biopsy: a mimicker of prostate cancer. *Am J Surg Pathol* 2006 Jul;30(7):866–870.

Stilmant MM, Freedlund MC, de las Moneras A, et al. Expanded role for fine needle aspiration of the prostate. A study of 335 specimens. *Cancer.* 1989 Feb;63(3):583–592.

Valdman A, Jonmarker S, Ekman P, et al. Cytological features of prostatic intraepithelial neoplasia. *Diagn Cytopathol* 2006 May;34(5):317–322.

Willems JS, Lowhagen T. Transrectal fine-needle aspiration biopsy for cytologic diagnosis and grading of prostatic carcinoma. *Prostate* 1981;2(4):381–395.

DUCTAL (ENDOMETRIOID) ADENOCARCINOMA

Alrahwan D, Staerkel G, Gong Y. Fine needle aspiration cytology of a metastatic duct carcinoma of the prostate: a case report. *Acta Cytol* 2006 Jul–Aug;50(4):469–472.

Masood S, Swartz DA, Meneses M, et al. Fine needle aspiration cytology of papillary endometroid carcinoma of the prostate. The grooved nucleus as a cytologic marker. *Acta Cytol* 1991 Jul–Aug;35(4):451–455.

SMALL CELL CARCINOMA

Caraway NP, Fanning CV, Shin HJ, et al. Metastatic small-cell carcinoma of the prostate diagnosed by fine-needle aspiration biopsy. *Diagn Cytopathol* 1998 Jul;19(1):12–26.

Parwani AV, Ali AZ. Prostatic adenocarcinoma metastases mimicking small cell carcinoma on fine-needle aspiration. *Diagn Cytopathol* 2002 Aug;27(2):75–79.

Shin HJ, Caraway NP. Fine-needle aspiration biopsy of metastatic small cell carcinoma from extrapulmonary sites. *Diagn Cytopathol* 1998 Sep;19(3):177–181.

OTHER TUMORS

Henkes DN, Stein N. Fine-needle aspiration cytology of prostatic embryonal rhabdomyosarcoma: a case report. *Diag Cytopathol* 1987 Jun;3(2):163–165.

Perez-Guillermo M, Acosta-Ortega J, Garcia-Solano J. Pitfalls and infrequent findings in fine-needle aspiration of the prostate gland. *Diagn Cytopathol* 2005;33(2):126–137.

Renshaw AA. Granter SR. Metastatic, sarcomatoid, and PSA- and PAP-negative prostatic carcinoma: diagnosis by fine-needle aspiration. *Diagn Cytopathol* 2000 Sep;23(3):199–201.

18

Lymph Nodes

Marilin Rosa and Shahla Masood

SPECIMEN TYPES IN LYMPH NODE CYTOPATHOLOGY

FINE-NEEDLE ASPIRATION OF LYMPH NODES

Definition
- Fine-needle aspiration (FNA) is a technique for obtaining cellular material using a 21- to 25- gauge needle

Uses of FNA in Lymph Node
- All palpable lymph nodes (LN) are amenable to aspiration
- Deep-seated lymphadenopathy (e.g., CT-guided FNA of retroperitoneal LN)
- Confirmation of clinical impression in infectious processes
- Diagnosis of a suspected malignancy (e.g. lymphoma, metastatic disease, etc.)
- Alternative procedure when surgical biopsy is not possible
- Staging purposes in patients with known malignancy

Advantages
- Cost-effectiveness
- Very low incidence of complications
- Minimal discomfort for the patient
- Rapid results and potential bedside diagnosis
- Provides cellular material for immunophenotyping and molecular diagnostic tests
- Preserve lymph nodes architecture if subsequent excision is necessary

Disadvantages
- Sampling error: Occur in deep-seated lymph nodes, nodal fibrosis, and partial involvement
- Impossible to evaluate architectural pattern

Complications
- Occasionally, hematoma formation, bleeding, or infection
- Infarct of the lymph node can occur

Technique
- A triple approach should be used for diagnosis: Clinical information, light microscopy, and ancillary studies
- After cleaning the skin, the palpable lymph node is immobilized between two fingers to avoid displacement of the targeted lymph node
- The aspiration can be done using a syringe holder, using the needle attached to a syringe or using a bare needle
- The material obtained should be gently smeared due to fragility of lymphocytes that could result in crushing artifact that precludes examination
- Slides can be stained using air-dried Romanowsky-type stains (modified Giemsa stain) and alcohol fixed Papanicolaou (PAP) stains. Romanowsky-type stain is preferred because it is the same stain used in bone marrow biopsy and highlights cytoplasmic details of cells and lymphoglandular bodies
- After initial evaluation, additional material can be procured for ancillary testing, for example, flow cytometry

Specimen Adequacy
- There are no specific requirements for a minimum number of cells; therefore a specimen is only considered adequate when it represents the lesion for which the biopsy has been performed when negative, at least 3 passes should have been done to rule out a false negative

FNA Report
▧ The final report should include all the following, if possible:
  ➤ Precise location
  ➤ Specimen type
  ➤ Technique used
  ➤ Diagnosis
  ➤ Ancillary studies
  ➤ Recommendations

IMPRINT CYTOLOGY OF LYMPH NODES

Definition
▧ After the LN is removed, in fresh state, it is bisected and the cut surfaces are gently touched onto clean glass slides

Uses of Imprint Cytology
▧ Intraoperative evaluation of sentinel lymph nodes
▧ Adjuvant technique in the evaluation of lymphoma

Advantages
▧ Imprint cytology is a simple, accurate, relatively quick, and inexpensive method
▧ Does not result in loss of nodal tissue
▧ When performed intraoperatively, allows most patients who require an axillary dissection to be identified and have one time surgery
▧ Allows evaluation of specimen adequacy before submitting fresh lymph nodes for flow cytometry
▧ Imprint cytology can reveal the presence of malignant cells that are missed by the standard H&E-stained paraffin sections

Disadvantages
▧ The most common reason for false-negative imprint result is the presence of small metastases away from the bisected surface of the node

Technique
▧ The surface of the LN is kindly touched with a glass slide. Smearing is not performed to avoid crushed artifact
▧ The touch imprinted slides can be air dried and stained with Romanowsky-type stains or alcohol fixed and stained with H&E

Pearl
▧ Pick-up of small metastases might be improved by multiple sectioning of the LN thus increasing the surface area of the node sampled by imprint cytology

NORMAL LYMPH NODE

Normal Histology
▧ The normal lymph nodes are bean shaped and located at sites throughout the body
▧ Their role is to process antigens present in lymph drained from most organs via the afferent lymphatics
▧ Lymph nodes have a fibrous capsule, cortex, medulla, and sinuses (subcapsular, cortical, and medullary)

- The sinuses contain macrophages, which take up and process antigens
- The lymph node cortex is divided into follicular and diffuse (paracortical) regions
- The medulla is divided into medullary cords and sinuses
- The medulla represents the zone for plasmacytoid lymphocytes, plasma cells, and immunoblasts separated by medullary sinuses
- The cortex is situated beneath the capsule and represents the zone for B cells and follicular dendritic cells (centroblast and centrocytes). It contains the follicles, which may contain germinal centers
- The paracortex represents the zone of T cells, which are suspended in nests of interdigitating reticulum cells

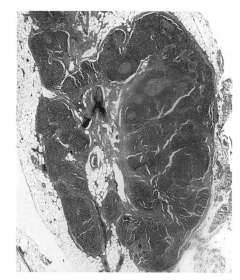

18-1. Normal anatomy of lymph nodes. Each lymph node is divided into two general regions, the capsule and the cortex, as seen in this figure. The capsule is an outer layer of connective tissue. Underlying the capsule is the cortex, the location of primary and secondary lymphoid follicles. The paracortex is the region surrounding and beneath the germinal centers. The medulla is located deep to the cortex/paracortex, and composed of medullary cords and medullary sinuses. Several afferent lymphatic vessels, which carry lymph into the node, enter the node on the convex side. The lymph moves through the lymph sinuses and enters an efferent lymphatic vessel, which carries the lymph away from the node. The efferent vessel leaves the node at an indented region called the hilum

Normal Components of LN Cytology Samples
- Small lymphocytes
  - Also known as mature, virgin, or unstimulated lymphocytes
  - Constitute the majority of the cells
  - Uniform in size and shape
  - Round nucleus with smooth membrane
  - Coarse dark chromatin
  - Inconspicuous nucleoli
  - A rim of scant blue cytoplasm
- Follicular center cells
  - Also known as lymphoblast
  - Found in follicular centers
  - Compose up to 16% of cells
  - Small or large size
  - Smooth nuclei (noncleaved) or irregular nuclei (cleaved)
  - Chromatin more opened than mature lymphocytes
- Centrocytes
  - Also known as small and large cleaved cells
  - Scant cytoplasm
  - Clefted to angulated nuclei
  - Coarse chromatin
  - Inconspicuous nucleoli
- Centroblasts
  - Large nuclei
  - Noncleaved membrane
  - One to three marginated prominent nucleoli
  - A rim of basophilic cytoplasm
- Immunoblast
  - Either B- or T-cell type
  - Large cells with large and round nucleoli
  - Prominent central macronucleoli
  - Abundant plasmacytoid cytoplasm
- Histiocytes
  - Comprise 1–8% of the cells
  - Located in the sinuses
  - Tingible body macrophages are specialized histiocytes that engulf debris and are located in follicular centers
- Lymphoglandular bodies
  - Fragments of lymphocyte cytoplasm
  - About the size of an intact lymphocyte
  - Uniform gray blue appearance
  - Marker of organized lymphoid tissue, benign or malignant
- Follicular center fragments
  - They represent fragments of lymph node follicles

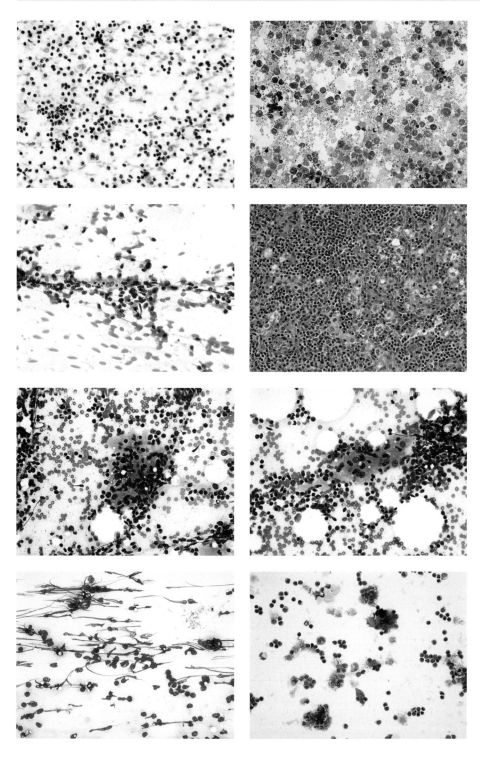

18-2. Normal lymphoid elements *(left)*. Seen in a benign lymph node, polymorphous population with predominance of small lymphocytes (modified Giemsa stain)

18-3. Lymphoglandular bodies *(right)*. Gray–blue fragments of lymphocyte cytoplasm. They are markers of organized lymphoid tissue (modified Giemsa stain)

18-4. Tingible body macrophage (center) *(left)*. A macrophage with cellular debris in its cytoplasm. The nucleus is kidney shaped and a conspicuous nucleolus is seen (Papanicolaou stain)

18-5. Tingible body macrophage *(right)*. (H&E)

18-6. Lymphohistiocytic aggregates *(left)*. Aggregates of lymphocytes admixed with histiocytes usually seen in benign processes (modified Giemsa stain)

18-7. Lymphohistiocytic aggregates *(right)*. Aggregates of lymphocytes admixed with histiocytes usually seen in benign processes (modified Giemsa stain)

18-8. and 18-9. Smearing artifact *(left* and *right)*. Lymphocytes are fragile cells that can be easily crushed during slide preparation precluding the examination of the smear (modified Giemsa stain)

➤ Composed of syncytial lymphohistiocytic aggregates, lymphocytes in variable degree of maturation, and tingible body macrophages
➤ Usually seen in benign processes
▦ Lymphohistiocytic aggregates
   ➤ They are aggregates of lymphocytes admixed with histiocytes
   ➤ Abundant syncytial cytoplasm
   ➤ Loose flat sheets or three-dimensional groups
   ➤ Usually seen in benign processes

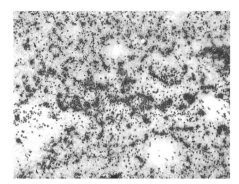 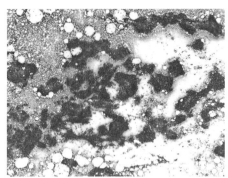

18-10. Dispersed cell pattern
(left). Seen in aspirates of lymph nodes (modified Giemsa stain)

18-11. Cohesive cell pattern
(right). Characteristic of metastatic carcinoma (modified Giemsa stain)

■ Plasma cells
  ➤ Represent about 0.1% of cells
  ➤ Located in the medulla
  ➤ Their increase is associated with syphilis, tuberculosis, toxoplasmosis, collagen-vascular disease, etc.
■ Neutrophils
  ➤ Commonly associated with infectious diseases
  ➤ Normally account for up to 2% of cells
■ Mast cells
  ➤ Constitute about 0.1% of the cells
■ Eosinophils
  ➤ Seen in nonspecific allergic conditions, parasitic diseases, etc.
  ➤ Constitute up to 0.3% of the cells
■ Basophils
  ➤ Constitute up to 0.2% of the cells
■ Capillaries
  ➤ Usually present in LN aspirates
■ Adipose tissue
  ➤ Fatty infiltration of a lymph node could cause enlargement and mimic malignancy clinically

PEARLS

★ The mixture of small lymphocytes, follicular center cells, and immunoblasts causes the "range of maturation" characteristic of reactive lymphadenopathy
★ The presence of tingible body macrophages is a clue for a benign process; however, they are also present in high, grade lymphomas
★ Lymphoglandular bodies are the hallmark of lymphoid nature of the aspiration; however, rarely they can be seen in other lesions including small cell carcinoma

PRACTICAL APPROACH TO LYMPH NODES ASPIRATES

Clinical Points
■ In the young population lymphadenopathy is frequently of reactive nature although lymphomas also occur
■ In the adult population, the presence of a malignant process, primary or metastatic is more probable

- In elderly people there is a strong chance of malignancy
- Some types of lymphomas are age specific
- Some lymphomas have a racial predominancy
- Disease progression
  - High-grade lymphomas grow in a rapid fashion whereas low-grade lymphomas present usually as indolent malignancy with a long course
  - Infectious processes are in general short lived
- Patient history
  - History of epithelial malignancy or lymphoma when metastasis is suspected
  - Patients with autoimmune or systemic diseases can have reactive lymphadenopathy
- Physical examination
  - To evaluate the size, consistency, mobility, and tenderness of the lymph node
- Localized swollen lymph nodes often have an infectious etiology, therefore the first step is to identify the possible focus of infection
- Generalized lymphadenopathy is frequently a sign of a hematological systemic disease, particularly in adults
- Lymphadenopathy persisting for more than one month requires invasive diagnostic procedures to rule out a malignant cause

Algorithms for Approach

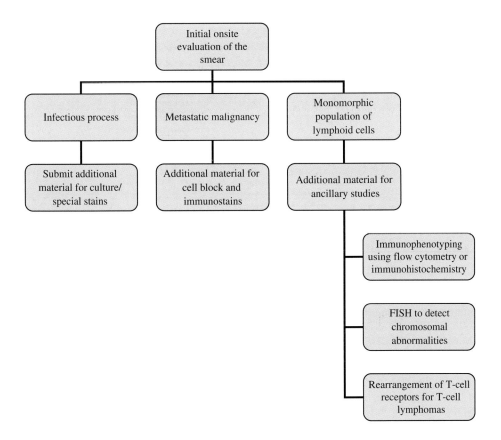

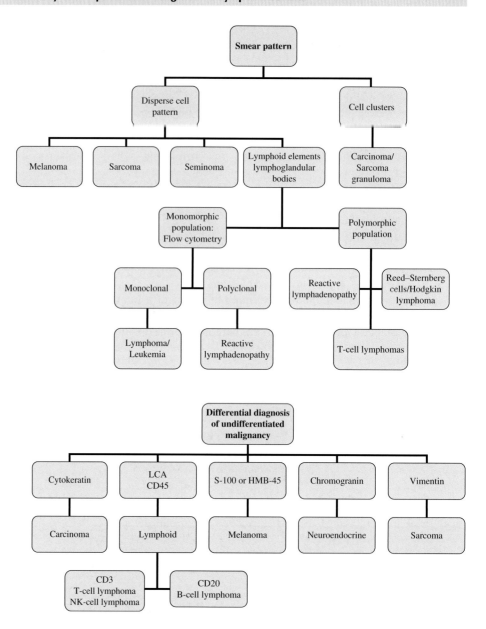

ANCILLARY TECHNIQUES FOR THE DIAGNOSIS OF LYMPHOID LESIONS

▦ The most commonly used ancillary techniques in lymphomas are immunohisto-chemistry, flow cytometry, Southern blot technique, polymerase chain reaction (PCR), and fluorescent in situ hybridization (FISH)

IMMUNOHISTOCHEMISTRY

▦ Immunohistochemistry demonstrates the presence of antigen using the corre-sponding antibody
▦ The antigen may be a CD marker or cell proliferation marker or protein product of an oncogene

Advantages of Immunohistochemistry
▦ It can be done on cytology smears and paraffin-embedded tissue
▦ The morphology of individual cells can also be visualized simultaneously

▓ Immunohistochemistry is a relatively inexpensive technique that can be easily performed in most laboratories

POLYMERASE CHAIN REACTION

▓ Polymerase chain reaction enables researchers to produce millions of copies of a specific DNA sequence in approximately two hours
▓ To get the amplified DNA from the test solution, four nucleotides are added along with the specific primers and DNA polymerase enzymes
▓ The primers are attached with the complementary DNA (cDNA) portions and extend toward the target DNA sequences with the help of polymerase enzymes and nucleotides. The PCR reaction is based on repetitive cycles to get amplified products of the specific DNA portions
▓ Once the amplification is complete, the amplified products are analyzed by gel electrophoresis and subsequently stained with a DNA-specific dye

Advantages of PCR
▓ Ability to use small fragments of DNA
▓ Short turnaround time
▓ Ability to analyze paraffin-embedded specimens

FLUORESCENCE IN SITU HYBRIDIZATION

▓ In the FISH technique, fluorescent-tagged DNA probes are used for the visualization of specific DNA sequences on metaphase or interphase nuclei
▓ This technique can be performed on frozen sections or paraffin-embedded tissue
▓ Multicolor FISH is very helpful for the detection of chromosomal translocations

Advantages of FISH
▓ Fluorescent in situ hybridization is a relatively cheap and rapid technique and can be done on archival material
▓ Tumor morphology can also be observed simultaneously in FISH
▓ It is very useful for assessing the genetic heterogeneity within a tumor

SOUTHERN BLOT TECHNIQUE

▓ In this technique, DNA is first extracted from fresh or frozen cells
▓ DNA is then cut into small pieces with the help of restricted endonuclease enzymes
▓ The small fragments of DNA are separated according to size by electrophoresis on agarose gel
▓ DNA fragments are then transferred to a nylon membrane, which represents the exact imprint of the DNA fragments on the gel
▓ The DNA fragments of interest are identified with the help of labeled probes
▓ The pattern of expression is visualized on X-ray by autoradiography or by development the color on the membrane
▓ Its used has decreased after the advent of PCR because more amount of DNA is necessary for analysis and it takes up to two weeks from the time a specimen is received to when a result is obtained

FLOW CYTOMETRY

▓ Flow cytometry uses the principles of light scattering, light excitation, and emission of fluorochrome molecules to generate specific multiparameter data from particles and cells
▓ Characterizes individual cells as they pass at high speed through a laser beam

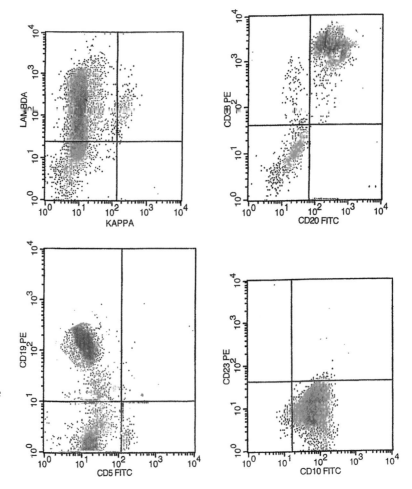

18-12. Flow cytometry of a malignant lymphoma. Showing the clonal population is positive for Lambda, CD20, CD38, CD19, and CD10, and negative for CD5. The tumor was morphologically and by flow cytometry consistent with diffuse large B-cell lymphoma

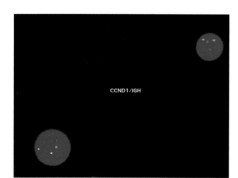

18-13. FISH/Mantle cell lymphoma. CCND1/IGH rearrangements (aka BCL1/IGH rearrangements) most often result from a t(11;14)(q13;q32) translocation exhibiting two fusion signals in addition to one green and one red signal. This abnormality is found in mantle cell lymphoma. A normal nucleus (right upper corner) is included as reference

▨ The morphological profile of a cell can be observed by combining forward light scatter (cell size) and orthogonal or side light scatter (cell surface granularity)

▨ A minimum of 10,000 events for each cell marker should be analyzed

▨ The optimal flow cytometry panel includes antibodies to kappa, lambda, CD3, CD5, CD10, CD19, CD20, CD23, and coexpression of CD10. This panel can be modified depending on the differential diagnosis

Value of Flow Cytometry in the Diagnosis of Lymphoproliferative Disorders on FNA

▨ The accuracy of FNA in diagnosing and classifying lymphomas has improved significantly using ancillary techniques that allow immunophenotyping

▨ If the suspicion of lymphoma arises after evaluation of the smears on-site, additional material should be submitted for flow cytometry studies in RPMI medium (RPMI was developed at Roswell Park Memorial Institute, hence the acronym RPMI)

▨ When compared with immunohistochemistry, flow cytometry allows for larger numbers of antigens to be tested and can improve the identification of dual antigen expression

▨ Compared to immunohistochemistry, flow cytometry has the advantage of being rapid and highly sensitive

▨ It is able to provide semiquantitative information regarding antigen density

Limitations of Flow Cytometry in the Diagnosis of Lymphoproliferative Disorders on FNA

▓ Tissue histology is lost and the detection of cytoplasmic and nuclear antigens is technically challenging, requiring permeabilization of the cells during specimen processing

▓ Cell suspensions may not be representative of the pathologic process due to fibrosis or abundant stromal elements

▓ Specimens must be processed shortly after collection which needs a careful planning and synchronization between the departments involved

▓ More accurate in classifying low-grade tumors, such as small lymphocytic lymphoma/chronic lymphocytic leukemia, and high-grade neoplasms

▓ Intermediate grade lymphomas are more difficult to classify

▓ Some oncologists would not treat a patient with a primary diagnosis and classification of lymphoma exclusively rendered on the basis of FNA

▓ Not useful in Hodgkin lymphomas

PEARLS

★ Molecular diagnostic tests are useful, but a negative result does not always exclude the possibility of lymphoma

★ Flow cytometry cannot be used to overrule convincing morphologic findings

NON-NEOPLASTIC LYMPH NODES

ACUTE LYMPHADENITIS

Clinical Features

▓ Clinically characterized by a red, hot, and tender area

▓ The most common causes are bacteria and their toxic products, and fungi (e.g., cryptococcus, histoplasma, and coccidioides)

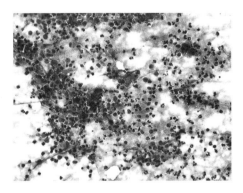 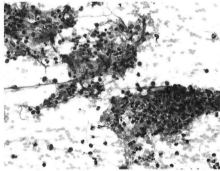

18-14. and 18-15. Acute lymphadenitis. *(left and right).* Mixed population of lymphocytes, neutrophils, macrophages, and necrotic debris (modified Giemsa stain)

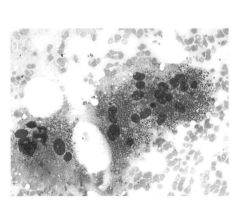 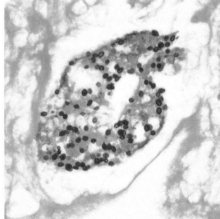

18-16. Histoplasma *(left).* Histiocytes containing numerous yeast of Histoplasma capsulatum (modified Giemsa stain)

18-17. Histoplasma *(right).* Special stain for fungi organism is positive in the cell block of the same case (GMS)

Cytologic Features

- Bacterial lymphadenitis
  - ➤ Hypercellular smears
  - ➤ Admixed population of lymphocytes and neutrophils
  - ➤ Cellular debris
  - ➤ Pus can be seen during aspiration
  - ➤ Microorganism can be seen directly in the smear
  - ➤ Late in the disease plasma cells and tingible body macrophages
- Fungal lymphadenitis
  - ➤ Neutrophilic or granulomatous infiltrate
  - ➤ Fungal organism can be seen

Special Stains and Immunohistochemistry

- Special stains for bacteria: Gram stain
- Special stains for fungi: Silver, PAS

Modern Techniques

- Culture is the gold standard diagnostic test

Differential Diagnosis

- Cat-scratch disease
  - ➤ Self-limited. Recent bite or cat scratch
  - ➤ Proliferation of monocytoid lymphocytes
  - ➤ Necrosis. Necrotizing granulomas
- Tuberculous lymphadenitis
  - ➤ Necrosis, granulomas, histiocytes, and neutrophils
  - ➤ Bacilli can be observed as negative images
- Rosai-Dorfman disease
  - ➤ Lymphadenopathy is bilateral and not tender
  - ➤ Small lymphocytes
  - ➤ Histiocytes with emperipolesis (phagocytosis of lymphocytes by histiocytes)
  - ➤ Can mimic lymphoma clinically
- Kikuchi lymphadenitis
  - ➤ Clinically simulates bacterial lymphadenitis due to enlargement and tenderness of LN
  - ➤ Necrotic debris and karyorrhexis
  - ➤ Histiocytes with angulated nuclei
  - ➤ Absence of neutrophils

PEARLS

★ In cases of infectious lymphadenitis part of the aspirated material should be submitted for cultures even if the patient is receiving antibiotics

★ All cases showing acute suppuration without granulomas or microorganisms identified by special stains should be reevaluated by follow-up FNA in order to establish a correct diagnosis

GRANULOMATOUS LYMPHADENITIS

Clinical Features

- Granuloma formation is a chronic inflammatory reaction involving antigen exposure and processing, T cells, macrophages, epithelioid cells, and giant cell activation, and granulomas formation
- Granuloma is considered as a defense mechanism against antigens, which stay in the organs without inactivation

- Granulomas are classified as noninfectious granulomas and infectious granulomas
- Generally present as multiple enlarged lymph nodes
- The clinical presentation varies according to the cause

Cytologic Features
- Cellular smears
- Mixture of lymphocytes, histiocytes, and plasma cells
- Clean or dirty background
- Aggregates of epithelioid histiocytes characterized by elongated, spindle cell nuclei with a "footprint" shape
- Multinucleated giant cells of foreign body type or Langhans type
- Granulomas composed of elongated epithelioid cells with abundant pale cytoplasm and giant cells with peripheral small nuclei

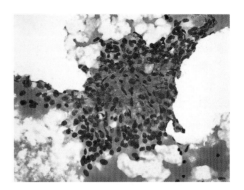

18-18. Noncaseous granulomatous inflammation. Aggregates of epithelioid histiocytes characterized by elongated, spindle cell nuclei mixed with lymphocytes and some plasma cells (modified Giemsa stain)

Sarcoidosis
- Sarcoidosis is a multisystemic disorder of unknown cause most commonly affecting the young and middle-aged adults
- Frequently presents with bilateral hilar lymphadenopathy, pulmonary infiltrates, and ocular and skin lesions
- The accepted diagnostic criteria for sarcoidosis include clinical–radiologic findings plus presence of granulomata in two or more organs with no agent known to cause a granulomatous response, and exclusion of other granulomatous diseases
- Cytologically characterized by granulomas, epithelioid histiocytes, multinucleated giant cells, lymphocytes, and absence of necrosis

Mycobacterial Granulomatous Lymphadenitis
- Includes *Mycobacterium tuberculosis* and atypical mycobacteria
- Clinical findings of tuberculosis include pyrexia, night sweats, recent travel to endemic areas, etc.
- Aspirates characterized by necrotic material, neutrophils, caseating granulomas
- Negative images of intra- and extracellular bacilli on DQ stain
- In *Mycobacterium avium* intracellular the bacilli are seen inside histiocytes

Lymphoma
- Granulomata may be encountered in both Hodgkin's disease and non-Hodgkin's lymphoma, particularly T-cell lymphoma
- Hodgkin's lymphoma is characterized by the classic Reed–Sternberg cells in a background of sarcoid-like granulomata, reactive lymphoid cells and occasional eosinophils

Other Causes of Granulomatous Inflammation
- Cat scratch disease: See bellow
- Post-vaccine granulomatous reaction
- Unknown etiology

Special Stains and Immunohistochemistry
- Mycobacteria: Acid-fast stain
- Lymphoma: Immunohistochemistry or flow cytometry according to morphologic features
- Metastasis: Immunohistochemistry directed to the suspected tumor

18-19. Noncaseous granulomatous inflammation *(left)*. Aggregates of epithelioid histiocytes characterized by elongated, spindle cell nuclei mixed with lymphocytes and some plasma cells (modified Giemsa stain)

18-20. Necrotizing granulomas *(right)*. Aggregates of epithelioid histiocytes intermixed with neutrophils and necrotic debris (Papanicolaou stain)

18-21. Necrotizing granulomas *(left)*. Aggregates of epithelioid histiocytes intermixed with neutrophils and necrotic debris (Papanicolaou stain)

18-22. Necrotizing granulomatous lymphadenitis *(right)*. Histologic appearance of the same case (H&E)

18-23. Necrotizing granulomatous lymphadenitis *(left)*. Special stain for acid fast is positive showing the small reddish bacilli (acid fast)

18-24. Granulomatous inflammation in lymphoma *(right)*. Granulomas can also be seen in malignant processes; therefore its presence does not always mean an infectious disease (modified Giemsa stain)

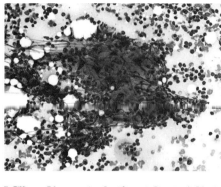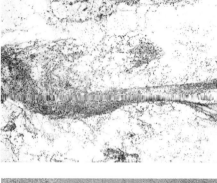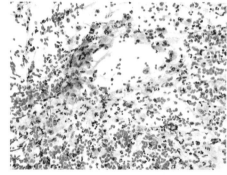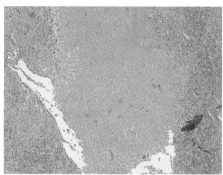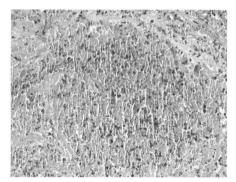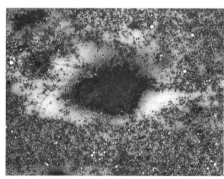

Modern Techniques
■ Atypical mycobacteria: Real-time PCR assay has shown a sensitivity of 72% for patients with lymphadenitis and a specificity of 100% for the detection of atypical mycobacteria

Differential Diagnosis
■ Metastasis
  ➤ Lymph nodes containing metastatic carcinoma may also show features of granulomata
  ➤ Metastatic nasopharyngeal carcinoma, seminoma, and malignant melanoma have been described
  ➤ Malignant cells or cluster are seen to be associated to the granulomatous reaction
■ Foreign body reaction
  ➤ Inflammation is absent
  ➤ Polarized light can reveal foreign body material
■ Spindle cells neoplasm
  ➤ Clinically a mass is almost always obvious
  ➤ Cytologically, the nuclei of the spindle cells in sarcoma are overtly malignant with coarse chromatin

★ The etiology of granulomatous disorders varies widely and the use of FNA with other ancillary tests (microbiological, immunohistochemical, radiological, biochemical, and special staining techniques) is very useful for obtaining a definitive diagnosis

★ In aspirates showing granulomas, infectious organisms must be always excluded with special stains or culture

CAT SCRATCH DISEASE

Clinical Features
▓ Cat scratch disease is a bacterial infection caused by the Gram-negative bacillus *Bartonella henselae*
▓ It has emerged as a relatively common and occasionally serious feline-associated zoonotic disease among children and adults
▓ Clinically, patients present with adenopathy, fever, malaise, history of feline contact, and a small cutaneous lesion at the site of inoculation of the germ

Cytologic Features
▓ Cellular smears
▓ Numerous neutrophils
▓ Variable-sized granulomas
▓ Necrotic background

Special Stains and Immunohistochemistry
▓ Polyclonal antibody-based IHC studies for the detection of *Bartonella henselae* can be performed when serologic and molecular studies are not available
▓ Warthin–Starry stain: Permits visualization of the small, slender, pleomorphic rods

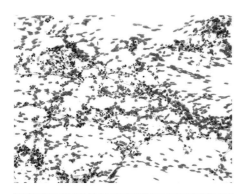

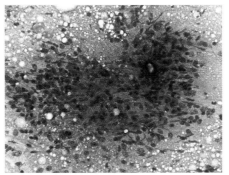

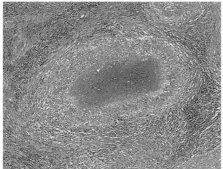

18-25. Cat scratch disease *(top, left)*. Presenting as acute lymphadenitis cytologically indistinguishable from other acute infectious processes (Papanicolaou stain)

18-26. Cat scratch disease *(top, right)*. Variable-sized granulomas in a necrotic background (modified Giemsa stain)

18-27. Cat scratch disease *(opposite)*.Necrotizing lymphadenitis with palisading of the histiocytes (H&E)

Modern Techniques

▨ Serologic testing is the standard method of diagnosis: A single elevated indirect immunofluorescence assay titer or enzyme immunoassay value for IgG or IgM antibodies are generally sufficient to confirm the disease. IgG levels rise during the first two months after onset of illness, followed by a gradual decline

▨ Polymerase chain reaction (PCR) and bacterial culture are available at reference laboratories

Differential Diagnosis

▨ Reactive lymphoid hyperplasia
➤ Early stages of cat scratch disease can have few granulomas and mimic reactive lymphoid hyperplasia
▨ Other lymphadenitis
➤ Cat scratch disease is cytologically indistinguishable from other suppurative granulomatous lymphadenitis, including *Chlamydia trachomatis* (lymphogranuloma venereum), *Yersinia enterocolitica* (mesenteric lymphadenitis), *Francisella tularensis* (tularemia), etc.
▨ Mycobacterial granulomatous lymphadenitis
➤ Late cases of cat scratch disease develop pink, amorphous appearance of the necrotic material closely resembling the caseation necrosis of tuberculosis
▨ Infection by pyogenic cocci
➤ The presence of a rim of histiocytes around the abscess favors cat scratch disease

PEARLS

☆ Because other organisms can produce identical cytomorphology, microbiological studies are necessary in order to make a specific diagnosis of cat scratch disease

REACTIVE HYPERPLASIA

Clinical Features

▨ Reactive hyperplasia, also known as chronic lymphadenitis, encompasses several entities; follicular hyperplasia, paracortical hyperplasia, and sinus histiocytosis
▨ Most cases of reactive hyperplasia are due to follicular hyperplasia
▨ It is common in children, often of viral etiology
▨ It is less common in adults and occurs in patients with systemic and immunologic diseases, including rheumatoid arthritis, syphilis, HIV lymphadenopathy, etc.

Cytologic Features

▨ Cellular smears
▨ Mixture of cells representing all areas of the lymph node (cortex, paracortex, medulla)
▨ Lymphocytes exhibiting various stages of maturation
▨ Small lymphocytes predominance
▨ Tingible body macrophages
▨ Lymphohistiocytic aggregates
▨ Plasma cell, eosinophils, neutrophils commonly seen
▨ Presence of mitosis
▨ Macrophages with melanin pigment: Dermatopathic lymphadenopathy

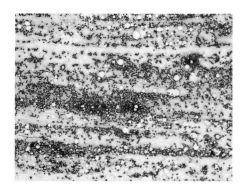

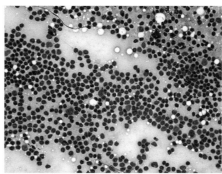

18-28. Reactive lymph node *(left)*. Cellular smear showing a polymorphous population of dispersed cells (modified Giemsa stain)

18-29. Reactive lymph node *(right)*. Polymorphous population showing lymphocytes in various stages of maturation, some plasma cells and tingible body macrophages (modified Giemsa stain)

Special Stains and Immunohistochemistry

▪ Immunohistochemistry with a panel of markers may help to exclude a lymphoproliferative disorder

Modern Techniques

▪ Flow cytometry is very helpful in difficult cases where the distinction between benign reactive hyperplasia and lymphoma is difficult

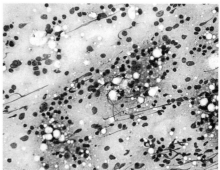

18-30. Reactive lymph node. Polymorphous population showing lymphocytes in various stages of maturation, some plasma cells and tingible body macrophages (modified Giemsa stain)

Differential Diagnosis

▪ Lymphoproliferative disorder
➤ Non-Hodgkin lymphomas, most commonly; follicular lymphoma, small lymphocytic lymphoma/chronic lymphocytic leukemia, MALT/lymphoma, and some types of T-cell lymphomas
➤ Lymphoma should be suspected when large immature lymphocytes are spread all over the smear
➤ Absence of range of maturation
➤ Absence of tingible body macrophages
▪ Hodgkin lymphoma
➤ Characterized by a polymorphic population of lymphocytes
➤ The clue for diagnosis is the presence of Reed–Sternberg cells
▪ Partial lymph node involvement by a malignant process
➤ Lymphoma or metastatic malignancy can partially involve lymph nodes resulting in false negative aspirates as a consequence of sampling error
▪ Rosai–Dorfman disease
➤ Lymphadenopathy is bilateral
➤ Small lymphocytes
➤ Histiocytes with emperipolesis (phagocytosis of lymphocytes by histiocytes)

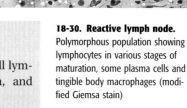

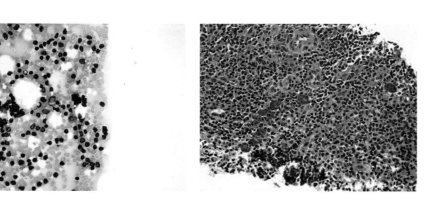

18-31. Reactive lymph node/Dermatopathic lymphadenopathy *(left)*. Nodal hyperplasia secondary to generalized dermatitis, particularly with exfoliation. Dermatopathic lymphadenopathy is characterized by a localized paracortical proliferation of histiocytes and deposition of melanin in the lymph nodes as seen in this picture. It has been associated with hematologic malignancies (modified Giemsa stain)

18-32. Dermatopathic lymphadenopathy *(right)*. Histologic section of the same case showing melanin pigment present in the cytoplasm of the macrophages (H&E)

★ The presence of a polymorphous population of lymphoid elements and tingible body macrophages are clues for the diagnosis of a benign process; however, do not exclude the possibility of lymphoma

★ When performing immediate evaluation of lymphoid aspirates always obtain additional material for flow cytometry studies, if needed

★ Because architectural pattern is not seen in FNA, some lymphadenopathies cannot be accurately diagnosed only by this method

LYMPHOPROLIFERATIVE DISORDER

HODGKIN LYMPHOMA

Clinical Features
- Accounts for about 30% of all lymphomas
- They usually arise in the lymph nodes of the cervical region
- More common in young adults
- Characterized by the presence of Reed–Sternberg cells or Hodgkin cells
- Hodgkin lymphoma can be classified as follows

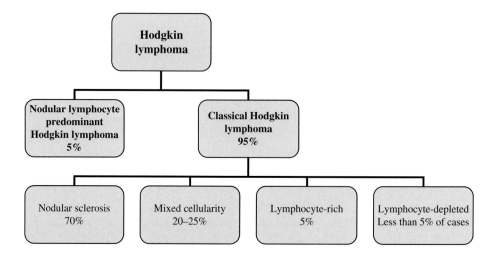

Cytologic Features
- Cellular aspirates
- Background of a polymorphous population similar to a reactive process
- Classic Reed–Sternberg cells
  - ➤ Bilobated, trilobated or multilobated
  - ➤ Prominent, inclusion-like nucleolus in each lobe or a single nucleus
  - ➤ Variable amounts of pale blue cytoplasm
  - ➤ Finely reticulated and clear chromatin pattern
- Hodgkin cells
  - ➤ Large mononucleated cells
  - ➤ Cytoplasmic characteristics, chromatin pattern, and nucleolar appearance are similar to those of classic Reed–Sternberg cells
- Popcorn cells
  - ➤ Nodular lymphocyte predominance Hodgkin lymphoma
  - ➤ Lobulated single nuclei
  - ➤ Scarce cytoplasm
  - ➤ Smaller size than classic Reed–Sternberg cells
- Clusters of histiocytes mimicking poorly formed granulomas

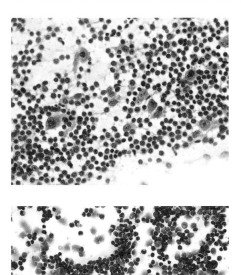

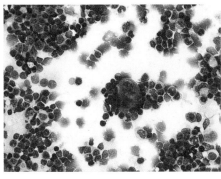

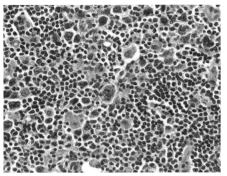

18-33. Hodgkin lymphoma
(top, left). Reed–Sternberg cells: Classic binucleated Reed–Sternberg cells displaying a large inclusion-like nucleolus in each lobe (H&E)

18-34. Hodgkin lymphoma
(top, right). Reed–Sternberg cells: Binucleated Reed–Sternberg cell showing prominent nucleoli (modified Giemsa stain)

18-35. Hodgkin lymphoma
(bottom, left). Reed–Sternberg variants (Hodgkin cells): Mononuclear variant of Reed–Sternberg cells with large prominent nucleoli (modified Giemsa stain)

18-36. Hodgkin lymphoma
(bottom, right). Histologic appearance of Hodgkin lymphoma. Reed–Sternberg cells and Hodgkin cells are seen in a reactive background including normally appearing lymphocytes and histiocytes (H&E)

Special Stains and Immunohistochemistry
▦ In classical Hodgkin lymphomas the Reed–Sternberg cells are typically CD30 and CD15 positive but CD45 negative
▦ Reed–Sternberg cells in nodular lymphocyte predominant Hodgkin lymphoma are positive for CD45 and pan B–cell markers (CD20 and CD19) but negative for CD30 and CD15

Modern Techniques
▦ Flow cytometry studies are not helpful in the distinction of reactive lymphoid hyperplasia from Hodgkin lymphoma, therefore is not used in the diagnosis of this type of lymphoma

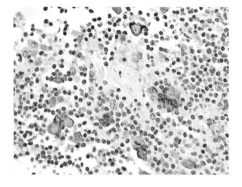

18-37. Hodgkin lymphoma. CD30 positive Reed–Sternberg cells

Differential Diagnosis
▦ Reactive lymphoid hyperplasia
➤ A careful search for Reed–Sternberg cells and its mononuclear variants avoid misdiagnosis of reactive lymphoid hyperplasia
▦ Anaplastic large cell lymphoma
➤ Smears from anaplastic large cell lymphoma tend to show more neoplastic cells than those from Hodgkin lymphoma where the neoplastic cells represent less than 10% of the total cell population
➤ Aggregation of tumor cells is more common in anaplastic large cell lymphoma
➤ Neoplastic cells in anaplastic large cell lymphoma are positive for ALK and EMA
➤ Gene rearrangement studies for T-cell receptors are helpful
▦ Acute lymphadenitis
➤ Necrosis and massive neutrophilic infiltrates may be prominent findings in smears from patients with Hodgkin lymphoma, mostly in the nodular sclerosing variant
➤ Few tumoral cells may be present in the smears
➤ Neoplastic cells can show degenerative-associated changes, which makes their recognition difficult as Hodgkin's-related cells

> ➤ A detailed search for the characteristic neoplastic cells is mandatory in these cases
> ▪ T-cell–rich variant of the diffuse B-cell lymphoma
> ➤ The neoplastic cells in T-cell–rich variant of the diffuse B-cell lymphoma are CD30 and CD15 negative
> ➤ The differential diagnosis in cytology is very difficult and excisional biopsy may be required for definitive differential diagnosis

PEARLS

★ Reed–Sternberg cells may be overlooked because they typically comprise a small percentage of the total cellular population and may be masked by the predominant polymorphous infiltrate

★ A definitive cytologic diagnosis of Hodgkin lymphoma requires the identification of classic Reed–Sternberg cells, Hodgkin cells, or both in a reactive background including normally appearing lymphocytes, eosinophils, histiocytes, and plasma cells

★ FNA has some limitations in the diagnosis of Hodgkin lymphomas including cases of partial lymph node involvement, absence of typical Reed–Sternberg cells in the aspirate, scant cellularity due to fibrosis, etc. Surgical biopsy is indicated when the cytologic diagnosis is equivocal

NON-HODGKIN LYMPHOMA (NHL)

Clinical Features
▪ They are subdivided in B-cell and T-cell types and have different presentation, treatment and prognosis

WORLD HEALTH ORGANIZATION CLASSIFICATION OF NON-HODGKIN LYMPHOMAS

B-Cell Neoplasms
▪ Precursor B-cell neoplasm
  ➤ Precursor B-lymphoblastic leukemia/lymphoma
▪ Mature (peripheral) B-cell neoplasms
  ➤ Chronic lymphocytic leukemia/small lymphocytic lymphoma
  ➤ B-cell prolymphocytic leukemia
  ➤ Lymphoplasmacytic lymphoma/Waldenstrom macroglobulinemia
  ➤ Splenic marginal zone B-cell lymphoma
  ➤ Nodal marginal zone lymphoma
  ➤ Extranodal marginal zone B-cell lymphoma of mucosa-associated lymphoid tissue (MALT) type
  ➤ Hairy cell leukemia
▪ Plasma cell neoplasms
  ➤ Myeloma
  ➤ Plasmacytoma
  ➤ Monoclonal immunoglobin deposition diseases
  ➤ Heavy chain diseases
▪ Follicular lymphoma
▪ Mantle cell lymphoma
▪ Diffuse large cell B-cell lymphoma
▪ Mediastinal (thymic) large B-cell lymphoma
▪ Intravascular large B-cell lymphoma
▪ Primary effusion lymphoma

▓ Burkitt's lymphoma/Burkitt's cell leukemia
▓ Lymphomatoid granulomatosis

T-Cell and Natural Killer Cell Neoplasms
▓ Precursor T cell neoplasm
➤ Precursor T-lymphoblastic lymphoma/leukemia
▓ Mature (peripheral) T cell and NK-cell neoplasms
➤ T cell prolymphocytic leukemia
➤ T-cell granular lymphocytic leukemia
➤ Aggressive NK-cell leukemia
➤ Adult T-cell lymphoma/leukemia
➤ Extranodal NK/T-cell lymphoma, nasal type
➤ Enteropathy-type T-cell lymphoma
➤ Hepatosplenic T-cell lymphoma
➤ Subcutaneous panniculitis-like T-cell lymphoma
➤ Blastic NK lymphoma
➤ Mycosis fungoides/Sézary syndrome
▓ Primary cutaneous CD30 positive T-cell lymphoproliferative disorders
➤ Primary cutaneous anaplastic large cell lymphoma
➤ Lymphomatoid papulosis
➤ Borderline lesions
▓ Peripheral T-cell lymphoma, unspecified
▓ Angioimmunoblastic T-cell lymphoma
▓ Anaplastic large cell lymphoma, T/null cell

Cytologic Features
▓ Cell size is one of the most important criteria in the diagnosis and classification of NHL
▓ Using small reactive lymphocyte nuclei as a standard, cytologically non-Hodgkin lymphomas can be classified in three groups
▓ Small size cells: Nuclei similar to or slightly larger than a small reactive lymphocyte
▓ Intermediate sized cells: The nuclei average 1.5 times the diameter of a small lymphocyte. Any lymphoma in between small and large cell morphology
▓ Large size cells: two times or more the diameter of a small lymphocyte
▓ For cytologic purposes the intermediate and large size groups may be combined

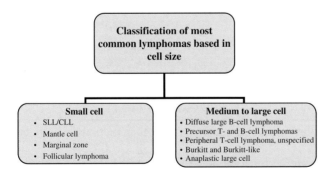

SMALL CELL LYMPHOMAS

SMALL LYMPHOCYTIC LYMPHOMA/CHRONIC LYMPHOCYTIC LEUKEMIA

Clinical Features
▓ It is a neoplasm of B cells involving the peripheral blood, bone marrow, and lymph nodes
▓ All patients with chronic lymphocytic leukemia have by definition involvement of bone marrow and peripheral blood at diagnosis

▓ When bone marrow and peripheral blood are not involved a diagnosis of small lymphocytic lymphoma is made
▓ Lymph node, liver, and spleen are more commonly involved
▓ Patient can be asymptomatic or present with fatigue, hemolytic anemia, hepatosplenomegaly, etc.

Cytologic Features
▓ Monomorphous small lymphocytes
▓ Scarce cytoplasm
▓ Slightly irregular nuclear outlines
▓ Clumped chromatin
▓ Inconspicuous nucleoli

MANTLE CELL LYMPHOMA

Clinical Features
▓ It is a B-cell lymphoma that comprises 3–10% of non-Hodgkin lymphomas
▓ Occurs in middle age to old patients
▓ Lymph nodes are the most common site of involvement followed by spleen and bone marrow
▓ The most common involved extranodal sites are the gastrointestinal tract and Waldeyer's ring
▓ Often present as stage III or IV with lymphadenopathy, hepatosplenomegaly, and bone marrow involvement
▓ Poor prognosis

Cytologic Features
▓ Monomorphous population of small to medium size lymphoid cells
▓ Scarce cytoplasm
▓ Irregular nuclear chromatin
▓ Nuclear membrane irregularities and indentations
▓ Small nucleoli
▓ Blastic variant
  ➤ Intermediate to large cells
  ➤ Large, irregular nucleoli

FOLLICULAR LYMPHOMA

Clinical Features
▓ It is a neoplasm of follicle center cells that displays a follicular pattern on histology
▓ Comprise about 35% of adult non-Hodgkin lymphomas
▓ It affects adults, mean age fifty-nine years
▓ Predominantly involves lymph nodes but also spleen, bone marrow, peripheral blood, and Waldeyer's ring
▓ Most patients have widespread disease at diagnosis but are usually asymptomatic
▓ Histologic grade correlates with prognosis
▓ Three different histologic grades according to the number of centroblasts per high-power field (hpf)
  ➤ Grade 1 (<5 centroblasts/hpf)
  ➤ Grade 2 (5–15 centroblasts/hpf)
  ➤ Grade 3 (>15 centroblasts/hpf)

Cytologic Features
- Small to irregular cleaved lymphocytes
- The size of the cleaved lymphocyte varies with the tumor grade
- Few tingible body macrophages
- Lymphoid cell aggregates

MARGINAL ZONE LYMPHOMA

Clinical Features
- It is an indolent low grade B-cell lymphoma
- It is subdivided into extranodal and nodal types
- Extranodal marginal zone lymphoma of mucosa associated lymphoid tissue (MALT lymphoma): Comprises 7–8% of all B-cell lymphomas and up to 50% of primary gastric lymphomas. Most common in adults, median age of years sixty-one. Slight preponderance in females. Strong association with autoimmune disorders and *Helicobacter pylori*–associated gastritis
- Nodal marginal zone B-cell lymphoma: It is rare, accounting for less than 2% of lymphoid neoplasms. Affects peripheral lymph nodes, occasionally bone marrow and peripheral blood

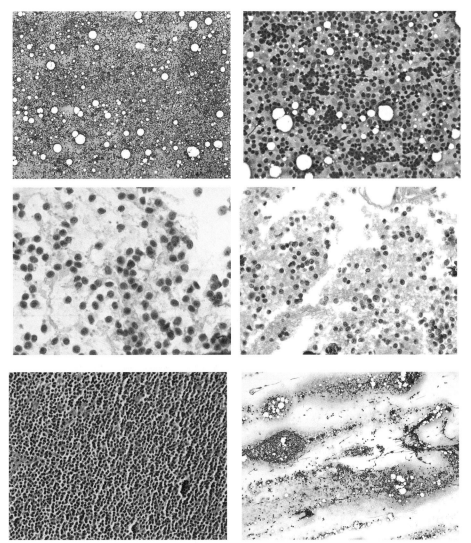

18-38. and 18.39. Small cell lymphomas/SLL/CLL *(top, left* and *right)*. Cellular aspirate characterized by a monomorphous population of small lymphocytes (modified Giemsa stain)

18-40. Small cell lymphomas/ SLL/CLL *(middle, left)*. The cells are round to oval and, for the most part, lack significant nuclear angularity or cleavage. The chromatin is coarse and clumped (Papanicoloau stain)

18-41. Small cell lymphomas/SLL/CLL (cell block) *(middle, right)*. The cells have scant cytoplasm, rounded nuclei, darkly clumped chromatin, and inconspicuous nucleoli (H&E)

18-42. Small cell lymphomas/ SLL/CLL *(bottom, left)*. Histologic appearance of a lymph node involved by SLL/CLL showing effacement of the normal architecture of the lymph node by a monomorphous population of small lymphocytes (H&E)

18-43. Small cell lymphomas/Follicular lymphoma, grade 1 *(bottom, right)*. Cellular smear of a lymph node involved by follicular lymphoma. At this low power magnification the malignant nature of the cells is not evident (modified Giemsa stain)

18-44. Small cell lymphomas/ Follicular lymphoma, grade 1 *(top, left)*. A case of follicular lymphoma, cytology preparation shows of small lymphocytes with scanty cytoplasm and irregular nuclei (centrocytes) mixed with a population of larger lymphocytes with scanty cytoplasm with rounded nuclei and single or multiple small nucleoli (centroblasts). The presence of a dual population does not mean normal range of maturation (modified Giemsa stain)

18-45. Small cell lymphomas/Mantle cell lymphoma *(top, right)*. Small to medium-sized lymphoid cells with markedly irregular nuclear contours. The nuclei have moderately dispersed chromatin and inconspicuous nucleoli (modified Giemsa stain)

18-46. Small cell lymphomas/ Marginal zone lymphoma *(bottom, left)*. Cellular smear showing a monomorphic population of small lymphocytes. Without the use of immunophenotyping ancillary techniques, it is difficult to distinguish it from other small cell lymphomas (modified Giemsa stain)

18-47. Small cell lymphomas/ Marginal zone lymphoma *(bottom, right)*. Lymphocytes with round to irregular nucleus. The monocytoid cells are characterized by more abundant cytoplasm. Numerous lymphoglandular bodies are seen in the background (modified Giemsa stain)

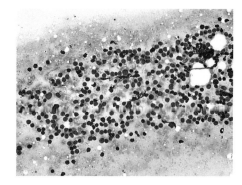 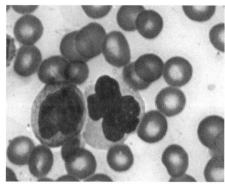

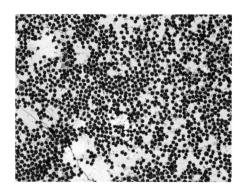 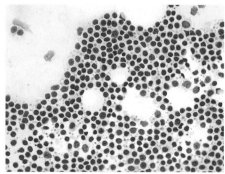

Cytology Features
- Small to medium-sized lymphocytes
- Background of polymorphous population
- Lymphocytes with round to irregular nucleus
- Monocytoid cells characterized by more abundant cytoplasm
- Plasma cells, follicular dendritic cells, immunoblasts, and lymphohistiocytic aggregates

Differential Diagnosis of Small Cell Lymphomas
- Reactive lymphoid hyperplasia
  - Presence of lymphohistiocytic aggregates and tingible body macrophages
  - Heterogenous population with predominance of small lymphocytes but presence of a range of lymphoid cells
  - The heterogenous cell population seen in marginal zone lymphoma makes it difficult to recognize as lymphoma; therefore, the definitive diagnosis rest on immunohistochemistry or flow cytometry
- Small cell carcinoma
  - Contains cell clusters
  - Nuclear molding
  - Extensive necrosis
  - Positive for cytokeratin
- Lymphocyte predominance Hodgkin lymphoma
  - Presence of Reed–Sternberg cells can be highlighted by immunohistochemistry
  - Flow cytometry reveals polyclonality in the small lymphocyte population

PEARLS

★ Small cell lymphomas can be overlooked when evaluating smears due to the lack of extremely atypical pleomorphic cells; however, attention should be paid to the monotony of the aspirate and additional material should be submitted for flow cytometry if there is clinical or cytological suspicion

MEDIUM TO LARGE LYMPHOMAS

DIFFUSE LARGE B-CELL LYMPHOMA

Clinical Features
- Constitutes a diffuse proliferation of large B-cells comprising 30–40% of adult non-Hodgkin lymphomas
- The median age is the seventh decade, but can be rarely be seen in children
- May present as nodal or extranodal disease. Most common extranodal site is gastrointestinal tract
- Many patients have disseminated disease at diagnosis
- It can arise de novo or as a transformation of a less aggressive lymphoma
- Histologically is characterized by complete effacement of the normal architecture of the lymph node

Cytologic Features
- Cellular smears
- Large cell population
- Variable number of tingible body macrophages
- In cases of mediastinal diffuse large B-cell lymphoma smears are hypocellular due to extensive fibrosis
- Variants
  - Centroblastic
  - Immunoblastic
  - T-cell/histiocyte rich
  - Lymphomatoid granulomatosis type
  - Anaplastic B cell
  - Plasmablastic

PRECURSOR T- AND B-CELL LYMPHOBLASTIC LYMPHOMAS

Clinical Features
- Aggressive lymphoma
- 90% are of T-cell derivation

Lymphoma	Clinical features
Precursor T-cell lymphoblastic leukemia/ lymphoblastic lymphoma	• Most frequent in adolescent males • Process is confined to a mass without bone marrow or blood involvement; the preferred term is lymphoblastic lymphoma • With bone marrow or peripheral blood involvement the preferred term is lymphoblastic leukemia • A mass lesion with 25% or fewer lymphoblasts in the bone marrow, the diagnosis of lymphoma is preferred • Precursor T-cell lymphoblastic leukemia presents with high leukocyte count, and a large mediastinal or other tissue mass • Precursor T-cell lymphoblastic lymphoma present as a fast-growing mediastinal mass. Other sites include lymph nodes, skin, liver, and spleen
Precursor B-cell lymphoblastic leukemia/ lymphoblastic lymphoma	• 75% of cases occur in children • Constitutes about 10% of cases of lymphoblastic lymphoma • When the process is confined to a mass without bone marrow or blood involvement; the preferred term is lymphoblastic lymphoma • When there is bone marrow or peripheral blood involvement the preferred term is lymphoblastic leukemia • A mass lesion with 25% or fewer lymphoblasts in the bone marrow, the diagnosis of lymphoma is preferred

(continued)

Table *(continued)*

Lymphoma	Clinical features
	• Most frequent sites of involvement in lymphoblastic lymphoma: skin, bone, lymph nodes and soft tissues • Most frequent sites of extramedullary involvement in lymphoblastic leukemia: central nervous system, lymph nodes, spleen, gonads, and liver • Clinical presentation includes bone marrow failure, lymphadenopathy, hepatosplenomegaly, arthralgias. Leukocyte count could be increased, decreased, or normal

Cytologic Features
- Cellular smears
- Monomorphic population of lymphoblasts
- Lymphoblasts are twice the size of a mature small lymphocyte
- Scarce to moderate cytoplasm
- Round to irregular nuclei
- Finely granular chromatin
- Small nucleoli
- Tingible body macrophages can be present

PERIPHERAL T-CELL LYMPHOMA, UNSPECIFIED

Clinical Features
- Comprise about half of peripheral T-cell lymphomas in Western countries
- Most frequent in adults, can occur in children
- Any site can be affected, but most commonly patient present with nodal involvement
- Patients often have generalized disease at diagnosis with liver, bone marrow, peripheral blood, and spleen involvement

Cytologic Features
- Cellular smears
- Polymorphous population of cells including intermediate and large lymphocytes, histiocytes, plasma cells, and eosinophils
- Irregular nuclear membranes

ANAPLASTIC LARGE CELL LYMPHOMA

Clinical Features
- A T-cell lymphoma that accounts for about 3% of adult non-Hodgkin lymphomas
- The cells are CD30 positive and the majority is positive for anaplastic large cell lymphoma kinase (ALK), but CD30 positive, ALK negative cases are also seen
- Frequently involve lymph nodes and extranodal sites
- Most common extranodal sites are skin, bone, and liver
- The majority of patients present with advanced stage at diagnosis

Cytologic Features

- Moderate to very cellular smears
- Intermediate to large cells with evident pleomorphism
- Horse-shoe nuclei
- Prominent nucleoli
- No tingible body macrophages

BURKITT LYMPHOMA

Clinical Features

- Highly aggressive B-cell lymphoma with high risk of central nervous system involvement
- Epstein–Barr virus (EBV) association is variable (see below)
- Three clinical variants are recognized
- Endemic
  - Most common malignancy of childhood in equatorial Africa
  - Peak incidence of four to seven years
  - The jaw or other fascial bones are the most common sites of presentation
  - Highly associated with EBV infection
- Sporadic
  - Mainly in children and young adults
  - The majority presents as abdominal masses with the ileocecal region as the most frequent site of involvement
  - 30% are associated with EBV infection
- Immunodeficiency associated
  - Primarily associated with HIV infection
  - More common in adults

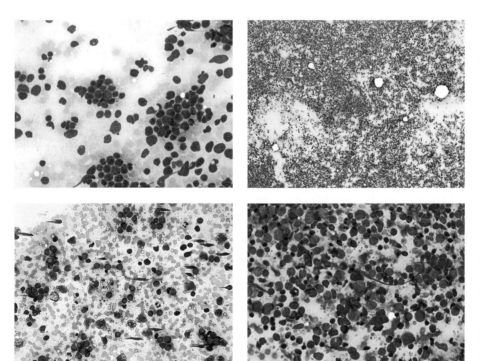

18-48. Intermediate cell lymphomas *(top, left)*. Follicular Grade 2. Small and medium-sized irregular cleaved lymphocytes. The size of the cleaved lymphocyte varies with the tumor grade (modified Giemsa stain)

18-49. Large cell lymphomas/ Diffuse large B-cell lymphoma *(top, right)*. Very cellular smear showing a large cell population (modified Giemsa stain)

18-50. Large cell lymphomas/Diffuse large B-cell lymphoma *(bottom, left)*. Numerous tingible body macrophages are seen also in high-grade lymphomas (modified Giemsa stain)

18-51. Large cell lymphomas/ Diffuse large B-cell lymphoma *(bottom, right)*. Cellular smear displaying large irregular cells. The bluish scant cytoplasm and the presence of numerous lymphoglandular bodies in the background aids in the differential diagnosis with small cell carcinoma (modified Giemsa stain)

18-52. Large cell lymphomas/ Diffuse large B-cell lymphoma/ Immunoblastic variant *(top, left).* Smear showing a few immunoblasts with a typical large, red, central nucleolus; relatively clear chromatin and abundant bluish red cytoplasm (DQ)

18-53. Large cell lymphomas/ Burkitt *(top, right).* Large lymphocytes showing the characteristic vacuolated cytoplasm (lipid vacuoles). Mitotic figures are also seen (modified Giemsa stain)

18-54. Large cell lymphomas/Burkitt *(bottom, left).* Large lymphocytes showing the characteristic vacuolated cytoplasm (lipid vacuoles). Mitosis figures are also seen (modified Giemsa stain)

18-55. Large cell lymphoma *(bottom, right).* Burkitt lymphoma with necrosis and acute inflammation, not to be confused with acute lymphadenopathy (modified Giemsa stain)

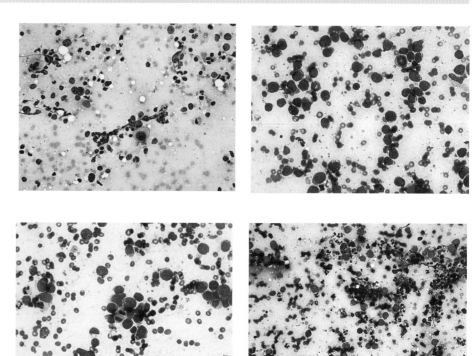

> Epstein–Barr virus is present in 25–40% of cases
> Nodal localization and bone marrow involvement

Cytologic Features
- Hypercellular smears
- Uniform intermediate sized cells
- Scant blue vacuolated cytoplasm
- Round nuclei
- Coarse chromatin
- Several nucleoli
- Abundant tingible body macrophages
- Dirty background due to apoptosis

Differential Diagnosis of Medium to Large Cell Lymphomas
- Reactive hyperplasia
  > Some cases of peripheral T-cell lymphomas and diffuse large B-cell lymphomas can simulate reactive hyperplasia
  > The presence of atypical cells, nuclear membrane irregularities are helpful to rule out reactive hyperplasia
  > Immunophenotype is confirmatory
- Granulocytic sarcoma/myeloid sarcoma
  > Tumor of immature myeloid cells
  > Occur in bone and extramedullary locations
  > Immunophenotyping is necessary (positive for CD13, CD33, and CD117)
  > Immunohistochemistry for myeloperoxidase is positive
- Histiocytic and dendritic neoplasm
  > Histiocytic sarcoma is morphologically indistinguishable from diffuse large B-cell lymphoma and anaplastic large cell lymphoma. It expresses the histiocytic marker CD68

➤ Dendritic cell sarcoma and Langerhans cell sarcoma express S-100 protein and CD1a
■ Non-lymphoid tumors
  ➤ Anaplastic large cell lymphoma can be confused with carcinoma in smears due to its propensity to form clusters, marked pleomorphism, and scant number of lymphoglandular bodies
  ➤ A panel of immunostains is very helpful in cases of undifferentiated neoplasm
  ➤ Anaplastic lymphomas are negative for CD45
■ Lymphoblastic lymphoma and Burkitt
  ➤ Should be differentiated from small round blue cell tumors of childhood
  ➤ Small round blue cell tumors do not have lymphoglandular bodies
  ➤ The cells in small round blue cell tumors tend to form clusters on the smears
  ➤ Neuroblastoma form rosettes and displays nuclear molding
  ➤ Rhabdomyosarcoma cells are more pleomorphic with more abundant cytoplasm
  ➤ Immunohistochemistry is confirmatory

PEARLS

★ Large B-cell lymphomas have been reported to show a significant rate of false negativity by flow cytometry analysis. Morphologic assessment of the material obtained by FNA may raise the suspicion of lymphoma in many cases, which are falsely negative by flow cytometry.

IMMUNOHISTOCHEMISTRY IN NON-HODGKIN LYMPHOMAS

Algorithm for the Diagnosis of Low-Grade Lymphomas

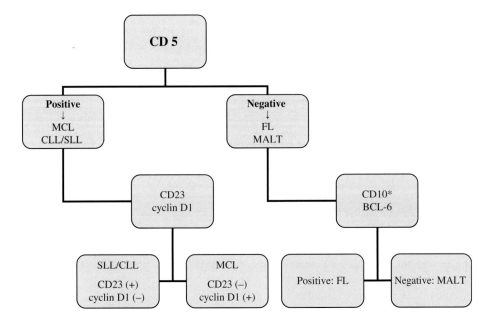

* Some cases of follicular lymphoma are CD10 negative
MCL: Mantle cell lymphoma, CLL/SLL: Chronic lymphocytic leukemia/small lymphocytic lymphoma, FL: Follicular lymphoma, MALT: marginal zone lymphoma of MALT type.

Markers Used in Immunohistochemistry

Antigen (Antibody)	Immune cells and/or tumor cells detected
CD20	B-cells, L&H cells, R-S cells +/−
CD79a	pre B-cells, B-cells, plasma cells
Kappa, Lambda	pre B-cells +/− (cytoplasmic), B-cells, plasma cells
CD3	Peripheral T-cell, thymocytes
CD45 (LCA)	All leukocytes
CD45Ro	Memory T-cells
CD43	T-cells, some B-cells, myeloid cells
CD15	Granulocytes, R-S cells
CD30	R-S cells, ALCL, immunoblasts
Myeloperoxidase	Myeloid cells
CD68	Histiocytes, myeloid cells
TdT	Lymphoblasts
MIB-1/Ki-67	Proliferation marker
Bcl-2	Follicular hyperplasia vs. follicular lymphoma germinal centers (−), Follicular lymphoma and other low grade lymphomas (+)
CD4, CD8	T-cell subsets
CD5	T-cells, CLL/SLL, mantle cell lymphoma
CD10 (CALLA)	Follicular lymphoma, follicle center cells, AILT
BCL6	Normal and neoplastic germinal center cells
IgD	Mantle cells, MCL, SMZL
CD21	Follicular dendritic cells, AILT
CD23	Follicular dendritic cells, CLL
CD1a	Langerhans cells, cortical thymocytes
CD56	NK cells, nasal T/NK-cell lymphoma, TCL
CD57	Cytotoxic T-cells, NK-cells
EMA	ALCL, plasma cells, L&H cells
CD34	Pluripotent hematopoietic stem cell
CD-99	Lymphoblastic lymphoma, Ewing's sarcoma
Cyclin D1	MCL, HCL (weak)
ALK	Anaplastic large cell lymphoma

EMA, epithelial membrane antigen; ALK, anaplastic lymphoma kinase; TCL, T-cell lymphoma; EBV, Epstein–Barr virus; ALCL, anaplastic large cell lymphoma; AILT, angioimmunoblastic T-cell lymphoma; SMZL, splenic marginal zone lymphoma; HCL, hairy cell leukemia.

Most Useful Markers for Lymphoma Classification
- Precursor lymphoblastic neoplasm: TdT
- Chronic lymphocytic leukemia/Small lymphocytic lymphoma: CD5, CD23
- Mantle cell lymphoma: Cyclin D1
- Follicular lymphoma: CD10/BCL-6
- Burkitt lymphoma: Ki-67 near 100%
- Plasma cell neoplasm: CD138
- Anaplastic large cell lymphoma: ALK, CD30
- Extranodal NK/T-cell lymphoma: CD56

Chromosomal Translocations in Non-Hodgkin Lymphomas

Lymphoma type	Translocation/ genetic alterations	Percentage affected	Protooncogene	Protooncogene function
Lymphoplasmacytic lymphoma	del(6)(q21) t(9;14)(p13;q32)*	Del(6)(q21) is most common in bone marrow based cases but is not specific	PAX-5*	Transcription factor regulating B-cell proliferation and differentiation
Follicular lymphoma	t(14;18)(q32;q21) 3q27 and/or BCL6	80–90% 5–15%, more common in Grade 3	BCL-2	Negative regulator of apoptosis
Mantle cell lymphoma	t(11;14)(q13;q32)	70%	Cyclin D1	Cell cycle regulator
MALT lymphoma	t(11;18)(q21;q21) t(1;14)(p22;q32)	50% rare	API2/MLT BCL-10	API2 has antiapoptotic activity
Diffuse large B-cell lymphoma	3q27 t(14;18)	30% 20–30%	BCL-6 BCL-2	BCL-6: Transcriptional repressor required for GC formation
Burkitt lymphoma	t(8;14)(q24;q32) t(2;8)(p12;q24) t(8;22)(q24;q11)	80% 15% 5%	c-MYC	Transcription factor regulating cell proliferation/growth
Anaplastic large T-cell lymphoma	t(2;5)(p23;q35)	60% adults 85% child	NPM/ALK	ALK is a tyrosine kinase

* Recent data proved that this translocation is rare if even found, and when found it is not specific.

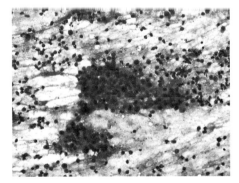
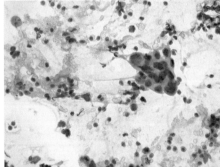
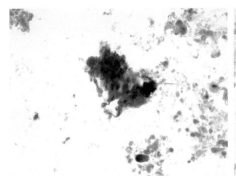
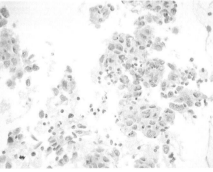

18-56. Metastatic ductal carcinoma of breast to the axillary lymph node *(top, left)*. Cluster of carcinoma cells in a background of necrosis. Crowding, overlapping, and prominent nucleoli are seen. With the presence of a carcinoma in the breast, no immunohistochemistry is necessary for the diagnosis (modified Giemsa stain)

18-57. Metastatic nonkeratinizing squamous cell carcinoma of lung to lymph nodes *(top, right)*. Cluster of carcinoma cells showing irregular borders and polygonal cells with dense cytoplasm. Keratin is not seen (Papanicolaou stain)

18-58. Metastatic keratinizing squamous cell carcinoma of lung to lymph nodes *(bottom, left)*. Cells with sharply demarcated, orangeophilic cytoplasm and pyknotic nuclei. Orange balls (keratin) and necrosis are also present (Papanicolaou stain)

18-59. Metastatic nonkeratinizing squamous cell carcinoma of lung to lymph nodes *(bottom, right)*. Negative for TTF-1. Although the majority of lung cancers are TTF-1 positive, squamous cell carcinoma of the lung is an exception, showing positivity only in about 20% of the cases

18-60. Metastatic melanoma
(top, left). Large pleomorphic cells with abundant cytoplasm and prominent nucleoli (modified Giemsa stain)

18-61. Metastatic melanoma
(top, right). Large cells with abundant cytoplasm, prominent nucleoli, and eccentric nuclei. An intranuclear pseudoinclusion is seen at the center (Papanicolaou stain)

18-62. Metastatic melanoma
(middle, left). S-100 immunohistochemistry performed in the cell block shows strong reactivity confirming the diagnosis of metastatic melanoma

18-63. Metastatic melanoma
(middle, right). Excisional biopsy of a lymph node showing partial replacement by a sheet of eosinophilic cells with abundant cytoplasm (H&E)

18-64. Metastatic neuroendocrine carcinoma to lymph node *(bottom, left)*. Smear showing loosely cohesive tumor cells. The tumor cells have large and pleomorphic nuclei with coarse chromatin. The nuclear/cytoplasmic ratio of the tumor cells is moderate. The salt-and-pepper chromatin is better appreciated in PAP-stained slides (modified Giemsa stain)

18-65. Metastatic neuroendocrine carcinoma to lymph node *(bottom, right)*. Smear showing loosely cohesive tumor cells. The tumor cells have large and pleomorphic nuclei with coarse chromatin. The nuclear/cytoplasmic ratio of the tumor cells is moderate. The salt-and-pepper chromatin is better appreciated in PAP-stained slides (modified Giemsa stain)

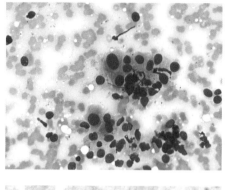 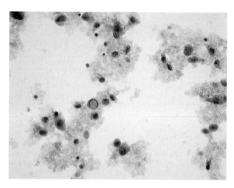
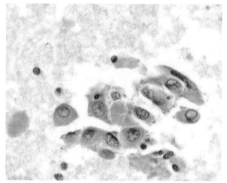 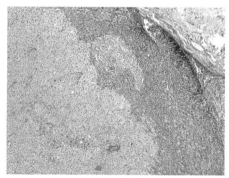
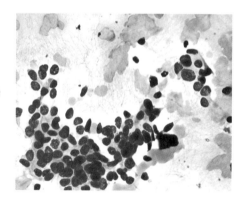 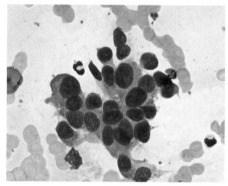

METASTATIC DISEASE TO LYMPH NODES

Clinical Features

- The strategic localization of lymph nodes throughout the body allows them to filter the lymph drained from most organs via the afferent lymphatics. This also makes them very susceptible to metastatic disease
- Metastatic disease can present in a patient with a previous diagnosis of cancer or in cases where no prior diagnosis have been established
- Most common culprits are carcinomas, melanomas, germ cell tumors, and less frequently sarcomas
- Sarcomas rarely metastasize to lymph nodes. When they do it, the most common are rhabdomyosarcoma, clear cell sarcoma, and synovial sarcoma
- According to the location the primary malignant tumor can be suspected
  - Cervical lymph nodes: Oral cavity, thyroid, skin of the face, larynx
  - Axillary lymph nodes: Breast and melanoma
  - Inguinal lymph nodes: Cervix, skin, vulva, anus, and rectum
  - Pelvic lymph nodes: Prostate, uterus, cervix
  - Mediastinal lymph nodes: Lung

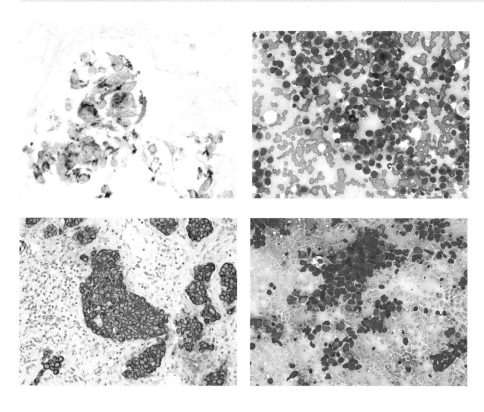

> Supraclavicular lymph nodes: Lung, prostate, gastrointestinal tract
> Retroperitoneal lymph nodes: Gastrointestinal tract, pancreas, gonads, kidney

Cytologic Features
▣ Carcinomas
  ➤ Usually two cell populations: Malignant cells in a background of lymphoid tissue
  ➤ Usually cellular smears
  ➤ Cells in clusters
  ➤ Necrosis variably present
  ➤ Absence of lymphoglandular bodies
  ➤ Cytologic clues for diagnosis of specific tumors
     • Irregularly shaped groups of polygonal cells with dense cytoplasm → nonkeratinizing squamous cell carcinoma
     • Cells with sharply demarcated, orangeophilic cytoplasm and pyknotic nuclei → Keratinizing squamous cell carcinoma
     • Signet ring cells → Lobular carcinoma of breast and gastric carcinomas
     • Dirty necrosis → Colon carcinomas
▣ Germ cell tumors
  ➤ Usually two cell populations: malignant cells in a background of lymphoid tissue
  ➤ Dispersed large malignant cells
  ➤ Abundant cytoplasm
  ➤ Lymphocytes may be part of the tumor
  ➤ Tigroid background
▣ Melanoma
  ➤ Usually two cell populations: Malignant cells in a background of lymphoid tissue
  ➤ Cellular smears
  ➤ Dispersed cells
  ➤ Abundant cytoplasm
  ➤ Eccentrically located nuclei

18-66. Metastatic neuroendocrine carcinoma to lymph node *(top, left)*. Cell block showing strong positivity for chromogranin, a neuroendocrine marker

18-67. Metastatic carcinoma of unknown primary to retroperitoneal lymph node *(top, right)*. Isolated malignant cells with moderately abundant cytoplasm and pleomorphism are seen in the slide. At first glance the discohesiveness of the tumor cells may cause the cytopathologist to entertain other malignant neoplasms characterized by a dispersed cell pattern (modified Giemsa stain)

18-68. Metastatic carcinoma of unknown primary to retroperitoneal lymph node *(bottom, left)*. Cytokeratin immunohistochemistry of the same case showing strong positivity, and confirms this tumor as carcinoma. Multiple additional stains failed to point out the site of the primary tumor

18-69. Metastatic small cell carcinoma to lymph node *(bottom, right)*. Highly pleomorphic large malignant cell showing irregular nuclear membranes, scant almost invisible cytoplasm, and molding. The differential diagnosis includes large cell lymphomas (modified Giemsa stain)

18-70. Metastatic carcinoma to lymph node *(below)*. Smear showing necrosis, acute inflammation and abundant macrophages, not to be confused with acute lymphadenopathy. A cluster of malignant epithelial cells is seen in the upper part of the smear (modified Giemsa stain)

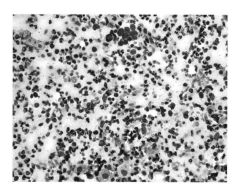

➢ Commonly binucleated
➢ Intranuclear inclusions
➢ Prominent nucleoli
➢ May have melanin pigment
➢ No lymphoglandular bodies
▣ Sarcoma
➢ Cytologic features depend of the specific tumor but usually the malignant cells have spindly nuclei with evident pleomorphism
➢ Exception is synovial sarcoma characterized by bland-appearing rounded cells

Special Stains and Immunohistochemistry
▣ Carcinomas
➢ Lung: Positive for CK7 and TTF-1
➢ Breast: Positive for GCDFP-15, Mammaglobin, ER, PR
➢ Pancreas: Positive for CK19, CK7
➢ Stomach: Positive for CDX2, CK7 > CK20
➢ Liver: Positive for AFP, Hep Par-1, Polyclonal CEA
➢ Colon: Positive for CK20, CEA, B72.3, CDX2, (CK7 negative)
➢ Prostate: Positive for PSA, PAP
➢ Thyroid: Positive for thyroglobulin, TTF-1, CK19 (papillary carcinoma), calcitonin (medullary carcinoma)
➢ Small cell carcinoma: Positive for chromogranin and synaptophysin
➢ Endometrial: Positive for ER, PR, negative for GCDFP-15, and mammaglobin
➢ Ovary: Positive for CA-125
▣ Germ cell tumors
➢ PLAP (seminoma)
➢ B-HCG (choriocarcinoma)
➢ AFP (yolk sac tumor)
➢ CAM 5.2 (Spermatocytic seminoma)
➢ CD30 (embryonal carcinoma)
▣ Melanoma
➢ S-100; HMB-45 and melan A
▣ Sarcomas
➢ Rhabdomyosarcoma: Positive for desmin and myogenin
➢ Clear cell sarcoma: Positive for S-100, HMB-45, A103
➢ Synovial sarcoma: Positive for EMA, CD99, vimentin
➢ Leiomyosarcoma: Positive for smooth muscle actin (SMA), desmin, h-caldesmon

Differential Diagnosis
▣ Granulomatous inflammation
➤ The presence of spindle cells and necrosis in some granulomatous diseases may be confused with spindle cell neoplasia, including sarcomas
➤ Clinically granulomatous inflammation present with generalized nonspecific symptoms and sarcoma usually present with a large mass
➤ The absence of overtly malignant features in granulomatous inflammation aids in the differential diagnosis
▣ Anaplastic large cell lymphoma
➤ Propensity to form clusters, marked pleomorphism, and scant number of lymphoglandular bodies
➤ A panel of immunostains may be necessary to differentiate anaplastic large cell lymphoma from carcinoma

⋆ When encounter with the possibility of a metastatic malignancy to a lymph node, additional cellular material should be submitted for cell block preparation and immunohistochemistry

⋆ Rarely sarcomas can appear deceptively bland cytologically; therefore always look for clinical history and use ancillary techniques for diagnosis in difficult cases

REFERENCES

FINE-NEEDLE ASPIRATION OF LYMPH NODES

Caraway NP, Kats RL. Lymph nodes. In: Koss LG, Melamed MR, eds. *Koss' Diagnostic Cytology and its Histopathological Bases*, 5th ed. Volume II. Philadelphia, 2006, pp. 1187–224.

Nasuti JF, Yu G, Boudousquie A, Gupta P. Diagnostic value of lymph node fine needle aspiration cytology: an institutional experience of 387 cases observed over a 5-year period. *Cytopathology.* 2000 Feb;11(1):18–31.

Wakely PE, Cibas ES. Lymph nodes. In: Cibas ES, Ducatman BS, eds. Cytology. *Diagnostic Principles and Clinical Correlates.* 2nd ed. Philadelphia, 2003, pp. 307–41.

IMPRINT CYTOLOGY OF LYMPH NODES

Cserni G. Effect of increasing the surface sampled by imprint cytology on the intraoperative assessment of axillary sentinel lymph nodes in breast cancer patients. *Am J Surg.* 2003; 69:419–23.

Nejc D, Pasz-Walczak G, Piekarski J, Pluta P, Sek P, Bilski A, Durczynski A, Berner A, Jastrzebski T, Jeziorski A. 94% accuracy of intraoperative imprint touch cytology of sentinel nodes in skin melanoma patients. *Anticancer Res.* 2008 Jan–Feb;28(1B):465–69.

Ravichandran D, Kocjan G, Falzon M, Ball RY, Ralphs DN. Imprint cytology of the sentinel lymph node in the assessment of axillary node status in breast carcinoma. *Eur J Surg Oncol.* 2004 Apr;30(3):238–42.

NORMAL LYMPH NODES

Caraway NP, Kats RL. Lymph nodes. In: Koss LG, Melamed MR, eds. *Koss' Diagnostic Cytology and its Histopathological Bases*, 5th ed. Volume II. Philadelphia, 2006, pp. 1187–224.

DeMay R. Lymph nodes. In: DeMay R, ed. *The Art and Science of Cytopathology. Aspiration Cytology*, Chicago, IL: ASCP Press, 1996, pp. 780–822.

Wakely PE, Cibas ES. Lymph nodes. In: Cibas ES, Ducatman BS, eds. *Cytology. Diagnostic Principles and Clinical Correlates*, 2nd ed. Philadelphia, 2003, pp. 307–41.

PRACTICAL AND ANCILLARY APPROACHES

Bagg A. Molecular diagnosis in lymphoma. *Curr Hematol Rep.* 2005 Jul;4(4):313–23.

Caraway NP, Kats RL. Lymph nodes. In: Koss LG, Melamed MR, eds. *Koss' Diagnostic Cytology and its Histopathological Bases*, 5th ed. Volume II. Philadelphia, 2006, pp. 1187–224.

Dey P, Amir T, Al Jassar A, Al Shemmari S, Jogai S, Bhat M G, Al Quallaf A, Al Shammari Z. Combined applications of fine needle aspiration cytology and flow cytometric immunphenotyping for diagnosis and classification of non Hodgkin lymphoma. *Cytojournal.* 2006 Oct 27;3:24.

Dunphy CH. Applications of flow cytometry and immunohistochemistry to diagnostic hematopathology. *Arch Pathol Lab Med.* 2004 Sep;128(9):1004–22.

Kaleem Z. Flow cytometric analysis of lymphomas: current status and usefulness. *Arch Pathol Lab Med.* 2006 Dec;130(12):1850–8.

Mourad WA, Tulbah A, Shoukri M, Al Dayel F, Akhtar M, Ali MA, Hainau B, Martin J. Primary diagnosis and REAL/WHO classification of non-Hodgkin's lymphoma by fine-needle aspiration: cytomorphologic and immunophenotypic approach. *Diagn Cytopathol.* 2003 Apr; 28(4):191–5.

Wakely PE, Cibas ES. Lymph nodes. In: Cibas ES, Ducatman BS, eds. *Cytology. Diagnostic Principles and Clinical Correlates*. 2nd ed. Philadelphia, 2003, pp. 307–41.

ACUTE LYMPHADENITIS

Caraway NP, Kats RL. Lymph nodes. In: Koss LG, Melamed MR, eds. *Koss' Diagnostic Cytology and its Histopathological Bases*, 5th ed. Volume II. Philadelphia, 2006, pp. 1187–224.

Kumar N, Jain S, Murthy NS. Utility of repeat fine needle aspiration in acute suppurative lesions. Follow-up of 263 cases. *Acta Cytol*. 2004 May–Jun;48(3):337–40.

Wakely PE, Cibas ES. Lymph nodes. In: Cibas ES, Ducatman BS, eds. *Cytology. Diagnostic Principles and Clinical Correlates*, 2nd ed. Philadelphia, 2003, pp. 307–41.

GRANULOMATOUS LYMPHADENITIS

Bruijnesteijn Van Coppenraet ES, Lindeboom JA, Prins JM, Peeters MF, Claas EC, Kuijper EJ. Real-time PCR assay using fine-needle aspirates and tissue biopsy specimens for rapid diagnosis of mycobacterial lymphadenitis in children. *J Clin Microbiol*. 2004 Jun;42(6): 2644–50.

Caraway NP, Kats RL. Lymph nodes. In: Koss LG, Melamed MR, eds. *Koss' Diagnostic Cytology and its Histopathological Bases*, 5th ed. Volume II. Philadelphia, 2006, pp. 1187–224.

Inoue Y, Suga M. Granulomatous diseases and pathogenic microorganism. *Kekkaku*. 2008 Feb;83(2):115–30.

Kishore PV, Paudel R, Paudel B, Palaian S, Mishra P. Sarcoidosis-three clinical vignettes with a short review. *JNMA J Nepal Med Assoc*. 2007 Oct–Dec;46(168):194–8.

Koo V, Lioe TF, Spence RA. Fine needle aspiration cytology (FNAC) in the diagnosis of granulomatous lymphadenitis. *Ulster Med J*. 2006 Jan;75(1):59–64.

Wakely PE, Cibas ES. Lymph nodes. In: Cibas ES, Ducatman BS, eds. *Cytology. Diagnostic Principles and Clinical Correlates*, 2nd ed. Philadelphia, 2003, pp. 307–41.

Wu JJ, Schiff KR. Sarcoidosis. *Am Fam Physician*. 2004 Jul 15;70(2):312–22.

CAT SCRATCH DISEASE

Caraway NP, Kats RL. Lymph nodes. In: Koss LG, Melamed MR, eds. *Koss' Diagnostic Cytology and its Histopathological Bases*, 5th ed. Volume II. Philadelphia, 2006: 1187–224.

Cat-scratch disease in children – Texas, September 2000 to August 2001. *Can Commun Dis Rep*. 2002 Apr 15;28(8):64–7.

Dalton MJ, Robinson LE, Cooper J, et al. Use of Bartonella antigens for serologic diagnosis of cat-scratch disease at a national referral center. *Arch Intern Med* 1995;155:1670–676.

Ferry JA, Harris NL. *Atlas of Lymphoid Hyperplasia and Lymphoma*. Philadelphia: W.B. Saunders, 1997, p. 17.

Lin YY, Hsiao CH, Hsu YH, Lee CC, Tsai HJ, Pan MJ. Immunohistochemical study of lymph nodes in patients with cat scratch disease. *J Formos Med Assoc*. 2006 Nov;105(11):911–7.

Wakely PE, Cibas ES. Lymph nodes. In: Cibas ES, Ducatman BS, eds. *Cytology. Diagnostic Principles and Clinical Correlates*, 2nd ed. Philadelphia, 2003, pp. 307–41.

REACTIVE HYPERPLASIA

Caraway NP, Kats RL. Lymph nodes. In: Koss LG, Melamed MR, eds. *Koss' Diagnostic Cytology and its Histopathological Bases*, 5th ed. Volume II. Philadelphia, 2006, pp. 1187–224.

DeMay R. Lymph nodes. In: DeMay R, ed. *The Art and Science of Cytopathology. Aspiration Cytology*. Chicago, IL: ASCP Press, 1996, pp. 780–822.

Wakely PE, Cibas ES. Lymph nodes. In: Cibas ES, Ducatman BS, eds. *Cytology. Diagnostic Principles and Clinical Correlates*, 2nd ed. Philadelphia, 2003, pp. 307–41.

HODGKIN LYMPHOMA

Chhieng DC, Cangiarella JF, Symmans WF, Cohen JM. Fine-needle aspiration cytology of Hodgkin disease: a study of 89 cases with emphasis on false-negative cases. *Cancer*. 2001 Feb 25;93(1):52–9.

Funamoto Y, Nagai M, Haba R, Ishikawa M, Kishida F, Kohno K, Matsunaga T, Kushida Y, Kobayashi S. Diagnostic accuracy of imprint cytology in the assessment of Hodgkin's disease in Japan. *Diagn Cytopathol*. 2005 Jul;33(1):20–5.

Stein H, et al. Hodgkin Lymphomas. In: Jaffe ES, Lee Harris N, Stein H, Vardiman W. eds. *Pathology and Genetics. Tumours of Haematopoietic and Lymphoid Tissues.* Lyon: IARC Press, 2001, pp. 238–53.

Vicandi B, Jiménez-Heffernan JA, López-Ferrer P, Gamallo C, Viguer JM. Hodgkin's disease mimicking suppurative lymphadenitis: a fine-needle aspiration report of five cases. *Diagn Cytopathol.* 1999 May;20(5):302–6.

Wakely PE, Cibas ES. Lymph nodes. In: Cibas ES, Ducatman BS, eds. *Cytology. Diagnostic Principles and Clinical Correlates,* 2nd ed. Philadelphia, 2003, pp. 307–341.

MARGINAL ZONE LYMPHOMA

Dey P. Role of ancillary techniques in diagnosing and subclassifying non-Hodgkin's lymphomas on fine needle aspiration cytology. *Cytopathology.* 2006 Oct;17(5):275–87.

Gong JZ, Williams DC, Jr, Liu K, Jones C. Fine-needle aspiration in non-Hodgkin lymphoma: evaluation of cell size by cytomorphology and flow cytometry. *Am J Clin Pathol.* 2002 Jun;117(6):880–8.

Jaffe ES, Lee Harris N, Stein H, Vardiman W. eds. *Pathology and Genetics. Tumours of Haematopoietic and Lymphoid Tissues.* Lyon: IARC Press 2001, pp. 127–129, 157–161, 162–170.

Mourad WA, Tulbah A, Shoukri M, Al Dayel F, Akhtar M, Ali MA, Hainau B, Martin J. Primary diagnosis and REAL/WHO classification of non-Hodgkin's lymphoma by fine-needle aspiration: cytomorphologic and immunophenotypic approach. *Diagn Cytopathol.* 2003 Apr;28(4):191–5.

Wakely PE, Cibas ES. Lymph nodes. In: Cibas ES, Ducatman BS, eds. *Cytology. Diagnostic Principles and Clinical Correlates,* 2nd ed. Philadelphia, 2003, pp. 307–41.

MEDIUM TO LARGE LYMPHOMAS

Dey P. Role of ancillary techniques in diagnosing and subclassifying non-Hodgkin's lymphomas on fine needle aspiration cytology. *Cytopathology.* 2006 Oct;17(5):275–87.

Jaffe ES, Lee Harris N, Stein H, Vardiman W. eds. *Pathology and Genetics. Tumours of Haematopoietic and Lymphoid Tissues.* Lyon: IARC Press, 2001, pp. 111–117,181–3, 230.

Wakely PE, Cibas ES. Lymph nodes. In: Cibas ES, Ducatman BS, eds. *Cytology. Diagnostic Principles and Clinical Correlates,* 2nd ed. Philadelphia, 2003, pp. 307–41.

IMMUNOHISTOCHEMISTRY IN NON-HODGKIN LYMPHOMAS

Dey P, Amir T, Al Jassar A, Al Shemmari S, Jogai S, Bhat M G, Al Quallaf A, Al Shammari Z. Combined applications of fine needle aspiration cytology and flow cytometric immunphenotyping for diagnosis and classification of non Hodgkin lymphoma. *Cytojournal.* 2006 Oct 27;3:24.

Dey P. Role of ancillary techniques in diagnosing and subclassifying non-Hodgkin's lymphomas on fine needle aspiration cytology. *Cytopathology.* 2006 Oct;17(5):275–87.

Harris NL, Stein H, Coupland SE, Hummel M, Favera RD, Pasqualucci L, Chan WC. New approaches to lymphoma diagnosis. *Hematol Am Soc Hematol Educ Program.* 2001: 194–220.

Jaffe ES, Lee Harris N, Stein H, Vardiman W. eds. *Pathology and Genetics. Tumours of Haematopoietic and Lymphoid Tissues.* Lyon: IARC Press, 2001, pp. 111–7,181–3, 230.

Tailor CR, Cote R. *Immunomicroscopy. A Diagnostic Tool for the Surgical Pathologist.* 3rd ed. Philadelphia: Elsevier, 2006, pp. 103–153.

METASTATIC DISEASE TO LYMPH NODES

Caraway NP, Kats RL. Lymph nodes. In: Koss LG, Melamed MR, eds. *Koss' Diagnostic Cytology and its Histopathological Bases,* 5th ed. Volume II. Philadelphia, 2006, pp. 1187–224.

Chen KT. Rhabdomyosarcoma in an adult presenting with nodal metastasis: a pitfall in fine-needle aspiration cytology of lymph nodes. *Diagn Cytopathol.* 2005 May;32(5): 303–6.

Rosa M, Chopra HK, Sahoo S. Fine needle aspiration biopsy diagnosis of metastatic prostate carcinoma to inguinal lymph node. *Diagn Cytopathol.* 2007 Sep;35(9):565–7.

Tailor CR, Cote R. *Immunomicroscopy. A Diagnostic Tool for the Surgical Pathologist*, 3rd ed. Philadelphia: Elsevier, 2006, pp. 379–95.

Wakely PE, Cibas ES. Lymph nodes. In: Cibas ES, Ducatman BS, eds. *Cytology. Diagnostic Principles and Clinical Correlates*, 2nd ed. Philadelphia, 2003, pp. 307–41.

19

FNA of the Gonads

Güliz A. Barkan and Eva M. Wojcik

OVARY

FOLLICULAR CYST

Clinical Features
- Solitary or multiple
- Usually asymptomatic or with mild vague pelvic pain

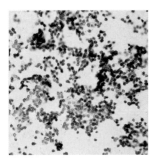

19-1. Follicular cyst. Hypercellular aspirate with loosely cohesive clusters of granulosa cells (Papanicolaou stain)

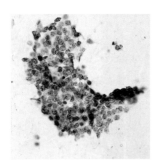

19-2. Follicular cyst. Granulosa cells with round to oval vesicular nuclei with scant cytoplasm forming a sheet (Papanicolaou stain)

■ Solitary luteinized follicle cyst could be seen in pregnancy or puerperium and could reach up to 25 cm

■ Multiple follicular cysts are seen in polycystic ovary disease and hyperstimulation syndrome

■ Unilocular with smooth thin wall and clear or cloudy serous/serosanguinous fluid

Cytologic Features

■ Hypo or hypercellular aspirate

■ Tight clusters and single granulosa cells containing round to oval vesicular nuclei with scant cytoplasm

■ Granular chromatin, small nucleoli, nuclear grooves

■ Rarely atypia and mitotic figures could be seen

■ Luteinized follicle cysts has similar cytologic features except for the ample, finely vacuolated cytoplasm

Special stains and Immunohistochemistry

■ Noncontributory

Modern Techniques for diagnosis

■ Cyst fluid estradiol (E2) content > 20 nmoL/L

Differential Diagnosis

■ Corpus luteum cyst
  ➤ Larger cells with ample foamy cytoplasm (luteinized cells)
  ➤ Macrophages
■ Cystic granulosa cell tumor
  ➤ Highly cellular aspirates
  ➤ Nuclei with pale, finely dispersed chromatin
  ➤ More frequent intranuclear grooves
■ Serous epithelial cysts
  ➤ Carcinoembryonic antigen (CEA) and CA-125 levels are higher, estradiol levels are low

PEARLS

★ Small cysts with no solid component that have low cellularity and are mostly composed of granulosa cells; these are likely to be benign follicular cysts

★ Cellular follicular cysts could be a potential pitfall

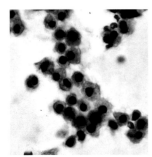

19-3. Corpus luteum cyst. Luteinized granulosa cells with granular chromatin, small chromocenters, and foamy cytoplasm (Papanicolaou stain)

CORPUS LUTEUM CYST

Clinical Features

■ Single, less than 6 cm

■ Unilocular

Cytologic Features

■ Hypo or hypercellular aspirate

■ Loose cell clusters of large granulosa cells and/or luteinized granulosa cells with abundant foamy/granular cytoplasm containing lipid

■ Eccentric small, pyknotic nuclei, and conspicuous nucleoli

■ Macrophages with hemosiderin and/or hematoidin pigment

■ Cytoplasmic hyaline globules and calcifications in pregnant patients

Special stains and Immunohistochemistry
- Noncontributory

Modern Techniques for diagnosis
- Noncontributory

Differential Diagnosis
- Follicular cyst
  - ➤ Granulosa cells have scant cytoplasm
  - ➤ At times the aspirate shows a high cellular smear containing atypical cells with high nuclear/cytoplasmic ratio, hyperchromasia prominent nucleoli and mitoses, mimicking malignancy
- Endometriotic cyst
  - ➤ Usually have three components, endometrial glandular and stromal cells as well as hemosiderin-laden macrophages

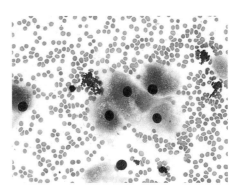

19-4. Corpus luteum cyst. Luteinized granulosa cells with abundant cytoplasm (modified Giemsa stain)

PEARLS

★ Precise classification may not be possible especially when only benign cyst fluid with macrophages are obtained; in such cases a differential diagnosis may be suggested

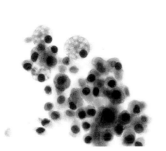
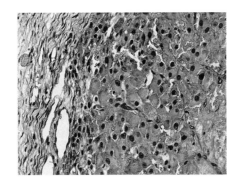

19-5. Hemorrhagic corpus luteum cyst *(left).* Luteinized granulosa cells and hemosiderin laden macrophages (Papanicolaou stain)

19-6. Hemorrhagic corpus luteum cyst *(right).* Cyst wall with luteinized granulosa cells (hematoxylin and eosin stain)

ENDOMETRIOTIC CYST

Clinical Features
- In women of reproductive age
- Associated with infertility
- Pain during menstrual cycle is the most common symptom
- Rarely it could be complicated by ascitis or perforation into the peritoneal cavity
- Dark brown – "chocolate" colored fluid

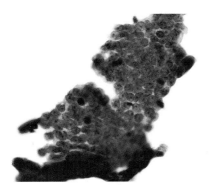
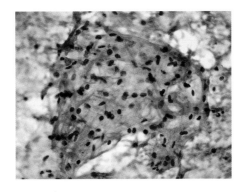

19-7. Endometriotic cyst *(left).* Endometrial glandular cells with slight nuclear atypia, nuclear enlargement, overlapping, and prominent nucleoli (Papanicolaou stain)

19-8. Endometriotic cyst *(right).* Cluster of hemosiderin laden macrophages (Papanicolaou stain)

Cytologic Features

■ Low cellularity

■ Three components: Endometrial stromal and glandular cells, and hemosiderin-laden macrophages

■ Rare epithelial atypia, slight nuclear enlargement, minimal nuclear overlap could be seen

Special Stains and Immunohistochemistry

■ Endometrial stromal cells are CD10 positive

Modern Techniques for diagnosis

■ Noncontributory

Differential Diagnosis

■ Hemorrhagic corpus luteum cyst
  ➤ Cytomorphologically identical to corpus luteum cysts especially in the absence of epithelial cells
■ Endometrial adenocarcinoma
  ➤ Atypia is more pronounced

PEARLS

★ At least two of the three cell types (stromal, glandular cells, and macrophages) should be seen to render a diagnosis of endometriotic cyst

SEROUS CYSTADENOMA AND CARCINOMA

Clinical Features

■ Serous tumors comprise 25% of all ovarian tumors

■ Approximately 60% of serous tumors are benign, 10% borderline, and 30% malignant

■ Benign serous tumor are bilateral 10–25% of cases, and they are partially or completely cystic, they are distinguished from a cortical inclusion cyst if >1 cm

■ In benign serous tumors the cyst wall is smooth, mostly without excrescences and the cyst is filled with clear fluid

■ Serous carcinomas are bilateral in 70% of the cases

■ Carcinomas mostly have both cystic and solid components

Cytologic Features

■ Serous cystadenoma
  ➤ Cohesive sheets and/or papillary clusters of uniform epithelial cells
  ➤ Moderate amount of cytoplasm, well-differentiated cell borders
  ➤ Finely granular chromatin, small nucleoli
  ➤ Occasional ciliated columnar cells, psammoma bodies, detached cilia

Serous Cystadenocarcinoma

■ Single cells, irregular clusters, papillary fragments of epithelium with cellular atypia

■ Scant cytoplasm and high nuclear/cytoplasmic (N:C) ratio

■ Cellular pleomorphism, with degree of atypia increasing as tumor becomes less differentiated

■ Coarse chromatin pattern

■ Rare psammoma bodies

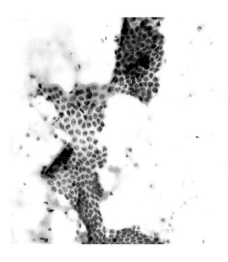
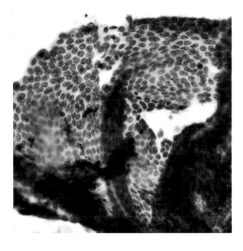

19-9. Serous cystadenoma *(left).* Sheet of benign glandular cells without atypia (Papanicolaou stain)

19-10. Serous cystadenoma *(right).* Sheet of benign glandular cells with rare nucleoli (Papanicolaou stain)

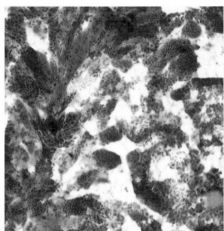
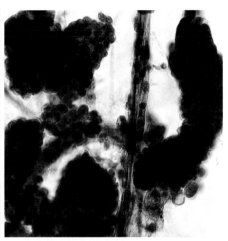

19-11. Papillary serous cystadenocarcinoma *(left).* Hypercellar smear with abundant papillary groups (Papanicolaou stain)

19-12. Papillary serous cystadenocarcinoma *(right).* Tight papillary clusters with scant cytoplasm, high N:C ratio, coarse hyperchromatic chromatin (Papanicolaou stain)

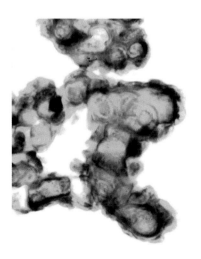
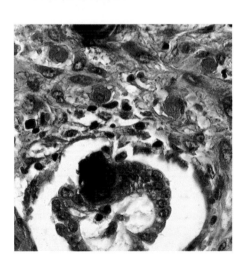

19-13. Papillary serous cystadenocarcinoma *(left).* Psammoma bodies showing concentric laminations (Papanicolaou stain)

19-14. Papillary serous cystadenocarcinoma *(right).* Large pleomorphic cell and prominent nucleoli arranged in a papillary configuration and psammoma bodies (hematoxylin and eosin stain)

Special Stains and Immunohistochemistry
- Cytokerating and Wilm's tumor (WT-1): Positive
- CK20: Negative

Modern Techniques for diagnosis
- Mutations of BRCA 1 and 2 is seen in familial cases of serous carcinoma
- CA-125 levels are elevated for serous cysts

Differential Diagnosis

■ Cortical inclusion cyst
  ➤ Essentially same cytomorphologic features as serous cystadenoma; however, size is < 1 cm
■ Cystadenofibroma
  ➤ Lesion has a solid component with benign spindled cells (stromal cells)
■ Endometrioid carcinoma
  ➤ It may resemble serous carcinoma. However, it shows scanty cytoplasm, nuclear crowding and micro-acini. Squamous differentiation may be present
■ Metastatic carcinoma
  ➤ Poorly differentiated metastatic carcinoma from a variety of organs, such as GI tract and breast may mimic cytologically a primary serous carcinoma

PEARLS

★ The role of FNA in the diagnosis of borderline lesions is limited because of its inability to evaluate stromal invasion

MUCINOUS CYSTADENOMA AND CARCINOMA

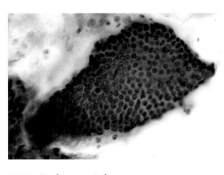

19-15. Mucinous cystadenoma.
Large sheet of uniform glandular epithelium in a background of thick mucin (Papanicolaou stain)

Clinical Features

■ Account for 15% of all ovarian tumors
■ About 80% are benign, 10% borderline, 10% malignant
■ Most common nonendocrine tumor associated with estrogenic and androgenic symptoms
■ Approximately 5% of mucinous have another component, namely dermoid cyst or Brenner tumor

Cytologic Features

■ Mucinous cystadenoma
  ➤ Abundant mucin
  ➤ Epithelial cells may resemble foamy macrophages
  ➤ Sheets of glandular cells in honeycomb arrangement, at the periphery of the sheets columnar appearance of the cells or their abundant foamy cytoplasm may be seen

Mucinous Cystadenocarcinoma

■ Presence of nuclear pleomorphism, hyperchromasia, prominent nucleoli, high N:C ratio, nuclear overlapping, and nuclear membrane irregularity point toward malignancy

19-16. Mucinous cystadenocarcinoma, well differentiated *(left).*
Group of columnar cells with slight nuclear enlargement, nuclear overlapping, and occasional prominent nucleoli in a background of mucin droplets (Papanicolaou stain)

19-17. Mucinous cystadenoma *(right).* Columnar cyst lining with pale cytoplasm and basally placed nuclei (Hematoxylin and Eosin stain)

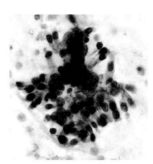

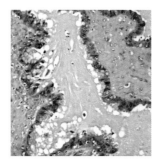

Special Stains and Immunohistochemistry
▥ Tumor cells express cytokeratin 8/18, cytokeratins 7 and 20, CEA, and epithelial membrane antigen (EMA)

Modern Techniques for diagnosis
▥ Serum CEA, CA19-9, and CA72.4 are elevated
▥ K-ras mutation is present

Differential Diagnosis
▥ Metastatic carcinoma
➤ Metastatic carcinoma from the colon has dirty necrosis, and the cells are columnar and stratified. Tumor cells are cdx-2 positive
➤ Metastatic cervical carcinoma is cytologically indistinguishable from primary ovarian carcinoma, however p16 positivity favors the former diagnosis

PEARLS
✶ Benign lesions are mostly paucicellular
✶ Mucinous tumors are distinguished from serous tumors by the presence of cytoplasmic vacuoles and the mucinous background
✶ Poorly differentiated mucinous tumors may have less mucin and therefore are difficult to differentiate from other epithelial neoplasms

BRENNER TUMOR

Clinical Features
▥ Accounts for 2–3% of ovarian neoplasms
▥ Most are benign and < 10% occur bilaterally
▥ May be an incidental finding in a patient with another type of ovarian tumor
▥ Occasionally associated with estrogenic or androgenic manifestations

Cytologic Features
▥ Epithelial and stromal elements
▥ Sheets and clusters of epithelial cells which are polygonal to round with abundant eosinophilic cytoplasm, uniform nuclei, and deep intranuclear grooves – "coffee bean nuclei"
▥ Globular, dense, homogenous eosinophilic hyaline structures "eosinophilic bodies" may be seen
▥ Stromal cells are usually isolated single cells
▥ Background is granular and fibrillary

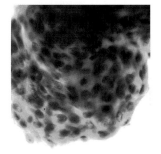 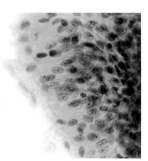 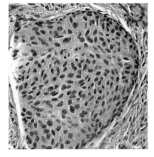

19-18. Brenner tumor *(left)*. Sheet of uniform epithelial cells with abundant eosinophilic cytoplasm and uniform nuclei (Papanicolaou stain)

19-19. Brenner tumor *(middle)*. Epithelial cells with abundant eosinophilic cytoplasm, uniform nuclei, and occasional deep intranuclear grooves (Papanicolaou stain)

19-20. Brenner tumor *(right)*. Epithelial island with a oval nucleus and eosinophilic cytoplasm (hematoxylin and eosin stain)

Special Stains and Immunohistochemistry
- Tumor cells frequently positive for serotonin and
- CK20: Negative

Modern Techniques for diagnosis
- Noncontributory

Differential Diagnosis
- Granulosa cell tumor
  - Scant, poorly defined, pale cytoplasm
  - Microfollicular pattern "Call-Exner bodies"
  - Tumor cells are negative for keratin
- Metastatic urothelial carcinoma
  - Lack nuclear grooves
  - CK20, p63 and CK5/6: Positive

PEARLS

★ Malignant Brenner tumor is difficult to diagnose based on cytology alone. They resemble urothelial carcinoma or nonkeratinizing squamous carcinoma

ENDOMETRIOID CARCINOMA

Clinical Features
- Accounts for 20% of ovarian carcinomas and is bilateral in 30% of the cases
- Approximately 30% is associated with endometriosis
- One of the most common primary neoplasms associated with endocrine manifestations

Cytologic Features
- Sheets and short strips of columnar cells with granular eosinophilic cytoplasm and eccentric nuclei and prominent nucleoli
- Numerous single columnar cells in a bloody background and hemosiderin-laden macrophages
- Tumor necrosis may be seen
- Squamoid differentiation could be present

Special stains and Immunohistochemistry
- Tumor cells are positive for EMA, CK7

Modern Techniques for diagnosis
- CA-125 levels are elevated

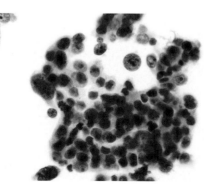 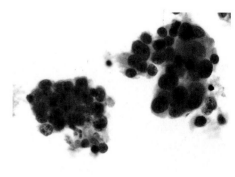

19-21. Endometriod carcinoma *(left).* Groups of columnar cells with granular eosinphilic cytoplasm and eccentric nuclei and prominent nucleoli and rare mitotic figure (ThinPrep, Papanicolaou stain)

19-22. Endometriod carcinoma *(right).* Groups of glandular columnar cells with granular eosinphilic cytoplasm and eccentric nuclei, coarse chromatin and prominent (ThinPrep, Papanicolaou stain)

Differential Diagnosis

■ Serous – mucinous cystadenoma
  ➤ Especially high-grade lesions are almost impossible to distinguish from one other

★ Cell block sections are helpful to see the similarity to endometrial glands

CLEAR CELL CARCINOMA

Clinical Features

■ Account for 5% of all surface epithelial cancers
■ Common in fifth to seventh decades
■ Rarely (2%) bilateral
■ Usually cystic

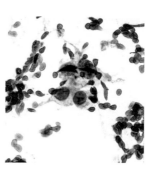

19-23. Clear cell carcinoma. Large cells with abundant, pale vacuolated cytoplasm, and prominent nucleoli. (Papanicolaou stain)

Cytologic Features

■ Tumor cells had abundant, pale, finely vacuolated cytoplasm with indistinct cytoplasmic membranes, round to oval eccentric nuclei with fine chromatin, prominent nucleoli
■ Basement membrane-like substance staining pink to purple-red in modified Giemsa stain preparations and frequently observed within the cancer cell clusters
■ Background with tumor diathesis

Special Stains and Immunohistochemistry

■ PAS with diastase confirms the presence of intracytoplasmic glycogen

Modern Techniques for Diagnosis

■ Noncontributory

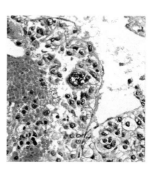

19-24. Clear cell carcinoma. Cell block section with large pleomorphic cells with indistinct cytoplasmic borders, abundant, vacuolated cytoplasm, and prominent nucleoli. (hematoxylin and eosin stain)

Differential Diagnosis

■ Metastatic clear cell carcinoma
  ➤ Clear cell carcinomas of the vagina, cervix, and endometrium as well other metastatic clear cell tumors including renal cell carcinoma are cytologically similar therefore clinical history is important as well as utilization of immunohistochemical markers (e.g. renal cell carcinoma marker is positive in renal cell carcinoma)

★ May be associated with ovarian or pelvic endometriosis

DYSGERMINOMA

Clinical Features

■ Most common primitive germ cell tumor
■ Account for 5% of all malignant ovarian tumors
■ Most common germ cell tumor
■ Highly radiosensitive

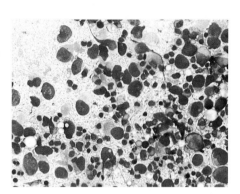 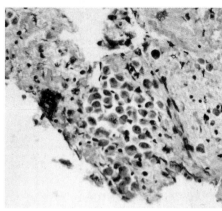

19-25. Dysgerminoma *(left)*. Large cell with high N:C ratio in a striped – "tigroid" background with small lymphocytes, plasma cells, and eosinophils (modified Giemsa stain)

19-26. Dysgerminoma *(right)*. Cell block section with single large pleomorphic cells with centrally located nucleolus. (hematoxylin and Eosin stain)

Cytologic Features
▦ Highly cellular aspirate
▦ Single tumor cells and loose syncytial clusters
▦ Large round central nucleus, high N:C ratio, centrally placed prominent nucleoli
▦ Striped background (especially on modified Giemsa stain), small mature lymphocytes, and rarely granulomas could also be seen

Special Stains and Immunohistochemistry
▦ PAS with or without diastase confirms the presence of glycogen in tumor cells
▦ Tumor cells are positive for placental alkaline phosphatase (PLAP) and vimentin

Modern Techniques for Diagnosis
▦ Very rarely alpha fetoprotein (AFP) and β human chorionic gonadotropin (β-hCG) elevated

Differential Diagnosis
▦ Lymphoma
  ➤ Lacks the striped background
  ➤ Lymphoglandular bodies are present

PEARLS

★ Single large cells in a characteristic "tigroid" background
★ Tigroid background could also be seen in other glycogen-rich neoplasms such as renal cell carcinoma, squamous cell carcinoma

OTHER GERM CELL TUMORS

For discussion of other germ cell tumors, please see the section "germ cell tumors of gonads."

GRANULOSA CELL TUMOR (ADULT AND JUVENILE TYPES)

Clinical Features
▦ Adult type granulosa tumor (95%) is much more common than the juvenile types (5%)
▦ Adult type typically occurs in the fifth decade; it is the most common ovarian neoplasm to secrete estrogen
▦ Most of the juvenile type occurs in the first three decades of life, if occurs before puberty could cause isosexual precocity

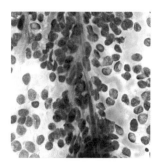 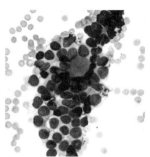 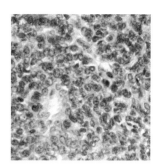

19-27. Granulosa cell tumor, adult type *(left).* Single cells and loosely cohesive clusters composed of small to medium sized monotonous cells with scant cytoplasm and occasional intranuclear grooves (modified Giemsa stain)

19-28. Granulosa cell tumor, adult type *(middle).* Microfollicular arrangement of granulosa cells arranged around a space containing eosinophilic fluid, "Call–Exner body" (modified Giemsa stain)

19-29. Granulosa cell tumor, adult type *(right).* Cell block section showing granulosa cells with scant cytoplasm, pale, uniform, oval, grooved nuclei (hematoxylin and eosin stain)

Cytologic Features

- **Adult type**
  - ➤ Hypercellular material with a clear background
  - ➤ Small to medium cells with scant cytoplasm, centrally placed round or oval monomorphic nuclei
  - ➤ Pale, finely dispersed chromatin with occasional nuclear grooves
  - ➤ Occasional microfollicular arrangement showing Call–Exner bodies
- **Juvenile type**
  - ➤ Loose clusters of cells with granular cytoplasm, round nuclei, fine chromatin, small to prominent nucleoli
  - ➤ No grooves, rare mitotic figures
  - ➤ Call–Exner bodies are usually not found

Special Stains and Immunohistochemistry

- Granulosa cells are positive for inhibin, vimentin, and S-100 protein

Modern Techniques for Diagnosis

- Cytogenetic studies reveal trisomy 12 for both adult and juvenile types

Differential Diagnosis

Differential diagnosis for adult type

- Follicular cysts
  - ➤ Coarse chromatin, nuclear degeneration
  - ➤ Lack of grooves
- Lymphoma
  - ➤ Dispersed single cells rather than clusters
- Carcinoid
  - ➤ Lacks nuclear grooves
  - ➤ Positive for neuroendocrine markers (chromogranin, synaptophysin, CD56)
- Brenner tumor
  - ➤ Diffuse positivity for cytokeratin
  - ➤ Clusters and sheets of uniform cells with conspicuous nucleoli and moderate amount of cytoplasm
  - ➤ Extracellular hyaline globules, usually surrounded by tumor cells

Differential Diagnosis for Juvenile Type

- Adenocarcinoma
  - ➤ Vimentin negative
  - ➤ Glandular appearance with more atypical nuclear changes
- Malignant germ cell tumors
  - ➤ Reactivity for AFP, placental alkaline phosphatase, and CEA (seen in yolk sac tumor and embryonal carcinoma)
  - ➤ See malignant germ cell tumor section

■ Large cell lymphoma
➤ Monomorphic population of single cells with scant amount of cytoplasm
➤ Lymphoglandular bodies
➤ Positivity for lymphoid markers
■ Melanoma
➤ Usually single cells with large amount of cytoplasm and prominent nucleoli
➤ Binucleation, multinucleation, intranuclear/cytoplasmic inclusions and melanin pigments
➤ HMB-45 and MART-1: Positive

PEARLS

★ Intranuclear grooves and Call–Exner bodies in the adult type of granulosa cell tumor
★ Adult granulosa cell tumor is associated with endometrial hyperplasia and carcinoma while the juvenile type is associated with Ollier's disease (enchondromatosis) and Mafucci Syndrome (enchondromatosis and hemangiomatosis)

FIBROMA/THECOMA

Clinical Features
■ Accounts for 4% of all ovarian tumors
■ Seen most commonly in the fourth to fifth decades

Cytologic Features
■ Hypocellular aspirate
■ Isolated spindled cells and loosely cohesive clusters with clear finely vacuolated cytoplasm, and granular chromatin

Special stains and Immunohistochemistry
■ Oil red-O confirms presence of lipid in tumor cells
■ Rare immunoreactivity for inhibin

Modern Techniques for Diagnosis
■ Noncontributory

Differential Diagnosis
■ Ovarian stromal hyperplasia
➤ Impossible to differentiate based on cytology alone

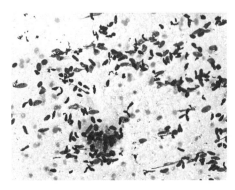
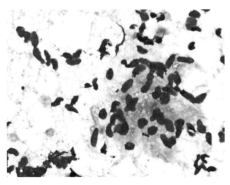

19-30. Fibroma/Thecoma *(left).* Spindled cell arranged singly and in loose clusters with clear finely vacuolated cytoplasm, and granular chromatin (modified Giemsa stain)

19-31. Fibroma/Thecoma *(right).* Spindled cell with indistinct cytoplasmic borders, clear finely vacuolated cytoplasm (modified Giemsa stain)

- Leiomyoma
  - ➤ Single spindle cells with uniform nuclei
  - ➤ SMA positive
- Metastatic endometrial stromal sarcoma
  - ➤ Hypercellular smear, spindle cell have higher N:C ratio, as well as nuclear hyperchromasia and mitotic figures

★ Rare monotonous spindled cells
★ Known associations are Meigs syndrome (ascitis and pleural effusion) and Gorlin syndrome (nevoid basal cell syndrome)

METASTATIC TUMORS

Clinical Features
- Most common tumors metastasizing to the ovaries are from the colon, stomach, breast, and GU tract
- Approximately 20% of all bilateral ovarian malignancies are metastatic

Cytologic Features
- Adenocarcinoma
  - ➤ Single cells, small clusters and sheets of cells with high N:C, ratio, hyperchromatic chromatin, prominent nucleoli. See specific chapters for further description
- Lymphoma
  - ➤ Mostly single cells with high N:C ratio and lymphoglandular bodies in the background

Special Stains and Immunohistochemistry
- Colon cancer; CK20 and CDX2 positive; CK7 negative
- Appendiceal carcinoma (mucinous variant): CK20, CDX2, and MUC2 positive, CK7 negative/positive
- Breast carcinoma: GCDFP and mammoglobin positive
- Lung carcinoma: TTF-1 positive
- Renal cell carcinoma: CD10 and renal cell carcinoma marker positive
- Urothelial carcinoma: CK8/18, p63 and CK5/6 positive, WT-1 negative

Modern Techniques for diagnosis
- Metastatic colon cancer has a high CEA level

Differential Diagnosis
- Primary ovarian carcinoma
  - ➤ Difficult to differentiate from metastatic carcinoma based on cytology only. Tumor markers could aid in the differential diagnosis

★ Most common tumors that metastasize to the ovaries are urogenital tract, colon, stomach, and breast
★ Metastatic signet ring cell carcinoma, most commonly from the stomach is known as Krukenberg tumor

TESTIS

Testicular FNAs performed for diagnosis of mass lesions are rather unusual and rare especially in the United States. Although there are reports of FNAs of various neoplastic and nonneoplastic lesions, majority of the literature of testicular FNAs are performed for infertility evaluation, and occasionally for scrotal masses. Still, one needs to be aware of the cytological features portrayed by different tumors to be able to evaluate the metastatic lesions

HYDROCELE

Clinical Features
■ Clear yellow fluid accumulation in tunica vaginalis
■ Transillumination of the testis demonstrates the presence of hydrocele

Cytologic Features
■ Hypocellular, rare macrophages, inflammatory cells, and benign/reactive mesothelial cells

Special Stains and Immunohistochemistry
■ Noncontributory

Modern Techniques for diagnosis
■ Noncontributory

Differential Diagnosis
■ Mesothelioma
  ➤ Malignant mesothelial cells are usually larger that their reactive counterparts with higher N:C ratio. Inflammation is usually not seen in the background. The tumor cells are positive for p53 and negative for desmin

PEARLS

★ Avoid interpreting reactive mesothelial cells as malignant

SPERMATOCELE

Clinical Features
■ Small cystic accumulation of semen in dilated efferent ducts or ducts of the rete testis

Cytologic Features
■ Spermatozoa, macrophages, and seminal vesicle cells in a proteinaceous background
■ Detached ciliary tufts may be seen

Special Stains and Immunohistochemistry
■ Noncontributory

Modern Techniques for Diagnosis
■ Noncontributory

Differential Diagnosis

- Seminoma
  - ➤ Seminal vesicle cells may be mistaken for seminoma cells (which do not have intracytoplasmic golden-brown pigment)
  - ➤ Spermatozoa and macrophages are not seen in seminoma

PEARLS

★ Seminal vesicle cells have a golden-brown pigment (on Papanicolaou stain), which helps in the differentiating them from neoplastic cells

HEMATOCELE

Clinical Features

- Accumulation of blood in tunica vaginalis
- Etiology: dircct trauma to testis, testicular torsion
- Red–brown fluid aspirated

Cytologic Features

- Intact or degenerated red blood cells and hemosiderin–laden macrophages

Special Stains and Immunohistochemistry

- Noncontributory

Modern Techniques for diagnosis

- Noncontributory

Differential Diagnosis

- Hematoma
  - ➤ Cannot be reliably distinguished from hematocele based on cytology alone

PEARLS

★ Glacial acetic acid could be used to distinguish peripheral blood elements from "old blood." When used as a fixative glacial acetic acid lyses intact erythrocytes but not degenerated erythrocytes

EPIDIDYMITIS AND ORCHITIS

Clinical Features

- Commonly related to urinary tract infections
- In younger men, the causative agent is generally *Chlamydia trachomatis* and Neisseria gonorrhea while in older men *Escherichia coli* and pseudomonas
- Granulomatous orchitis could be infectious (tuberculosis, mycotic infection), autoimmune, or due to sarcoidosis

Cytologic Features

- Acute and/or chronic inflammatory cells and fibroblasts could be seen
- Granulomas in case of granulomatous orchitis

Special Stains and Immunohistochemistry
■ AFB and GMS stains to identify the etiologic organisms

Modern Techniques for Diagnosis
■ PCR for identification of the organisms, especially for *Mycobacterium tuberculosis*

Differential Diagnosis
■ Leukemic involvement
➤ Lymphocytes are atypical and usually lack acute inflammatory cells
■ Abscess formation
➤ Suppurative inflammation

PEARLS

★ When faced with an aspirate of inflammatory cells obtain microbiologic culture
★ In some tumors (such as seminoma) granulomas could be seen; therefore a diligent search for tumor cells is warranted if granulomas are seen

ADENOMATOID TUMOR

Clinical Features
■ Most common tumor of the paratesticular tissue
■ Most common in third to fourth decade of life

Cytologic Features
■ Epithelioid sheets and multilayered clusters of bland, monotonous cells with round or ovoid, eccentric nuclei containing small, central nucleoli
■ Binucleation and intranuclear inclusions may be seen
■ Paranuclear clearing with a pink coloration (modified Giemsa stain) or a clear vacuole-like area (Papanicolaou stain) and abundant cellularity with a background of naked nuclei and stromal fragments

Special Stains and Immunohistochemistry
■ Tumor cells are strongly reactive for cytokeratin, EMA, and calretinin

Modern Techniques for Diagnosis
■ Noncontributory

Differential Diagnosis
■ Mesothelioma
➤ Malignant mesothelial cells are usually larger that their reactive counterparts with higher N:C ratio. Inflammation is usually not seen in the background. The tumor cells are p53 positive and desmin negative

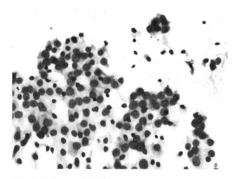

19-32. Adenomatoid tumor.
Sheet of bland, monotonous cells with round to ovoid, eccentric nuclei containing small, central nucleoli (modified Giemsa stain)

PEARLS

★ Adenomatoid tumor arising in other genitourinary system locations (bladder, prostate, uterus, fallopian tube, and ovary) have the same cytomorphological features

LYMPHOMA

Clinical Features
▓ Most common after the fifth decade
▓ Leukemic involvement of the testis is rare in the older age group but could been seen in children and adolescents

Cytologic Features
▓ Single atypical lymphoid cells with high N:C ratio and lymphoglandular bodies in the background

Special stains and Immunohistochemistry
▓ Lymphoid markers on immunohistochemistry

Modern Techniques for diagnosis
▓ Flow cytometry analysis
▓ Gene rearrangement studies

> **Differential Diagnosis**
> ▪ Seminoma
> ➤ Background with small lymphocytes, plasma cells and rare granulomas in addition to tigroid striping
> ➤ N:C ratio lower in seminoma compared to lymphoma
> ➤ PLAP and c-kit positive, negative for lymphoma markers

PEARLS

✶ Collection of material in RPMI or another media amenable for flow cytometry analysis

LEYDIG CELL TUMOR

Clinical Features
▓ Most common testicular stromal tumor
▓ Occurs in all age groups
▓ Patients present with gynecomastia and testicular swelling
▓ Children may present with isosexual precocity
▓ Tumors may produce testosterone and estrogen

Cytologic Features
▓ Large, monomorphic cells found singly or in loosely cohesive clusters
▓ Round nuclei with smooth nuclear borders, fine chromatin
▓ Reinke's crystalloids (rentangular, long crystals) can be seen in intra- or extracytoplasmic locations
▓ Background composed of granular material reminiscent of seminoma

Special stains and Immunohistochemistry
▓ Vimentin and inhibin: Positive
▓ PLAP and EMA: Negative

Modern Techniques for diagnosis
▓ Noncontributory

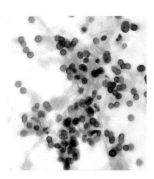

19-33. Sertoli/leydine cell tumor. Large, monomorphic cells with round nuclei, smooth nuclear borders, fine chromatin, and prominent nucleoli. One cell intracytoplasmic with rectangular crystal (Reinke's cystalloid) (Papanicolaou stain)

Differential Diagnosis

■ Seminoma/Dysgerminoma
  ➤ Tigroid background, cells are mostly found singly
  ➤ PLAP and c-kit are: Positive

PEARLS

★ Electron microscopy: Reinke's crystals
★ 10–15% associated with cryptorchidism

SERTOLI CELL TUMOR

Clinical Features
■ Rare
■ Rarely in children under ten years old

Cytologic Features
■ Glandular cells with oval nuclei, irregular chromatin, and prominent nucleoli
■ Large calcifying sertoli cell tumor has large polygonal tumor cells with abundant granular/vacuolated cytoplasm, and prominent nucleoli
■ Malignant Sertoli–Leydig cell tumors could have heterologous differentiation

Special Stains and Immunohistochemistry
■ Oil red-o highlights the lipid content of the tumor cells
■ Vimentin and keratin: Positive
■ Inhibin: Positive/negative

Modern Techniques for Diagnosis
■ Noncontributory

Differential Diagnosis

■ Metastatic renal cell carcinoma
  ➤ Transgressing vessels among the tumor cells
  ➤ CD10 and renal cell carcinoma marker positive

PEARLS

★ Associated with androgen insensitivity and Peutz-Jegher syndrome
★ Large cell calcifying variant of Sertoli cell tumor is associated with Carney syndrome

SEMINOMA

Clinical Features
■ Most common germ cell tumor of the testis
■ Highly radiosensitive
■ Painless enlargement of the testis
■ Mostly presents at an earlier clinical stage, confined to the testis

Cytologic Features
■ Highly cellular aspirates composed of mostly single cells and occasional syntitial clusters of tumor cells with clear/granular cytoplasm, centrally placed nucleus and prominent nucleoli
■ The background has small lymphocytes, plasma cells, and may also have granulomas

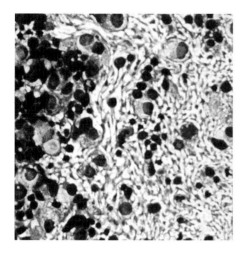
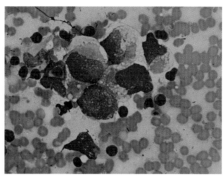

19-34. Seminoma *(left)*. Single cells and rare clusters of tumor cells with clear/granular cytoplasm centrally placed nucleus and prominent nucleoli in a "tigroid" background (modified Giemsa stain)

19-35. Seminoma *(right)*. Cells granular vacuolated cytoplasm, cytoplasm centrally placed nucleus, and in a background of lymphocytes and plasma cells (modified Giemsa stain)

▪ "Tigroid" background – stripes due to smearing artifact of the highly glycogen laden cells, seen especially in modified Giemsa stain smears
▪ Necrosis, hemorrhage, and mitotic figures may be seen

Special Stains and Immunohistochemistry
▪ CD117 and PLAP: Positive
▪ CD30 and pancytokeratin: Focally positive

Modern Techniques for diagnosis
▪ Noncontributory

Differential Diagnosis
▪ Other neoplasms with tigroid background
➤ Ewings/PNET, renal cell carcinoma, squamous cell carcinoma are also high in glycogen, therefore producing a tigroid background. However, the clinical scenarios, cytomorphological and immunohistochemical profiles are different
▪ Embryonal carcinoma
➤ Cohesive highly pleomorphic cells with coarse chromatin and prominent nucleoli
➤ No tigroid background
➤ Cytokeratin and CD30: Positive
➤ C-kit: Negative
▪ Poorly differentiated adenocarcinoma
➤ Acinar formation and nuclear polarity
➤ Cytokeratin: Positive
➤ Mucin: May be positive
▪ Lymphoma
➤ Mostly single cells
➤ No tigroid background
➤ Positive for lymphoma markers, and flow cytometry analysis demonstrates lymphoid nature of the neoplasm
▪ Melanoma
➤ Binucleation, multinucleation, intranuclear inclusions, and intracytoplasmic melanin pigment
➤ Mart-1, HMB-45, and S-100: Positive

PEARLS

★ Increased incidence in infertile patients

SPERMATOCYTIC SEMINOMA

Clinical Features
- One of the most common testicular tumor in elderly men
- Most common in the fifth decade and later

Cytologic Features
- Three populations of cells: Small, medium, and large, with a preponderance of medium-sized cells showing visible nucleoli
- Lacks characteristic background features of seminoma (lymphocytes, eosinophils, granulomas, and tigroid striping)

Special Stains and Immunohistochemistry
- AFP, hCG, CEA, LCA, and CD30: Negative
- Unlike classical seminoma tumor cells are negative for PLAP

Modern Techniques for diagnosis
- Noncontributory

Differential Diagnosis
- Seminoma
  - Tigroid background, as well as the presence of lymphocytes, eosinophils, granulomas
  - PAS with or without diastase shows the presence of glycogen
  - PLAP positive
- Lymphoma
  - Uniform population of lymphoid cells with scant cytoplasm
  - Presence of lymphoglandular bodies
  - Lymphoid markers are positive

PEARLS
- ★ Spermatocytic seminoma is not associated with cryptoorchism or intratubular germ cell neoplasia, unlike classical seminoma
- ★ Never associated with other germ cell tumors

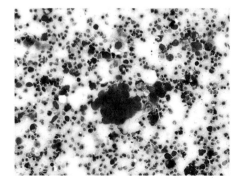

19-36. Embryonal carcinoma. Single cells and cohesive clusters of epithelioid cells with granular/vacuolated cytoplasm, indistinct cell borders, large nuclei with coarse chromatin, irregular nucleoli (modified Giemsa stain)

EMBRYONAL CARCINOMA

Clinical Features
- Testis
  - Embryonal carcinoma is a component of nearly all nonseminomatous germ cell tumors
  - Most common in the second to third decade
  - Presents with testicular swelling associated with pain
- Ovary
  - Rare, 3% of malignant ovarian germ cell neoplasms
  - Usually found as a component of mixed germ cell tumor
  - Most patients are prepubertal, median age twelve years

Cytologic Features
- Cellular smears
- Cohesive clusters of epithelioid cells with granular/vacuolated cytoplasm, indistinct cell borders

- Large nuclei with coarse chromatin, irregular nucleoli
- Numerous mitotic figures and necrosis can be seen

Special Stains and Immunohistochemistry
- PLAP, pancytokeratin, and CD30: Positive
- AFP and hCG: Focally positive
- CEA, EMA, and C-KIT: Negative

Modern Techniques for diagnosis
- Isochromosome 12p

Differential Diagnosis
- Seminoma/Dysgerminoma
  - ➤ Mostly discohesive cells, in a classical tigroid background
  - ➤ Usually the background of the smear contains small mature lynphocytes
  - ➤ Cells are smaller than of embyonal carcinoma
- Poorly differentiated carcinoma
  - ➤ Poorly differentiate large carcinoma and adenocarcinoma can mimic embryonal carcinoma

---

PEARLS

⋏ Elevated serum levels of hCG (in 60% of the patients) and AFP, as the disease advances serum levels of LDH as well as PLAP also increases

YOLK SAC TUMOR

Clinical Features
- Testis
  - ➤ Most common testicular tumor in children
  - ➤ In prepubertal children it is in pure form whereas in postpubertal patients the tumor is in mixed form
- Ovary
  - ➤ Occurs in second to third decade
  - ➤ Fast growing tumor with sudden onset of abdominal pain caused by tumor rupture
  - ➤ Extraovarian spread common at time of diagnosis

Cytologic Features
- Large, irregular cohesive groups forming three-dimensional structures and papillae
- Large cells with abundant vacuolated cytoplasm with irregular nucleoli, coarse chromatin, and prominent nucleoli
- Schiller–Duval bodies: Glomeruloid structures formed by invagination of tumor cells into an empty space
- Hyalin globules large round PAS-positive, AFP-containing, intracytoplasmic inclusions
- Abnormal mitotic figure can be seen
- Lymphocytes, plasma cells, macrophages, as well as mucinous material could be seen in the background

Special stains and Immunohistochemistry
- PAS with diastase highlights hyaline bodies
- AFP and cytokeratin: Positive

- PLAP: Focally positive
- EMA and CD30: Negative

Modern Techniques for diagnosis
- Frequent abnormalities in chromosomes 1p, 6q, and 3q

Differential Diagnosis
- Embryonal carcinoma
  - Less cohesive, lacks papillary clusters
  - More prominent nucleoli
  - CD30: Positive

PEARLS

- Elevated serum AFP levels

CHORIOCARCINOMA

Clinical Features
- Testis
  - Most common in the second and third decade
  - Very rare in pure form
- Ovary
  - Very rare in pure form
  - Typically occurs in children and young adults
  - Clinical presentation mimics an ectopic pregnancy due to elevated hCG levels

Cytologic Features
- Biphasic cyto and syncytiotrophoblasts
- Syncytiotrophoblasts are large, pleomorphic, multinucleated bizarre cells, with hyperchromatic nuclei, prominent nucleoli and abundant eosinophilic cytoplasms
- Cytotrophoblasts are loose clusters and single small cells, with indistinct cell borders, pale vacuolated cytoplasm pleomorphic vesicular nucleoli and inconspicuous nucleoli
- Spindled cells could also be seen

Special Stains and Immunohistochemistry
- Syncytiotrophoblasts are hCG positive but cytotrophoblasts are mostly negative
- Syncytiotrophoblasts are positive for inhibin and EMA
- Both syncytiotrophoblasts and cytotrophoblasts are positive for cytokeratin and CEA
- PLAP is positive in 50% of all tumors

Modern Techniques for diagnosis
- Noncontributory

Differential Diagnosis
- Mixed germ cell tumors/other germ cell tumors with syncytiotrophoblastic cells (seminoma and embryonal carcinoma)
  - Lack cytotrophoblastic cells
- Seminoma
  - Classical background features; tigroid striping, lymphocytes, plasma cells, eosinophils

➤ C-kit: Positive
➤ It may contain scattered syncytiotrophoblastic cells
■ Embryonal carcinoma
➤ CD30: Positive
■ Poorly differentiated carcinoma
➤ Do not have a biphasic pattern
➤ Do not have elevated β-hCG levels

★ Elevated serum β-hCG levels. Due to the biochemical similarity of hCG and TSH occasionally patients could present with symptoms of thyrotoxicosis

TERATOMA

Clinical Features
■ Testis
➤ Second most common germ cell tumor of infancy
➤ May be seen in postpubertal age group
■ Ovary
➤ Most common ovarian neoplasm
➤ Usually occur in the reproductive years
➤ Most cases present with a pelvic mass with or without pain, one forth of the cases are asymptomatic
➤ This lesion is rarely aspirated since it is radiologically diagnostic due to the presence of heterologous elements

Cytologic Features
■ Mature squamous cells admixed with vacuolated cells of presumed sebaceous origin
■ Ciliated cells, detached ciliary tufts and mucinous cells could be seen

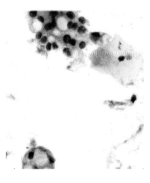

19-37. Mature cystic teratoma.
Mature squamous cells admixed with vacuolated cells of sebaceous origin (Papanicolaou stain)

Special stains and Immunohistochemistry
■ Noncontributory

Modern Techniques for Diagnosis
■ Noncontributory

Differential Diagnosis
■ Immature teratoma
➤ Presence of immature or malignant components: neural cells (i.e., neuroblasts), epithelial/mesenchymal malignancies (e.g., squamous cell carcinoma, osteosarcoma)

★ Rarely MCT could undergo malignant transformation to squamous cell carcinoma
★ If benign follicular cells are seen a variant of MCT, struma ovarii, should be suspected
★ Immature elements should be reported
★ Pure teratomas of the testis (with or without immature elements) in postpubertal patients have a high incidence of metastasis unlike pure teratomas of the ovary which can only metastasize if immature elements are present

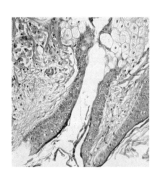

19-38. Mature cystic teratoma.
Oophorectomy section revealing mature squamous lining and underlying squamous epithelium (hematoxylin and eosin stain)

REFERENCES

FOLLICULAR CYST

Ganjei P. Fine-needle aspiration cytology of the ovary. *Clin Lab Med* 1995;15:705–26.

Mulvany NJ, Ostor A, Teng G. Evaluation of estradiol in aspirated ovarian cystic lesions. *Acta Cytol* 1995 Jul–Aug;39(4):663–8.

Mulvany NJ. Aspiration cytology of ovarian cysts and cystic neoplasms. A study of 235 aspirates. *Acta Cytol* 1996;4:911–20.

Pinto MM, Bernstein LH, et al. Measurement of CA125, CEA and AFP in ovarian cyst fluid: a diagnostic adjunct to cytology. *Diag Cytopathol* 1990;6:160–3.

Ramzy I, Delaney M., Rose P. Fine-needle aspiration of ovarian masses II correlative cytologic and histologic study of nonneoplastic cysts and noncelomic epithelial neoplasms. *Acta Cytol* 1979;23:185–93.

Selvaggi S. Cytology of nonneoplastic cysts of the ovary. *Diag Cytopathol* 1990;6:77–85.

Wojcik EM, Selvaggi S. Fine-needle aspiration of the cystic ovarian lesions. *Diag Cytopathol* 1994;11:9–14.

CORPUS LUTEUM CYST

Ganjei P. Fine-needle aspiration cytology of the ovary. *Clin Lab Med* 1995;15:705–26.

Ramzy I, Delaney M., Rose P. Fine-needle aspiration of ovarian masses II correlative cytologic and histologic study of celomic epithelial neoplasms. *Acta Cytol* 1979;23:185–93.

Selvaggi S. Cytology of nonneoplastic cysts of the ovary. *Diag Cytopathol* 1990;6:77–85.

Wojcik EM, Selvaggi S. Fine-needle aspiration of the cystic ovarian lesions. *Diag Cytopathol* 1994;11:9–14.

ENDOMETRIOTIC CYST

Ganjei P. Fine-needle aspiration cytology of the ovary. *Clin Lab Med* 1995;15:705–26.

Ramzy I, Delaney M., Rose P. Fine-needle aspiration of ovarian masses II correlative cytologic and histologic study of nonneoplastic cysts and noncelomic epithelial neoplasms. *Acta Cytol* 1979;23:185–93.

Selvaggi S. Cytology of nonneoplastic cysts of the ovary. *Diag Cytopathol* 1990;6:77–85.

Wojcik EM, Selvaggi S. Fine–needle aspiration of the cystic ovarian lesions. *Diag Cytopathol* 1994;11:9–14.

SEROUS CYSTADENOMA AND CARCINOMA

Athanassiadou P, Grapsa D. Fine needle aspiration of borderline ovarian lesions. Is It useful? *Acta Cytol* 2005;49:278–85.

Ganjei P. Fine-Needle aspiration cytology of the ovary. *Clin Lab Med* 1995;15:705–26.

Selvaggi S. Cytology of nonneoplastic cysts of the ovary. *Diag Cytopathol* 1990;6:77–85.

Wojcik EM, Selvaggi S. Fine-needle aspiration of the cystic ovarian lesions. *Diag Cytopathol* 1994;11:9–14.

MUCINOUS CYSTADENOMA AND CARCINOMA

Ganjei P. Fine-needle aspiration cytology of the ovary. *Clin Lab Med* 1995;15:705–26.

Ramzy I, Delaney M. Fine-needle aspiration of ovarian masses I correlative cytologic and histologic study of celomic epithelial neoplasms. *Acta Cytol* 1979;23:97–104.

Vang R, Gown AM, Farinola M, Barry TS, Wheeler DT, Yemelyanova A, Seidman JD, Judson K, Ronnett BM. p16 expression in primary ovarian mucinous and endometrioid tumors and metastatic adenocarcinomas in the ovary: utility for identification of metastatic HPV-related endocervical adenocarcinomas. *Am J Surg Pathol* 2007;31:653–63.

Wojcik EM, Selvaggi S. Fine–needle aspiration of the cystic ovarian lesions. *Diag Cytopathol* 1994;11:9–14.

BRENNER TUMOR

Ganjei P. Fine-needle aspiration cytology of the ovary. *Clin Lab Med* 1995;15:705–26.

Wojcik EM, Selvaggi S. Fine-needle aspiration of the cystic ovarian lesions. *Diag Cytopathol* 1994;11:9–14.

ENDOMETRIOID CARCINOMA

Ganjei P. Fine-needle aspiration cytology of the ovary. *Clin Lab Med* 1995;15:705–26.

Ramzy I, Delaney M. Fine-needle aspiration of ovarian masses I correlative cytologic and histologic study of celomic epithelial neoplasms. *Acta Cytol* 1979;23:97–104.

Wojcik EM, Selvaggi S. Fine–needle aspiration of the cystic ovarian lesions. *Diag Cytopathol* 1994;11:9–14.

CLEAR CELL CARCINOMA
Atahan S, Ekinci C, Içli F, Erdoğan N. Cytology of clear cell carcinoma of the female genital tract in fine needle aspirates and ascites. *Acta Cytol* 2000;44:1005–9.
Ganjei P. Fine-needle aspiration cytology of the ovary. *Clin Lab Med* 1995;15:705–26.

DYSGERMINOMA
Ganjei P. Fine-needle aspiration cytology of the ovary. *Clin Lab Med* 1995;15:705–26.
Ramzy I, Delaney M., Rose P. Fine-needle aspiration of ovarian masses II correlative cytologic and histologic study of nonneoplastic cysts and noncelomic epithelial neoplasms. *Acta Cytol* 1979;23:185–93.

GRANULOSA CELL TUMOR
Ganjei P, Nadji M. Aspiration cytology of ovarian neoplasms. A review. *Acta Cytol* 1984;28:329–32.
Ganjei P. Fine-needle aspiration cytology of the ovary. *Clin Lab Med* 1995;15:705–26.
Ramzy I, Delaney M, Rose P. Fine-needle aspiration of ovarian masses II correlative cytologic and histologic study of nonneoplastic cysts and noncelomic epithelial neoplasms. *Acta Cytol* 1979;23:185–93.

FIBROMA / THECOMA
Ganjei P, Nadji M. Aspiration cytology of ovarian neoplasms. A review. *Acta Cytol* 1984;28:329–32.

METASTATIC TUMORS
Ganjei P. Fine-Needle aspiration cytology of the ovary. *Clin Lab Med* 1995;15:705–26.
Ramzy I, Delaney M, Rose P. Fine-needle aspiration of ovarian masses II correlative cytologic and histologic study of nonneoplastic cysts and noncelomic epithelial neoplasms. *Acta Cytol* 1979;23:185–93.

HYDROCELE
Pérez-Guillermo M, Sola Pérez J. Aspiration cytology of palpable lesions of the scrotal content. *Diagn Cytopathol* 1990;6:169–77.

SPERMATOCELE
Pérez-Guillermo M, Sola Pérez J. Aspiration cytology of palpable lesions of the scrotal content. *Diagn Cytopathol.* 1990,0.109–77.

HEMATOCELE
Pérez-Guillermo M, Sola Pérez J. Aspiration cytology of palpable lesions of the scrotal content. *Diagn Cytopathol.* 1990;6:169–77.

EPIDIDYMITIS AND ORCHITIS
Pérez-Guillermo M, Sola Pérez J. Aspiration cytology of palpable lesions of the scrotal content. *Diagn Cytopathol* 1990;6:169–77.

ADENOMATOID TUMOR
Braini G, et al. Adenomatoid tumor of the epididymis: cytologic diagnosis by fine-needle aspiration. *Pathologica* 1992;84:377–82.
Pérez-Guillermo M, Thor A, Löwhagen T. Paratesticular adenomatoid tumors. The cytologic presentation in fine needle aspiration biopsies. *Acta Cytol* 1989;33:6–10.
Pérez-Guillermo M, Sola Pérez J. Aspiration cytology of palpable lesions of the scrotal content. *Diagn Cytopathol* 1990;6:169–77.

LYMPHOMA
Suh YK, Shin H: Fine-needle aspiration biopsy of granulocytic sarcoma: a clinicopathologic study of 27 cases. *Cancer* 2000;90:364–72.

LEYDIG CELL TUMOR
Jain M, Aiyer HM, Bajaj P, Dhar S. Intracytoplasmic and intranuclear Reinke's crystals in a testicular Leydig-cell tumor diagnosed by fine-needle aspiration cytology: a case report with review of the literature. *Diagn Cytopathol.* 2001;25:162–4.

Pérez-Guillermo M, Sola Pérez J. Aspiration cytology of palpable lesions of the scrotal content. *Diagn Cytopathol.* 1990;6:169–77.

SERTOLI CELL TUMOR

Pettinato G, Insabato L, De Chiara A, Latella R. Fine needle aspiration cytology of a large cell calcifying Sertoli cell tumor of the testis. *Acta Cytol* 1987;31:578–82.

Watson B, Siegel CL, Ylagan LR. Metastatic ovarian Sertoli-cell tumor: FNA findings with immunohistochemistry. *Diagn Cytopathol.* 2003;29:283–6.

SEMINOMA

Balslev E, Francis D, Jacobsen GK. Testicular germ cell tumors. Classification based on fine needle aspiration biopsy. *Acta Cytol* 1990;34:690–4.

García-Solano J, Sánchez-Sánchez C, Montalbán-Romero S, Sola-Pérez J, Pérez-Guillermo M. Fine needle aspiration (FNA) of testicular germ cell tumours; a 10-year experience in a community hospital. *Cytopathology* 1998;9:248–62.

Pérez-Guillermo M, Sola Pérez J. Aspiration cytology of palpable lesions of the scrotal content. *Diagn Cytopathol* 1990;6:169–77.

SPERMATOCYTIC SEMINOMA

Pérez-Guillermo M, Sola Pérez J. Aspiration cytology of palpable lesions of the scrotal content. *Diagn Cytopathol* 1990;6:169–77.

EMBRYONAL CARCINOMA

Balslev E, Francis D, Jacobsen GK. Testicular germ cell tumors. Classification based on fine needle aspiration biopsy. *Acta Cytol* 1990;34:690–4.

García-Solano J, Sánchez-Sánchez C, Montalbán-Romero S, Sola-Pérez J, Pérez-Guillermo M. Fine needle aspiration (FNA) of testicular germ cell tumours; a 10-year experience in a community hospital. *Cytopathology.* 1998;9:248–62.

YOLK SAC TUMOR

Balslev E, Francis D, Jacobsen GK. Testicular germ cell tumors. Classification based on fine needle aspiration biopsy. *Acta Cytol.* 1990;34:690–4.

García-Solano J, Sánchez-Sánchez C, Montalbán-Romero S, Sola-Pérez J, Pérez-Guillermo M. Fine needle aspiration (FNA) of testicular germ cell tumours; a 10-year experience in a community hospital. *Cytopathology* 1998;9:248–62.

Pérez-Guillermo M, Sola Pérez J. Aspiration cytology of palpable lesions of the scrotal content. *Diagn Cytopathol* 1990;6:169–77.

CHORIOCARCINOMA

Balslev E, Francis D, Jacobsen GK. Testicular germ cell tumors. Classification based on fine needle aspiration biopsy. *Acta Cytol.* 1990;34:690–4.

García-Solano J, Sánchez-Sánchez C, Montalbán-Romero S, Sola-Pérez J, Pérez-Guillermo M. Fine needle aspiration (FNA) of testicular germ cell tumours; a 10-year experience in a community hospital. *Cytopathology.* 1998;9:248–62.

Pérez-Guillermo M, Sola Pérez J. Aspiration cytology of palpable lesions of the scrotal content. *Diagn Cytopathol* 1990;6:169–77.

TERATOMA

Ganjei P. Fine-Needle aspiration cytology of the ovary. *Clin Lab Med* 1995;15:705–726.

Pérez-Guillermo M, Sola Pérez J. Aspiration cytology of palpable lesions of the scrotal content. *Diagn Cytopathol* 1990;6:169–77.

20

Cytopathology of the Central Nervous System

Anil V. Parwani and Syed Z. Ali

Central neurocytoma

Pineocytoma

Pineoblastoma

Medulloblastoma

Primitive neuroectodermal tumor (PNET)

Metastatic neoplasms

INTRODUCTION

Cytopathological evaluation of central nervous system (CNS) lesions not only requires a good understanding of the general concepts of cytopathology, but also needs an adequate knowledge of various neurological diseases and neuroanatomy. The cytopathologist must be able to correlate the clinical and radiological information and have a good understanding of clinicopathologic entities and their anatomical locations in the CNS.

Stereotactically guided needle aspiration with intraoperative CT monitoring is a particularly valuable technique in the diagnosis of intracranial lesions that are not amenable to resection. This minimally invasive diagnostic modality ensures an accurate sampling of intracerebral lesions with the least risk of damage to the native brain tissue. Finally, touch preparations and smears during intraoperative evaluation of CNS lesions need an enhanced understanding of the cytomorphology of these various lesions.

In this chapter, we will review the cytopathology of the commonly encountered nonneoplastic and neoplastic diseases of the brain. We will review benign and reactive conditions of the CNS, which may be seen in CT-guided needle biopsies. In the nonneoplastic category, emphasis will be placed on HIV-related infections as well as certain pseudotumoral space-occupying lesions. In the neoplastic category, cytomorphology of primary and metastatic brain tumors will be presented according to the cell of origin as well as a discussion of the differential diagnosis based on the predominant phenotype.

The role of ancillary studies such as immunoperoxidase staining and molecular studies will be highlighted. Wherever applicable, corresponding radiological studies and tissue correlation with surgical biopsy will also be presented.

STEREOTACTIC NEEDLE BIOPSY TECHNIQUE

Three-dimensional coordinates of the lesion are determined by preoperative CT scanning, and the needle is directed to the target via computer-assisted guidance through a tiny burr-hole. Several samples are commonly needed to establish the diagnosis. Specimens consist of varying sized tissue fragments or fluid in cases of cystic lesions. On-site evaluation is performed by the cytopathologist with assistance of a cytopreparatory technician. In each sample, a small tissue fragment is picked up and spread on two slides by the crush or squash technique. One of the slides is fixed in 95% ethyl alcohol for Papanicolaou or H&E staining; the other is air dried and stained with modified Giemsa stain for immediate evaluation. The larger tissue fragments from the remaining specimen are fixed in 10% NB formalin. Immediate microscopic evaluation of the modified Giemsa–stained material at the time of aspiration serves several useful purposes:

▪ Assurance of adequate diagnostic material
▪ Proper handling of specimens if special studies (e.g., flow cytometry, electron microscopy) are needed

IMPORTANT CONSIDERATIONS

When assessing the cytomorphology of CNS lesions, the following questions must be considered:

(1)   Is this *smear abnormal?*
Beware of the normal cellular constituents of the brain tissue. A thick smear may look falsely hypercellular. Watch for neuronal cells, such as large pyramidal cells (cortical or deeper gray matter sampling), choroid plexus fragments (ventricular sampling) and macrophages.

(2)   Is this tissue *neoplastic?*
Reactive astrocytes, macrophage-rich lesions, and lymphomononuclear infiltrates may make a benign smear look abnormally hypercellular and atypical. Necrosis (radiation induced, infection related) may also on occasion lead to a false-positive diagnosis.

(3)   What *type of tumor* is this?
In the brain, one would, in most cases, be dealing with a malignant neoplasm, most often of astrocytic origin. Close attention to cytomorphology, with help from ancillary techniques such as IPOX and ultrastructural studies (in undifferentiated or difficult to classify tumors) and past medical history (in metastatic neoplasms), can be extremely helpful.

(4)   What is the *cytohistologic grade* of the tumor?
This is often the most difficult question to answer with the limited sampling of a stereotactic biopsy. The question usually comes up when evaluating astrocytic tumors. A Ki-67 (MIB-1) immunostaining along with close attention to the cytomorphologic features is extremely helpful. Less often encountered but more difficult to grade are other neoplasms such as tumors of neuronal origin (e.g., pineocytoma vs. pineoblastoma, etc.).

PROGRESSIVE MULTIFOCAL LEUKOENCEPHALOPATHY (PML)

Clinical Features
▨ A fatal progressive demyelinating disease of the brain caused by infection of the oligodendrocytes by papova/polyoma virus (JC virus) infection
▨ Usually reactivation of a latent infection acquired during childhood
▨ Usually seen in AIDS patients and other severely immunocompromised patients
▨ Although multifocal, it may present as a solitary lesion simulating a brain neoplasm, in particular malignant glioma
▨ Cytopathic effect in oligodendrocytes leads to demyelination

Cytologic Features
▨ Hypercellularity
▨ Abundant macrophages
▨ Occasional atypical reactive astrocytes, hyperchromatic and pleomorphic
▨ Scattered atypical cells (oligodendroglial) with enlarged, darkly stained nuclei
▨ Effaced, smudgy and glassy chromatin – "virally infected cells"
▨ Occasionally, intranuclear eosinophilic inclusions
▨ Lymphocytic infiltration can also be seen

Special Stains and Immunohistochemistry
▨ Positive immunostaining with SV-40 (antibody against Polyoma virus)

Modern Techniques for Diagnosis
▨ In situ hybridization can also be performed
▨ Indirect immunofluorescence

20-1. Progressive multifocal leukoencephalopathy (PML) *(top, left).* The smear is hypercellular, with numerous macrophages with round to oval nuclei in a fibrillary background. Hypercellularity is also caused by reactive glial cells, lymphocytes and virally infected oligodendroglial cells (Papanicolaou stain)

20-2. Progressive multifocal leukoencephalopathy (PML) *(top, right).* The smear shows hypercellularity with pleomorphic cells, many macrophages, and other chronic inflammatory cells. This picture may resemble malignant glioma. The distinctively large cells with smudgy nuclei are infected oligodendrocytes (Papanicolaou stain)

20-3. Progressive multifocal leukoencephalopathy (PML) *(bottom, left).* Hypercellular smear with numerous inflammatory cells, histiocytes, and pleomorphic smudgy nuclei, some of which are infected by Polyoma virus. Two such cells are evident in the center of the field with hyperchromatic nuclei and effaced chromatin (Papanicolaou stain)

20-4. Progressive multifocal leukoencephalopathy (PML) *(bottom, right).* Immunostaining of the infected cells with antibody against the SV-40 antigen (IPOX)

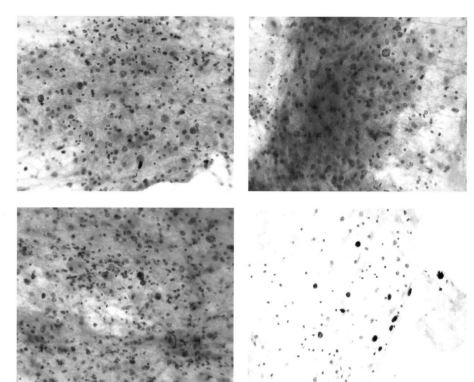

Differential Diagnosis

- Glioma
- Demyelinating diseases
- Cerebral Infarct
- Oligodendroglioma

PEARLS

- ★ Presence of macrophages is important in leading to an accurate diagnosis
- ★ Eosinophilic or basophilic intranuclear inclusions are seen in atypical oligodendrocytes
- ★ Destruction of axons, atypical for demyelinating diseases, is also seen in PML
- ★ A negative result with JC virus PCR does not rule out PML

SUBACUTE SCLEROSING PANENCEPHALITIS

Clinical Features

- Chronic persistent infection of the central nervous system
- Causative agent is an altered form of the measles virus
- Typically presents in the first two decades of life
- Behavioral changes including irritability, memory loss
- Neurological deterioration
- Often with a prior history of measles infection
- Both gray and white matters are usually involved

Cytologic Features

- Variable number of macrophages
- Intranuclear inclusions may be identifiable
- Inflammation and necrosis

Special Stains and Immunohistochemistry
▦ Marked elevation of measles IgG antibodies in CSF

Modern Techniques for Diagnosis
▦ Measurement of specific antibodies by enzyme-linked immunosorbent assay

Differential Diagnosis
▪ Viral encephalitis

PEARLS

★ Key to diagnosis is the clinical history, typical electroencephalographic (EEG) findings (periodic complexes with high-voltage diphasic waves occurring synchronously throughout the recording), and elevated serum and CSF antimeasles antibody titers
★ Inclusion bodies in oligodendroglia, neurons, and astrocytes may be seen

HERPESVIRUS

Clinical Features
▦ Most frequent cause of viral encephalitis in nonimmunocompromised patients, also seen in AIDS patients, often fatal
▦ Olfactory hallucinations, personality changes
▦ Temporal lobe disease
▦ Rarely aspirated
▦ Caused by types 1 and 2 herpes simplex virus

Cytologic Features
▦ Characteristic intranuclear inclusions and ground-glass nuclei may be seen
▦ Multinucleated cells
▦ Bloody CSF

Special Stains and Immunohistochemistry
▦ Positive staining with anti-HSV antibodies

Modern Techniques for Diagnosis
▦ Multiplex PCR assay for HSV

Differential Diagnosis
▪ Cytomegalovirus (has both intranuclear and cytoplasmic inclusions)
▪ Toxoplasmosis
▪ Other viral infections

PEARLS

★ Herpes virus often shows multinucleation with molding of nuclei

CYTOMEGALOVIRUS (CMV)

Clinical Features
▦ Most common opportunistic infection of the brain in AIDS
▦ Form gray matter microglial nodules (rarely mass lesions)
▦ Rarely aspirated (mostly incidentally noticed)

Cytologic Features
▦ Characteristic large cells and intranuclear and intracytoplasmic inclusions
▦ Predilection for ependymal and subependymal zones

Special Stains and Immunohistochemistry
▦ Positive staining with anti-HSV antibodies

Modern Techniques for Diagnosis
▦ Multiplex PCR assay for CMV
▦ DNA microarray

Differential Diagnosis
■ Herpes virus
■ Toxoplasmosis
■ Viral syndrome
■ Brain abscess

PEARLS

★ Ependymal and subependymal areas are the most involved zones

MOLLARET MENINGITIS

Clinical Features
▦ A rare form of meningitis, which is self-limiting, aseptic, and mild
▦ Recurrent episodes of headache and fever, separated by symptom-free episodes
▦ Photophobia
▦ Associated with herpes simplex type 2 viruses
▦ Recently Mollaret-like cells have been detected in patients with West Nile virus infections

Cytologic Features
▦ Marked monocytosis
▦ Characteristic Mollaret cells with a bean shape and bilobed nuclei
▦ Mollaret cells are activated monocytes
▦ Mollaret cells have enlarged nuclei and cerebriform nuclear contours
▦ Degenerated monocytes can give an appearance of "ghost cells"
▦ Background cells are mostly small lymphocytes

Special Stains and Immunohistochemistry
▦ Noncontributory

Modern Techniques for Diagnosis
▦ PCR assays for viral agents such as HSV-2

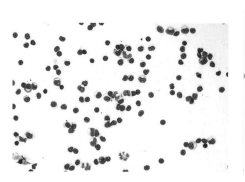
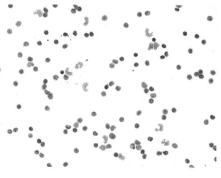

20-5. *(left).* CSF with hypercellularity and scattered activated monocytes (modified Giemsa stain)

20-6. Mollaret meningitis *(right).* CSF with increased cellularity and scattered activated monocytes some of which have the characteristic morphology of a "footprint in sand" (modified Giemsa stain)

Differential Diagnosis
- Inflammatory and infectious diseases of the CNS
- Lymphoproliferative disorder

★ Mollaret cells have deep nuclear clefts, leading to their characteristic "footprint" appearance
★ The clinical picture and the CSF cytology are diagnostic of Mollaret meningitis

TOXOPLASMOSIS

Clinical Features
- Caused by an obligate intracellular protozoal parasite, *Toxoplasma gondii*
- Common opportunistic infection in AIDS patients
- Clinically and radiologically can be confused with malignant lymphoma
- Most common cause of a focal brain lesion in patients with AIDS
- Patients with ring-enhancing lesions are usually treated empirically for this infection

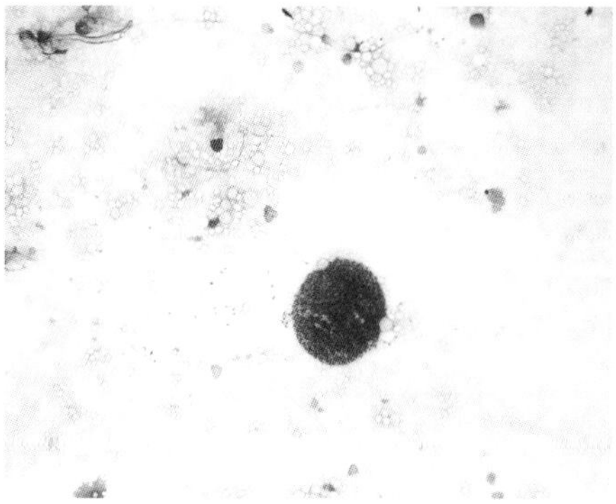

Cytologic Features
- Abundant macrophages
- Polymorphous lymphoid cells
- Reactive astrocytosis
- Typical cysts containing oval or crescent-shaped bradyzoites, which are best seen in air-dried Romanowsky-stained (e.g., modified Giemsa stain) preparations

20-7. Toxoplasmosis. Large pseudocyst with innumerable organisms (modified Giemsa stain)

Special Stains and Immunohistochemistry
- Anti-*Toxoplasma* antibodies can be used for identification of organisms

Modern Techniques for Diagnosis
- PCR assays for viral agents such as HSV-2
- Indirect immunofluorescent antibody studies

Differential Diagnosis
- Cerebral vasculitis
- CNS lymphoma
- HIV encephalopathy
- HIV dementia
- Other (non-HIV) forms of dementia
- Cerebrovascular disease
- Neurosyphilis

★ Space-occupying lesions, usually bilateral in the basal ganglia region
★ On computed tomography (CT) scan may mimic malignant lymphoma

CYSTICERCOSIS

Clinical Features
- Infection caused by the pork tapeworm, *Taenia solium*
- Transmission by fecal–oral route

- Acquired by accidentally swallowing pork tapeworm eggs
- Intracranial hypertension due to obstructive hydrocephalus
- Seizures and headaches are the most common symptoms
- Can present as a single enhancing cystic mass
- Common cause of encephalitis in Latin American immigrants

Cytologic Features
- Mixed inflammatory cells including eosinophils
- Abundant macrophages, giant cells, and necrosis may be present
- Fragments of the wall of the larva may be seen as amorphous eosinophilic structures
- In tissue sections: Sections of larva surrounded by fibrous capsule and granulation tissue with acute and chronic inflammation

Special Stains and Immunohistochemistry
- Noncontributory

Modern Techniques for Diagnosis
- Multiplex PCR assay
- Newer enzyme-linked immunoelectrotransfer blot (EITB) is preferred to ELISA

Differential Diagnosis
- Metastatic diseases, which characteristically lodge at the corticomedullary junction
- Cerebral abscesses

PEARLS

- Single enhancing brain lesions, mostly as a result of neurocysticercosis or tuberculosis, are a common cause of seizures
- Serology is the most useful of laboratory tests

PSEUDOTUMORAL MACROPHAGE-RICH LESIONS

Pseudotumoral macrophage-rich lesions include cerebral infarct, PML, and demyelinating diseases. This category of lesions shares the common feature of a predominant histiocytic infiltrate. An understanding of the neuroanatomy and careful correlation of the cytological findings with radiologic imaging is critical for an accurate diagnosis of these lesions, because these lesions may mimic primary or metastatic tumors of the brain.

PEARLS FOR DIAGNOSIS OF PSEUDOTUMORAL MACROPHAGE-RICH LESIONS

- During cytological evaluation of these lesions, an accurate identification of histiocytes is crucial and avoids a false-positive diagnosis
- Immunostaining for macrophages (i.e., KP-1 [CD68] HAM56) is often extremely helpful in demonstrating the cell of origin of the infiltrate

SUBACUTE CEREBRAL INFARCTION

Clinical Features
- Rarely aspirated (only when there is an atypical clinical presentation and/or prominent surface ring enhancement on CT scans)
- Radiological appearance consistent with the distribution of the lesion in the territory of a vascular supply

Cytologic Features
▥ Hypercellular with abundant finely granular or foamy macrophages, often hemo-siderin laden
▥ Vascular proliferation, often with tangled clumps of fine capillaries and/or atypical mitotically active endothelial cells
▥ Hematoidin crystals
▥ Coagulative necrosis

Special Stains and Immunohistochemistry
▥ Noncontributory

Modern Techniques for Diagnosis
▥ Noncontributory

Differential Diagnosis
■ Vascular disorders (arterial ischemia and venous infarctions)
■ Neoplasms
■ Infectious and demyelinating diseases
■ Metabolic–toxic alterations

PEARLS

⋆ Cytologically this lesion may mimic a neoplastic, inflammatory, and demyelinating process

DEMYELINATING DISEASE (MULTIPLE SCLEROSIS)

Clinical Features
▥ Multicentric foci of demyelination (plaques), rarely solitary, usually paraventricular
▥ Unknown etiology
▥ More common in patients who lived first decade of life in northern latitudes
▥ Relapsing, asymmetric limb weakness, paresthesias, optic neuritis
▥ Radiologic appearance: Bright foci on MRI, seen adjacent to the lateral ventricle "capping of the ventricle"
▥ Progressive decline leading to death

Cytologic Features
▥ Hypercellular
▥ Abundant vacuolated macrophages (uniform round nuclei, vacuolated cytoplasm, distinct cell borders) sometimes lipid laden, and often containing Luxol fast blue (LFB) material in the cytoplasm
▥ Reactive astrocytosis with array of processes
▥ Increase in the number of mature lymphocytes

Special Stains and Immunohistochemistry
▥ Immunostaining with SM-31 (phosphorylated neurofilament) may demonstrate intact neuronal processes in cell block or tissue sections (in contrast to cerebral infarct, where the latter immunostaining is lost)
▥ CD-68 to demonstrate the presence of histiocytes

Modern Techniques for Diagnosis
▥ Lumbar puncture to show increased CSF immunoglobulins seen as multiple oligo-clonal bands on electrophoresis

Differential Diagnosis
- May resemble glioma due to richness of histiocytes
- Oligodendroglioma is in the differential because the macrophages may mimic the appearance of oligodendrocytes (uniform, round nuclei, and cytoplasmic vacuolization)
- Acute disseminated encephalomyelitis
- Systemic lupus erythematosus
- Lyme disease
- HIV-associated myelopathy
- Neurosyphillis
- Progressive multifocal leukoencephalopathy – immunosuppressed patients

PEARLS

- ★ Perivascular inflammation (mostly T-cell lymphocytes) and demyelination
- ★ Granular astrocytoma may resemble demyelinating disease

ARTERIOVENOUS MALFORMATION (AVM)

Clinical Features
- Most commonly discovered in young adults aged twenty to forty years
- Usually detected in patients as the result of a seizure or hemorrhage
- Usually large lesions

Cytologic Features
- Usually in lateral cerebral hemispheres, rarely biopsied
- Numerous vessels of varying caliber, often thick-walled capillaries
- Hemorrhagic background, often with hemosiderin-laden macrophages

Special Stains and Immunohistochemistry
- Noncontributory

Modern Techniques for Diagnosis
- Noncontributory

Differential Diagnosis
- Normal vessels of subarachnoid may give the false appearance of an AV malformation

PEARLS

- ★ The diagnosis of AV malformations is aided by correlation with angiographic and intraoperative findings

CRANIOPHARYNGIOMA

Clinical Features
- Rare extraaxial slow-growing tumors arising in the region of the sella turcica and suprasellar space
- Comprise 3–5% of all intracranial tumors
- Benign tumors prone to recurrences

▨ Three forms: Adamantinomatous (pediatric type), papillary (adult type), and mixed
▨ Adamantinomatous type most commonly has a cystic appearance
▨ Suprasellar cystic and solid lesions
▨ Papillary type is often present in the third ventricle
▨ Thought to be derived during embryogenesis from Rathke's pouch epithelial tissues
▨ Clinical symptoms due to optic chiasm and/or pituitary gland compression often accompanied by headaches

Cytologic Features
▨ Adamantinomatous type
  ➤ Cystic fluid with an appearance of "motor oil"
  ➤ Aspirate has a thick viscous quality
  ➤ Keratinized squamous cells
  ➤ Wet keratin
  ➤ Background of degenerated cellular and keratinaceous debris, macrophages
  ➤ Cholesterol clefts
  ➤ Anucleate squames, calcified debris
  ➤ Multinucleated giant cells
  ➤ Fragments of basaloid epithelial cells
▨ Papillary type (also known as ciliated craniopharyngioma)
  ➤ Solid sheets of squamous epithelium
  ➤ Monomorphic squamous cells
  ➤ Small epithelial whorls may be present
  ➤ Cell block preparations may show prominent cores of fibrovascular stroma

Special Stains and Immunohistochemistry
▨ Typical immunoreactivity for keratin

Modern Techniques for Diagnosis
▨ Noncontributory

Differential Diagnosis
■ Epidermoid cyst
■ Rathke cleft cyst
■ Metastatic squamous carcinoma

PEARLS

★ The key to identification of adamantinomatous type of craniopharyngioma is the identification of sheets of cohesive epithelial cells and "wet keratin" nodules

---

RATHKE'S CLEFT CYST

Clinical Features
▨ An intrasellar or suprasellar cyst primarily affecting adults
▨ Usually incidental autopsy findings
▨ Clinical presentation may include headaches and visual disturbances

Cytologic Features
▨ Thin-walled structures
▨ Squamous cells in a granular background
▨ Often contains mucus in the background
▨ Cuboidal and/or ciliated columnar epithelium

Special Stains and Immunohistochemistry
- Typical immunoreactivity for keratin (CK20)
- Variable positivity with carcinoembryonic antigen (CEA)

Modern Techniques for Diagnosis
- Noncontributory

Differential Diagnosis
- Epidermoid cyst
- Papillary craniopharyngioma

PEARLS

- ★ Squamous metaplasia may be the predominant finding and may lead to misdiagnosis
- ★ The key is the location and the identification of mucus in the preparation

EPIDERMOID CYST

Clinical Features
- Most often located at the cerebellopontine angle less commonly in suprasellar region or brain stem
- Ectodermal malformations in the developing brain
- The cyst is only symptomatic when it attains a considerable size
- Usually uniloculated

Cytologic Features
- Often fragments of the cyst wall consisting of keratinizing squamous epithelium
- May see flaky type of keratin
- Isolated discohesive keratinized squamous cells
- Clean background
- Parakeratotic cells

Special Stains and Immunohistochemistry
- Typical immunoreactivity for keratin

Modern Techniques for diagnosis
- Noncontributory

Differential Diagnosis
- Craniopharyngioma
- Rathke cleft cyst
- Endodermal cyst

PEARLS

- ★ Radiological appearance of keratinous debris makes the diagnosis of epidermoid cyst easier

COLLOID CYST OF THE THIRD VENTRICLE

Clinical Features
- Endodermally derived mucus-filled, epithelial-lined cysts in the anterosuperior third ventricle (near the foramen of Monro)

■ Young to middle age

■ Intermittent obstruction to CSF flow causes headaches, incontinence, and personality changes

■ Radiologic appearance: *Characteristic;* smooth surfaced cyst with intrinsically bright signal on nonenhanced T1-weighted MRI

Cytologic Features

■ Amorphous, proteinaceous, and dense colloid-like material

■ Isolated cuboidal to columnar cells

■ Fragments of pseudostratified ciliated columnar cells

■ Goblet cells

■ Lack of metaplastic squamous cells (cf. other benign cysts)

■ Rare psammoma bodies (? choroid plexus contamination by the needle), or filamentous masses of nucleoprotein

Special Stains and Immunohistochemistry

■ The epithelial lining of the cyst is immunopositive for cytokeratins

Modern Techniques for Diagnosis

■ Noncontributory

Differential Diagnosis

■ Can rarely see fragments of normal choroid plexus and may lead to a "neoplastic" diagnosis

PEARLS

★ Radiological appearance and location of the lesion is highly characteristic

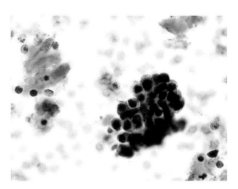

20-8. Colloid cyst. Amorphous, dense, proteinaceous "colloid-like" material with small monolayered fragment of epithelial cells. The location and the characteristic radiological appearance is diagnostic for colloid cyst of the third ventricle (modified Giemsa stain)

LOW-GRADE ASTROCYTOMA

Clinical Features

■ Usually in cerebral hemispheres of young to middle-aged adults or brain stem in children

■ Produce nonspecific symptoms of mass effect, seizures, and neurologic deficits

■ On computed tomography (CT), appear as ill-defined areas of low density with their epicenters in the white matter

Cytologic Features

■ Hypercellularity

■ Slight anisonucleosis

■ Fibrillary background

■ Infiltration of surrounding brain tissue (tissue sections)

■ Aggregation around neurons (satellitosis) (tissue sections and cytologic preparations)

Special Stains and Immunohistochemistry

■ S-100 protein immunoreactive

■ Cytoplasmic positivity with GFAP

■ Low Ki-67 proliferation (less than 5%)

Modern Techniques for Diagnosis

■ P53 mutations may be detected

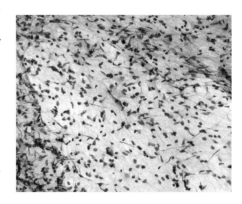

20-9. Low-grade astrocytoma. Smear shows increased cellularity with round to oval and spindled glial nuclei in a prominent fibrillary background. An assessment of cellularity in a cytologic smear is often misleading and is largely dependent on the thickness of the smear (Papanicolaou stain)

20-10. Low-grade astrocytoma
(top, left). Hypercellular smear with a prominent fibrillary background (Papanicolaou stain)

20-11. Low-grade astrocytoma
(top, right). Mildly increased cellularity with small uniform neoplastic glial cells in a prominent fibrillary background The neoplastic cells have elongated, slightly pleomorphic nuclei (modified Giemsa stain)

20-12. Reactive gliosis
(bottom, left). Polymorphous glial cells with numerous gemistocytes in a fibrillary background. There is mildly increased cellularity and numerous fine branching capillaries (modified Giemsa stain)

20-13. Reactive gliosis
(bottom, right). Round to oval polymorphous glial cells embedded in a fibrillary background with fine branching capillaries (modified Giemsa stain)

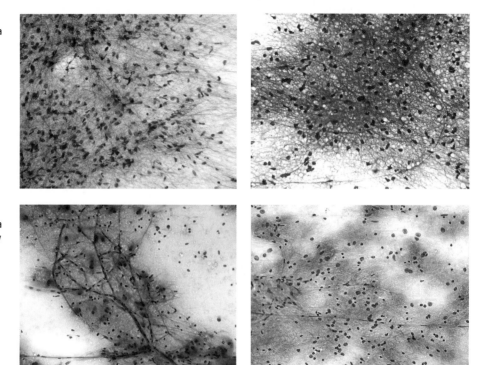

- Gain in a portion of chromosome 7
- Loss of chromosome 19q

Differential Diagnosis
- Glioblastoma
- Oligodendroglioma
- Abscess
- Metastatic disease
- Infarct
- Demyelinating disease

PEARLS

★ A contrast-enhancing ring lesion virtually rules out the diagnosis of an astrocytoma
★ Low-grade astrocytomas can be difficult, sometimes impossible, to differentiate from reactive gliosis
★ Evidence of diffuse involvement (the presence of increased cellularity in multiple aspirates from different levels), presence of calcifications, and mitoses can be helpful
★ Irregular distribution of cells in the brain tissue is difficult to assess in cytologic preparations and small tissue fragments of needle aspirations
★ The diagnosis and decisions about treatment in these cases are made usually after careful evaluation of the pathologic, radiologic, and clinical findings

ANAPLASTIC ASTROCYTOMA

Clinical Features
- Grade III infiltrating astrocytoma
- Majority affect the cerebral hemispheres

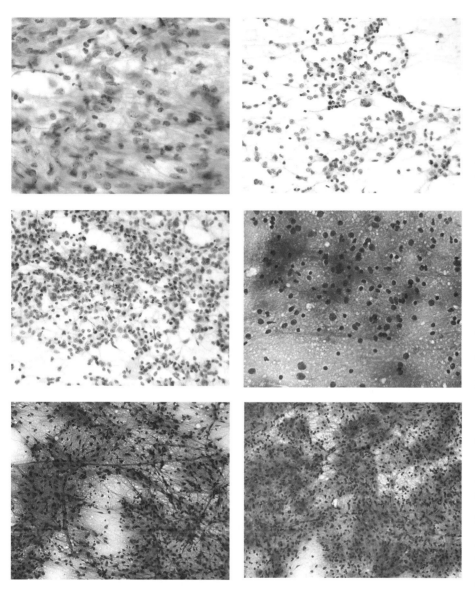

20-14. Anaplastic astrocytoma *(top, left).* Higher magnification showing round to oval nuclei, aniso-nucleosis, fine nuclear chromatin and inconspicuous nucleoli in a fibrillary background (Papanicolaou stain)

20-15. Anaplastic astrocytoma *(top, right).* Cellular smear with numerous round to oval nuclei of neoplastic astrocytes. Occasional clusters of neoplastic cells are also evident. There are no mitosis or karyorrhectic nuclei (Papanicolaou stain)

20-16. Anaplastic astrocytoma *(middle, left).* Diffusely cellular smear with pleomorphic neoplastic astrocytes with round to oval hyperchromatic nuclei. Occasional gemistocytes, fine capillaries are present (Papanicolaou stain)

20-17. Anaplastic astrocytoma *(middle, right).* Moderately cellular smear with diffusely scattered, pleomorphic astrocytes in a fibrillary background (modified Giemsa stain)

20-18. Anaplastic astrocytoma *(bottom, left).* Hypercellular smear with pleomorphic population of neoplastic glial cells, numerous fine-branching capillaries in a prominent fibrillary background (modified Giemsa stain)

20-19. Anaplastic astrocytoma *(bottom, right).* Hypercellular smear with loose clusters and single malignant astrocytic nuclei embedded in a thick fibrillary background (modified Giemsa stain)

- Patients are usually a decade older than the well-differentiated astrocytomas
- Surface ring-enhancing pattern of GBM is not seen on radiologic scans

Cytologic Features
- Increased cellularity with definite atypia
- Hyperchromasia
- Small elongated cells with bipolar processes
- Fibrillar background
- Moderate to marked nuclear pleomorphism
- Occasional mitotic figures
- Gemistocytic appearance accompanied by small hyperchromatic cells may be seen
- Invasion of surrounding brain tissue (tissue sections)
- Satellitosis (tissue sections and cytologic preparations)

Special Stains and Immunohistochemistry
- S-100 protein immunoreactive
- Cytoplasmic positivity with GFAP

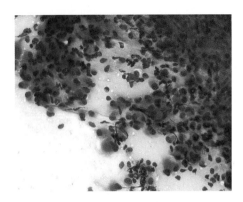

20-20. Anaplastic astrocytoma with gemistocytic features.
Hypercellular smear with numerous crowded clusters of neoplastic astrocytes. Majority of the cells have eccentric nuclei with prominent globoid and glassy-appearing cytoplasm (modified Giemsa stain)

■ Ki-67 proliferation index is variable and is often in between that seen in low grade astrocytoma and glioblastoma

Modern Techniques for Diagnosis
■ Mutations in PTEN
■ Expression of the mutant EGFRvIII protein is prognostically unfavorable

Differential Diagnosis
■ Reactive gliosis, particularly when dealing with paucicellular material
■ Demyelinating disease, such as PML, where there is atypia and marked nuclear pleomorphism
■ Oligodendroglioma
■ Gliomatosis cerebri

PEARLS

★ The presence of multinucleated astrocytes/histiocytes should point to a reactive, macrophage-rich lesion
★ Anaplastic astrocytoma can only be differentiated from glioblastoma multiforme by the absence of necrosis and marked endothelial proliferation
★ Absence of these features, on the other hand, does not entirely rule out glioblastoma multiforme because of the limitations of sampling

GLIOBLASTOMA MULTIFORME (GBM)

Clinical Features
■ Most common glioma
■ Involves cerebral hemispheres in adults and brain stem in children
■ Seen in all age groups (most frequent after the fifth decade)
■ On CT, appears as a central area of low density surrounded by a ring of contrast enhancement
■ On MRI, glioblastomas typically have an enhancing ring or rim in postcontrast T1-weighted images
■ Presenting symptomatology more abrupt than well-differentiated astrocytomas (although similar in characteristics)

Cytologic Features
■ Extreme hypercellularity
■ Marked pleomorphism
■ Presence of fine processes surrounding clumps of cells usually "bipolar"
■ Nuclei have evenly dispersed chromatin
■ Multinucleated cells
■ Cellular necrosis
■ Endothelial/vascular proliferation
■ Palisading of tumor cells around the necrotic area (tissue sections)
■ Invasion of surrounding brain tissue (tissue sections)

Special Stains and Immunohistochemistry
■ Immunoreactive for GFAP, vimentin, and S-100 protein

Modern Techniques for Diagnosis
■ Losses on chromosomes 6, 10, 15, 18, and Y chromosome and gains of chromosome 7 can be detected by cytogenetics

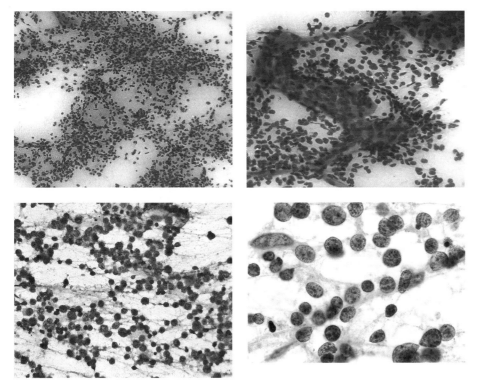

20-21. Glioblastoma multiforme *(top, left).* Hypercellular smear with pleomorphic malignant glial cells. A distinction from a pleomorphic astrocytoma requires microvascular proliferation and presence of cellular necrosis (modified Giemsa stain)

20-22. Glioblastoma multiforme *(top, right).* Smear shows pleomorphic round to oval malignant nuclei with focal microvascular (endothelial) proliferation. A fibrillary background is more often absent in GBM smears (modified Giemsa stain)

20-23. Glioblastoma multiforme *(bottom, left).* Smear shows hypercellularity with a uniform population of relatively small round nuclei with numerous karyorrhectic cells and a suggestion of background necrosis. Cytomorphologic distinction from other small round blue cell neoplasms including non-Hodgkin lymphoma and oligodendroglioma can be challenging and clinical and radiologic correlation becomes pivotal (modified Giemsa stain)

20-24. Glioblastoma multiforme *(bottom, right).* Higher magnification shows pleomorphic and hyperchromatic round and oval nuclei of the malignant glial cells. (Papanicolaou stain)

▓ Deletions and mutations of p16 and PTEN, loss of heterozygosity of chromosome 17p, p53 mutations

▓ Amplifications of MDM2 and EGFR

Differential Diagnosis

▓ Anaplastic astrocytoma versus glioblastoma multiforme

▓ Metastatic cancer vs. Glioblastoma multiforme particularly when the glioblastoma is highly cellular with monomorphous small cells

▓ Glioblastoma multiforme Versus benign lesions associated with necrosis and cellular atypia (e.g., infarct and other macrophage-rich lesions, radiation necrosis)

PEARLS

★ Poorly differentiated metastatic carcinoma can be difficult to differentiate from high-grade gliomas

★ Demonstration of glial fibrillary acidic protein (GFAP) by immunoperoxidase staining establishes the glial origin of the tumor, but undifferentiated cells of glioblastoma may not show positive staining

★ With a limited sample, negative results do not rule out GBM. Worthwhile to remember that GBM may often show immunoexpression for cytokeratins compounding the diagnostic difficulty

★ In contrast to astrocytomas, metastatic tumors are usually well demarcated from the adjacent brain tissue

★ The presence of necrosis alone should be evaluated with great caution. In some cases (i.e., infarct and radiation necrosis), necrotic material may also be associated with atypical cellular (astrocytic) proliferation

★ Histiocytes, which are present in infarcts, are usually absent in gliomas

★ Clinical history and clinical/radiological evaluation with close follow-up are needed in problematic cases

PILOCYTIC ASTROCYTOMA

Clinical Features
- Well-circumscribed, cystic neoplasm
- Common in children and young adults
- Slow growing tumor with excellent prognosis
- Some tumors are associated with neurofibromatosis type 1
- Most common form of astrocytoma in the visual system and cerebellum
- Relatively circumscribed, often cystic, common in children and young adults

Cytologic Features
- Slender, long, bipolar cytoplasmic processes, brightly eosinophilic on H&E stain
- Uniform, bland, elongated nuclei
- Intracytoplasmic Rosenthal fibers, eosinophilic granular bodies (EGB)

Special Stains and Immunohistochemistry
- Immunoreactive with GFAP, negative for neuroendocrine markers
- EGBs are immunoreactive for alpha-1-antichymotrypsin and alpha-1-antitrypsin
- Ki-67 proliferative index is very low (1–2%)

Modern Techniques for Diagnosis
- Loss of NF1 alleles are seen in patients with pilocytic astrocytomas associated with neurofibromatosis type 1

Differential Diagnosis
- Reactive gliosis
- Diffuse astrocytoma
- Ganglion cell tumors
- Pleomorphic xanthoastrocytoma

PEARLS
★ Cytopathological diagnosis becomes challenging when trying to differentiate between pilocytic tumors and diffuse astrocytomas
★ Characteristic findings such as Rosenthal fibers, EGBs, microcystic changes are sometimes helpful when present

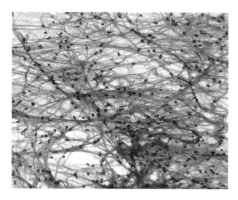
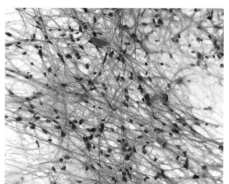

20-25. Pilocytic astrocytoma *(left)*. Uniform oval to spindled nuclei embedded in a brightly eosinophilic fibrillary background. Numerous elongated, slender pencil-shaped nuclei are also seen (H&E)

20-26. Pilocytic astrocytoma *(right)*. Eosinophilic granular bodies (EGB) associated with occasional Rosenthal fibers are seen in association with fine, spindled, and fusiform nuclei (H&E)

GLIOMATOSIS CEREBRI

Clinical Features
- Gliomatosis cerebri is extensive, diffusely infiltrating glioma
- Usually seen in adults but children may also be affected
- MRI demonstrates a diffuse increase in the T2 signal
- Involves greater part of a cerebral hemisphere, often both sides of the brain in continuity
- Symptoms include seizures, personality changes, and aphasia
- Most often not curable by surgical resection

Cytologic Features
- Widely infiltrating, lack of inclination to form a distinct mass
- Variable cellularity, often normocellular or even paucicellular
- Angiotropism, perineuronal satellitosis (in cell block sections, tissue cores)
- Degree of cytological atypia is variable
- Hyperchromatic, oval to elongated nuclei, scant cytoplasm
- Lack of significant pleomorphism, endothelial proliferation, or necrosis

Special Stains and Immunohistochemistry
- Elongated cellular processes are positive for GFAP
- Immunoreactive for Ki-67 (MIB-1) with low to moderate expression

Modern Techniques for Diagnosis
- No unique molecular profile
- Mutations in p53 have been reported

Differential Diagnosis
- May be difficult to distinguish from reactive gliosis

PEARLS

✴ This is a difficult lesion to diagnose because of the variable cytological atypia with the diagnostic spectrum from a classic well-differentiated lesion to one that is grade III and has significant nuclear hyperchromatism and atypia with mitosis

SMALL CELL GBM

Clinical Features
- Morphologic subtype of GBM, with the same poor prognosis
- Not a neuroendocrine neoplasm

Cytologic Features
- Hypercellular
- Predominance of small, round to oval, and hyperchromatic cells
- Slightly elongated nuclei
- Nuclear molding and/or "crush" artifact
- Mitosis/karyorrhexis
- Close, but false cytopathologic resemblance to small cell carcinoma

Special Stains and Immunohistochemistry
- Variably positive for GFAP, negative for neuroendocrine markers,
- High Ki-67 proliferative index

Modern Techniques for diagnosis
- Amplification of EGFR

Differential Diagnosis
- Oligodendroglioma is in the differential but small GBM neoplastic cells do not have the uniform round nuclei of oligodendrogliomas
- Ependymoma

PEARLS

★ Focally increased mitotic activity and necrosis may be helpful in the diagnosis, particularly when the smears may show predominantly bland cytology with small cells which may suggest a more "reactive" diagnosis

GLIOSARCOMA

Clinical Features
- Contain both malignant glial and mesenchymal elements
- Rare subtype of GBM (<2%)
- Shares the same bad prognosis as GBM

Cytologic Features
- Hypercellular
- High-grade morphological features
- Often dimorphic with glial and sarcomatous elements (predominance of the latter cell type)
- Glial component is astrocytic often with gemistocytes
- The sarcomatous component may be undifferentiated, rhabdoid, chondroid, and osteoblastic
- Spindle cells in fasciculation and/or bizarre pleomorphic histiocytoid cells and multinucleated tumor cells, occasional "strap-shaped" and "rhabdoid" cells
- Perivascular aggregation with marked endothelial proliferation
- High mitosis/karyorrhexis often with necrosis

Special Stains and Immunohistochemistry
- Epithelial component is positive for cytokeratins
- Glial component is positive for GFAP
- Vimentin positivity in the sarcomatous component with more specific staining for muscle markers such as smooth muscle actin has been described

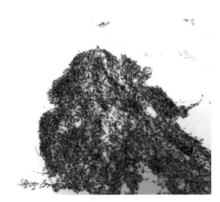
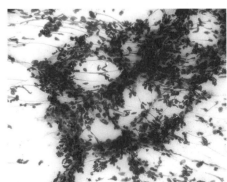

20-27. Gliosarcoma *(left)*. Large cohesive fragment of malignant glial cells with oval to spindled nuclei in a vague perivascular arrangement (Papanicolaou stain)

20-28. Gliosarcoma *(right)*. Hypercellular smear with pleomorphic oval to spindled nuclei set in a prominent branching cordlike perivascular arrangement (modified Giemsa stain)

Modern Techniques for Diagnosis
- p53 mutations

Differential Diagnosis
- Glioblastoma with an intense mesenchymal reaction
- Glioblastoma with dural involvement and desmoplastic response
- Pure primary or metastatic sarcoma
- Metastatic carcinoma

PEARLS

⭐ Presence of a predominant sarcomatous/mesenchymal component requires a distinction of gliosarcoma from other primary and metastatic spindle cell lesions

EPENDYMOMA

Clinical Features
- Arise throughout the neuroaxis
- Large intraventricular or periventricular masses
- Frequently calcified on radiology scans
- Supratentorial ependymomas are frequently associated with a cyst
- Usually well-circumscribed
- Intracranial lesions more common in children, spinal in adults

Cytologic Features
- Uniform monomorphic cells, often with a flat, luminal cytoplasmic edge
- Small, round, hyperchromatic nuclei and well-preserved small amount of cytoplasm
- Cords and papillary-like structures around eosinophilic fibrovascular cores
- True ependymal rosettes

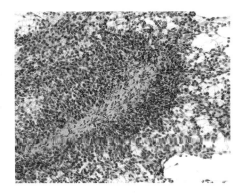

20-29. Ependymoma. Touch imprint of an avascular core of a papillary structure surrounded by small, uniform, ependymal cells. These cells have round nuclei and pale fragile cytoplasm (H&E)

Special Stains and Immunohistochemistry
- Positive staining for GFAP (prominent in fibrillar areas including perivascular pseudorosettes) and S-100 protein (positive but not diffusely strong as compared to a schwannoma)
- Variable staining with EMA and cytokeratins

Modern Techniques for Diagnosis
- Frequent loss of the chromosomal arm 22q
- Spinal ependymomas are seen in patients with neurofibromatosis 2 (NF2)

Differential Diagnosis
- Schwannoma (diffuse strong reactivity for S-100 protein)
- Meningioma (EMA positive, GFAP negative)
- Pilocytic astrocytoma, particularly in tumors from the fourth ventricle and the spinal cord
- Oligodendroglioma (cellular ependymoma with clear cells)
- Medulloblastoma particularly when assessing a markedly cellular ependymoma
- Central neurocytoma

★ Ependymomas frequently present with diagnostic challenges, particularly when evaluating spinal lesions

★ Correlation with key radiological findings and the presence of additional cytomorphological clues such as high grade appearance, may prevent a diagnostic pitfall

MYXOPAPILLARY EPENDYMOMA

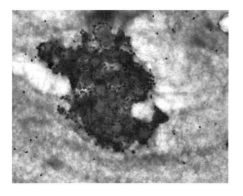

20-30. Myxopapillary ependymoma. Large tumor fragment with uniform ependymal cells surrounding a well-formed globule of metachromatic material. This appearance is reminiscent of an adenoid cystic carcinoma (modified Giemsa stain)

Clinical Features
■ Rare variant, which occurs in the presacral or postsacral regions, and rarely in the sacrum
■ A high incidence of loss on 13q14-q31 in adults

Cytologic Features
■ Cells with rounded nuclei, with delicate, open chromatin
■ Typically amphophilic cytoplasm
■ Cohesion and a tendency for perivascular arrangement
■ Frequently have a myxoid background
■ Hyaline globules surrounded by tumor cores
■ Perivascular myxoid material is present

Special Stains and Immunohistochemistry
■ Positive staining for GFAP, vimentin and S-100 protein
■ Usually negative staining with cytokeratins

Modern Techniques for Diagnosis
■ Deletions of chromosome 11q
■ Rearrangement of chromosome 1p has been described

Differential Diagnosis
■ Metastatic adenocarcinoma (adenocarcinoma may have mucin and papillary architecture)
■ Chordoma
■ Paraganglioma

★ The mucinous matrix in myxopapillary ependymomas is present near or in the walls of the blood vessels

★ Correlation with key radiological findings and the presence of cytomorphological clues such as the pseudopapillary architecture, perivascular mucin and round structures or "balloons" (reticulin positive) are helpful in rendering a correct cytological diagnosis

MENINGIOMA

Clinical Features
■ Meningiomas account for approximately 20% of all primary intracranial neoplasms
■ A neoplasm derived from meningothelial (arachnoidal cells)
■ Typically occur in adults but children are occasionally affected
■ Most common location is the intracranial meninges
■ Multiple histological types, some with unfavorable prognosis (Grade II or III)

Cytologic Features

▓ Classic features include lobules, whorls, or psammoma bodies
▓ Neoplastic meningothelial cells have slightly oval nuclei with occasional intranuclear vacuoles
▓ Neoplastic cells do not have a clearly identifiable cytoplasmic border
▓ Nuclei have delicate chromatin and small nucleoli
▓ Intranuclear pseudoinclusions are occasionally present

Special Stains and Immunohistochemistry

▓ Positive staining with EMA (membranous pattern)

Modern Techniques for Diagnosis

▓ In NF2-associated tumors, inactivation of the NF2 gene on chromosome 22q12 occurs
▓ Cytogenetic assays may detect loss or monosomy of chromosome 22
▓ Molecular-based assays such as PCR may also detect these abnormalities

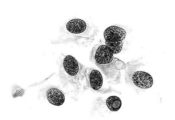

20-31. Meningioma. Neoplastic cells with uniform round to oval nuclei and fragile cytoplasm. A rare intranuclear inclusion is also present (H&E)

Differential Diagnosis

▪ Inflammatory pseudotumors (sarcoidosis, plasma cell granuloma)
▪ Schwannoma
▪ Solitary fibrous tumors (lack of whorls/psammoma bodies; positive for CD34 and Bcl-2 and negative for EMA)
▪ Hemangiopericytoma (staghorn vascular channels)
▪ Hemangioblastoma
▪ Pilocytic astrocytomas (GFAP positive)
▪ Metastatic carcinoma

PEARLS

✶ The differential diagnosis of meningioma is broad and includes both neoplastic and non-neoplastic entities
✶ Well-differentiated meningiomas may present as metastatic disease to the lung, which on cytological smears may present with a diagnostic dilemma. Careful look back at the clinical history is the key to avoiding a diagnostic pitfall

CHOROID PLEXUS PAPILLOMA/CARCINOMA

Clinical Features

▓ Papillary neoplasms derived from the choroid plexus epithelium
▓ Usually seen in children, arise in the lateral, and less often, third ventricle
▓ Uncommon in adults where the favored location is the fourth ventricle
▓ Produce hydrocephalus with its usual signs and symptoms
▓ On radiology, discrete, contrast-enhancing intraventricular lesions

Cytologic Features

▓ Hypercellular with cohesive cell clusters
▓ Papillary fragments of columnar epithelial cells, often crowded/stratified around well-formed fibrovascular cores
  ➢ Scattered naked nuclei in the background
  ➢ Occasional prominent nuclear grooves
  ➢ Carcinoma cells are less cohesive and more atypical

20-32. Choroid plexus papilloma. Well-developed fibrovascular cores surrounded by neoplastic epithelium. Numerous discohesive neoplastic cells are present in the smear background (modified Giemsa stain)

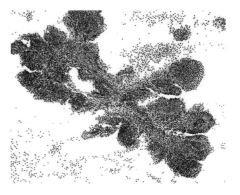

Special Stains and Immunohistochemistry

▧ Positive staining with cytokeratins, EMA, vimentin, and transthyretin (prealbumin)

▧ Immunostaining for p53 is more prominent in carcinomas as compared to papillomas

Modern Techniques for Diagnosis

▧ FISH or comparative genomic hybridization of papillomas may show gains of chromosomes 5,7,9,12,15, and 18 and loss of chromosomes 21 and 22

▧ Carcinomas may have gains of chromosomes 1, 4, and 14 and loss of chromosomes 5, 15, and 18

▧ FISH for diagnosis of abnormalities in the INI1 gene (to distinguish from atypical teratoid/rhabdoid tumors)

Differential Diagnosis

■ Normal choroid plexus (epithelium of the neoplasms is more complex and more cellular)

■ Papillary ependymoma

■ Metastatic carcinoma

■ Atypical rhabdoid/teratoid tumors (EMA-positive rhabdoid cells)

■ Germ cell tumors (immunohistochemistry can help resolve the diagnosis)

PEARLS

✶ When trying to distinguish from an intraventricular focus of metastatic carcinoma, use immunohistochemistry to resolve the diagnosis. However, if it looks clearly malignant with significant cytological atypia, it more likely to be a metastatic carcinoma

ATYPICAL TERATOID/RHABDOID TUMORS (AT/RT)

Clinical Features

▧ Highly aggressive neoplasm of uncertain origin with a unique cytogenetic profile

▧ Almost all patients are under two years of age

▧ Characterized by large, rapidly enlarging tumors contrast enhancing with hemorrhage and necrosis

▧ Most common location – posterior intracranial fossa

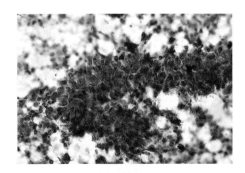

20-33. Atypical teratoid/rhabdoid tumors. Large collection of neoplastic cells with prominent perivascular aggregation (H&E)

Cytologic Features

▧ Hypercellularity with tissue fragments and single cells

▧ Neoplastic cells show pleomorphism, perivascular aggregation around branching vessels – "papillary-like"

▧ Large round "plasmacytoid" cells, characteristic "rhabdoid" cells, and cells with reniform nuclei are seen

▧ "Rhabdoid" cells have brightly eosinophilic cytoplasm with or without fibrillary globoid inclusion, large eccentrically placed nuclei with single prominent nucleoli

▧ Few cases with predominance of high N/C ratio, primitive "neuronal-appearing" cells

▧ Prominent nuclear "crush" artifact

▧ Pleomorphic, multinucleated giant cells

▧ Apoptosis, mitoses, necrosis, and dystrophic calcification

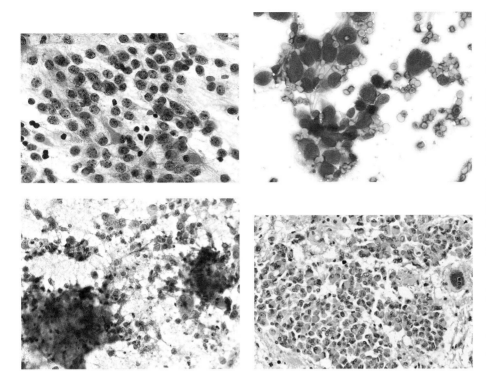

20-34. Atypical teratoid/rhabdoid tumors *(top, left)*. Higher magnification showing malignant cells with a round nuclei and high nuclear to cytoplasmic ratio (H&E)

20-35. Atypical teratoid/rhabdoid tumors *(top, right)*. Large pleomorphic malignant cells with eccentric nuclei and occasional binucleation. Macronucleoli are not evident in this preparation (H&E)

20-36. Atypical teratoid/rhabdoid tumors *(bottom, left)*. Pleomorphic malignant cells with high nuclear to cytoplasmic ratios, occasional prominent nucleoli, eosinophilic cytoplasm and focal necrosis (H&E)

20-37. Atypical teratoid/rhabdoid tumors *(bottom, right)*. Histopathologic appearance of an AT/RT with predominance of "rhabdoid" cells. The "rhabdoid" cell have a brightly eosinophilic cytoplasmic inclusion, eccentric nucleus and prominent nucleolus (H&E)

Special Stains and Immunohistochemistry

▓ Positive staining shows reactivity with EMA, GFAP, cytokeratins, and less frequently with actin, NF, and chromogranin

Modern Techniques for Diagnosis

▓ FISH assays can be used to detect 22q deletions in AT/RTs

Differential Diagnosis

▓ Medulloblastoma/PNET
▓ Gemistocytic astrocytoma
▓ Choroid plexus carcinoma

PEARLS

✷ It is important to recognize that even though the term "rhabdoid" is used to describe this rare tumor, this may be a rare finding in cytological preparations
✷ Some of these tumors may predominantly contain small cells and it may be difficult to distinguish from a small round blue cell tumor such as medulloblastoma

GERM CELL TUMORS

Clinical Features

▓ Most arise in the midline, pineal gland, or suprasellar location
▓ Males two times more likely than females to develop germ cell tumors
▓ Rarely in lateral basal ganglia or thalamus
▓ Most intracranial germ cell tumors are well circumscribed and contrast enhancing

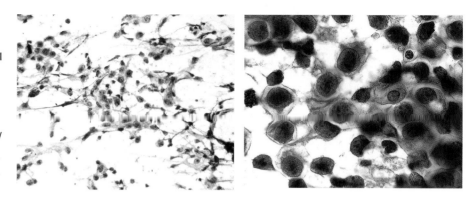

20-38. Seminoma *(left).* Bimodal population of large neoplastic germ cells and few background lymphocytes, the latter showing nuclear crush artifact (Papanicolaou stain)

20-39. Seminoma *(right).* Loosely cohesive tumor cells with large nuclei, macronucleoli, surrounded by relatively clear cytoplasm and a well-developed cell membrane (H&E)

▦ There are five subtypes: germinoma, yolk sac tumor, embryonal carcinoma, teratoma, and choriocarcinoma
▦ Most frequent subtype is germinoma
▦ Extremely radiosensitive (germinoma)
▦ Nongerminomatous tumors metastasize widely with poor outcome

Cytologic Features
▦ Large, often pleomorphic cells, singly and in small nests
▦ Biphasic appearance with scattered background lymphocytes (often with crush artifact)
▦ Neoplastic cells with large prominent single nucleoli, well-formed, often clear cytoplasm
▦ Prominent frothy background, particularly on modified Giemsa stain, resembling "tigroid" appearance of a gonadal seminoma
▦ Diagnostic Schiller–Duval bodies in yolk sac tumors

Special Stains and Immunohistochemistry
▦ Positive staining for placental alkaline phosphatase (PLAP), CKIT, CD30, AFP, HCG (depending on the germ cell tumor type) and negative for cytokeratins

Modern Techniques for Diagnosis
▦ Noncontributory

Differential Diagnosis
▦ Parenchymal tumors such as pineocytoma and pineoblastoma-positive CSF beta-hCG, and/or alpha-fetoprotein levels exclude pineal parenchymal tumors and suggest the presence of a germ cell neoplasm

PEARLS

★ Subtyping of the cytological material with the help of ancillary studies such as IPOX is important in the management of patients and may lead to design of appropriate therapeutic regimens
★ Pineal calcification on skull radiographs is a useful clue to the diagnosis of a germ cell tumor

LYMPHOMA

Clinical Features
▦ Primary CNS lymphoma is usually a B-cell lymphoma
▦ Occur more frequently in HIV-positive patients

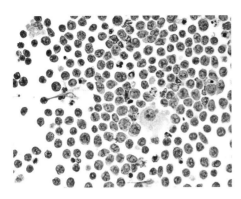 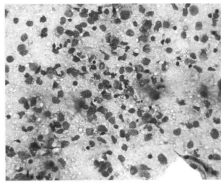

20-40. Non-hodgkin lymphoma *(left).* CSF with markedly increased cellularity with large malignant nuclei showing prominent irregularity of nuclear membranes (Papanicolaou stain). Non-Hodgkin lymphoma, large cell type

20-41. Non-hodgkin lymphoma *(right).* Large nuclei with macronucleoli and irregular nuclear membranes (modified Giemsa stain). Non-Hodgkin lymphoma, large cell type

▓ Systemic lymphoma – leptomeningeal involvement; primary CNS lymphoma – deep-seated parenchymal masses
▓ Mostly supratentorial
▓ Mostly fatal within two years of diagnosis

Cytologic Features
▓ May be primary or secondary
▓ Almost exclusively have B-cell lineage
▓ Hypercellular smears
▓ Single cells
▓ Round, reniform, or convoluted nuclei with prominent nucleoli and vesicular chromatin
▓ Discrete cell borders
▓ Frequent apoptosis
▓ Occasional plexiform capillaries
▓ Necrosis

Special Stains and Immunohistochemistry
▓ Phenotyping by flow cytometry or immunostaining for lymphoma markers (CD3, CD20 etc)

Modern Techniques for Diagnosis
▓ Clonal studies may be useful
▓ In situ hybridization

20-42. Non-hodgkin lymphoma. Uniform population of large nuclei with macronucleoli. There are numerous karyorrhectic nuclei (Papanicolaou stain). Non-Hodgkin lymphoma, large cell type

Differential Diagnosis
■ Glioblastoma (lymphomas can have an infiltrating appearance but lack pseudo-palisading and vascular proliferation)
■ Anaplastic oligodendroglioma

PEARLS

★ Plasmacytoid cytological features may help to differentiate some diffusely infiltrating lymphomas from gliomas

OLIGODENDROGLIOMA

Clinical Features
▓ Primarily affects the cerebral hemisphere, frontal lobe in particular
▓ Adults are more commonly affected

▓ Frequently calcified on imaging
▓ Usually a long history of seizures
▓ Due to their infiltrative nature, not considered resectable

Cytologic Features
▓ Hypercellular with discohesive monotonous bland cells
▓ Round uniform nuclei with small amount of cytoplasm
▓ Clearly defined nucleoli, speckled chromatin
▓ Microgemistocytes
▓ Arborizing capillaries with perivascular sleeves of tumor cells
▓ Calcifications
▓ Background of the smears may be fibrillar

Special Stains and Immunohistochemistry
▓ Occasional membranous staining for Leu-7, variable positivity for GFAP

Modern Techniques for Diagnosis
▓ PCR assay for 1p/19q deletion

Differential Diagnosis
■ Astrocytoma
■ Macrophage-rich lesions (infarct, demyelinating disease)
■ CNS lymphoma
■ Glioblastoma (particularly in the diagnosis of high-grade oligodendroglioma)

PEARLS

★ When evaluating a high-grade oligodendroglioma, the smears may have discohesive, well-defined, and relatively small cells that can mimic a metastatic carcinoma and/or lymphoma

CENTRAL NEUROCYTOMA

Clinical Features
▓ Supratentorial mass protruding into the ventricle near the midline
▓ Also termed as, central neuroblastoma or differentiated neuroblastoma
▓ Cause signs and symptoms of increased intracranial pressure
▓ Mostly in young to middle-aged adults
▓ Often calcified on radiology scans

20-43. Oligodendroglioma *(left).*
A monotonous population of round to oval nuclei. Numerous fine capillaries are seen in the smear background (Papanicolaou stain)

20-44. Oligodendroglioma *(right).*
Uniform population of round to oval nuclei with scant amount of fragile cytoplasm. The nuclei lack prominent nucleoli. Fibrillary background is rarely seen (modified Giemsa stain)

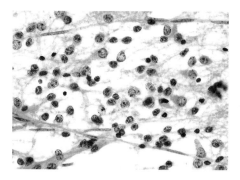
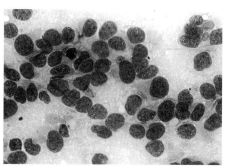

Cytologic Features
▣ Streams of uniform cells in a fibrillar background
▣ Perivascular pseudorosettes
▣ Round uniform nuclei with "salt-and-pepper" chromatin pattern
▣ Delicate cytoplasm
▣ Calcifications

Special Stains and Immunohistochemistry
▣ Immunoreactive for NSE and synaptophysin, nonreactive for GFAP

Modern Techniques for Diagnosis
▣ These tumors do not have the 1p/19q deletion of oligodendroglioma
▣ Comparative genomic hybridization has shown gains on chromosomes 2p, 10q, and 18q

Differential Diagnosis
▣ Oligodendroglioma
▣ Ependymoma

PEARLS

★ Because of the cytological features of monotonous appearing cells with perinuclear halos, a potential diagnostic pitfall is calling these oligodendrogliomas. The latter are distinctly synaptophysin negative

PINEOCYTOMA

Clinical Features
▣ Contrast-enhancing masses in the posterior third ventricle
▣ Occurs in mid- to late adulthood
▣ Arise from pineocytes or pineal parenchymal cells
▣ Leads to hydrocephalus and change in mental status

Cytologic Features
▣ Rosette formations with fibrillar zones (pinocytomatous rosettes)
▣ Pale round or oval nuclei
▣ Arborizing capillaries with tumor angiotropism
▣ Ganglion cells may be rarely seen

Special Stains and Immunohistochemistry
▣ Immunoreactive with NSE and synaptophysin, nonreactive with GFAP
▣ Ki-67 proliferation index is low

Modern Techniques for Diagnosis
▣ Noncontributory

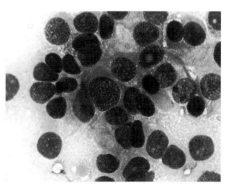

20-45. Pineocytoma. Neoplastic cells with round to oval nuclei. Occasional cells have relatively abundant cytoplasm. A partial rosette formation is seen at 3:00 o'clock (modified Giemsa stain)

Differential Diagnosis
▣ Normal pineal tissue
▣ Pineal cyst

★ Cytological preparations from normal pineal parenchyma can be mistaken for a pineal neoplasm. Always include it in the differential

PINEOBLASTOMA

Clinical Features
- Typically occurs in children
- Radiographic contrast enhancement
- Locally invasive tumor, most often fatal
- Rapid recurrence and wide dissemination is characteristic
- WHO Grade IV tumor

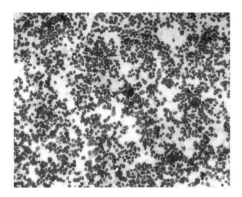

Cytologic Features
- Hypercellular
- Small cells with hyperchromatic crowded nuclei
- Varying mitotic activity
- Flexner–Wintersteiner rosettes (tumor cells radially surrounding a small lumen)
- Hemorrhage and necrosis are common

Special Stains and Immunohistochemistry
- Immunoreactive with synaptophysin, chromogranin, and neurofilament protein
- May be immunoreactive for retinal S-antigen

Modern Techniques for Diagnosis
- Most common cytogenetic findings are gains of 1q and losses of 22

20-46. Pineoblastoma. Hypercellular smear with diffuse proliferation of small round blue cells with occasional nuclear molding and rare crush artifact (modified Giemsa stain)

Differential Diagnosis
- Pineal parenchymal tumor of intermediate differentiation
- Medulloblastoma

★ Flexner–Wintersteiner rosettes are more likely to be seen in pineoblastomas as compared to medulloblastomas

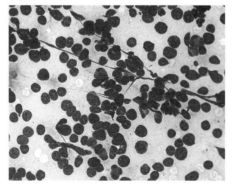
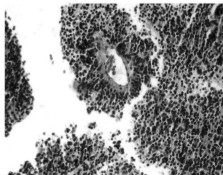

20-47. Pineoblastoma *(left).* Higher magnification of smear from twenty to fifty showing hypochromatic small round blue cells with foci of nuclear molding and crush artifact (modified Giemsa stain)

20-48. Pineoblastoma *(right).* Cell block preparation shows prominent perivascular proliferation of malignant small round blue cells (H&E)

MEDULLOBLASTOMA

Clinical Features
▨ Medulloblastoma (MB) is a small cell tumor of the cerebellum, accounting for approximately 30% of pediatric intracranial neoplasms
▨ Most likely original from external granular layer of the cerebellum
▨ Considered a distinct clinicopathologic entity, undifferentiated or with varying types of differentiation
▨ Most often seen in the first two decades of life
▨ Radiological appearance: Contrast-enhancing, vermian, or cerebellar hemispheric mass
▨ Histologically staged largely by the presence or absence of metastases

Cytologic Features
▨ Hypercellular
▨ Hyperchromatic with rosetting, nuclear molding
▨ Degree of pleomorphism and apoptosis varies with tumor grade
▨ Occasional "carrot-shaped" cells
▨ Mitosis/karyorrhexis
▨ Usually lacks calcification

Special Stains and Immunohistochemistry
▨ Synaptophysin positive
▨ Fibrillar areas are GFAP positive
▨ Few cases are positive for retinal S-antigen

Modern Techniques for Diagnosis
▨ Molecular based assays can be helpful in evaluating for cytogenetic abnormalities
▨ The most common finding is the complete or partial loss of chromosome 17p

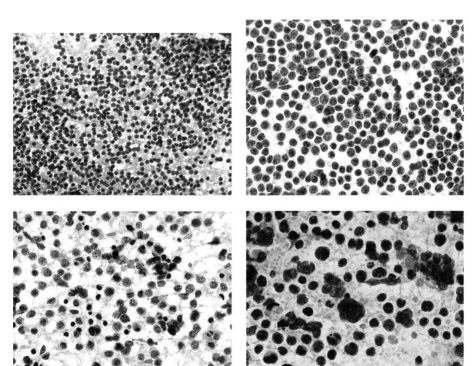

20-49. Medulloblastoma, low grade *(top, left).* Hypercellular smear with a uniform population of small round blue cells (H&E)

20-50. Medulloblastoma, low grade *(top, right).* Hypercellular smear showing the malignant small round blue cells at higher magnification. The degree of atypia may be variable even within the same preparation (H&E)

20-51. Medulloblastoma, high grade *(bottom, left).* Hypercellular smear with numerous small round blue cells with high nuclear to cytoplasmic ratios. There is occasional cell to cell molding. Numerous karyorrhectic nuclei are also present (H&E)

20-52. Medulloblastoma, high grade *(bottom, right).* Hypercellular smear with increased degree of cytologic atypia and pleomorphism and a high mitotic activity. In general, higher grade lesions such as this one will have increased nuclear size, prominent nucleoli, frequent nuclear molding, nuclear pleomorphism/angulation and increased number of mitoses/karyorrhexis (H&E)

Differential Diagnosis

■ Normal internal granule cell layer (can be misdiagnosed as neoplastic)
■ Atypical teratoid/rhabdoid tumor (in infants mostly)
■ Metastatic small cell carcinoma
■ Ependymoma

PEARLS

★ Higher grade lesions will have increased nuclear size, more prominent nucleoli, more nuclear molding, pleomorphism/angulation and increased number of mitoses/karyorrhexes
★ Higher grade lesions will also have an increased formation of tight cellular nests and multinucleated cells with peripherally placed nuclei

PRIMITIVE NEUROECTODERMAL TUMOR (PNET)

Clinical Features

■ Malignant tumor of primitive undifferentiated cells
■ Cellular embryonal tumor
■ Unsettled histogenesis
■ Includes a variety of primary CNS tumors
■ PNETs of the CNS can be subdivided into infratentorial PNETs (medulloblastoma is the prototype) and supratentorial PNETs

Cytologic Features

■ Pleomorphic, hyperchromatic cells with indented or pointed nuclei
■ Fine chromatin, inconspicuous nucleoli, and nuclear molding
■ Occasional granular eosinophilic cytoplasmic inclusions
■ Formation of Homer-Wright rosettes

Special Stains and Immunohistochemistry

■ Synaptophysin positive

Modern Techniques for Diagnosis

■ The most common finding is the complete or partial loss of chromosome 17p

Differential Diagnosis

■ Atypical teratoid/rhabdoid tumor (in infants mostly)
■ Metastatic small cell carcinoma
■ Desmoplastic infantile ganglioglioma

20-53. Primitive neuroectodermal tumor *(left)*. Neoplastic cells with round to oval nuclei, and hyperchromasia with fine nuclear chromatin. The nucleoli are inconspicuous. Occasional mitotic figures are seen (Papanicolaou stain)

20-54. Primitive neuroectodermal tumor *(right)*. Neoplastic cells in loose fragments with bare naked nuclei. Individual cells have uniform oval nuclei with hyperchromasia. The nucleoli are inconspicuous (modified Giemsa stain)

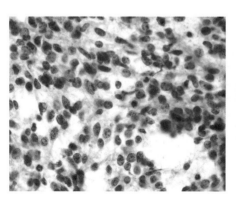
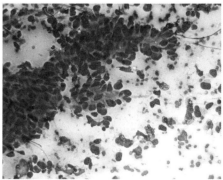

★ Medulloblastoma is the most common PNET of the CNS

★ Based on location and histologic features, these tumors can be classified as medulloblastomas, medulloepitheliomas, neuroblastoma, retinoblastoma, pineoblastoma, and ependymoblastoma

METASTATIC NEOPLASMS

Clinical Features

▦ Carcinoma of lung, breast, bladder, prostate, ovary, and melanoma are among the more common metastatic tumors

▦ Adults are commonly affected

▦ Usually involves the cerebral hemispheres

▦ Usually multiple lesions but can be single

▦ Well circumscribed

Cytologic Features

▦ CSF findings

➤ Malignant cells are much larger than normal cellular constituents of the CSF

➤ Metastatic tumors can be seen in aggregates with cellular disorder and nuclear crowding

➤ Primary CNS tumors such as GBM and medulloblastomas may be seen in the CSF

➤ Melanoma cells are large, single cells, with large eccentric nuclei with macronucleoli

➤ Melanoma cells may have characteristic pigment

➤ Adenocarcinoma may be shed in single pleomorphic cells such as lung carcinoma with irregular chromatin and prominent nucleoli

▦ Needle biopsy findings

➤ Cytologic preparations from aspirates are usually very cellular

➤ Tissue fragments usually present (carcinomas)

➤ Characteristic cytologic features according to the type of tumor such as lung

➤ Epithelial neoplasms are in sheets and may have glandular appearance

➤ Pigment may be seen in malignant melanomas

➤ Mucin may be seen in mucin-producing tumors

➤ Metastatic renal cell carcinomas will have clear cytoplasm

➤ Colonic origin adenocarcinoma will have typical elongated nuclei and columnar appearance

➤ Small cell carcinomas show characteristic crush artifact, high nuclear to cytoplasmic ratios, and nuclear molding

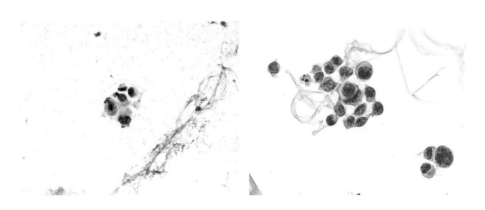

20-55. Metastatic glioblastoma multiforme *(left)*. Loose cluster of large pleomorphic malignant cells with scant and wispy cytoplasmic processes and eccentric nuclei with macronucleoli. A definite diagnosis in such cases requires an adequate clinical history (Papanicolaou stain)

20-56. Metastatic medulloblastoma *(right)*. Uniform population of small round blue cells with high nuclear to cytoplasmic ratios, and fine dusty chromatin. Occasional nuclear molding is also present (Papanicolaou stain)

20-57. Metastatic melanoma, CSF *(left)*. Dispersed population of malignant cells. The presence of prominent nucleoli and pigment formation are helping features in making the diagnosis of metastatic melanoma (Papanicolaou stain)

20-58. Metastatic adenocarcinoma of the lung *(right)*. Fragment of pleomorphic cells with a glandular architecture (modified Giemsa stain)

20-59. Metastatic melanoma, FNA *(left)*. Malignant cells with large eccentric nuclei and macronucleoli (modified Giemsa stain)

20-60. Metastatic adenocarcinoma *(right)*. Malignant gland-forming tumor with mucin production (Mucicarmine)

20-61. Metastatic undifferentiated carcinoma small cell type *(left)*. Tissue fragment of malignant cells with high nuclear to cytoplasmic ratios and prominent nuclear molding (Cell block, H&E)

20-62. Metastatic undifferentiated carcinoma, small cell type *(right)*. Malignant cells are immunoreactive for synaptophysin

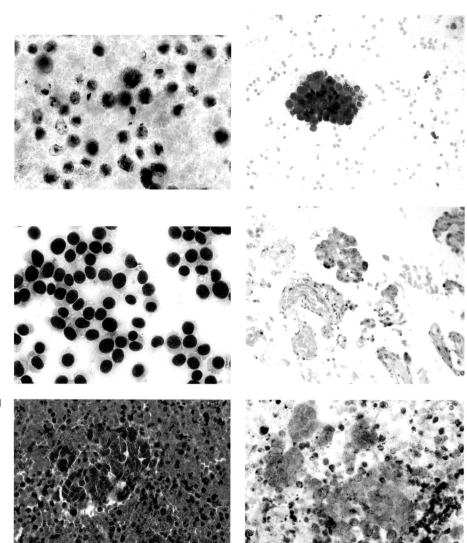

Special Stains and Immunohistochemistry
■ Immunostaining for epithelial markers (cytokeratins, EMA) or specific monoclonal antibodies are helpful in determining the type and origin of the tumor
■ Small cell carcinomas originating in the lung are immunoreactive for cytokeratins and less frequently for synaptophysin and chromogranin
■ GFAP immunostaining can help distinguish glioblastoma from a metastatic process

Modern Techniques for Diagnosis
■ Depends on the tumor type

Differential Diagnosis
■ Glioblastoma with epithelioid morphology
■ Gliosarcoma
■ Anaplastic oligodendroglioma

★ The presence of monomorphous epithelial cytological features

★ Metastatic lesions tend to have a lobular architecture

★ Metastatic disease into the cerebral cortex has an affinity for the gray–white junction

★ Metastatic sarcomas are extremely rare

★ Primary CNS lesions will have a more infiltrative appearance

REFERENCES

INTRODUCTION

Crain BJ, Bigner SH, Johnston WW. Fine needle aspiration biopsy of deep cerebrum. A comparison of normal and neoplastic morphology. *Acta Cytol* 1982;26(6):772–8.

Fratkin JD, Ward MM, Roberts DW, Sullivan MM. CT-guided stereotactic biopsy of intracranial lesions: correlation between core biopsy and aspiration smear. *Diagn Cytopathol* 1986;2(2): 126–32.

Liwnicz BH, Henderson KS, Masukawa T, Smith RD. Needle aspiration cytology of intracranial lesions. A review of 84 cases. *Acta Cytol* 1982;26(6):779–86.

Louis DN, Ohgaki H, Wiestler OD, Cavenee WK, Burger PC, Jouvet A, et al. The 2007 WHO classification of tumours of the central nervous system. *Acta Neuropathol (Berl)* 2007 Aug;114(2):97–109.

Mouriquand C, Benabid AL, Breyton M. Stereotaxic cytology of brain tumors. Review of an eight-year experience. *Acta Cytol* 1987;31(6):756–64.

Seliem RM, Assaad MW, Gorombey SJ, Moral LA, Kirkwood JR, Otis CN. Fine-needle aspiration biopsy of the central nervous system performed freehand under computed tomography guidance without stereotactic instrumentation. *Cancer.* 2003 Oct 25;99(5): 277–84.

Silverman JF. Cytopathology of fine-needle aspiration biopsy of the brain and spinal cord. *Diagn Cytopathol* 1986;2(4):312–9.

PROGRESSIVE MULTIFOCAL LEUKOENCEPHALOPATHY

Aksamit AJ. Review of progressive multifocal leukoencephalopathy and natalizumab. *Neurologist* 2006;12(6):293–8.

Andreula C. Cranial viral infections in the adult. *Eur Radiol* 2004;14 Suppl. 3:E132–44.

Berger JR, Houff S. Progressive multifocal leukoencephalopathy: lessons from AIDS and natalizumab. *Neurol Res* 2006;28(3):299–305.

Boriskin YS, Rice PS, Stabler RA, Hinds J, Al-Ghusein H, Vass K, Butcher PD. DNA microarrays for virus detection in cases of central nervous system infection. *J Clin Microbiol* 2004;42(12): 5811–8.

Cajulis RS, Hayden R, Frias-Hidvegi D, Brody BA, Yu GH, Levy R. Role of cytology in the intraoperative diagnosis of HIV-positive patients undergoing stereotactic brain biopsy. *Acta Cytol* 1997;41(2):481–6.

Gordon H. Hidvegi D, et al. Cytomorphology of progressive multifocal leukoencephalopathy (PML): Review of sixteen cases occurring in HIV-positive patients. *Diagn Cytopathol* 1996;14(1):4–9.

SUBACUTE SCLEROSING PANENCEPHALITIS

Andreula C. Cranial viral infections in the adult. *Eur Radiol* 2004;14 Suppl. 3:E132–44.

Boriskin YS, Rice PS, Stabler RA, Hinds J, Al-Ghusein H, Vass K, Butcher PD. DNA microarrays for virus detection in cases of central nervous system infection. *J Clin Microbiol* 2004;42(12): 5811–8.

Cole AJ, Henson JW, Roehrl MH, Frosch MP. Case records of the Massachusetts General Hospital. Case 24-2007. A 20-year-old pregnant woman with altered mental status. *N Engl J Med* 2007;357(6):589–600.

Duman O, Balta G, Metinsoy M, Haspolat S. Unusual manifestation of subacute sclerosing panencephalitis: case with intracranial high-pressure symptoms. *J Child Neurol* 2004;19(7): 552–5.

Ishida H, Ayata M, Shingai M, Matsunaga I, Seto Y, Katayama Y, Iritani N, Seya T, Yanagi Y, Matsuoka O and others. Infection of different cell lines of neural origin with subacute sclerosing panencephalitis (SSPE) virus. *Microbiol Immunol* 2004;48(4):277–87.

Prashanth LK, Taly AB, Ravi V, Sinha S, Arunodaya GR. Adult onset subacute sclerosing panencephalitis: clinical profile of 39 patients from a tertiary care centre. *J Neurol Neurosurg Psychiatry* 2006;77(5):630–3.

Wight C, Jin L, Nelson CS, Cosby SL, Padfield CJ. Case report: an autopsy-proven case of fulminant subacute sclerosing panencephalitis. *Neuropathol Appl Neurobiol* 2003;29(3):312–6.

HERPESVIRUS

Boivin G. Diagnosis of herpesvirus infections of the central nervous system. *Herpes* 2004;11 Suppl. 2:48A–56A.

Boriskin YS, Rice PS, Stabler RA, Hinds J, Al-Ghusein H, Vass K, Butcher PD. DNA microarrays for virus detection in cases of central nervous system infection. *J Clin Microbiol* 2004;42(12): 5811–8.

Cajulis RS, Hayden R, Frias-Hidvegi D, Brody BA, Yu GH, Levy R. Role of cytology in the intraoperative diagnosis of HIV-positive patients undergoing stereotactic brain biopsy. *Acta Cytol* 1997;41(2):481–6.

Eza D, Cerrillo G, Moore DA, Castro C, Ticona E, Morales D, Cabanillas J, Barrantes F, Alfaro A, Benavides A and others. Postmortem findings and opportunistic infections in HIV-positive patients from a public hospital in Peru. *Pathol Res Pract* 2006;202(11):767–75.

Grover D, Newsholme W, Brink N, Manji H, Miller R. Herpes simplex virus infection of the central nervous system in human immunodeficiency virus-type 1-infected patients. *Int J STD AIDS* 2004;15(9):597–600.

Hobson-Peters J, O'Loughlin P, Toye P. Development of an internally controlled, homogeneous polymerase chain reaction assay for the simultaneous detection and discrimination of herpes simplex virus types 1 and 2 and varicella-zoster virus. *Mol Cell Probes* 2007;21(1): 24–30.

Kimberlin DW. Management of HSV encephalitis in adults and neonates: diagnosis, prognosis and treatment. *Herpes* 2007;14(1):11–16.

CYTOMEGALOVIRUS

Cajulis RS, Hayden R, Frias-Hidvegi D, Brody BA, Yu GH, Levy R. Role of cytology in the intraoperative diagnosis of HIV-positive patients undergoing stereotactic brain biopsy. *Acta Cytol* 1997;41(2):481–6.

Eza D, Cerrillo G, Moore DA, Castro C, Ticona E, Morales D, Cabanillas J, Barrantes F, Alfaro A, Benavides A and others. Postmortem findings and opportunistic infections in HIV-positive patients from a public hospital in Peru. *Pathol Res Pract* 2006;202(11):767–75.

Griffiths P. *Cytomegalovirus infection of the central nervous system.* 2004;11 Suppl. 2:95A–104A.

Tarrago D, Quereda C, Tenorio A. Different cytomegalovirus glycoprotein B genotype distribution in serum and cerebrospinal fluid specimens determined by a novel multiplex nested PCR. *J Clin Microbiol* 2003;41(7):2872–7.

MOLLARET MENINGITIS

Chan TY, Parwani AV, Levi AW, Ali SZ. Mollaret's meningitis: cytopathologic analysis of fourteen cases. *Diagn Cytopathol* 2003;28(5):227–31.

Haynes BF, Wright R, McCracken JP. Mollaret meningitis. A report of three cases. *JAMA* 1976;236(17):1967–9.

Kwong YL, Woo E, Fong PC, Yung RW, Yu YL. Mollaret's meningitis revisited. Report of a case with a review of the literature. *Clin Neurol Neurosurg* 1988;90(2):163–7.

Picard FJ, Dekaban GA, Silva J, Rice GP. Mollaret's meningitis associated with herpes simplex type 2 infection. *Neurology* 1993;43(9):1722–7.

Procop GW, Yen-Lieberman B, Prayson RA, Gordon SM. Mollaret-like cells in patients with West Nile virus infection. *Emerg Infect Dis* 2004;10(4):753–4.

Teot LA, Sexton CW. Mollaret's meningitis: case report with immunocytochemical and polymerase chain reaction amplification studies. *Diagn Cytopathol* 1996;15(4):345–8.

TOXOPLASMOSIS

Holtkamp M, Okuducu AF, Klingebiel R, Ploner CJ. Cerebral toxoplasmosis in a patient with common variable immunodeficiency. *Neurology* 2004;63(11):2192–3.

Cajulis RS, Hayden R, Frias-Hidvegi D, Brody BA, Yu GH, Levy R. Role of cytology in the intra-operative diagnosis of HIV-positive patients undergoing stereotactic brain biopsy. *Acta Cytol* 1997 Mar–Apr;41(2):481–6.

Lanjewar DN, Surve KV, Maheshwari MB, Shenoy BP, Hira SK. Toxoplasmosis of the central nervous system in the acquired immunodeficiency syndrome. *Indian J Pathol Microbiol* 1998 Apr;41(2):147–51.

Sell M, Klingebiel R, Di Iorio G, Sampaolo S. Primary cerebral toxoplasmosis: a rare case of ventriculitis and hydrocephalus in AIDS. *Clin Neuropathol* 2005 May–Jun;24(3):106–11.

CYSTICERCOSIS

Garcia HH, Gonzalez AE, Gilman RH. Diagnosis, treatment and control of *Taenia solium* cysticercosis. *Curr Opin Infect Dis* 2003;16(5):411–9.

Ito A, Takayanagui OM, Sako Y, Sato MO, Odashima NS, Yamasaki H, Nakaya K, Nakao M. Neurocysticercosis: clinical manifestation, neuroimaging, serology and molecular confirmation of histopathologic specimens. *Southeast Asian J Trop Med Public Health* 2006;37 Suppl. 3:74–81.

Saenz B, Ruiz-Garcia M, Jimenez E, Hernandez-Aguilar J, Suastegui R, Larralde C, Sciutto E, Fleury A. Neurocysticercosis: clinical, radiologic, and inflammatory differences between children and adults. *Pediatr Infect Dis J* 2006;25(9):801–3.

Serpa JA, Moran A, Goodman JC, Giordano TP, White AC, Jr. Neurocysticercosis in the HIV era: a case report and review of the literature. *Am J Trop Med Hyg* 2007;77(1):113–7.

Silver SA, Erozan YS, Hruban RH. Cerebral cysticercosis mimicking malignant glioma: a case report. *Acta Cytol* 1996;40(2):351–7.

PSEUDOTUMORAL MACROPHAGE-RICH LESIONS

Alvarez-Lafuente R, Garcia-Montojo M, De Las Heras V, Bartolome M, Arroyo R. JC virus in cerebrospinal fluid samples of multiple sclerosis patients at the first demyelinating event. *Mult Scler* 2007;13(5):590–5.

Charil A, Filippi M. Inflammatory demyelination and neurodegeneration in early multiple sclerosis. *J Neurol Sci* 2007;259(1–2):7–15.

Dutta R, Trapp BD. Pathogenesis of axonal and neuronal damage in multiple sclerosis. *Neurology* 2007;68(22 Suppl3):S22–31; discussion S43–54.

Fabriek BO, Zwemmer JN, Teunissen CE, Dijkstra CD, Polman CH, Laman JD, Castelijns JA. In vivo detection of myelin proteins in cervical lymph nodes of MS patients using ultrasound-guided fine-needle aspiration cytology. *J Neuroimmunol* 2005;161(1–2): 190–4.

Karceski S. Multiple sclerosis: what have we learned? *Neurology* 2007;68(9):E9–10.

Lassmann H. Multiple sclerosis: is there neurodegeneration independent from inflammation? *J Neurol Sci* 2007;259(1-2):3–6.

Rolak LA, Fleming JO. The differential diagnosis of multiple sclerosis. *Neurologist* 2007;13(2): 57–72.

ARTERIOVENOUS MALFORMATION

Mandybur TI, Nazek M. Cerebral arteriovenous malformations. A detailed morphological and immunohistochemical study using actin. *Arch Pathol Lab Med* 1990;114(9):970–3.

Ondra SL, Troupp H, George ED, Schwab K. The natural history of symptomatic arteriovenous malformations of the brain: a 24-year follow-up assessment. *J Neurosurg* 1990;73(3): 387–91.

Yamada S, Brauer FS, Colohan AR, Won DJ, Siddiqi J, Johnson WD, Yamada SM, Rouse GA, Lonser RR, Iacono RP and others. Concept of arteriovenous malformation compartments and surgical management. *Neurol Res* 2004;26(3):288–300.

CRANIOPHARYNGIOMA

Daneshbod Y, Monabati A, Kumar PV, Taghipoor M, Bedayat GR. Intraoperative cytologic crush preparation findings in craniopharyngioma: a study of 72 cases. *Acta Cytol* 2005;49(1): 7–10.

Fraioli MF, Contratti F, Fraioli C. Craniopharyngioma. *J Neurosurg* 2007;106(6 Suppl):517–9.

Izumoto S, Suzuki T, Kinoshita M, Hashiba T, Kagawa N, Wada K, Fujimoto Y, Hashimoto N, Saitoh Y, Maruno M, et al. Immunohistochemical detection of female sex hormone receptors in craniopharyngiomas: correlation with clinical and histologic features. *Surg Neurol* 2005; 63(6):520–5; discussion 525.

Louis DN, Ohgaki H, Wiestler OD, Cavenee WK, Burger PC, Jouvet A, et al. The 2007 WHO classification of tumours of the central nervous system. *Acta Neuropathol (Berl)* 2007 Aug;114(2):97–109.

Mincione GP, Mincione F, Mennonna P. Cytological features of a craniopharyngioma. *Pathologica* 1991;83(1084):191–6.

Parwani AV, Taylor DC, Burger PC, Erozan YS, Olivi A, Ali SZ. Keratinized squamous cells in fine needle aspiration of the brain. Cytopathologic correlates and differential diagnosis. *Acta Cytol* 2003;47(3):325–31.

Sato K, Oka H, Utsuki S, Kondo K, Kurata A, Fujii K. Ciliated craniopharyngioma may arise from Rathke cleft cyst. *Clin Neuropathol* 2006;25(1):25–8.

RATHKE'S CLEFT CYST

Louis DN, Ohgaki H, Wiestler OD, Cavenee WK, Burger PC, Jouvet A, et al. The 2007 WHO classification of tumours of the central nervous system. *Acta Neuropathol (Berl.* 2007 Aug;114(2):97–109.

Naylor MF, Scheithauer BW, Forbes GS, Tomlinson FH, Young WF. Rathke cleft cyst: CT, MR, and pathology of 23 cases. *J Comput Assist Tomogr* 1995;19(6):853–9.

Parwani AV, Taylor DC, Burger PC, Erozan YS, Olivi A, Ali SZ. Keratinized squamous cells in fine needle aspiration of the brain. Cytopathologic correlates and differential diagnosis. *Acta Cytol* 2003;47(3):325–31.

Shimoji T, Shinohara A, Shimizu A, Sato K, Ishii S. Rathke cleft cysts. *Surg Neurol* 1984;21(3):295–310.

Sidhu M, Suri VS, Singh D, Tatke M, Kumar S. Histological analysis of cystic tumour like lesions of central nervous system. *Indian J Pathol Microbiol* 2002;45(1):7–14.

EPIDERMOID CYST

Parwani AV, Taylor DC, Burger PC, Erozan YS, Olivi A, Ali SZ. Keratinized squamous cells in fine needle aspiration of the brain. Cytopathologic correlates and differential diagnosis. *Acta Cytol* 2003;47(3):325–31.

Sidhu M, Suri VS, Singh D, Tatke M, Kumar S. Histological analysis of cystic tumour like lesions of central nervous system. *Indian J Pathol Microbiol* 2002;45(1):7–14.

Silverman JF, Timmons R, Harris LS. Fine needle aspiration cytology of primary epidermoid cyst of the brain. *Acta Cytol* 1985;29(6):989–93.

Gao PY, Osborn AG, Smirniotopoulos JG, Harris CP. Radiologic-pathologic correlation. Epidermoid tumor of the cerebellopontine angle. *AJNR Am J Neuroradiol* 1992 May–Jun;13(3):863–72.

Louis DN, Ohgaki H, Wiestler OD, Cavenee WK, Burger PC, Jouvet A, et al. The 2007 WHO classification of tumours of the central nervous system. *Acta Neuropathol (Berl.* 2007 Aug;114(2):97–109.

Seliem RM, Assaad MW, Gorombey SJ, Moral LA, Kirkwood JR, Otis CN. Fine-needle aspiration biopsy of the central nervous system performed freehand under computed tomography guidance without stereotactic instrumentation. *Cancer* 2003 Oct 25;99(5):277–84.

COLLOID CYST OF THE THIRD VENTRICLE

Armao D, Castillo M, Chen H, Kwock L. Colloid cyst of the third ventricle: imaging-pathologic correlation. *AJNR Am J Neuroradiol* 2000;21(8):1470–7.

Lach B, Scheithauer BW. Colloid cyst of the third ventricle: a comparative ultrastructural study of neuraxis cysts and choroid plexus epithelium. *Ultrastruct Pathol* 1992;16(3):331–49.

Maqsood AA, Devi IB, Mohanty A, Chandramouli BA, Sastry KV. Third ventricular colloid cysts in children. *Pediatr Neurosurg* 2006;42(3):147–50.

Parwani AV, Fatani IY, Burger PC, Erozan YS, Ali SZ. Colloid cyst of the third ventricle: cytomorphologic features on stereotactic fine-needle aspiration. *Diagn Cytopathol* 2002;27(1):27–31.

Seliem RM, Assaad MW, Gorombey SJ, Moral LA, Kirkwood JR, Otis CN. Fine-needle aspiration biopsy of the central nervous system performed freehand under computed tomography guidance without stereotactic instrumentation. *Cancer.* 2003 Oct 25;99(5):277–84.

LOW-GRADE ASTROCYTOMA

Burger PC. Pathology of brain stem astrocytomas. *Pediatr Neurosurg.* 1996;24(1):35–40.

Daumas-Duport C, Scheithauer B, O'Fallon J, Kelly P. Grading of astrocytomas. A simple and reproducible method. *Cancer* 1988 Nov 15;62(10):2152–65.

Coons SW, Johnson PC, Pearl DK. The prognostic significance of Ki-67 labeling indices for oligodendrogliomas. *Neurosurgery* 1997 Oct;41(4):878–84;discussion 84–5.

Louis DN, Ohgaki H, Wiestler OD, Cavenee WK, Burger PC, Jouvet A, et al. The 2007 WHO classification of tumours of the central nervous system. *Acta Neuropathol (Berl)* 2007 Aug;114(2):97–109.

Mai M, Huang H, Reed C, Qian C, Smith JS, Alderete B, et al. Genomic organization and mutation analysis of p73 in oligodendrogliomas with chromosome 1 p-arm deletions. *Genomics* 1998 Aug 1;51(3):359–63.

Marshall LF, Jennett B, Langfitt TW. Needle biopsy for the diagnosis of malignant glioma. *Jama* 1974;228(11):1417–8.

Silverman JF. Cytopathology of fine-needle aspiration biopsy of the brain and spinal cord. *Diagn Cytopathol* 1986;2(4):312–9.

Smith JS, Alderete B, Minn Y, Borell TJ, Perry A, Mohapatra G, et al. Localization of common deletion regions on 1p and 19q in human gliomas and their association with histological subtype. *Oncogene* 1999 Jul 15;18(28):4144–52.

Smith AR, Elsheikh TM, Silverman JF. Intraoperative cytologic diagnosis of suprasellar and sellar cystic lesions. *Diagn Cytopathol* 1999;20(3):137–47.

ANAPLASTIC ASTROCYTOMA

Aldape KD, Ballman K, Furth A, Buckner JC, Giannini C, Burger PC, Scheithauer BW, Jenkins RB, James CD. Immunohistochemical detection of EGFRvIII in high malignancy grade astrocytomas and evaluation of prognostic significance. *J Neuropathol Exp Neurol* 2004;63(7):700–7.

Louis DN, Ohgaki H, Wiestler OD, Cavenee WK, Burger PC, Jouvet A, et al. The 2007 WHO classification of tumours of the central nervous system. *Acta Neuropathol (Berl)* 2007 Aug;114(2):97–109.

Silverman JF. Cytopathology of fine-needle aspiration biopsy of the brain and spinal cord. *Diagn Cytopathol* 1986;2(4):312–9.

Smith AR, Elsheikh TM, Silverman JF. Intraoperative cytologic diagnosis of suprasellar and sellar cystic lesions. *Diagn Cytopathol* 1999;20(3):137–47.

Smith JS, Tachibana I, Passe SM, Huntley BK, Borell TJ, Iturria N, O'Fallon JR, Schaefer PL, Scheithauer BW, James CD and others. PTEN mutation, EGFR amplification, and outcome in patients with anaplastic astrocytoma and glioblastoma multiforme. *J Natl Cancer Inst* 2001;93(16):1246–56.

Tihan T, Davis R, Elowitz E, DiCostanzo D, Moll U. Practical value of Ki-67 and p53 labeling indexes in stereotactic biopsies of diffuse and pilocytic astrocytomas. *Arch Pathol Lab Med* 2000 Jan;124(1):108–13.

GLIOBLASTOMA MULTIFORME

Belda-Iniesta C, de Castro Carpeno J, Casado Saenz E, Cejas Guerrero P, Perona R, Gonzalez Baron M. Molecular biology of malignant gliomas. *Clin Transl Oncol* 2006 Sep;8(9):635–41.

Louis DN, Ohgaki H, Wiestler OD, Cavenee WK, Burger PC, Jouvet A, et al. The 2007 WHO classification of tumours of the central nervous system. *Acta Neuropathol (Berl)* 2007 Aug;114(2):97–109.

Marshall LF, Jennett B, Langfitt TW. Needle biopsy for the diagnosis of malignant glioma. *Jama* 1974;228(11):1417–8.

Silverman JF. Cytopathology of fine-needle aspiration biopsy of the brain and spinal cord. *Diagn Cytopathol* 1986;2(4):312–9.

Smith AR, Elsheikh TM, Silverman JF. Intraoperative cytologic diagnosis of suprasellar and sellar cystic lesions. *Diagn Cytopathol* 1999;20(3):137–47.

Smith JS, Tachibana I, Passe SM, Huntley BK, Borell TJ, Iturria N, O'Fallon JR, Schaefer PL, Scheithauer BW, James CD and others. PTEN mutation, EGFR amplification, and outcome in patients with anaplastic astrocytoma and glioblastoma multiforme. *J Natl Cancer Inst* 2001;93(16):1246–56.

Tihan T, Davis R, Elowitz E, DiCostanzo D, Moll U. Practical value of Ki-67 and p53 labeling indexes in stereotactic biopsies of diffuse and pilocytic astrocytomas. *Arch Pathol Lab Med* 2000 Jan;124(1):108–13.

PILOCYTIC ASTROCYTOMA

Forsyth PA, Shaw EG, Scheithauer BW, O'Fallon JR, Layton DD, Jr., Katzmann JA. Supratentorial pilocytic astrocytomas. A clinicopathologic, prognostic, and flow cytometric study of 51 patients. *Cancer* 1993 Aug 15;72(4):1335–42.

Gajjar A, Bhargava R, Jenkins JJ, Heideman R, Sanford RA, Langston JW, et al. Low-grade astrocytoma with neuraxis dissemination at diagnosis. *J Neurosurg* 1995 Jul;83(1):67–71.

Kleihues P, Burger PC, Scheithauer BW. The new WHO classification of brain tumours. *Brain Pathol* 1993 Jul;3(3):255–68.

Silverman JF. Cytopathology of fine-needle aspiration biopsy of the brain and spinal cord. *Diagn Cytopathol* 1986;2(4):312–9.

Teo JG, Ng HK. Cytodiagnosis of pilocytic astrocytoma in smear preparations. *Acta Cytol* 1998 May–Jun;42(3):673–8.

Tihan T, Davis R, Elowitz E, DiCostanzo D, Moll U. Practical value of Ki-67 and p53 labeling indexes in stereotactic biopsies of diffuse and pilocytic astrocytomas. *Arch Pathol Lab Med* 2000 Jan;124(1):108–13.

GLIOMATOSIS CEREBRI

Bae JY, Choi BO, SunWoo IN, Kim DI, Cho SH, Kim TS. Diffuse cerebrospinal gliomatosis with extensive leptomeningeal spread. *Yonsei Med J* 2000 Aug;41(4):517–21.

Herrlinger U, Felsberg J, Kuker W, Bornemann A, Plasswilm L, Knobbe CB, et al. Gliomatosis cerebri: molecular pathology and clinical course. *Ann Neurol* 2002 Oct;52(4):390–9.

Kim DG, Yang HJ, Park IA, Chi JG, Jung HW, Han DH, et al. Gliomatosis cerebri: clinical features, treatment, and prognosis. *Acta Neurochir (Wien)* 1998;140(8):755–62.

Kros JM, Zheng P, Dinjens WN, Alers JC. Genetic aberrations in gliomatosis cerebri support monoclonal tumorigenesis. *J Neuropathol Exp Neurol* 2002 Sep;61(9):806–14.

Silverman JF. Cytopathology of fine-needle aspiration biopsy of the brain and spinal cord. *Diagn Cytopathol* 1986;2(4):312–9.

Louis DN, Ohgaki H, Wiestler OD, Cavenee WK, Burger PC, Jouvet A, et al. The 2007 WHO classification of tumours of the central nervous system. *Acta Neuropathol (Berl)* 2007 Aug;114(2):97–109.

Peretti-Viton P, Brunel H, Chinot O, Daniel C, Barrie M, Bouvier C, et al. Histological and MR correlations in gliomatosis cerebri. *J Neurooncol* 2002 Sep;59(3):249–59.

Vates GE, Chang S, Lamborn KR, Prados M, Berger MS. Gliomatosis cerebri: a review of 22 cases. *Neurosurgery* 2003 Aug;53(2):261–71; discussion 71.

SMALL CELL GBM

Louis DN, Ohgaki H, Wiestler OD, Cavenee WK, Burger PC, Jouvet A, et al. The 2007 WHO classification of tumours of the central nervous system. *Acta Neuropathol (Berl)* 2007 Aug;114(2):97–109.

GLIOSARCOMA

Actor B, Cobbers JM, Buschges R, Wolter M, Knobbe CB, Lichter P, et al. Comprehensive analysis of genomic alterations in gliosarcoma and its two tissue components. *Genes Chromosomes Cancer* 2002 Aug;34(4):416–27.

Hayashi K, Ohara N, Jeon HJ, Akagi S, Takahashi K, Akagi T, et al. Gliosarcoma with features of chondroblastic osteosarcoma. *Cancer* 1993 Aug 1;72(3):850–5.

Louis DN, Ohgaki H, Wiestler OD, Cavenee WK, Burger PC, Jouvet A, et al. The 2007 WHO classification of tumours of the central nervous system. *Acta Neuropathol (Berl)* 2007 Aug;114(2):97–109.

Meis JM, Ho KL, Nelson JS. Gliosarcoma: a histologic and immunohistochemical reaffirmation. *Mod Pathol* 1990 Jan;3(1):19–24.

Ozolek JA, Finkelstein SD, Couce ME. Gliosarcoma with epithelial differentiation: immunohistochemical and molecular characterization. A case report and review of the literature. *Mod Pathol* 2004 Jun;17(6):739–45.

Parwani AV, Berman D, Burger PC, Ali SZ. Gliosarcoma: cytopathologic characteristics on fine-needle aspiration (FNA) and intraoperative touch imprint. *Diagn Cytopathol* 2004 Feb;30(2):77–81.

Reis RM, Konu-Lebleblicioglu D, Lopes JM, Kleihues P, Ohgaki H. Genetic profile of gliosarcomas. *Am J Pathol* 2000 Feb;156(2):425–32.

Reis RM, Martins A, Ribeiro SA, Basto D, Longatto-Filho A, Schmitt FC, et al. Molecular characterization of PDGFR-alpha/PDGF-A and c-KIT/SCF in gliosarcomas. *Cell Oncol* 2005;27(5-6):319–26.

Shintaku M, Miyaji K, Adachi Y. Gliosarcoma with angiosarcomatous features: a case report. *Brain Tumor Pathol* 1998;15(2):101–5.

EPENDYMOMA

Kleihues P, Burger PC, Scheithauer BW. The new WHO classification of brain tumours. *Brain Pathol* 1993 Jul;3(3):255–68.

Kumar PV. Nuclear grooves in ependymoma. Cytologic study of 21 cases. *Acta Cytol* 1997;41(6):1726–31.

Louis DN, Ohgaki H, Wiestler OD, Cavenee WK, Burger PC, Jouvet A, et al. The 2007 WHO classification of tumours of the central nervous system. *Acta Neuropathol (Berl.* 2007 Aug;114(2):97–109.

Rodriguez FJ, Scheithauer BW, Robbins PD, Burger PC, Hessler RB, Perry A, et al. Ependymomas with neuronal differentiation: a morphologic and immunohistochemical spectrum. *Acta Neuropathol (Berl)* 2007 Mar;113(3):313–24.

Sanford RA, Gajjar A. Ependymomas. *Clin Neurosurg* 1997;44:559–70.

Sanford RA, Kun LE, Heideman RL, Gajjar A. Cerebellar pontine angle ependymoma in infants. *Pediatr Neurosurg* 1997 Aug;27(2):84–91.

Scheithauer BW, Bruner JM. Central nervous system tumors. *Clin Lab Med* 1987 Mar;7(1): 157–79.

MYXOPAPILLARY EPENDYMOMA

Bardales RH, Porter MC, Sawyer JR, Mrak RE, Stanley MW. Metastatic myxopapillary ependymoma: report of a case with fine-needle aspiration findings. *Diagn Cytopathol* 1994;10(1): 47–53.

Kleihues P, Burger PC, Scheithauer BW. The new WHO classification of brain tumours. *Brain Pathol* 1993 Jul;3(3):255–68.

Kumar ND, Misra K. Fine needle aspiration cytodiagnosis of subcutaneous sacrococcygeal myxopapillary ependymoma. A case report. *Acta Cytol* 1990 Nov–Dec;34(6):851–4.

Kulesza P, Tihan T, Ali SZ. Myxopapillary ependymoma: cytomorphologic characteristics and differential diagnosis. *Diagn Cytopathol* 2002 Apr;26(4):247–50.

Louis DN, Ohgaki H, Wiestler OD, Cavenee WK, Burger PC, Jouvet A, et al. The 2007 WHO classification of tumours of the central nervous system. *Acta Neuropathol (Berl)* 2007 Aug;114(2):97–109.

Ng WK, Khoo US, Ip P, Collins RJ. Fine needle aspiration cytology of myxopapillary ependymoma. A case report. *Acta Cytol* 1998;42(4):1022–6.

Pohar-Marinsek Z, Frkovic-Grazio S. Fine needle aspiration (FNA) cytology of primary subcutaneous sacrococcygeal myxopapillary ependymoma. *Cytopathology* 1998 Dec;9(6): 415–20.

MENINGIOMA

Baisden BL, Hamper UM, Ali SZ. Metastatic meningioma in fine-needle aspiration (FNA) of the lung: cytomorphologic finding. *Diagn Cytopathol* 1999;20(5):291–4.

Gill SS, Bharadwaj R. Cytomorphologic findings of hemangiopericytoma of the meninges: a case report. *Indian J Pathol Microbiol* 2007 Apr;50(2):422–5.

Louis DN, Ohgaki H, Wiestler OD, Cavenee WK, Burger PC, Jouvet A, et al. The 2007 WHO classification of tumours of the central nervous system. *Acta Neuropathol (Berl)* 2007 Aug;114(2):97–109.

McCullough JB, Evans AT, Vaughan-Jones R, Hussein KA. Fine needle aspiration (FNA) of a nasal meningioma: a case report. *Cytopathology* 1996 Feb;7(1):56–60.

Parwani AV, Mikolaenko I, Eberhart CG, Burger PC, Rosenthal DL, Ali SZ. Rhabdoid meningioma: cytopathologic findings in cerebrospinal fluid. *Diagn Cytopathol* 2003;29(5): 297–9.

Perry A, Jenkins RB, Dahl RJ, Moertel CA, Scheithauer BW. Cytogenetic analysis of aggressive meningiomas: possible diagnostic and prognostic implications. *Cancer* 1996 Jun 15;77(12): 2567–73.

Perry A, Stafford SL, Scheithauer BW, Suman VJ, Lohse CM. Meningioma grading: an analysis of histologic parameters. *Am J Surg Pathol* 1997 Dec;21(12):1455–65.

Riemenschneider MJ, Perry A, Reifenberger G. Histological classification and molecular genetics of meningiomas. *Lancet Neurol* 2006 Dec;5(12):1045–54.

Spitz DJ, Reddy V, Selvaggi SM, Kluskens L, Green L, Gattuso P. Fine-needle aspiration of scalp lesions. *Diagn Cytopathol* 2000 Jul;23(1):35–8.

Tan LH. Meningioma presenting as a parapharyngeal tumor: report of a case with fine needle aspiration cytology. *Acta Cytol* 2001 Nov–Dec;45(6):1053–9.

CHOROID PLEXUS PAPILLOMA/CARCINOMA

Barreto AS, Vassallo J, Queiroz Lde S. Papillomas and carcinomas of the choroid plexus: histological and immunohistochemical studies and comparison with normal fetal choroid plexus. *Arq Neuropsiquiatr* 2004 Sep;62(3A):600–7.

Buchino JJ, Mason KG. Choroid plexus papilloma. Report of a case with cytologic differential diagnosis. *Acta Cytol* 1992 Jan–Feb;36(1):95–7.

Due-Tonnessen B, Helseth E, Skullerud K, Lundar T. Choroid plexus tumors in children and young adults: report of 16 consecutive cases. *Childs Nerv Syst* 2001 Apr;17(4–5):252–6.

Hasselblatt M, Bohm C, Tatenhorst L, Dinh V, Newrzella D, Keyvani K, et al. Identification of novel diagnostic markers for choroid plexus tumors: a microarray-based approach. *Am J Surg Pathol* 2006 Jan;30(1):66–74.

Louis DN, Ohgaki H, Wiestler OD, Cavenee WK, Burger PC, Jouvet A, et al. The 2007 WHO classification of tumours of the central nervous system. *Acta Neuropathol (Berl)* 2007 Aug;114(2):97–109.

Strojan P, Popovic M, Surlan K, Jereb B. Choroid plexus tumors: a review of 28-year experience. *Neoplasma* 2004;51(4):306–12.

ATYPICAL TERATOID/RHABDOID TUMORS

Bouffard JP, Sandberg GD, Golden JA, Rorke LB. Double immunolabeling of central nervous system atypical teratoid/rhabdoid tumors. *Mod Pathol* 2004 Jun;17(6):679–83.

Chen ML, McComb JG, Krieger MD. Atypical teratoid/rhabdoid tumors of the central nervous system: management and outcomes. *Neurosurg Focus* 2005 Jun 15;18(6A):E8.

Dang T, Vassilyadi M, Michaud J, Jimenez C, Ventureyra EC. Atypical teratoid/rhabdoid tumors. *Childs Nerv Syst* 2003 Apr;19(4):244–8.

Gessi M, Giangaspero F, Pietsch T. Atypical teratoid/rhabdoid tumors and choroid plexus tumors: when genetics "surprise" pathology. *Brain Pathol* 2003 Jul;13(3):409–14.

Louis DN, Ohgaki H, Wiestler OD, Cavenee WK, Burger PC, Jouvet A, et al. The 2007 WHO classification of tumours of the central nervous system. *Acta Neuropathol (Berl)* 2007 Aug;114(2):97–109.

Ogino S, Cohen ML, Abdul-Karim FW. Atypical teratoid/rhabdoid tumor of the CNS: cytopathology and immunohistochemistry of insulin-like growth factor-II, insulin-like growth factor receptor type 1, cathepsin D, and Ki-67. *Mod Pathol* 1999 Apr;12(4):379–85.

Parwani AV, Stelow EB, Pambuccian SE, Burger PC, Ali SZ. Atypical teratoid/rhabdoid tumor of the brain: cytopathologic characteristics and differential diagnosis. *Cancer* 2005;105(2):65–70.

Zarovnaya EL, Pallatroni HF, Hug EB, Ball PA, Cromwell LD, Pipas JM, et al. Atypical teratoid/rhabdoid tumor of the spine in an adult: case report and review of the literature. *J Neurooncol* 2007 Aug;84(1):49–55.

GERM CELL TUMORS

Baehring J, Vives K, Duncan C, Piepmeier J, Bannykyh S. Tumors of the posterior third ventricle and pineal region: ependymoma and germinoma. *J Neurooncol* 2004 Nov;70(2):273–4.

Crawford JR, Santi MR, Vezina G, Myseros JS, Keating RF, LaFond DA, et al. CNS germ cell tumor (CNSGCT) of childhood: presentation and delayed diagnosis. *Neurology* 2007 May 15;68(20):1668–73.

Gindhart TD, Tsukahara YC. Cytologic diagnosis of pineal germinoma in cerebrospinal fluid and sputum. *Acta Cytol* 1979 Jul–Aug;23(4):341–6.

Louis DN, Ohgaki H, Wiestler OD, Cavenee WK, Burger PC, Jouvet A, et al. The 2007 WHO classification of tumours of the central nervous system. *Acta Neuropathol (Berl)* 2007 Aug;114(2):97–109.

Mishima K, Kato Y, Kaneko MK, Nakazawa Y, Kunita A, Fujita N, et al. Podoplanin expression in primary central nervous system germ cell tumors: a useful histological marker for the diagnosis of germinoma. *Acta Neuropathol (Berl)* 2006 Jun;111(6):563–8.

Ng HK. Cytologic diagnosis of intracranial germinomas in smear preparations. *Acta Cytol* 1995;39(4):693–7.

Parwani AV, Baisden BL, Erozan YS, Burger PC, Ali SZ. Pineal gland lesions: a cytopathologic study of 20 specimens. *Cancer* 2005;105(2):80–6.

Sawamura Y, Ikeda J, Shirato H, Tada M, Abe H. Germ cell tumours of the central nervous system: treatment consideration based on 111 cases and their long-term clinical outcomes. *Eur J Cancer* 1998 Jan;34(1):104–10.

Sarkar C, Deb P, Sharma MC. Recent advances in embryonal tumours of the central nervous system. *Childs Nerv Syst* 2005 Apr;21(4):272–93.

Schneider DT, Zahn S, Sievers S, Alemazkour K, Reifenberger G, Wiestler OD, et al. Molecular genetic analysis of central nervous system germ cell tumors with comparative genomic hybridization. *Mod Pathol* 2006 Jun;19(6):864–73.

LYMPHOMA

Batchelor T, Loeffler JS. Primary CNS lymphoma. *J Clin Oncol* 2006;24(8):1281–8.

Sherman ME, Erozan YS, Mann RB, Kumar AA, McArthur JC, Royal W, Uematsu S, Nauta HJ. Stereotactic brain biopsy in the diagnosis of malignant lymphoma. *Am J Clin Pathol* 1991;95(6):878–83.

Bromberg JE, Breems DA, Kraan J, Bikker G, van der Holt , B, Smitt PS, et al. CSF flow cytometry greatly improves diagnostic accuracy in CNS hematologic malignancies. *Neurology* 2007 May 15;68(20):1674–9.

Louis DN, Ohgaki H, Wiestler OD, Cavenee WK, Burger PC, Jouvet A, et al. The 2007 WHO classification of tumours of the central nervous system. *Acta Neuropathol (Berl)* 2007 Aug;114(2):97–109.

Plasswilm L, Herrlinger U, Korfel A, Weller M, Kuker W, Kanz L, et al. Primary central nervous system (CNS) lymphoma in immunocompetent patients. *Ann Hematol* 2002 Aug;81(8): 415–23.

Tani E, Costa I, Svedmyr E, Skoog L. Diagnosis of lymphoma, leukemia, and metastatic tumor involvement of the cerebrospinal fluid by cytology and immunocytochemistry. *Diagn Cytopathol* 1995 Feb;12(1):14–22.

Tani E, Liliemark J, Svedmyr E, Mellstedt H, Biberfeld P, Skoog L. Cytomorphology and immunocytochemistry of fine needle aspirates from blastic non-Hodgkin's lymphomas. *Acta Cytol* 1989 May–Jun;33(3):363–71.

Yu GH, Montone KT, Frias-Hidvegi D, Cajulis RS, Brody BA, Levy RM. Cytomorphology of primary CNS lymphoma: review of 23 cases and evidence for the role of EBV. *Diagn Cytopathol* 1996 Mar;14(2):114–20.

OLIGODENDROGLIOMA

Agulnik M, Mason WP. Recent advances in the treatment of oligodendrogliomas. *Curr Neurol Neurosci Rep* 2006 May;6(3):212–7.

Coons SW, Johnson PC, Pearl DK. The prognostic significance of Ki-67 labeling indices for oligodendrogliomas. *Neurosurgery* 1997 Oct;41(4):878–84; discussion 84–5.

Kleihues P, Burger PC, Scheithauer BW. The new WHO classification of brain tumours. *Brain Pathol* 1993 Jul;3(3):255–68.

Law ME, Templeton KL, Kitange G, Smith J, Misra A, Feuerstein BG, Jenkins RB. Molecular cytogenetic analysis of chromosomes 1 and 19 in glioma cell lines. *Cancer Genet Cytogenet* 2005;160(1):1–14.

Louis DN, Ohgaki H, Wiestler OD, Cavenee WK, Burger PC, Jouvet A, et al. The 2007 WHO classification of tumours of the central nervous system. *Acta Neuropathol (Berl)* 2007 Aug;114(2):97–109.

Mut M, Guler-Tezel G, Lopes MB, Bilginer B, Ziyal I, Ozcan OE. Challenging diagnosis: oligodendroglioma versus extraventricular neurocytoma. *Clin Neuropathol* 2005 Sep–Oct;24(5): 225–9.

Nguyen GK, Johnson ES, Mielke BW. Comparative cytomorphology of pituitary adenomas and oligodendrogliomas in intraoperative crush preparations. *Acta Cytol* 1992 Sep–Oct;36(5): 661–7.

Stupp R, Hegi ME. Neuro-oncology: oligodendroglioma and molecular markers. *Lancet Neurol* 2007 Jan;6(1):10–12.

Trost D, Ehrler M, Fimmers R, Felsberg J, Sabel MC, Kirsch L, et al. Identification of genomic aberrations associated with shorter overall survival in patients with oligodendroglial tumors. *Int J Cancer* 2007 Jun 1;120(11):2368–76.

CENTRAL NEUROCYTOMA

De Tommasi A, D'Urso PI, De Tommasi C, Sanguedolce F, Cimmino A, Ciappetta P. Central neurocytoma: two case reports and review of the literature. *Neurosurg Rev* 2006 Oct;29(4): 339–47.

Jacques TS, Galloway MJ, Scaravilli F. Cerebrospinal fluid findings in central neurocytoma. *Cytopathology* 2006 Oct;17(5):301–3.

Jay V, Edwards V, Hoving E, Rutka J, Becker L, Zielenska M, et al. Central neurocytoma: morphological, flow cytometric, polymerase chain reaction, fluorescence in situ hybridization, and karyotypic analyses. Case report. *J Neurosurg* 1999 Feb;90(2):348–54.

Louis DN, Ohgaki H, Wiestler OD, Cavenee WK, Burger PC, Jouvet A, et al. The 2007 WHO classification of tumours of the central nervous system. *Acta Neuropathol (Berl)* 2007 Aug;114(2):97–109.

Mut M, Guler-Tezel G, Lopes MB, Bilginer B, Ziyal I, Ozcan OE. Challenging diagnosis: oligodendroglioma versus extraventricular neurocytoma. *Clin Neuropathol* 2005 Sep–Oct;24(5): 225–9.

Ng HK. Cytologic features of central neurocytomas of the brain. A report of three cases. *Acta Cytol* 1999;43(2):252–6.

Tong CY, Ng HK, Pang JC, Hu J, Hui AB, Poon WS. Central neurocytomas are genetically distinct from oligodendrogliomas and neuroblastomas. *Histopathology* 2000 Aug;37(2):160–5.

PINEOCYTOMA

Fevre-Montange M, Champier J, Szathmari A, Wierinckx A, Mottolese C, Guyotat J, et al. Microarray analysis reveals differential gene expression patterns in tumors of the pineal region. *J Neuropathol Exp Neurol* 2006 Jul;65(7):675–84.

Fevre-Montange M, Champier J, Szathmari A, Brisson C, Reboul A, Mottolese C, et al. Histological features and expression of enzymes implicated in melatonin synthesis in pineal parenchymal tumours and in cultured tumoural pineal cells. *Neuropathol Appl Neurobiol* 2007 Oct 29.

Jouvet A, Saint-Pierre G, Fauchon F, Privat K, Bouffet E, Ruchoux MM, et al. Pineal parenchymal tumors: a correlation of histological features with prognosis in 66 cases. *Brain Pathol* 2000 Jan;10(1):49–60.

Louis DN, Ohgaki H, Wiestler OD, Cavenee WK, Burger PC, Jouvet A, et al. The 2007 WHO classification of tumours of the central nervous system. *Acta Neuropathol (Berl)* 2007 Aug;114(2):97–109.

Parwani AV, Baisden BL, Erozan YS, Burger PC, Ali SZ. Pineal gland lesions: a cytopathologic study of 20 specimens. *Cancer* 2005;105(2):80–6.

PINEOBLASTOMA

Baehring J, Vives K, Duncan C, Piepmeier J, Bannykyh S. Tumors of the posterior third ventricle and pineal region: ependymoma and germinoma. *J Neurooncol.* 2004 Nov;70(2): 273–4.

Fauchon F, Jouvet A, Paquis P, Saint-Pierre G, Mottolese C, Ben Hassel M, et al. Parenchymal pineal tumors: a clinicopathological study of 76 cases. *Int J Radiat Oncol Biol Phys* 2000 Mar 1;46(4):959–68.

Jouvet A, Saint-Pierre G, Fauchon F, Privat K, Bouffet E, Ruchoux MM, et al. Pineal parenchymal tumors: a correlation of histological features with prognosis in 66 cases. *Brain Pathol* 2000 Jan;10(1):49–60.

Kumar P, Tatke M, Sharma A, Singh D. Histological analysis of lesions of the pineal region: a retrospective study of 12 years. *Pathol Res Pract* 2006;202(2):85–92.

Louis DN, Ohgaki H, Wiestler OD, Cavenee WK, Burger PC, Jouvet A, et al. The 2007 WHO classification of tumours of the central nervous system. *Acta Neuropathol (Berl)* 2007 Aug;114(2):97–109.

Parwani AV, Baisden BL, Erozan YS, Burger PC, Ali SZ. Pineal gland lesions: a cytopathologic study of 20 specimens. *Cancer* 2005;105(2):80–6.

MEDULLOBLASTOMA

Eberhart CG, Cohen KJ, Tihan T, Goldthwaite PT, Burger PC. Medulloblastomas with systemic metastases: evaluation of tumor histopathology and clinical behavior in 23 patients. *J Pediatr Hematol Oncol* 2003 Mar;25(3):198–203.

Eberhart CG, Tihan T, Burger PC. Nuclear localization and mutation of beta-catenin in medulloblastomas. *J Neuropathol Exp Neurol* 2000 Apr;59(4):333–7.

Gershon TR, Becher OJ. Medulloblastoma: therapy and biologic considerations. *Curr Neurol Neurosci Rep* 2006 May;6(3):200–6.

Law ME, Templeton KL, Kitange G, Smith J, Misra A, Feuerstein BG, Jenkins RB. Molecular cytogenetic analysis of chromosomes 1 and 19 in glioma cell lines. *Cancer Genet Cytogenet* 2005;160(1):1–14.

Louis DN, Ohgaki H, Wiestler OD, Cavenee WK, Burger PC, Jouvet A, et al. The 2007 WHO classification of tumours of the central nervous system. *Acta Neuropathol (Berl)* 2007 Aug;114(2):97–109.

Min HS, Lee YJ, Park K, Cho BK, Park SH. Medulloblastoma: histopathologic and molecular markers of anaplasia and biologic behavior. *Acta Neuropathol (Berl)* 2006 Jul;112(1): 13–20.

Riazmontazer N, Daneshbod Y. Cytology of desmoplastic medulloblastoma in imprint smears: a report of 2 cases. *Acta Cytol* 2006 Jan–Feb;50(1):97–100.

PRIMITIVE NEUROECTODERMAL TUMOR

Louis DN, Ohgaki H, Wiestler OD, Cavenee WK, Burger PC, Jouvet A, et al. The 2007 WHO classification of tumours of the central nervous system. *Acta Neuropathol (Berl)* 2007 Aug;114(2):97–109.

METASTATIC NEOPLASMS

Aragon-Ching JB, Zujewski JA. CNS metastasis: an old problem in a new guise. *Clin Cancer Res* 2007 Mar 15;13(6):1644–7.

Batchelor T, Loeffler JS. Primary CNS lymphoma. *J Clin Oncol* 2006;24(8):1281–8.

Louis DN, Ohgaki H, Wiestler OD, Cavenee WK, Burger PC, Jouvet A, et al. The 2007 WHO classification of tumours of the central nervous system. *Acta Neuropathol (Berl)* 2007 Aug;114(2):97–109.

Nguyen TD, Abrey LE. Brain metastases: old problem, new strategies. *Hematol Oncol Clin North Am* 2007 Apr;21(2):369–88.

Taillibert S, Laigle-Donadey F, Chodkiewicz C, Sanson M, Hoang-Xuan K, Delattre JY. Leptomeningeal metastases from solid malignancy: a review. *J Neurooncol* 2005 Oct;75(1): 85–99.

Tani E, Costa I, Svedmyr E, Skoog L. Diagnosis of lymphoma, leukemia, and metastatic tumor involvement of the cerebrospinal fluid by cytology and immunocytochemistry. *Diagn Cytopathol* 1995 Feb;12(1):14–22.

Weil RJ, Palmieri DC, Bronder JL, Stark AM, Steeg PS. Breast cancer metastasis to the central nervous system. *Am J Pathol* 2005 Oct;167(4):913–20.

Weil RJ, Lonser RR, Quezado MM. CNS manifestations of malignancies: case 2. Skull and brain metastasis from tibial osteosarcoma. *J Clin Oncol* 2005 Jun 20;23(18):4226–9.

Yu GH, Montone KT, Frias-Hidvegi D, Cajulis RS, Brody BA, Levy RM. Cytomorphology of primary CNS lymphoma: review of 23 cases and evidence for the role of EBV. *Diagn Cytopathol* 1996 Mar;14(2):114–20.

Index